SCIENTIFIC WORKS

EDICIONES UNIVERSAL, Miami, Florida, 1983

DAVID R. IRIARTE

SCIENTIFIC WORKS

- - EDICIONES UNIVERSAL

P.O. Box 450353 (Shenandoah Station)
Miami, Florida, 33145., U.S.A.

Library of Congress Catalog Card No.: 82-82544

I.S.B.N.: 0-89729-316-9

Cover pictures by: Valery Rísquez's printing.

Printed by: Ortex Corp., Miami, Fl. U.S.A.

To my daughter Evangelina for her decisive cooperation in the publication and proofreading of this book, as in the previous one published in Madrid in 1981, entitled "Trayectoria de una Vida."

Also I would like to thank Le Petit Laboratories for their fine advices and suggestions.

PREFACE

We have wanted at this stage in our lives, to leave the most interesting scientific works published in english, the language that takes possession of the first place in the spoken and written communication in the world.

Thus, as we have succeeded in having our books and pamphlets distributed all over in Academies, Libraries, Institutes, Universities of different countries, separated by large geographical distances, and placed in the hands of scientists and researchers of the wide universal panoram, we understand that english is the language that reaches all corners and that it is spreading day by day, being a necessity of modern man.

It is said that 800.000.000 people speak Chinese, but we have read that there are more than one thousand dialects; that 400.000.000 speak english. The United States, England, Australia, New Zealand, South Africa, Canada, have that language as maternal tongue; that 270.000.000 speak Russian, but we know a great part of Russia speaks different languages; equally, that 200.000.000 speak Spanish. Castilian would be the fourth spoken language in the world.

In a first trip to Greece, in the environment in which we moved, about the time of the french influence in the Balkan countries, our scarce ability in the language of Racine and Voltaire permitted us to act without difficulty. In a last journey to Hellas, prevailed the english. Not excluding the inextinguishable vestiges of the Albion, now existed the luxurious Hilton and American Embassy occupying a block, with its thorny group of receiving and emitting antennas that were seen from different places in Athens where we met young physicians who had done post-graduate work in the United States.

In the long tour to the Far East we listened everywhere to the Anglo-Saxon tongue, in every place that we visited, observing that the Asiatic, mainly the Japanese, were interested in learning english. The french language that became international and was called the "diplomatic language", was heard twice: first, a girl guide, addressing while in Japan a group of french tourists; and later, in the dining of the well known María Isabel in Mexico-City, during a discussion of seemingly Antillian gentleman.

Our language, today, is studied with dedication in the United States, and in some areas, as Miami, is almost compared with English. We found it necessary, to locate an scholastic Spanish speaking person as we did in Tokio, or as the one appointed to us, a very well trained cicerone named Wanda, in Praga.

The well remembered teacher, Conde Flores, said: "that the cases not published were as if they had not existed at all". We would say: "that not to have published in english, or at least, not to have an explicit summary in that language, is as if not published at all".

The bibliographies of most works of present time we would say, an 80%, are written in English.

This translation has been made by us, and although imperfect, it has been made possible by the medical terminology used and by being myself the author. In other fields, perhaps, we would not have dared to enter into this matter.

This one is our ninth book. Someone said once that it was necessary to write several books in order to obtain the equivalent of one. There is a need to write and to publish. We write for pleasure, because we believe on approaches happiness, if this probability exists. We are not the true writer; for him the literary creation is the meaning of his life.

We realize, without presumption, that the fact of bringing forth this book, pioneers many things in our country:

1.- For the first time, we found Leishman bodies in the heart of a patient with the Chagas disease.
2.- We practiced, for the first time, the Machado-Guerreiro test in the diagnosis of the Chagas disease, and helped in the work of other researchers.
3.- For the first time, we tried to break the old scaffolding that existed about Carate, which claimed that the pinta of Cuba and the Carate from Mexico, Venezuela, Colombia, Ecuador and Brazil, were two diseases completely different, and giving to the treponema found by Sáenz, Grau-Triana and Armenteros in a Cuban patient, the name of Treponema iriartei.
4.- The author was one of the first in the world, since 1931, to describe the principle and evolution of Carate.
5.- For the first time, the author found a human case of Sodoku.
6.- For the first time, with the collaboration of Cuenca, we utilized electrocardiograms in animals inoculated with Sch. cruzi.
7.- With the collaboration of Briceño Rossi, we found, for the first time, the spirochete of Carate; our country was the second in Latin-América to find it after León i Blanco found it in Mexico.
8.- Ample chemical study about the fruit of the bread-fruit tree was performed, for the first time.
9.- For the first time, we found the hemipterous Corizus sidae as the transmissor of the flagelliase in plants.
10.- For the first time, in vivo, we found in a patient, with the collabora-

tion of Rodríguez, the fungus Paracoccidioides brasiliensis, cited before by O'Daly in authopsies.

11.- For the first time, we found the otomycosis in Venezuela. With the collaboration of Montemayor, two species of Penicillium: Ochraceus and terreus var. flocconosa, were found in Venezuela.

12.- For the first time, we did an ample study, with the collaboration of Montemayor, on the fungi in the tonsils in relation with the actinomycosis, including the classification of the fungi.

13.- We found, for the first time, in the látex of Codiaem variegatum Blume, a protozoan (amoeba) besides the leptomonas davidi.

14.- We performed an experimental infection, for the first time, of Triatoma capitata (Usinger) specimens (1939), with a Sch. cruzi human strain.

15.- For the first time, we found Leishman bodies in the histopathological cuttings of guinea pigs inoculated with human strain and with intestinal parasites of R. prolixus infected with the mentioned strain.

16.- We found two news insects of the family Reduviidae: Spiniger rubropictus H.S. and Brontostoma notata Stal.

17.- We found a hyperparasite of the cheliferidae family living on Psammolestes arthuri in the nests of Phalecodomus rufifrons inornatus Ridway.

18.- For the second time in the world, we found the tick Amblyomma curruca Schultze living on an armadillo (Dasypus) in the zone of San Casimiro (State of Aragua). The site where the first tick specimen was caught is unknown.

19.- After Hase, the author wrote the most complete biological essay on Triatominae specimens.

20.- With the collaboration of Ballou and his wife, we wrote a complete description on Psammolestes arthuri, after the original works of Pinto (1926) and Pinto and Lent (1935).

21.- We did the first histopathological studies on inoculated animals with Trypanosoma venezuelense, found by Rangel in 1905 and classified by Mesnil in 1910 with the collaboration of Koppish of the Tropical School of the University of Puerto Rico.

22.- With the collaboration of Salas, we wrote the most extensive work on the Granuloma venereum, with the presence of the Kalimmato bacterium granulomatis.

23.- We found the first case, with the collaboration of Gedeón, of Rhinoscleroma, with the characteristic cells of Mikulicks and the capsulated diplo-bacillus of Frisch.

24.- With the collaboration of Edgar Anzola, we made the second scientific film; this one on the Chagas disease. The first film was made by Iturbe and Anzola on the equine trypanosomiasis "derrengadera".

25.- For the first time, in 1940, we had suspicions of the existence of Bilharziosis mansoni in the East of the country, mainly in the State of Sucre, with the finding of eggs in patients of that region, corroborated by hepatic biopsies studied by Potenza and by shells of Planorbidae collected by Luttermosser.

26.- In doing a most extensive work on Ceratoponidae, the author found these three species, of which C. stellifer, new in Venezuela. Cited other genus: Atrichopogon and Lasiohelea.

27.- An insect of the Ceratoponidae family has been called, in honor of the author, Culicoides iriartei; classification done by Irving Fox, in a specimen from La Salina, State of Zulia.

28.- In a most extensive work on Simuliidae, the author has found twelve species in the country, some of them for the first time: haematopotum, bicoloratum, sanguineum, limbatum.

29.- One of these Arthropoda has been called in honor of the author, Simulium iriartei; classification made by Luis Vargas, Martínez and A. Díaz Nájera, in a mosquito from Mexico.

30.- In Psichodidae, we have found four species. By the year 1944 there were fourteen found in Venezuela.

31.- In 1943 we presented a list of 140 specimens. In 82 of them we gave genus an specie; in 55 we gave the genus; in 1, the subfamily and in 2, only the family. This list included arthropoda, molluscs, birds, mammalians.

32.- We made the first attempts to transmit Trypanosoma venezuelense, employing triatominae, of the genus Eutriatoma (maculata) and Rhodnius (prolixus).

33.- For the first time, we found a new specie of horsefly Tabanus subruber Bell; and a new specimen of Harpagopyga, possibly in the world, like the Harpagopyga divergens Curr.

34.- In 1936, we detected the presence of the Eutriatoma maculata in five States; it had never been found infected, according to the opinion of César Pinto; later, experimental infection was obtained with Sch. cruzi by Díaz and Torrealba.

35.- We had already made some publications in 1929 on leishmaniosis, and since the year 1942 we have spoken about the oto-rhino-laryngologic lesions of this disease.

36.- In 1942, we made an ample publication on yaws in Venezuela.

37.- We had suspicions of the presence of spirochetosis gallinarum in hens in Caracas and Ciudad Bolívar. Later we found the Argas persicus.

38.- We made Commentaries about the Laphygma frugiperda (S.A.), which was causing havocs in Caracas and the States of Aragua and Carabobo.

39.- We made Commentaries on the Statistics of serological and coprological tests in persons from middle and high social classes, in a private laboratory.

40.- In close collaboration with Gutiérrez Alfaro and Díaz Ungría, we did a most extensive bibliographical list about the Parasitology in Venezuela, since 1926 to 1955.

SCIENTIFIC WORKS

by

DAVID R. IRIARTE

Doctor in Medical Sciences (Caracas - Venezuela).

Ex-Professor of Bacteriology and Parasitology in Central University of Venezuela.

Honorary and Retired Professor in Central University of Venezuela.

Member of National Academy of Medicine (Caracas - Venezuela).

Corresponding Member Academy of Medicine of State Zulia (Venezuela).

Corresponding Member Academy of Medicine (Bogotá - Colombia).

Laureate Academy of Medicine (Paris - France).

Member Royal Society of Tropical Medicine (London - England).

Member Société of Pathologie Exotique (Paris - France).

Corresponding Member Tropical Medicine Society "Carlos Finlay" (Havana - Cuba).

Corresponding Member Natural Sciences Society (México City - Mexico).

Founder Laboratory of Clínica Luis Razetti (Caracas - Venezuela).

Co-founder and Co-director Bulletin of Laboratory Clínica Luis Razetti (Caracas - Venezuela).

Foreign Honorary Member Argentina Medical Association (Buenos Aires - Argentina).

Ex-Director Gaceta Médica de Caracas (Caracas - Venezuela).

Prize Alejandro Próspero Reverend (Caracas - Venezuela).

Prize José Gregorio Hernández (Caracas - Venezuela).

Prize Monbinne (Paris - France).

Member United States Public Health Society

Member American Association for the Advancement of Science (U.S.A.)

Member American Association of Tropical Medicine (U.S.A.)

Member American Society of Parasitologists (U.S.A.

Member Aerospace Medical Association (U.S.A.)

Member Space Medicine Branch (U.S.A.)

MORE RESEARCH PARASITOLOGICAL AND ENTOMOLOGICAL ABOUT THE CHAGAS' DISEASE

CHAPTER I

In the State Sucre we have made research about reduviidae in the surroundings of Cumaná: farmer Bordones, agricultural grange, around the airport, etc. In this last region, in a hut, we have found larves and nymphs hided in sleeping mats and in old basket. In the roof we did not find insects, probably, because it was made with palms of coconut (C. nucifera L.), not good for living the hemipteres. In six of the insects (2 nymphs and 4 larves) found one of these infected in fresh and panoptical (16.66 % infection).

Not withstanding, this low percentage, living three children in the hut, we did the examination of the blood in fresh and thick drop with negative result and inquired about the sign Chagas-Mazza Romaña, being unknown. In this place we examined the blood of an armadillo (D. novemcinctus) and a rabipelado (Didelphis aurita) with null result. Equally, we examined eight nests of pespé (Icteridae. Icterus nigrogularis heliolides Clark) not finding triatomidae. According Mazzotti and Brumpt in nests of calandrias, possibly the same bird by the type of the nest, not finding

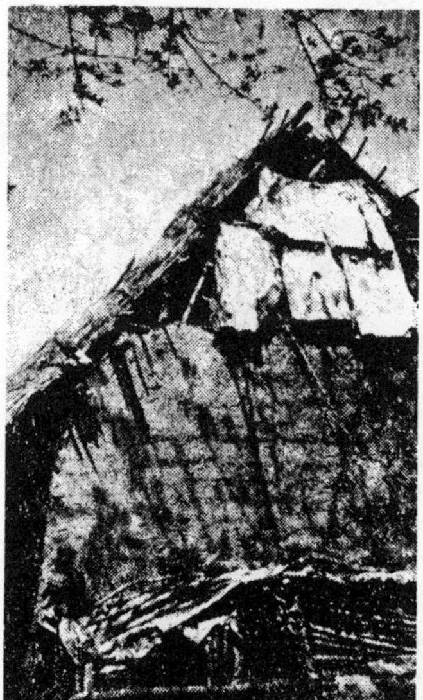

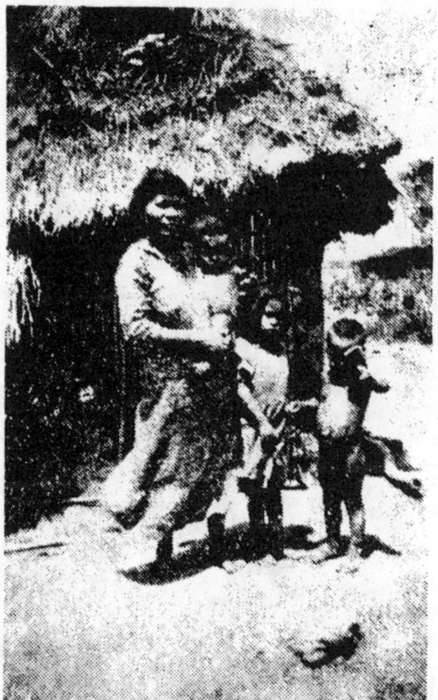

insects. Search in nests of pericos were negative.

Let refer about wild rats and cockroach in nests of Myopsilta monacha cotorra (Wiell). We did not find nests of cucaracheros. Summaring: in these short investigations in the surroundings of Cumaná we can say that the reduviidae are scarce and with low average of infection and so the human infection must be rare.

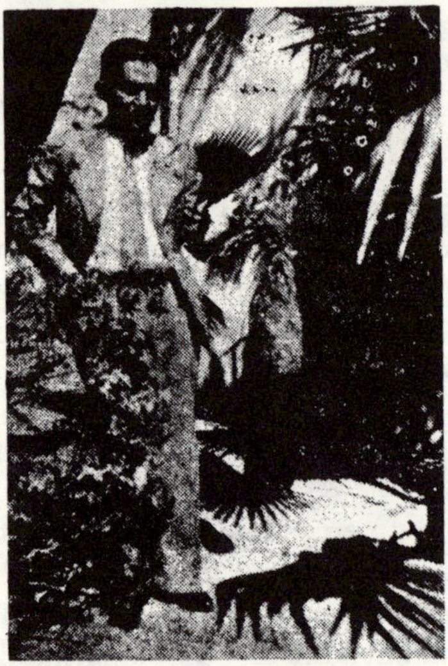

Nest of pespé

Research done in Margarita island, in Porlamar (El Morro), La Asunción, Los Hatos, San Juan, Juan Griego, has not been possible to find triatomidae. In the village El Tirano, at border of the sea, some persons told us to know them, but was impossible to get specimens, even offering reward. In general aspect the fauna in the island is very poor. The rainings are scarce and then the sickness of Chagas must be very rare.

In 13 specimens received from Rio Chico (State Miranda) of R. prolixus in their three stages, none infection.

In trip to Guarenas looking for triatomidae, these kind of insects are rare, because the houses have roof tiles and the species adaptable to this lodging are unknown for us, in accord Mazza and his school (Argentine) and Talice and others in Uruguay. Only we have seen some huts of caña amarga (Hynerium saggittatum) and sugar cane top (Sacharum of-

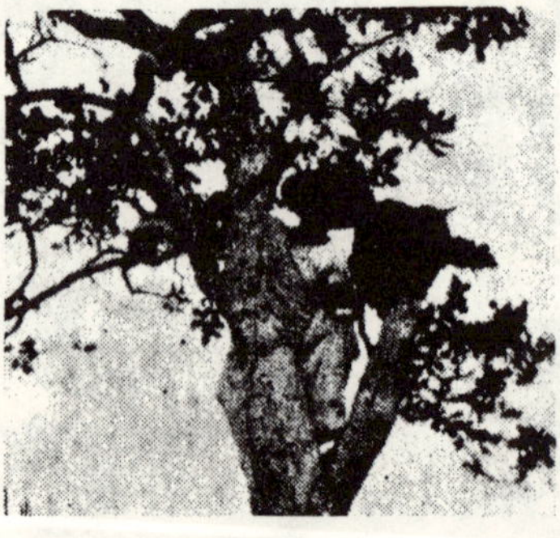

Nest of perico

ficinarum L.), lodging not convenient for the life of prolixus. Where it lives very well is in the gamelot (Panicum maximum), because the eggs go glue to the leaves and break when the hut is done. The reduviidae seeks more the hierba de guinea, because being the grass for feed, in those pasture grounds for cattle and echinus, the feeding is near and sure. Scarcely, in one of the huts made with caña amarga we found four specimens of R. prolixus and nymphs dead. Showing to the rural people the collection of insects that we carry in our trips, the natives said to know the R. prolixus, but had doubts about the E. maculata.

An armadillo of that region has been examined the blood in fresh with negative result. Living on an armadillo (Dasypus) of the zone San Casimiro (State Aragua) we had caught a tick (Amblyoma curruca Schultze), that for second time had been found in the world, being unkwnown the place of the first finding.

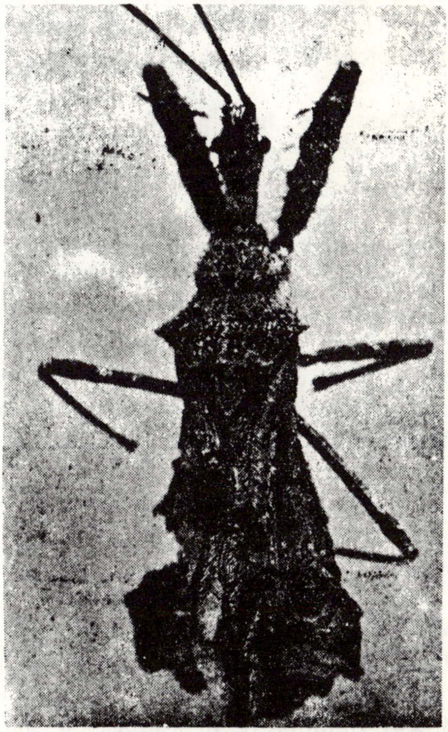

Insect caught in the road from Caracas to Santa Lucía (State Miranda).

An example of P. geniculatus dead 24 hours before, brought from a farmer near Guarenas, in the intestinal liquid we have found numerous metacyclic forms that we have inoculated a white mouse. Other specimen, caught in El Calvario (Caracas - Dto. Federal) with, probably, several days died, was negative.

Summary: The insects from Rio Chico undamaged; in Guarenas scarce trypanosomas; test of a Dasypus negative and finding of one Panstrongylus geniculatus with infection.

From the surroundings of Maturin (State Monagas) we have received two specimens of R. prolixus (nymph and adult). The first undamaged, but the second showed a strong percentage of metacyclic intestinal forms. This finding (50%) suggest an epidemiological survey in State Monagas.

* * *

In Maracaibo (State Zulia) in a house of the center of the town, where there is a pigeon house, we have caught a triatomidae, several specimens, for which we have been very interesting. Either in this region has been found the Spiniger rubropictus H.S., classified by Barber in Washington. Lent, of the Brazil, believes is an insect of the genus Triatoma, taking in account the biologycal details and photos in work published about the affair. The systematical studies made about the samples concluded in the classification of E. maculata. It seems to be is the first time that it has been in State Zulia. The specimens of rubropictus were caught in the surroundings of Maracaibo.

There are very interesting details about these hemipterous from Maracaibo. We have placed two females inside different tubes N° 1 and 2. Observing the oviposition, on 1-8-40, the number 1, had 9 eggs and for the following day one more. The number 2, on 1-8-40, had 3 eggs. On 1-12-40, the number 1, has 4 more and the number 2, the same account.

The eggs have not mucilagous substance, but sometimes are glue to the walls of the tube for the gummy evacuations. Are very nimbles, joining often and sick the pigeon when are near. However, have had an high mortality, perhaps, the influence of height, climate, the temperature in Caracas, was commonly lower 20 degrees. This thought is not sure, because these class of animals support winters as has been seen in Illinois State (U.S.A.), and heights of 4.000 meters as has observed Niño in the bolivians mountains. The change between Maracaibo and Caracas must have effects. This point is disputable.

Of the lot brought were examined 6 adults and 4 nymphs and the intestinal liquid was negative.

Coming again on the oviposition, on 1-18-40, the number 1 had 4 eggs more and number 2 had 2 more. The number 2 died and continue studying the number 1. On 1-17-40 has 6 eggs more and on 2-4-40, 5 more; on 2-7-40, 1 more. For 2-11-40 has 34 eggs. Summarily: in 33 days, 34 eggs, an average of 1 daily, without relation with the feeding that was given 1-18-40 and 1-24-40, blood of pigeon.

On 2-8-40, appeared in the tube the first larves; the incubation has been of 30 days that seems long, perhaps the influence of the factors that we have announced before. The incubation time, more or less is of two weeks, mainly for R. prolixus.

Introducing inside the ice-box in order to observe the effect of the cold, we have seen that the lowest temperature supported is of 9° degrees; lower, the insect presents lethargy and dead. Taking off of the ice-box the

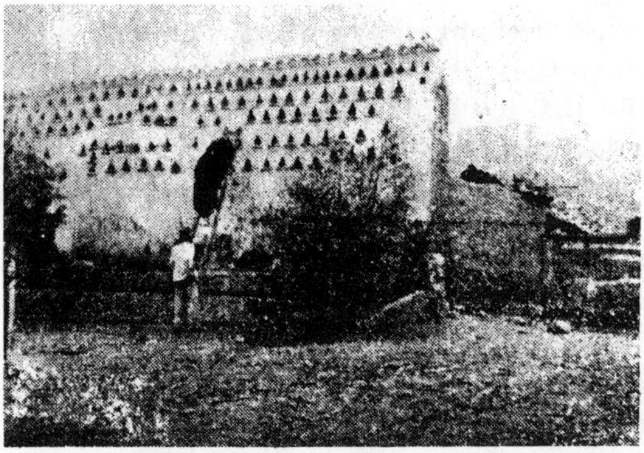

Looking for triatomidae in the pigeon house of a farmer near Caracas.

tube and putting it inside the stove to 35° degrees, inmediately the insects revive.

The same female number 1 introduced inside the ice-box at 9 a.m., to 9:15 was in lethargy, pick up and put it inside the stove to 35° degrees, to 12 meridiem, was in excellent conditions. Looked newly at 4 p.m. had 9 eggs, the following day 5 more and two days after 6 more. This increase of the oviposition we do not know if it is the influence of the heat or cold. Putting the tube to the ambient of the laboratory the oviposition stopped quickly.

Putting inside a tube 14 eggs of E. maculata and in another one 19 eggs of R. prolixus, we saw that in first, 9 eggs gave good rearings and 5 eggs an immature incubation; while that all the eggs of R. prolixus had a normal maturity, excepted one. In the E. maculata 35.75% not good incubation, while in R. prolixus was an average of bad incubation only of 7.14%. Lefting eggs of maculata and prolixus in the frigidaire to 9° degrees, none incubation in both, and taking and taking off, either in the stove to 35° degrees, neither the temperature of the laboratory, the incubation was null.

The action of the low temperature is felt by E. maculata not only in the ice-box, but also to ambiental temperature of the laboratory, of more or less, 20° degrees in January 1940, and so, we saw a female in lethargy stage and put it in the stove, 35° degrees, and inmediately revived; any time after sucked the pigeon and did an abundant meal and oviposition of 3 eggs, that was stopping. This a fact that the temperature has influence on the oviposition, because, we have observed that the effect of the feeding is none.

After to stay in the cold the maculata it seems on recovery rapidly in about thirty minutes, while the prolixus delay more time. The larval stage is more sensitive to the cold, and so, of a group of 14 larves, only 3 revived, the others died, nevertheless the help of the stove.

Feeding specimens of E. maculata and R. prolixus of this manner: 6 tubes with each 4 larves of R. prolixus and 4 tubes with each one 4 larves of E. maculata. The larves of R. prolixus of the total of 24, only 2 not fed in the pigeon, while with the maculata: 4 abundant meal, 5 not fed and the others 7 middling. This trial verify less voracity of the maculata, because, it is not possible to think in adaptation. Its ancestors are rearings accustom to live in pigeon houses and for that to blood of doves, while the rearings of prolixus are descending of rhodnius brought of the interior of the country caught in huts of straw and accostumed to human blood or mammalians (dogs, cats, pigs, etc.).

After an abundant meal on see that the blood is divided in two parts: one clear, anterior, that should be serum, and the other, often rear, redish, that should be red cells; in others cases, notwithstanding, after a large meal the abdomen is always clear and in some opportunities red.

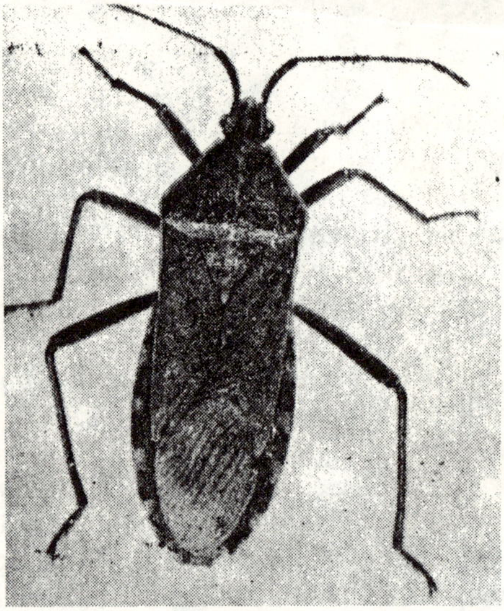

Leptoglossus gonagra F.
(Coroidae family)

In the way to Santa Lucía in one of the houses with roof of zinc inhabited by workers of M.O.P. we caught an hemiptere. In Caracas on fed with blood of pigeon during ten minutes; unfortunately was attacked by ants and destroyed. We found on the abdomen several files of eggs, that were put inside the stove, 35° degrees, without to obtain incubation. This fact is very interesting, are hemipterous suckers of blood that could coming to be accidental transmissors of the Chagas' disease. In Brazil, Castro Ferreira and Dean have published works about Clerada apicicornis as probable transmissor of this sickness.

In the States Miranda and Guárico we have done investigations in Villa de Cura and San Juan de los Morros. In the first place, in a village near 2 or 3 kilometers called Los Colorados seized a lot of R. prolixus in a typical hut where inhabited father, mother and three boys of short age. The examination of the blood of the children and a dog gave negative result.

For catching the reduviidae is convenient to seek in the internal part of the roof avoiding the action of the sun. The ideal site must be far from the kitchen avoiding the heat and near the dormitories. In this lot we found an average of the 25% infected. In the external part of the roof we have seized a phytophagous insect in abundance. In this trip we have examined two house pigeons and several nests of hens with negative result. Also, examined 5 nests of cucaracheros, finding in two triatomidae (psamolestes); in one of the nests we seized, and was the occasion with the greatest abundance (10 adults, 2 nymphs and 3 larves). Rapidly we knew when the nest was or not inhabited and was the presence of wasps, that without doubt contributed to the absence of birds and reduviidae.

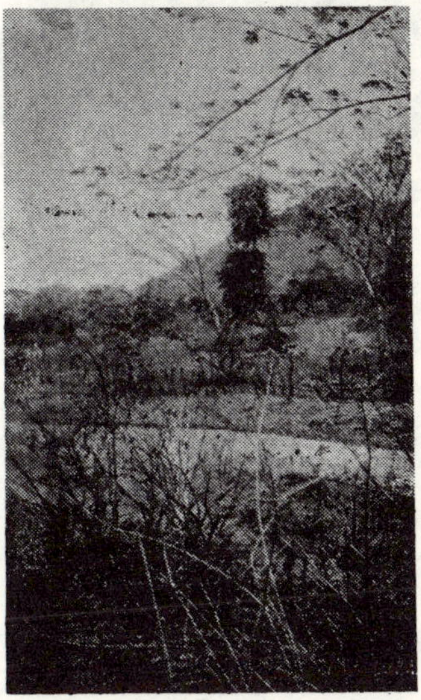

Nests of "cucarachero".

In San Juan de los Morros, easiness in the road to Ortiz in the huts of the borders of the way caught R. prolixus. In a hut far, around 100 meters from the road, we observed the exodus of a family (father, mother, daughter), so was the abundance of insects. Testing the blood of the daughter (child), dog and cat gave negative result. The capture in this hut was very abundant in R. prolixus, made in roof, old bags, pieces of cloth hanging of roof and walls. The percentage of infection of these insects was

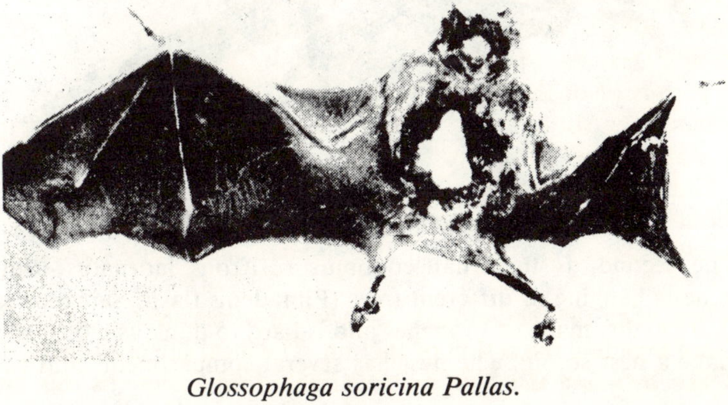

Glossophaga soricina Pallas.

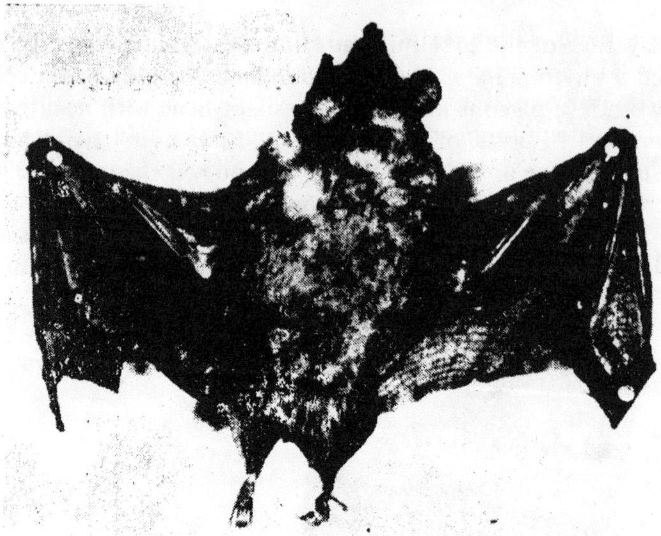

Desmodus rotundus Geoffroy.

very high, almost 100% and perhaps should be the highest seen till now.

In Trapichito, farmer near San Mateo (State Aragua) we have caught in the old house of the sugar mill 19 specimens of bats: 16 specimens of Desmodus rotundus Geoffroy and 3 specimens of Glossophaga soricina Pallas. In none of them we have found flagellates by test of the blood in fresh. The rearing of these animals was not possible.

In this same region we caught two exemplaries of cucarachero (housing and mountaineer). The first is the Troglodytes musculus clarus (Berlepsch and Hartert) and is small, place in the fissures of the walls or either between roof and walls; perhaps, these conditions are not well for living psammolestes in it.

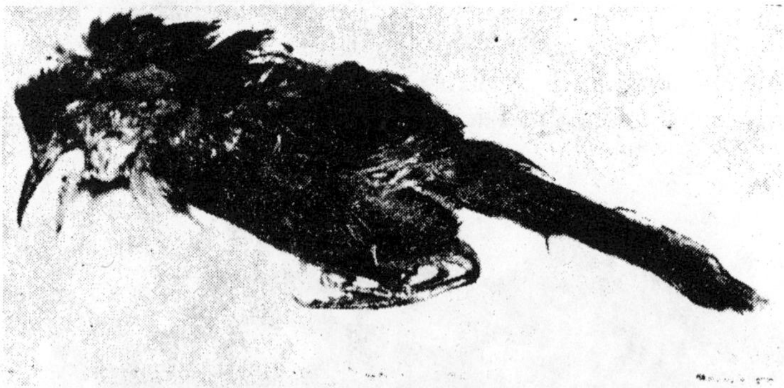

Phallecodomus rufifrons inornatus Ridgway.

The second, is the Phallecodomus rufifrons inornatus Ridgway, whose nests hanging of different trees (Piptadenis flava, Samanca samán Jacq.) are highs, made of branches and is hard to think as a bird so small can make a nest so big. The nest has several compartments and two entrances: one main, lateral, and another toward above, that we do not know if it will be an entrance of escape or belonging to the upper compartment. Accompanying the P. arthuri we have found a scorpion that possibly profit the psammolestes for transportation, and also an another coleopterous, for the first time. In all the invertebrates found in these nests we have found intestinal flagellates.

The feeding of the P. arthuri is very difficult employing pigeons, guinea pigs, men. We have made a dispositive looking for the natural ambient and so, we have introduced inside a large container of glass, pieces of paper, feathers of bird, pieces of wood and besides a pigeon; doing the assay day and night with negative result. Changing the pigeon for a little bird called "chirulí", we have got some stings. The biology of this insect is difficult, and only we could arrive till a second moulting and also to see a nymph seized arrives to adult stage, but to observe all the evolution of the triatomidae has been impossible. Is very sensitive to the feeding and outside things, and so: 12 larves are put at 6 p.m. near the chirulí inside the

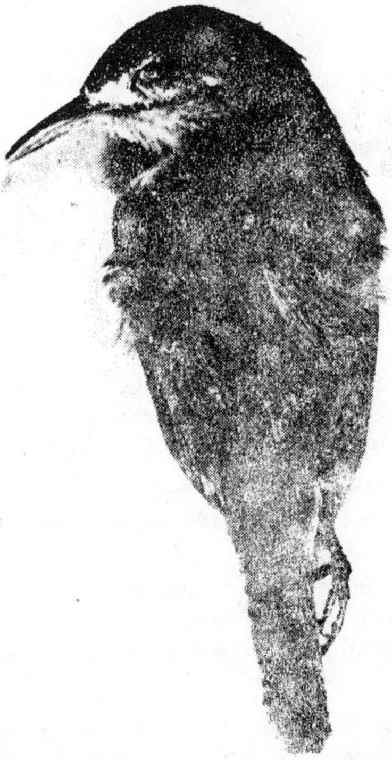

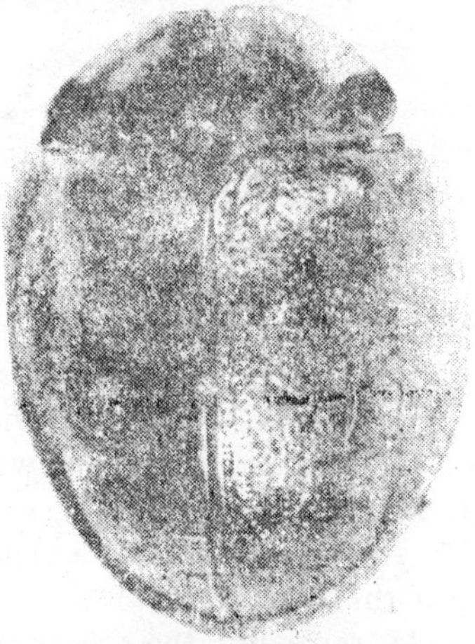

Coleopterous

Troglodytes musculus clarus (Berlepsch y Hartert).

dispositive described before; to the following morning only 5 were alives and only one had sucked.

A female of P. arthuri had in a tube did on a piece of wood an oviposition of 23 eggs, like a package of cigarettes, glue to the object by mucilaginous substance of which are covered; are of five elements; are operculated, having the operculum in the free end that is more narrow,

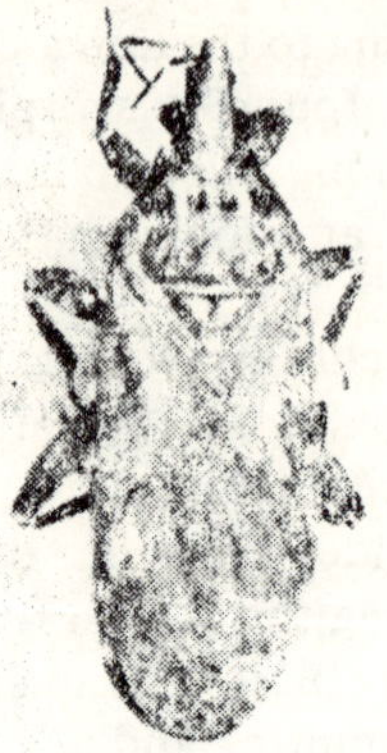

Psammolestes arthuri,
adult and male.

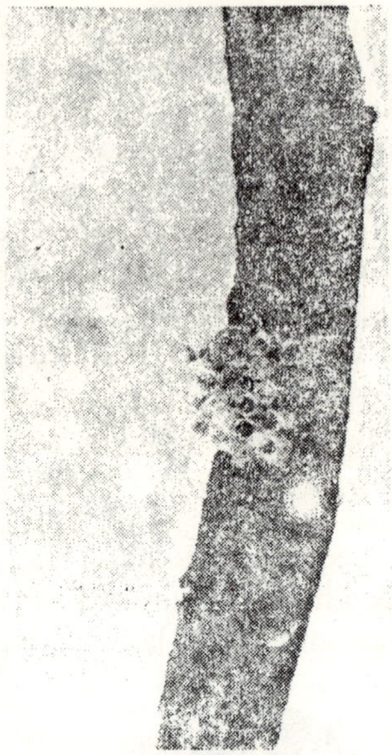

Eggs of Psammolestes
arthuri.

different to the others that is enlarged, as a base; with the development of the incubation the operculum is seen better.

The cells of the walls of the eggs are polygonals (penta); sometimes ronds. The incubation it seems shorter that we have seen in the genus triatoma, being of 11 days, starting comes out the first larves. In cold at 10° degrees produces lethargy of the animal and the incubation is stopped. The average of size of an egg, is: lenght, including the operculum, 1.5 m.m.; operculum, 0.1 m.m.; width, in end not operculated 0.7 m.m.; width, middle part, 0.6 m.m.; width, operculated end, 0.5 m.m.

It seems to be that the first classification of psammolestes was made in 1926, for César Pinto, in an specimen sent by Tejera to Professor Lutz, giving it the name Eutriatoma arthuri. Pinto accompanied by Lent, the year 1935, reviewing the same specimen found callosities situated behind the eyes, and for this detail was included in the genus Psammolestes (Bergroth 1911).

Pinto it seems, could not do a wide description for to have only one exemplary and perhaps damaged. At following, we give the original description of Pinto, taken of the work of del Ponte and after the make it by us, working with several specimens.

Description of Pinto: "especie pequeña de 1.5 cm. de largo. Cabeza muy corta, de 3 mm. de largo. Antenas insertas cerca de los ojos; primer artejo antenal corto, que llega casi hasta la extremidad apical de la cabeza; 2°, 3° y 4° artejos casi del mismo tamaño y todos ellos de color castaño. Cabeza del mismo color, presentando sin embargo, una estría longitudinal más clara, colocada en la parte central. Ojos negros; ocelos claros. Rostro recto, 3, articulado, llegando el primer artículo hasta cerca del tubérculo antenífero; el segundo artículo es el más largo de todos, llegando hasta el límite toraco-cefálico; el 3° es del mismo largo del 1°. La suma de los artículos 1° y 3° es menor que el largo del 2° artículo. Borde anterior del pronoto en forma de media luna, de concavidad anterior y más estrecho que el mesonoto; las partes laterales del pronoto son salientes y más oscuras que el resto del tórax; existen dos líneas paralelas de color castaño claro y que llegan hasta el mesonoto; estas líneas son de color más claro que el resto del tórax y salientes. Ancho máximo del mesonoto: 5 mm.; éste es castaño y distintamente separado del pronoto por dos excavaciones laterales, con granulaciones oscuras e irregularmente esparcidas; los bordes postero-laterales del mesonoto por dos excavaciones laterales, con granulaciones oscuras e irregulares de color castaño y oscuro en el ápice. Corio castaño. Membrana un poco más oscura. Cara ventral de color castaño irregularmente salpicada de negro. Las patas son de color castaño y las tibias son más oscuras. Todos los fémures son inermes''.

In this description we have had the help kindly of Dr. Charles Ballou and his wife, entomologist, working with the Ministry of Agriculture and Breeding.

Our description, now: especie mediana de 12 a 14 mm. de largo y 4.3 a 5 mm. de ancho. Cabeza lampiña, un poco más corta que el pronoto. Antenas insertas medio distintas entre los ojos y la extremidad anterior de la cabeza; primer artejo corto, castaño oscuro; segundo, cuatro veces más largo que el primero, castaño claro con el tercio distal oscuro; tercero, un poco más largo que el segundo, castaño oscuro; cuarto, un poco más corto que el segundo, castaño oscuro en las extremidades y castaño en el medio. Cabeza castaña en el disco, negruzca en los lados y a veces con una estría longitudinal más clara en el centro, aspecto ventral negruzco. Ojos grandes, negruzco-rojizos, colocados delante de un lóbulo que los separa de los ocelos, que se encuentran un poco afuera de la línea que marca el margen interior de los ojos: Rostro recto, primer segmento más corto y llegando un poco más atrás del tubérculo antenífero; segundo segmento 1.5 veces más largo que el primero y tercero juntos, llegando hasta el tórax; tercer

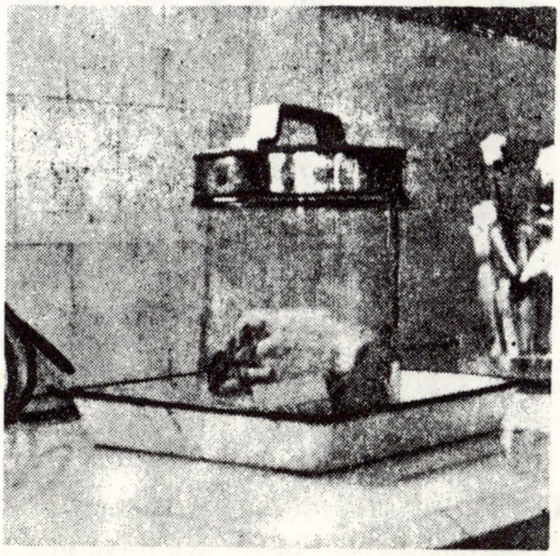

Special dispositive made for feeding of the P. arthuri.

segmento llegando hasta la parte anterior de las cavidades coxales. Pronoto con estrechamiento arriba separándolo en dos lóbulos, el posterior dos veces más largo que el anterior, sin angostamiento lateral; lóbulo posterior dividido póstero-longitudinalmente en tres partes por estrías elevadas que salen del lóbulo anterior; el espacio entre las dos estrías más ancho que entre las estrías y las márgenes laterales con una elevación en cada lado cerca del ángulo humeral. Todo el pronoto cubierto de vello castaño; ángulos laterales anteriores producidos en forma de dientes, oscuro en las márgenes laterales y en una línea central que se extiende desde el borde anterior hasta el centro. Conexivo estrecho de color marrón oscuro en las tres cuartas partes anteriores de cada segmento y claro en el cuarto posterior. Hemelitros de color castaño claro. Cara inferior de color castaño oscuro, irregularmente salpicada de negro y con vello de color castaño claro. Las patas son inermes, de color castaño, con las tibias negras, excepto en las bases que son castaño claras y todas las patas tienen vello, rojizo en las tibias y castaño en los otros artejos.

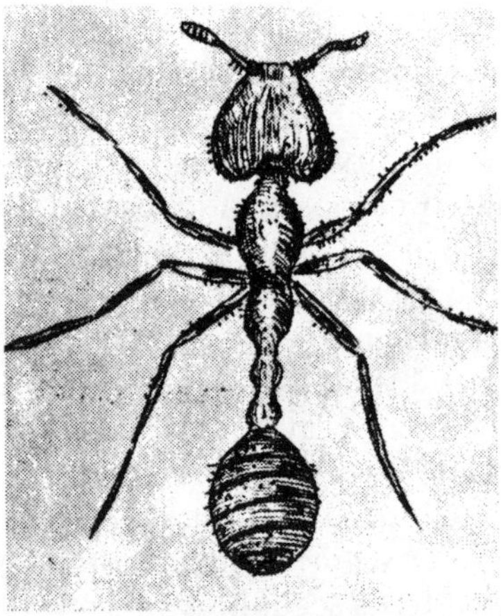

Monomorium pharaonensis L.
(drawing)

In the surroundings of Caracas we have caught a specimen of the genus Brontostoma, specie notata, Stal., predaceous insect that sometimes could be hematophagous and to be an accidental transmissor of the Sch. cruzi. Besides, we seized another species yet without classification. Ballou, in the entomological collection of the Ministry of Agriculture and Breeding has Brontostoma discus, seized in the interior of the country.

Finishing with this Chapter we will tell that there are specimens that suck rapidly and fill the abdomen, but there are others that prick several times without extract blood.

During the pricking, we can walk all the laboratory and the insect continue the suction. The piece of filter paper that we put inside of the tube or bottle, is useful for absorbing the evacuation and supporter of the insect, mainly in the moments of the sting.

Research with exemplaries of R. prolixus and E. maculata pricking rats or guinea pigs infected with T. venezuelense, never we have got success. However, feeding virgins specimens on rats or guinea pigs infected with T. cruzi (human or coming from intestinal liquid) the infection appear, nevertheless, the parasite has disappeared of the peripheric blood in the moment of the sucking.

In the tests with venezuelense sacrificing the insect half an hour after the meal, yet, it is possible to see scarce mobiles trypanosomas; some hours after, none, there is a true lysis of the parasites.

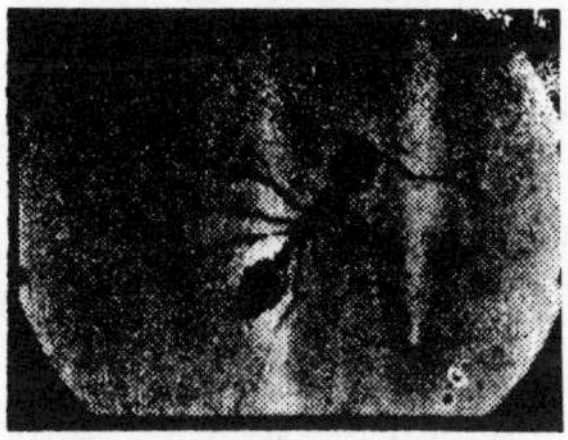

Monomorium pharaonensis L.
(microphoto)

CHAPTER II

The rearings of the triatomidae is necessary to take care and to watch over: change the pieces of paper; to take out the specimens dead and remainders of the moulting; avoid the clue of the larves to the wall of tube or bottle, either a larve or nymph very full after an abundant meal, remain trapped between a piece of paper and wall. But, the great care must be about the ants; these are the true enemy of the reduviidae.

Some hymenopterous have not any relation with the man, either are scarces or live far from the human dwelling. Few species are harmful, chiefly in the tropical countries, but some are profitables destroying numerous harmful insects.

Researchers have worked about the last fact. Professor Hase, absent some days of the farmer Puerto La Cruz (State Miranda) where had investigations, found the rearings of P. geniculatus, R. pictipes and E. cuspidatus, attacked by ants that destroyed much of its.

Later, returning to Germany in the bout the material was attacked equally for the argentine ant Irimidomirinex humilis Mayru.

We, some time ago, have made observations about this problem, finding at the beginning ants of the genus Solenopsis, without arrive to the species; after, we have caught, either attacking the rearings or near of its, specimens of Monomorium pharaonensis L., Brachymyrmex sp., Paratrechina longicornis Latr., Tapinoma melanocephalum F., Crematogaster brevispinosa, Pheidole sp.

The three firsts we have seen are rammers, mainly the Monomorium pharaonensis L. as we observed in several occasions. This ant is a domestic species, very common, it seems of African origin, not only in tropical sites, but also in places as New York and on says do ravages in the bouts.

The Brachymyrmex sp. is also very common in our laboratory and in several occasions we have found it on ours rearings of reduviidae.

The Paratrechina longicornis Latr. or Prenolepis (Nylandera) longicornis Latr. is called crazy ant by its reckless movements. It seems to be from India origin, has been found in tropical sites, but also in places as New York. Many times doing a xenodiagnosis a larve of R. prolixus has fallen to the floor and rapidly is attacked by these hymenopterous.

The rest of the ants noted in the former list, not withstanding, we have not yet proofs of to be rammers, but have been found near the rearings. One of them belonging to the genus Pheidole, either we have appointed the genus Solenopsis as rammer, both of the sub-family Myrmicinae. Pheidole megacephala of Fabricius, that perhaps, may be our species, is very abundant in tropical and sub-tropical regions, living in the soil, under the leaves or in the roots, being highly predaceous, because Illingworth in Hawaii and Simmonds in the island Fiji have demonstrated its importance in the control of the domestic fly.

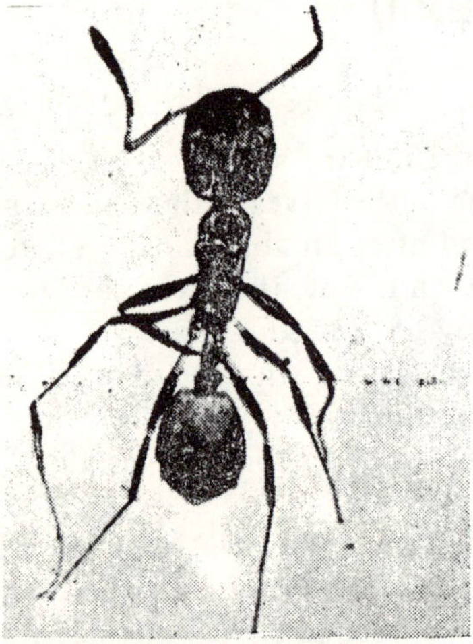

Brachymyrmex sp.

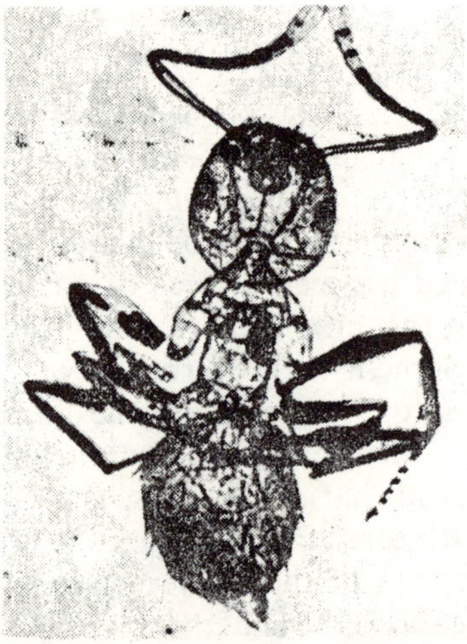

Crematogaster brevispinosa.

In the nests of cucarachero with the presence of ants and wasps we have not found psammolestes. Putting ants rammers in tubes or bottles with specimen of triatomidae in the three stages and the attack is not produced; the liberty of the nature is necessary. Possible will be different the attack to captives insects to the attack being in free nature.

It is very curious studying the biology of the triatomidae how these animals take in account the danger of approaching of the ants. Reveal afraid; continuous movements of the body; changes of places inside the tube or bottle; movements of the antennas; but the inimicals start for the legs, fixing the insect and continue after for the body. In 48 hours all the work is finished and the rearing destroyed.

We have not seen attack on the eggs, but some researchers have suspicions.

The hymenopterous seems to be very useful in the fight in the nature against the Chagas' disease, specially about to the transmissors. The struggle is hard, because these animals support prolonged fastings; wide changes of temperature and height and the biologycal struggle should be sure and economical. Today is very employed in animals and plants.

CHAPTER III

The xeno-diagnosis was devised by Professor Brumpt not only for the Chagas' disease, but, also as a method discovering the development of the parasite in virgin transmissors, being difficult find it through of others procedures. It is a culture *in vivo*. So, referring to Chagas' disease, often we see that the tests as direct examination in fresh, by smears, thick drop, inoculations to animals, guinea pigs, mice, being negative; however, with the xeno is easy find trypanosomiasis, either old.

The heritage transmission must be difficult, but it is admitted by researchers as M. Mayer. We have long time working with these hemipterous, sometimes, we take the eggs after the oviposition, washing and putting in new tubes; either leaving in the same container of the rearing in contact with infected specimens, taking out the larves to new tubes. Never, we could find intestinal flagellates.

The xeno is a good test of diagnosis for Chagas' disease, but, it is necessary do it in appropriated ambients. Doing it in hospitals or surveys is very complicated. In the first, the patient is filling a bed during six weeks and always there are scarcety of its; in the second, this people changes often of sites, break the tubes, loose the insects; in summary: indisciplined people. According to Brumpt, sometimes, eight days after the starting the xenodiagnosis may be positive.

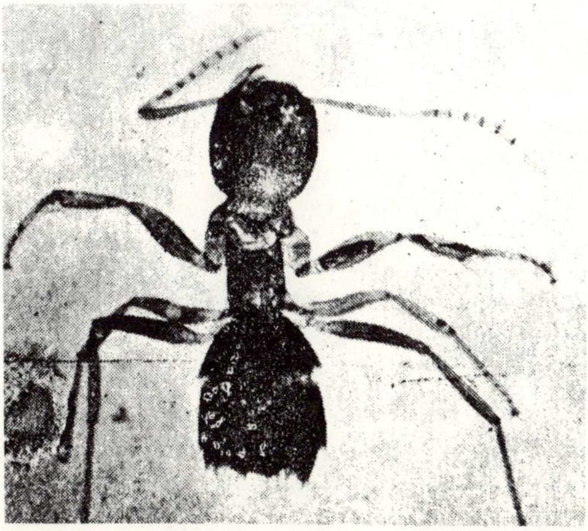

Paratrechina o Prenolepis (Nylanderia) longicornis (Latr.)

We present here 35 xenodiagnosis: 33 in hospital and 2 in private patients. They were submitted to a questionnaire.
Hall________ Bed________ Name________ Age________ Sex________ Race________ Employ________ Place of birth________ Is or has been rural people?________ Has lived in huts?________ Do you know the reduviidae?________ How are called in your region?________ Beginning of the sickness________ Symptoms of chronic Chagas' disease________ Tests of laboratory________.

We utilizes specimens (larves and nymphs) of R. prolixus and E. maculata) looking for the receptivity of both. These insects are rearings obtained in the laboratory and controlled to verify the indemnity.

Commonly we used 5 or 6 specimens for each test owned to the scarcity of the rearings. Sometimes, for mortality or others motives, we add new specimens and the time of the proof was prolonged. The insects were put inside test tubes with a piece of filter paper absorbing the evacuations and a plug of cotton.

During the proofs the insects have been inside the stove to 35°, leaving the door semi-open in order to change the internal ambient. The tubes inside the stove avoid the attack of the ants and we believe should be better to the life and infection of the reduviidae.

We should wished to have given 4 or 5 meals pricking the patient, but in an ambient of hospital is very difficult. In summary: 1 or 2 meals stinging the patient and one time a week sucking the pigeon, because the fasting sterilize the infected rearings, as we have verified. The reduviidae takes the infection at any stage. We have employed larves and nymphs because are more voraceous and are more handly.

The lapse of time to kill the insects has been more than one month: 45, 53, 54, 55 days. When the xeno start with larves finish with nymphs; when begin with nymphs finish with adults. We present here 24 xenos done with R. prolixus and 11 with E. maculata.

Name — ?

Age — The lowest was of 12 and the highest 50 years.

From 1 to 20 years	12
From 20 to 30 years	13
From 30 to 40 years	7
From 40 to 50 years	3

Sex - M - 27 F - 8

Race - Native 26 - White 4 - Indian 5

Place of birth - 14 States, so: Falcón 2, Guárico 6, Lara 7, Aragua 2, Miranda 5, Cojedes 2, Sucre 1, Portuguesa 2, Trujillo 2, Yaracuy 2, Anzoátegui 2, Monagas 1, Barinas 1.

Is or has been rural people?

Everything, except 2, have had relation with the rural zones. One, knows the triatomidae and the another, unknowns the insects. 15, always have lived in rural places and 18, have lived in rural zones a period of time between 1 to 15 years.

Do you know the triatomidae?

28 know the insects and 7 told unknown (in this answer there is something of prudery).

How are called in your region?

Only 21 of them answered this question: 8 say chipitos; others 8 call chupones; 1 tell pitos, and 3 chipos - The remainder gave, indistinctly, the names chupón or chipo, but chiefly chupón.

Symptoms chronic Chagas' disease

Deep anemia 12, Adenopathy 4, Nervous troubles 2, Edemas 9, Fever 10, Splenomegaly 15, Cardiac troubles 10, Hepatomegaly 6, Ascites 8.

In 28 of these xenodiagnosis has been possible to do control with the reaction of Machado-Guerreiro; in the others, we could not do it. In the hospital are things very difficult.

The antigen for the test of Machado is prepared with organs of puppies (mainly spleens), inoculated and with strong infection of cruzi, making maceration in distillable water and glycerine with 0,5% of carbolic acid. After two or three days in the ice-box, is taked the liquid that float, coming to be the antigen.

This antigen, we have used diluted 1 x 10 or 1 x 20 in saline solution physiological taking care not using high doses because have anticomplement action; frequently must be employed 0.2, because 0.4 either presents the former action.

As hemolytic serum we have used the anti-sheep, red cells of sheep and complement of guinea pigs to 1/3. Known the serum and complement; the dosage of it is as follow:

Tube 5	Antigen 1/100	Complement	S. Saline	Hemo- Serum	R. cells 1/8
1	0.1	0.5	1.4	1 c.c.	1 c.c.
o	0.2	0.5	1.3	1 c.c.	1 c.c.
3	0.3	0.5	1.2	1 c.c.	1 c.c.
4	0.4	0.5	1.1	1 c.c.	1 c.c.
5	0.5	0.5	1.0	1 c.c.	1 c.c.
6	0.6	0.5	0.9	1 c.c.	1 c.c.
7	0.7	0.5	0.8	1 c.c.	1 c.c.
8	0.8	0.5	0.7	1 c.c.	1 c.c.
9	0.9	0.5	0.6	1 c.c.	1 c.c.
10	1.0	0.5	0.5	1 c.c.	1 c.c.
11	1.0	0.5	1.5	1 c.c.	1 c.c.
12	1.0	0.5	1.0	1 c.c.	1 c.c.

Of these 28 reactions, in three: One, gave a positivity of + + + + +, another one of + + +, and the third of +. We should have: one, with a clear positivity and another one with a middle positivity. It was two with anticomplement action.

The patient of strong positivity has lived always in rural zones, in huts and knows the reduviidae. Others details in his history, are: epileptic attacks, hookworm in the feces and Wassermann and Kahn negatives.

The patient with the middle positivity has been lived all his life in rural zones in huts. Symptoms actually: cardiac troubles, light splenomegaly. Hookworm in feces. Kahn negative. In the 28 cases referring serology for syphilis: 18 were positives and 10 negatives. In the patients with Machado-Guerreiro positive, we increase the number of insects and were very carefully in the microscopic examination.

Summary: twenty four times both procedures were in accord; twice, not in accord (xenos negative and Machado positive) and in two others cases was anticomplement action, probably by the antigen.

One of the private xeno was made to a lady of the State Trujillo that live in the center of that town. This patient found, occasionally, three specimens of reduviidae in her home, possible carried by the washerwoman. This detail is very important, something similar to the bedbugs.

For several motives the test Machado-Guerreiro loose sphere of action today. It is not a specific test, but of group, and so, a leishmaniosic patient, sickness very frequently between us, could gives a positive test.

TRYPANOSOMIASIS CRUZI OR CHAGAS' DISEASE IN VENEZUELA

(Fragments of the conference red in the Clínica Luis Razetti)*

I am going to tell two words about an endemic that seems to be more abundant than really it is and probably produce terrible ravages in the interior of the country at side the malaria and the hookworm. I am referring to the Chagas' disease.

We know that since the studies of Dr. Tejera several years ago, reporting two cases in the borders of the States Zulia and Trujillo and after a new case in the State of Miranda, none person had spoken of new finding, not withstanding the investigations of Pino Pou in the surroundings of Barinas; Victor Raúl Soto in Falcón, catching reduvidae that Dr. Rísquez Jr. showed in the lessons of parasitology; Levy Romero and us finding in Maracaibo an insect belonging the genus Triatoma.

As you see in this collection of reduvidae there are specimens of Maracaibo, Coro, Ciudad Bolívar and Barcelona, four States of different regions of the country. The insects of the first site have been examined, not presenting infection; only the exemplar of Maracaibo has been classified for Barber of the Columbia University as *Spiniger rubropictus* H.S., who wrote us referring this specie has none relation with Chagas' disease and it feeds blood of doves and hens, places where it lives often.

We had the opportunity to stay two days in Zaraza and to accompany Dr. Torrealba in his investigations, eulogized labor in that far an poor region.

The insects collected by Torrealba have not been classified till now, but its seems are Rhodnius prolixus. Torrealba with the quiet life of those villages, taked a rest lying in a hammock, and suddenly felt a sting and captured a R. prolixus; happily for Torrealba, the insect had not time to make the evacuation. These invertebrates are called "chupones" in Zaraza; "chipitos" or "quipitos" in Coro and in Maracaibo "pitos" or "mamatetas"

Long time ago in those lands of Anzoátegui several physicians have observed patients with fever, deep anemia, edemas, splenomegaly, that not improved neither the antimalarics, nor the intestinal vermicides and thinking in Kala-azar, treat to them with tartar emetic and improved inmediately, disappearing the fever.

* Published in Caracas Médico (3) 139-148 — 1934

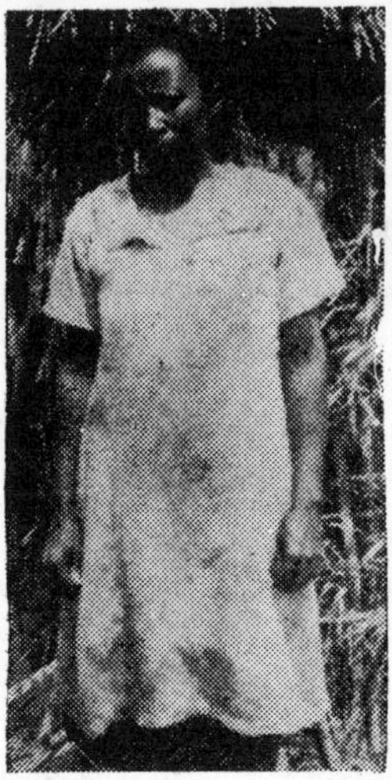

Woman with strong anemia, continuous fever, anxiety, cardiac troubles, edemas, etc. Xeno-diagnostic 100% positive. After 60 centigrams of tartar emetic dropped to 25%.

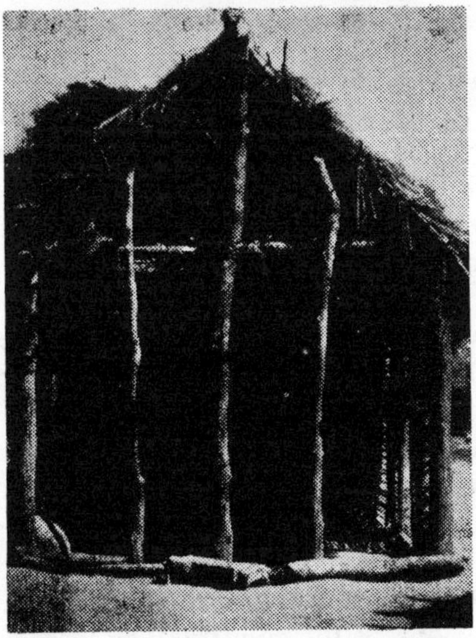

Typical hut of the surroundings of Zaraza, called also "caney". In the roof of these huts are very abundant the reduviidae.

Torrealba had seized numerous insects and in my presence searching in the straw of the roof found by hundreds of these animals in their three stages, demostrating a great ability for run and hide. One, of each three, presented infection or 33%, and one nymph examined in that moment showed 10 or 12 trypanosomas by microscopic field.

The trypanosomas at the beginning of the test are very actives and one or two hours after the movement goes disappearing and then is easy to see the flagellum and centrosoma in real end of the body; Torrealba has got to see them till 72 hours after the death of the insect alives in the intestinal liquid, as has been verified by us.

We have noted than in the larve after it born the evacuation is gummy, capable of joining to the wall of the containers. In the rearing of Triatoma we have not seen this observation. According to Torrealba the color of the eggs always should be white. Our investigations showed to us the white after the oviposition, but later goes taking a pink color in relation with the fecundation.

The hatching has a lapse of time of two or three weeks; the moulting are five and who wish know about the biology of these reduviidae please to read the interesting work of Professor Hasse of Berlín, investigations made during his stay in Venezuela in the farms Puerto La Cruz and Ocumare de la Costa.

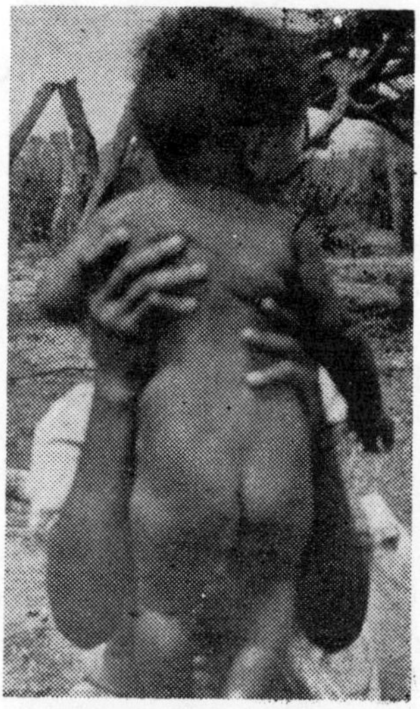

Child, one year and a half old, showing in back and legs numerous punctures produced by the stings of the insects.

Torrealba, tired of thinking the trypanosoma in those anemic patients, intended the xenodiagnostic, obtaining a positivity of 25%. As you will see by the photos of this woman, presented an aspect of deep anemia, continuous fever, nervosity, edemas, cardiac troubles, with cardiac blowing, intermissions, giving a xenodiagnostic of 100% (twelve indemnes invertebrates after twelve eatings, all presented metacycle trypanosomas). In this case the tartar emetic employed by Torrealba per os and enemas not in hight amounts improved the patient and the xenodiagnostic felt down to 20%.

Torrealba inoculated dogs, armadillos, oposums and one fox, with the intestinal containing of Rhodnius prolixus. In none of these animals contamined saw trypanosomas, notwithstanding in some of them has seen the death twenty days after, cheefly in the dogs that loose the appetite and weight, anxiety, weekness, paralysis of the posterior legs. In the heart, muscle, liver and spleen have been found leishmaniasic bodies.

The inoculation in a mouse was positive obtaining good microscopic preparations, better that those made with the intestinal liquid of the reduviidae. He had not rearing of white mice. It is necessary have in mind the Trypanosoma lewisi.

COMMENTARY TO THE DR. TORREALBA' WORK ABOUT CHAGAS DISEASE*

Chagas' disease is a nosological problem for the country, as has been mentioned by Professor Mazza relating to Argentine, and I suppose it is not as thought a colleague, because I told and wrote: "We know that it is an ailment decimating the country at side the malaria and hookworm, and if the first is curable with quinine and atebrine and the second with thymol and tetrachloride of carbono, for the trypanosomiasis cruzi there is not secure treatment".

If the Chagas' disease has not been found newly between us since the discovery of Tejera, is not necessary to think that is not abundant in the nation. Salas and us published in the year 1926 a communication about Granulome venereal with autochthonous cases, and today, after eight years nobody has pronounced a word more referring this problem, without to indicate the disease is not frequent in Venezuela.

All the persons that have found reduviidae in different regions of the country (Levy Romero, Víctor Raúl Soto, Pino Pou and us) going always seeking the finding of the trypanosoma in the blood of the inhabitants of those sites, the results have been negative, whether that the parasite scarcely is seen in the circulating blood and only the test of the thick drop gives a percentage not very flattering.

In Zaraza (Guárico - State) Dr. Torrealba had had the same lack, but after, employing the method of xeno-diagnostic, obtaining a percentage of 25% of positive results. Torrealba has found a percentage of infection in the reduviidae of 33%, (a specimen of each three is infected), percentage low in relation with the results in Argentine, relating a Triatoma infestans that has arrived to 60%. Torrealba has verified a far as that the trypanosomas can lives till 70 hours after extracted of the intestine of the insects, as we could appreciate during our stay in Zaraza.

In the plains of Guárico and Anzoátegui States some physicians had noted patients with deep anemia, fever, hepatic and splenomegaly, troubles of heart, etc., that no improved neither the antimalarial, nor the vermicides and thinking in cases de kala-azar applied tartar-emetic remarking notable improvement in health. Probably have been chronic cases of Chagas. It seems, the same has succeeded in Argentine and Romaña has discovered many chronic cases by inoculations and test of Machado-Guerreiro in patients with suspicious to be infected.

The tartar emetic without to be a specific medicine is one the few resources. Torrealba has uses it by enemas, not injections, and mentioned a case that gave 60% of xeno-diagnostic positive results before tartar emetic and only 25% after treatment. Tejera, it seems, to be glad with the

* Published in the Gaceta Médica de Caracas 1934 - pages 297-298

results that had obtained.

I wish to refer three new notions of the Argentine's school; two of them are very interesting and the third almost exactly original. The first, try about the domestic animals considerate as deposits of virus. Chagas was the first that found a cat infected; after, Emmanuel Díaz was in the same way, but has been the Professor Maza in Argentine and his adjunts, who have demonstrated that the puppies are the great deposit of virus and have show the nosologic importance in accord with the type of life of the rural people. The puppies have been found in the houses living acute cases of trypanosomiasis.

The second notion on refer about the reproduction of the Schyzotrypanum cruzi in the blood. Chagas by first time saw trypanosomas with two flagellums, two blefaroplastos and one nucleos. Subsequently, Emmanuel Díaz, one of the authors that has worked abundantly in this field has seen trypanosomas with the look, but he thinks are crithidias, that some times try leave the endocelular situation, but never any division in the circulatory blood. Has been the argentine's school who has found many of these forms and gives the opinion that there is a truly reproduction in the blood, and so, the schyzotrypanum cruzi on reproduce in the tissues and blood. So, the schyzotrypanum cruzi should loose its peculiar process of reproduction.

The third notion, original of Mazza and his school, on refer to the nodules of histiocites in the liver of the dogs by inoculations with T. cruzi.

Souza Campos had spoken of Sch. cruzi reproduction in the cells of the reticulo-endotelial system, as liver, lungs, kidneys, etc. Subsequently, Díaz had demonstrated that not only the reproduction in these places, but also in neuroglia and muscular fibres, flat and striated. The same investigator proved that he called biological blockade by inoculation of S. cruzi, in which the elements of the system loose the coloidopexis.

The nodules of Mazza have been denominated endotelial nodules, and certainly take birth in the cells of Kupffer, integring parts of the radiated capillary vessels. The histo-pathologycal studies of these formations is a field arid and hard.

Lastly, I will relate something with regards to reduviidae. In different trips to the interior of the country I collected insects in several States. Classified by Barber are Rhodnius prolixus and Triatoma maculata. R. prolixus is the reduviidae found by Torrealba, with a highest percentage infection. Triatoma maculata seems to be very common in the country, but till now it has not been found infected in the nature according to Pinto. We have not infected it, and for that reason we have thought that the genus Rhodnius will be the main transmissor between us as is accepted by Tejera and Torrealba.

For this exposition you will the importance of the Chagas' disease as a nosological problem, and I profit to send congratulations to Dr. Torrealba, to whom recently the National Academy of Medicine brought his nomination as Corresponding member.

PRESENCE OF THE TRIATOMA MACULATA IN VENEZUELA (ERICHSON 1848)

The subject of the reduviidae and the Chagas' disease is an affair up today for us. We know is a sickness to decimate the country at side the malaria and the hookworm. If the first cure with quinine and atebrine and the second with thymol and carbon tetrachloride, for the Chagas' disease till today there is not a specific treatment.

Trips done lastly to the interior of the country permitted us the seizure of reduviidae in Coro, Barcelona, Zaraza, Ciudad Bolívar, Barinas, El Morro de Barcelona and Pampán.

These insects have been sent to the Department of Agriculture in Washington, where Dr. Barber had the kindness doing the classification.

The insects from Valera, Morro de Barcelona and Zaraza belong to the genus Rhodnius, specie prolixus Stal. With this finding verified, the genus and specie of the insect found by Torrealba with high infection has been verified by us. In Brazil has been found infected another specie Rhodnius brumpti.

The specimens of the others four regions found without infections, belong to the genus Triatoma, specie maculata Stal.

The triatominae have, according to Pinto, the following genus: Triatoma Laporte 1832, Eratyrus Stal 1859, Rhodnius Stal 1859, Belminus Stal 1859, Adricomius Distant 1903, Linshcosteus Distan 1904 and

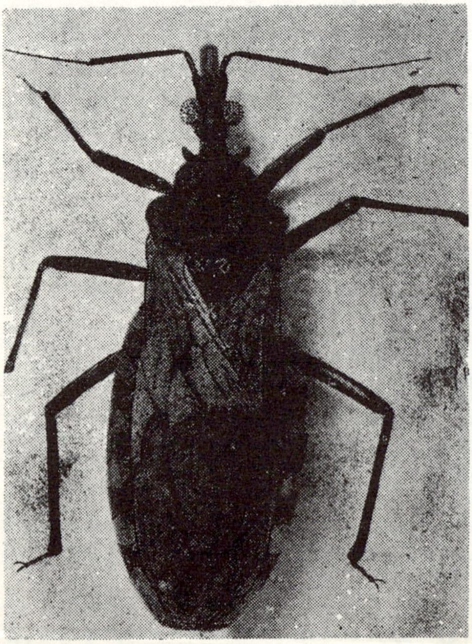

Triatoma maculata Stal. specimen seized in the surroundings of Coro.

Eutriatoma Pinto 1926. Besides, there are around of 80 species in all the world.

The description made by Pinto of the Triatoma maculata is the following:

Son: Chinche mosca abigarrada Stoll 1878
Conorhinus maculatus Erichson 1848
Conorhinus maculatus Stal 1859, 1868, 1872
Conorhinus maculatus Walker 1873
Conorhinus maculatus Let and Sew 1896

Cabeza obscura - Tórax obscuro con manchas blancas. Abdomen kaki. Conexivo con grandes manchas obscuras. Los tres pares de patas obscuras con una espuma en cada extremidad del fémur. Longitud 21 m.m. Anchura 9 m.m.

Brazil: Piauhy, Ceará, Rio Grande del Norte, Parahyba, Pernambuco and Bahía.

Venezuela and Guayana Inglesa.

* * *

We do not know if the reduviidae hematophagous by us in Maracaibo, classified for Barber as belonging to the genus Spiniger could to be include between the triatomidae, and Pinto stamp maculata in Venezuela and the do it Brumpt referring dimidiata and geniculata.

Up today, that we know, in the venezuelan scientific literature has not been classified none insect belonging to the genus Triatoma. According this assertion, only four insects belonging the family triatomidae: Rhodnius prolixus Stal, Triatoma maculata Stal and if it is permitted: Spiniger rubropictus H.S.

Triatoma maculata has not been found infected in nature. The following scheme of Pinto show that still year 1930 have been found with infection: nine insects of the genus Triatoma, two of the genus Rhodnius and one of the genus Eratyrus.

Triatomidae

1 - Triatoma megista (Burmeister) C. Chagas
2 - Triatoma sordida (Stal) Neiva
3 - Triatoma geniculata (Latreille) C. Chagas
4 - Triatoma infestans (Klug) Neiva, Carini and Maciel
5 - Triatoma vitticeps (Stal) Neiva
6 - Triatoma rubrovaria (Blanchard) Gaminara
7 - Triatoma brasiliensis (Neiva) Pinto
8 - Triatoma chagasi (Brumpt, Gomes) Brumpt, Gomes
9 - Triatoma dimidiata (Latreille) Segovia and Hustado
10 - Rhodnius prolixus (Stal) Brumpt and González Lugo
11 - Rhodnius brumpti (Pinto) Pinto
12 - Eratyrus cuspidatus (Stal) Tejera

For all this documentation, an insect very abundant in four and far regions of the country we have not been it found infected. It seems that the main transmissor of the Chagas' disease between us is the genus Rhodnius, as has been verified by Tejera and Torrealba and not the genus Triatoma.

SUMMARY

The study of the family Reduviidae and Chagas' disease is very important actually among us and aroused local interest. It is an illness which is decimating our country besides malaria and hookworm.

Several trips to the interior of the country permitted us collecting some lots of reduvids bugs from Coro, Barcelona, Zaraza, Ciudad Bolivar, Valera, el Morro de Barcelona i Pampán.

We have sent these insects to the Agriculture Department of Washington, where Dr. Barber has had the courtesy to classify them.

The specimens from Valera, Morro de Barcelona i Zaraza have resulted to belong genus Rhodnius, specie prolixus Stal. This demostrates that the insect found by Torrealba with high average of infection in the surroundings of Zaraza and comprobated by us, is the Rhodnius prolixus Stal.

The specimens from the other localities belong to the genus Triatoma, specie maculata Stal.

We do not know if the reduvid bug found by us in Maracaibo and classified as Spiniger rubropictus H.S. belong to the Reduviidae' family and can be included in the genus Triatoma. We believe that at present there are in Venezuela four insects belonging to the Reduviidae' family: Rhodnius prolixus Stal, Eratyrus cuspidatus Stal, Triatoma maculata Stal and if it be permitted Spiniger rubropictus H.S.

We can assure that the insect found in four regions of the country has not been met infected according to Pinto, nor by us.

This proves that the principal transmitter of the trypanosomiasis cruzi in Venezuela is the genus Rhodnius and not the genus Triatoma.

BIBLIOGRAFIA

1-Núñez Tovar.-Nota sobre dos conorhinus.-Anales Dirección de Sanidad.-1919.

2-Tejera.-Primer caso de tripanosomosis americana en el Estado Miranda.-Anales de Sanidad Nacional.-1919.

3-Tejera.-La tripanosomiasis americana o enfermedad de Chagas en Venezuela.-1919.

4-Quintini.-Nota sobre un conorhinus capturado en Caracas. Gaceta Médica de Caracas.-1920.

5-Brumpt.-Précis de Parasitologie.-1927.

6-Torrealba.-Pequeñas observaciones sobre Rhodnius prolixus y tripano-

somosis en el Distrito Zaraza (Guárico).-Gaceta Médica de Caracas.-1933.
7-Oramas.-Reduvídeos hematófagos de Venezuela.-1934.
8-Pino-Pou.-Enfermedad de Chagas en Barinitas.-Gaceta Médica de Caracas.-1927.
9-Pinto.-Arthropodes parasitos e transmissores de doencas. Río de Janeiro.-1930.
10-Brumpt y González Lugo.-Bull-Soc.-Path. Exotique.-1913.
11-Hase.-Resultado de algunas investigaciones parasitológicas en Venezuela.-1931.
12-Clark y Dunn.-Experimental Studies on Chagas' disease in Panama-20th annual report.-United Fruit Company.-1931.
13-Cecilio Romaña.-Investigaciones sobre la enfermedad de Chagas.-Buenos Aires.-1934.
14-Salvador Mazza, Jorg y Romaña.-Investigaciones sobre la enfermedad de Chagas.-Buenos Aires.-1934.
15-Iriarte.-Pequeña nota sobre el insecto Spiniger rubropictus H.S.-Folleto.-1931.
16-Iriarte.-Tripanosomiasis cruzi o enfermedad de Chagas en Venezuela.-Caracas Médico.-1934.

Trabajo del Laboratorio de la "Clínica Luis Razetti".

EXPERIMENTAL INFECTION BY SCHYZOTRYPANUM CRUZI OF TRIATOMA CAPITATA (USINGER 1939)*

The last year kindly we received of the colombian colleague Benjamín Otalora R. working in the Ministry of Health in Bogotá, two alives specimens, male and female, of Triatoma capitata. This specie only has been till today noted in Departments Boyacá and Santander in Colombia and was captured in Landazuri, Málaga and San Andrés, from 1.300 till 2.000 meters of height, according Otalora.

Is an insect (rudiviidae) very pretty, of dark color, with hemelitres and connective lightly red, strong, voracious, the female do ovipositions often and the eggs have an incubation of thirty one days as minimum according my observations. The invertebrate adapting itself easy to the climate and altitude of Caracas (24 c. degrees and around 900 meters height).

As Otalora has occuped enough of its biology of this insect and has been a field very known for us, we think should be more interesting to get the infection, because has been found living in lands at side four frontiers.

In effect, with blood of mice infected with Schizotripanum cruzi kindly provided by National Institute of Hygiene began a test with twenty virgen larves born in the Laboratory, giving them a weekly meal, experience prolonged since 19-10-42 to 9-1-43, obtaining an infection of 25%. The intestinal liquid of these insects diluted with saline solution inoculated in the peritoneum of white mice, some days after, appeared trypanosomas in the blood of these. We believe, for the first time, is obtained the experimental infections of this specie.

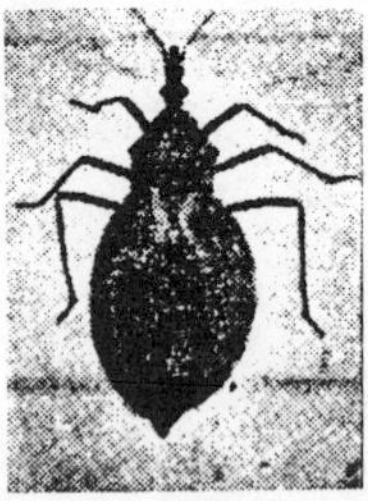

Triatoma capitata
Usinger 1939.

* Published in "Boletín del Laboratorio de la Clínica Luis Razetti" - Año VI - mayo 1943 -Vol. III - N° 10.

LITTLE COMMUNICATION ABOUT THE INSECT SPINIGER RUBROPICTUS H.S.*

In a trip that we did to Perijá seeking with eagerness the insect called "pito", and in each hut where we arrived, performed a survey on the roofs, walls, fissures, floors, but never we could to get a sample. When asked to the day laborers or rural people they showed us a harmless, phytophagous, black color, flattish insect to which they assigned the role of transmissor of the leishmaniosis.

Some time after of our return an old friend, the engineer Germán Valbuena, coming from lands of Perijá, brought us two dead examplaries of an insect with the characteristics of a reduviidae. Lastly, a client and old patient brought us five alives specimens captured in a farmer located one hour from Maracaibo and found i in a hole - pigeon (dovecot).

One of these specimens sent to Washington has been classified by Dr. Barber as Spiniger rubropictus H.S. Notwithstanding to travel almost all the country in several trips, only in the State Zulia we have seen this insect. In the answer Dr. Barber wrote us saying the difference is difficult with a Triatoma and add that Spiniger has none relation with trypanosomiasis.

The insect it seems very common in those zones and has been possible to get exemplaries in the surroundings of the town Maracaibo, as El Milagro, and is called "mamateta".

The animal is very easy to maintain it in the Laboratory, breeding them with a guinea pig, during sting five or ten minutes, and sometines at the end expelling a dark liquid; are nimbles, joining often, no rearing during our investigations.

This insect really not forget it, sucking blood is a reduviidae. Perhaps, some insects found by Soto in Falcón and Pino Pou in Zaraza may be specimens of Spiniger rubropictus H.S.

* Published in Maracaibo (S. Zulia) Pamphlet 1931.

THE SEMICENTENNIAL ANNIVERSARY OF THE CHAGAS' DISEASE*

At the present time is celebrating in Brazil, where our country sent a choice delegation, and possible also in universities and scientific centers, the fifty anniversary of the sickness that has the name of its discoverer CARLOS CHAGAS.

This anniversary was necessary remember it in all the medical science of the world, because is one of the principal rural disease and about the treatment of it we can say as told in 1936: "if the malaria is curable with quinine and atebrine and the hookworm with tymol and carbon tetrachloride, for the trypanosomiasis cruzi there is not a sure treatment".

Chagas was curious, complete and brilliant in the study about this disease. Doing antimalarial campaign in the construction of the railroad in the State of Minas Geraes, called his attention the abundance in the houses of an insect hematophageous that the natives named "barbeiro", attacking the persons during the night, in the darkness, chiefly in the face, and that on the light, escaped rapidly toward its hiding places. Making the examination of the intestinal liquid found numerous *flagellates*, insects that sent to Rio de Janeiro, by inoculations or stings gave positive results in monkeys, guinea pigs, dogs and rabbits. Thinking that the man could to be infected and to a host in reserve, everything was verified, but before, doing tests animals found the infection in cats. Of all these findings published a notable monography in 1909, where did a complete study meticulous, sagacious, perhaps influenced by the teaching of his german professors Von Provazek, Hartmann and Lutz, scientific work that today we have the pleasure to show you and is one of most esteemed and rare acquisitions of my humble library.

When you read it any lack was finish in his "Nova entidade morbida do homem (rezumo geral de estudios etiolojicos e clinicos" in 1911, describing forms cardiacs, nervous, myxedematous, pseudo-myxedematous.

The life of Chagas, born may 25th 1879, was an active labor without stops, continue, backbreaking, that was in accord with his courage and spirit. For a while he was at side Professor Oswaldo Cruz, being his follower and worshiper, entering to the Institute as Assistant and after as Chief of Service, arriving to the death of the Master to occupy the Direction of it, in the year 1917.

Chagas created a new nosologic chapter, without preceding, neither co-workers: discovered a parasite; accused as transmissor of disease an insect, fact that nobody had thought; described a cycle of intracellular

* Work red in the meeting of National Academy of Medicine (10-29-59)

reproduction, unkwnon still then, changing appreciations referring pathogenesis, histopathology and symptomatology, and established the solid basis of the prophylaxis arriving to fill a site between the great benefactors of the mankind.

Eurico Villela told about him: "labor of so size, large in courage and space, with a dedication without border lines, labor without rest, day and night, without selfishness; sacrificing his youthfulness; with a moral temper fighting in inhospitable places of the *hinterland brasileiro* and dangerous amazonian plains; only possible realize it with great altruism and pity for the human suffering".

XENODIAGNOSIS AND MACHADO—GUERREIRO' TEST IN CHAGAS' DISEASE*

The xenodiagnosis was conceived by Professor Brumpt, not only for the Chagas' disease, but as a test discovering the development of the parasite in virgins transmissors; it is a culture *in vivo*. Referring to trypanosomiasis cruzi, sometimes, the examination of the blood in fresh, smears, thick drop or inoculations in guinea pigs, mice, giving negative result, with the xeno is possible to see trypanosomas.

The hereditary transmission in the reduviidae it seems impossible; M. Mayer thinks it is true. Never, we have observed it. We have put in due place washed eggs after the oviposition or leaving its in the container of the rearing with infected specimens R. prolixus; taking the larves, the examination of the intestinal liquid always has been negative. The xenodiagnosis is an excellent method for the dignosis of Chagas' disease, chiefly if you work suitable in the laboratory, politeness in the patients and that if they may to wait six weeks for the result. Not withstanding, is possible to see parasites eight days after the infective meal.

In the hospitable medium the sick will be occupying a bed during forty five days where there is scarcity and at home often not observe all the advises and suggestions.

We present here 35 xenodiagnosis: 33, made in the hospital and two in private clients. All were negative. The patients have been submitted to the followed survey:

Room________ Bed________ Name________ Sex________ Race________
Employ________ Place of birth________ Are or were rural people?______
Have you lived in hut?________ Do you know the reduviidae?________
How are called in your region?________ When started the present nosological picture?________ Symptoms more specials in relation with chronic Chagas?________ Laboratory tests________.

We have utilized insects (larves or nymphs) of R. prolixus or E. maculata, observing the receptivity of both. Before the beginning of the test we did the control of the specimens about infection.

Almost always we employed five or six invertebrates in each process. Rarely, when more of the 50% dead, we put new animals into the test tube, prolonging the time of the xeno.

All the time of these trials we have placed the into the stove to 35 c. degrees, opening a little the door in order to renew the air, because the door closed many of them dead. The placement in the stove avoid the pursuit of the ants and besides the temperature will help the development of the infection.

* Published in the "Boletín del Laboratorio de la Clínica Luis Razetti - Año II - N° 5 - Vol. II. agosto 1941.

The entrance and going often of the patients in the hospital do very difficult the feeding of the insects, and almost always only do two meals. The rest of the test we fed the reduviidae with blood of doves and utilized larves and nymphs being them more voracious and more fitted for the trial and received one meal weekly. The long abstinence sterilize the infected rearings.

The time employed in the trial is at least of one month or 45, 53, 54, 54 days. We exposed 24 xenodiagnosis made with R. prolixus and 11 with E. maculata.

Age between 12 and 50 years

1 to 20 years	12
20 to 30 years	13
30 to 40 years	2
40 to 50 years	3

Sex: Male 26 - Female 8

Race: Hybrid 26 - White 4 - Indian 5

Place of birth: Belong to 14 States, so:

Falcón 2, Guárico 6, Lara 7, Aragua 2, Miranda 5, Cojedes 2, Sucre 1, Portuguesa 2, Trujillo 2, Yaracuy 2, Anzoátegui 2, Monagas 1, Barinas 1.

Are or were you rural people? Have you lived in huts?

Everybody, with exception of two, know the rural lands and one of them has seen before reduviidae. Have lived always in the country 15 and 18 have lived between 1 to 18 years.

Do you know the reduviidae?

28 know them, but 7 say are unknowned for them; in this there is something of modesty.

How are called in your region?

8 call "chipitos", another 8 "chupones", 1 says "pitos" and 4 "chipos". "Chupon" is the word more used.

Symptoms annotated:

Deep anemia	12 times
Adenopathy	4 "
Nervous troubles	2 "
Edemas	9 "
Fever	10 "
Splenomegaly	15 "
Cardiac troubles	10 "
Hepatomegaly	6 "
Ascites	8 "

We could verify 28 xenodiagnosis with the Machado-Guerreiro test. The antigen for these test was prepared with the organs of little dogs (mainly spleens) inoculated and with strong infection of S. cruzi in distillable water and glycerine with 0.5% carbolic acid; three days in the ice box, taking the liquid that float and this portion is the antigen.

The antigen must be used diluted to 1/10 or 1/20 in physiological saline solution and in very small amount (0.2). As hemolytic serum the anti-sheep, red cells of sheep and complement of guinea pig to 1/3. Well known the hemolytic serum and the complement for the antigen you follow the under picture.

Test tubes	Antigen 1/100	Complement	S. Saline	Serum Hemolytic	R. cells
1	0.1	0.5	1.4	1 c.c.	1 c.c.
2	0.2	0.5	1.3	1 c.c.	1 c.c.
3	0.3	0.5	1.2	1 c.c.	1 c.c.
4	0.4	0.5	1.1	1 c.c.	1 c.c.
5	0.5	0.5	1.0	1 c.c.	1 c.c.
6	0.6	0.5	0.9	1 c.c.	1 c.c.
7	0.7	0.5	0.8	1 c.c.	1 c.c.
8	0.8	0.5	0.7	1 c.c.	1 c.c.
9	0.9	0.5	0.6	1 c.c.	1 c.c.
10	1.0	0.5	0.5	1 c.c.	1 c.c.
11	1.0	0.5	1.5	1 c.c.	1 c.c.
12	1.0	0.5	1.0	1 c.c.	1 c.c.

Of these 28 tests, in three: one, gave positivity + + + + +; one, + + + and the third --. We have with clear result: strong and medium.

The patient with clear positivity has lived all his life in the country and knows, perfectly, the reduviidae, having as symptom epileptic attacks. Eggs of necator in feces. W. and K. negatives. The other one has been also a rural people, living in huts. Symptomatology: cardiac troubles; light splenomegaly; necator in the feces; K. negative. In 28 cases, referring the serology for syphilis: 18 were negatives and in the xenos, with Machado-Guerreiro positive, we had a special case. The Machado-Guerreiro test is not specific, is a test of group.

Summary: 24 times both tests were in accord, twice in discordance, (xeno negative and M.G. positive) in another two cases the result was anti-complementary reaction.

One of the private xenos was made in a patient of the town Trujillo, who has lived in the center of the city; lastly, found three reduviidae that she believes carrying its in the clean laundry, because the laundress lives in huts of the surroundings of the city. It is something similar to the bugs.

STUDIES ABOUT CHAGAS' DISEASE IN VENEZUELA*

CHAPTER I

The Schizotrypanosis cruzi or Chagas' disease, possible must be a problem extended to all America, since United States to Patagonia, either in these places have been found the insects transmissors. The fight against these insects by biological conditions (large abstinences of three and four months, heights till of 4.000 meters) is very difficult, remembering the fight against the glossinas transmissors of the sleeping sickness.

As before, we continue believing that the Chagas' disease at side the malaria and the hookworm, are the triad nosological devastating the interior of Venezuela. The first is worse because it has no treatment. The Bayer 205 with action on the majority of trypanosomas, about the cruzi its power is null; the success of the tartar emetic and arsenic are poors. Today are making assays with the 7.602.

We have suspicions that the good results obtained for many colleagues in the interior with the antimony salts in certain cases with fever, cardiac troubles, splenomegaly, deep anemia, may be chronic cases of Chagas. It is possible that a large part of the patients going to Caracas with troubles cardiac and in whom the therapy cardiological is null, may be bearers of lesions myocardic *Chagosas.*

The evolution of the S. cruzi rare and special, distroying organs very important even nervous system, as has been exposed for the argentine school.

ıs so the abundance of reduviidae in the interior of the country, that in occasions we have caught in a hut seventeen insects in fifteen minutes. In the intestinal liquid of these reduviidae we have found a 60 % of infection to trypanosomas metacyclics in some places. Rangel since 1905 comm enting the discoveries of Dutton and Castellani, wrote: "Perhaps, so many pernicious fevers of the "Llanos", not studied yet, can be owned to flagellates of this genus".

CHAPTER II

The year 1909, when Chagas did his discovery considered the parasite found belonging to the genus Trypanosoma Gruby 1843. Some time after seeing the multiplication schizogonic, doing it in the heart of vertebrate, resulting elements evolving inside the red cells arriving the adult stage, created a new genus Schizotrypanum, multiplication not seen in trypano-

* Work prized by the Board of Trustees "Premio José Gregorio Hernández".

somas discovered before. In that time Hartmann and Vianna described forms of reproduction of the same parasite type "leishmanias".

Machado and others, after, accused multiplication gametogony in other trypanosomas of invertebrates suggested, either as Chagas had forgotten the genus Schizotrypanum comes again to the old name of Trypanosoma cruzi.

Studies of the couple Delanoe and also Aragao, 1912-1913, finding forms of reproduction schizogonic in animal without former infection for

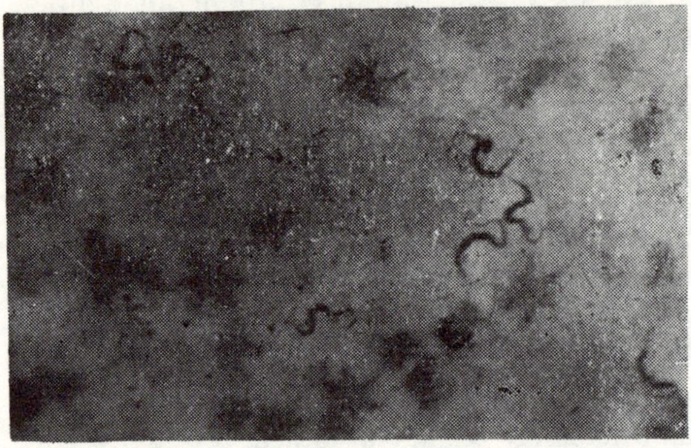

Schizotrypanum cruzi - Blood of rat - Thick drop.

trypanosomas, concluded that those elements didn't have any relation with homoflagellates, but were forms evolved of Pneumocystis carinii Delanoe and parasites of the genus Klosiella of Stevenson.

In summary, the reproduction of Trypanosoma cruzi is different to others trypanosomas; reproduction in the tissues with leishmaniosic forms and not the multiplication in the blood by binary division. The created word of the wise brazilian "Schizotrypanum" has not been taken in its original meaning, now then, by etymology, in greek language signify divide and not schizogony.

Have been described examples of binary division in the blood and forms of leishmania in the reproduction in others trypanosomas, but are sporadic cases without the biological definition of cruzi. Peruzzi, in 1928, said: "these manifestations of cellular invasion it seems to be relations opposite accidentals with the protoplasma disturbed for a degenerative process and not are the procedure of evolution real, cyclical, intracellular, characteristic of others trypanosomas."

The year 1921, the discovery of Chatton and Courrier of a trypanosoma in the bats doing the reproduction in the organs by leishmanoid forms as the S. cruzi, has given a big support to maintain the genus Schizotrypanum. This last parasite is called S. pipistrelli of Chatton and Courrier that will be possibly the T. vespertilionis of Bataglia, saw in 1904.

According to Díaz the genus Schizotrypanum must be situated, in the classification of Trypanosomidae, between leishmania and trypanosoma, more than protozoologist Minchin, since the year 1912, said:

"schizotrypanosoma establish an important bridge between a typical trypanosoma of the blood as T. lewisi and a parasite of the tissues, as the varying species of leishmania."

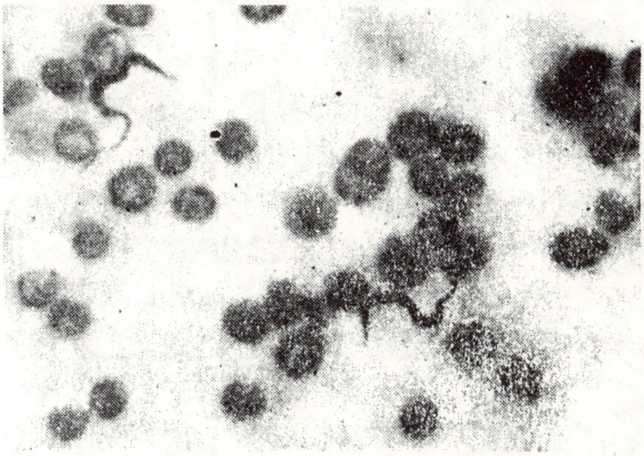

Schizotrypanum cruzi - Smear of blood of rat -Large magnification.

The opinions of the protozoologists Wenyon, Craig, Knowles, Minchin, etc., are disagreeing.

The picture following:

Family Trypanosomidae

A - Flagellates whose host is only invertebrate. The infection is contaminant and the transmission through cysts.

- a - leptomonads
- b - crithidias
- c - herpetomonads

B - Flagellates that have vertebrate and invertebrate hosts. The infection is made by contamination or inoculation. There are no cysts. Are parasites of the blood and tissues.

a - flagellates that reproduce in the tissues of the vertebrate below forms of leishmanias.

1 - flagellates in which the form more advanced in the insect is the type leptomonads. Infection of the vertebrate is contaminant and by inoculation. In the vertebrate the parasite have the form leishmanoid.

2 - flagellates that in the transmissor and in the vertebrate arrive the form trypanosoma. Evolution in the rear part of the insect. Transmission for contamination.

S c h i z o t r y p a n u m

b - flagellates that in the vertebrate do not suffering evolving intracellular. The development is made in the blood chiefly below forms of Trypanosoma. The form more advanced in the transmissor is of the type trypanosoma. Transmission by contamination or inoculation.

T r y p a n o s o m a

We, humbly, when see for the first time the notable book of Wenyon, we daringly to include the *Phytomonas* in the diagram.

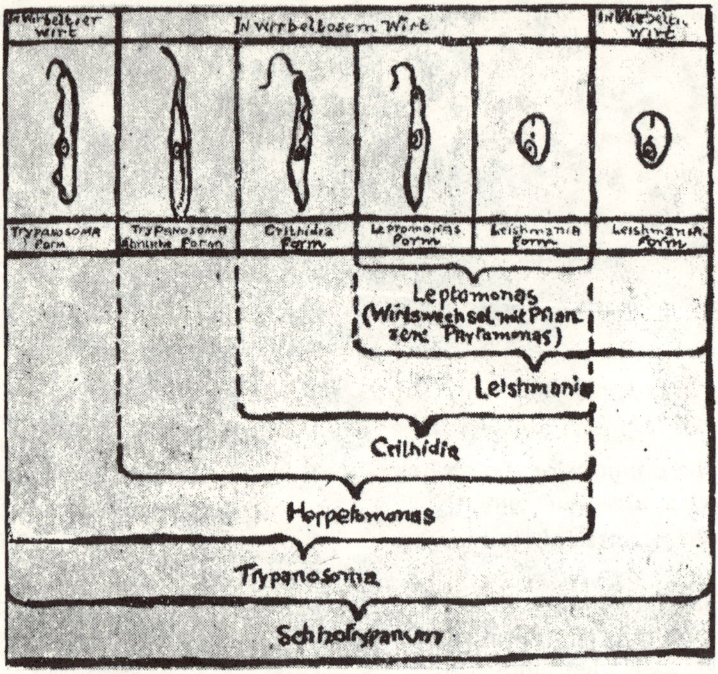

CHAPTER III

In investigations in the interior of the country we have examined persons, chiefly children, living in huts sheltering reduviidae and also the domestic animals, sinking intermediary hosts.

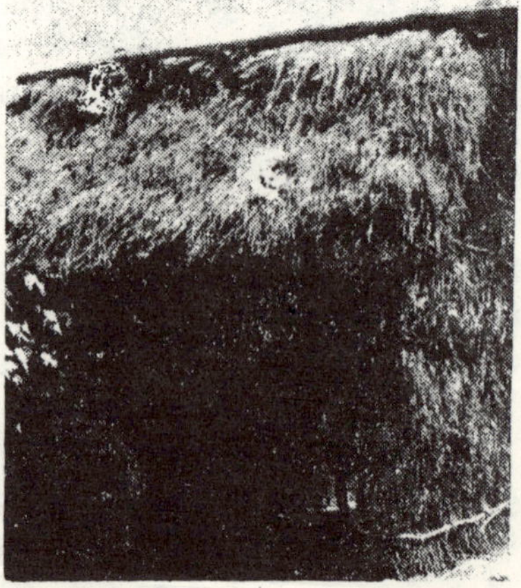

Typical hut of the venezuelan rural people.

In surveys, region of the State Guarico, about 11 huts, with roof and walls of straw, examined the blood of twelve children in fresh between slides, with ages of eight and nine months, giving negative results. In another region, examined seven children of ages very low and the result of the blood was negative. In both places examined ten dogs and two pigs, and all was negative. We think that going on a mission with good equipment, the percentage of persons and animals must be high, seeing the poor life and promiscuity.

Testing a little girl of ten months of age that had one month and a half had trypanosomas in the blood. We appreciate edema of the face, light splenomegaly and polimicroadenopathy. Seeing the photo we can appreciate the following, expressing a boy with enlarged splenomegaly, thin, face of an old man, etc., that probably will be victim of the others sickness either named: malaria and hookworm.

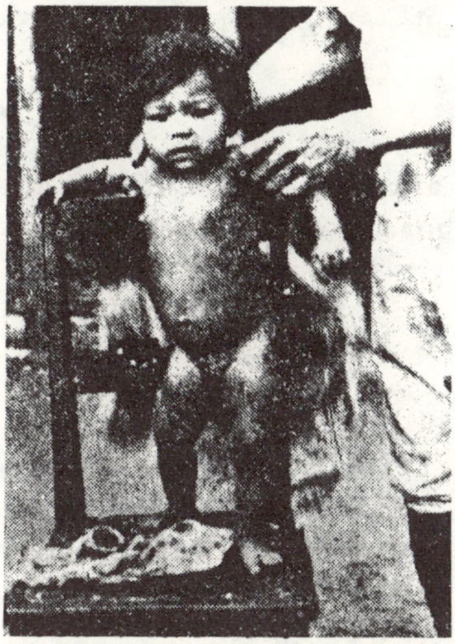

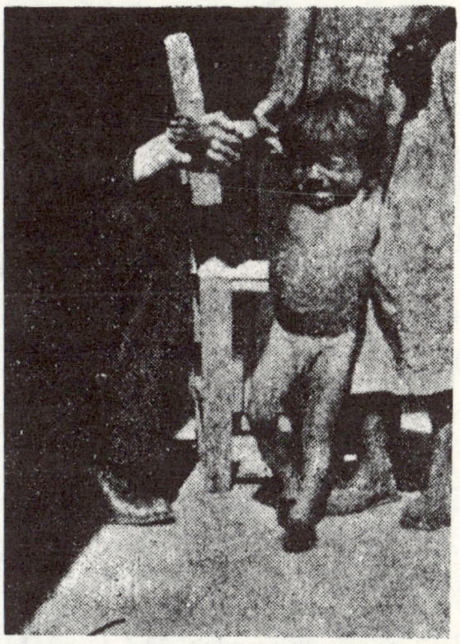

Doing them a differential count white blood, one, demonstrated a very true mononucleosis, characteristic of the Chagas' disease and the other one, light mononucleosis, perhaps malaric and also light eosinophilia, possibly by intestinal parasitism.

From the interior of the country came a patient whose history is the following: 38 years old, born in Los Llanos, single, 59 k. weight, light edema legs and eyelids, cardiac troubles.

Tests of the apparatus circulatory gave Mx 15, Mn 10 and Md 11.5; arrhythmia; systolic blowing; enlarged the abdomen; widening of the liver; spleen Boyd 3; light ascites.

Differential count:

Lymphocytes	39%
Mono-small	6%
Mono-medium	1%

Mono-large	4%
Neutrocytes	41%
Eosinophiles	3%
Basophilous	2%
Transition	4%
Red cells	4.524.000
White cells	4.500
Hemoglobin	80%
Urea	0.37
Sugar	0.80
Creatinine	1 mlg.
Wassermann	positive (+ + + + +)
Kahn	positive (+ + + +)
Metabolism basal	- 10%
Urine	light albumin & sugar
Feces	no eggs parasites

The orthodiagram gave: arch mediun enlarged, large heart and possible arteritis of the lungs. Electro-cardiogram: fibrillation auricle; bad corveying intraventricle (low voltage, leveling of T., increasing of W.S.; hooks in the branches of the complex ventricle.

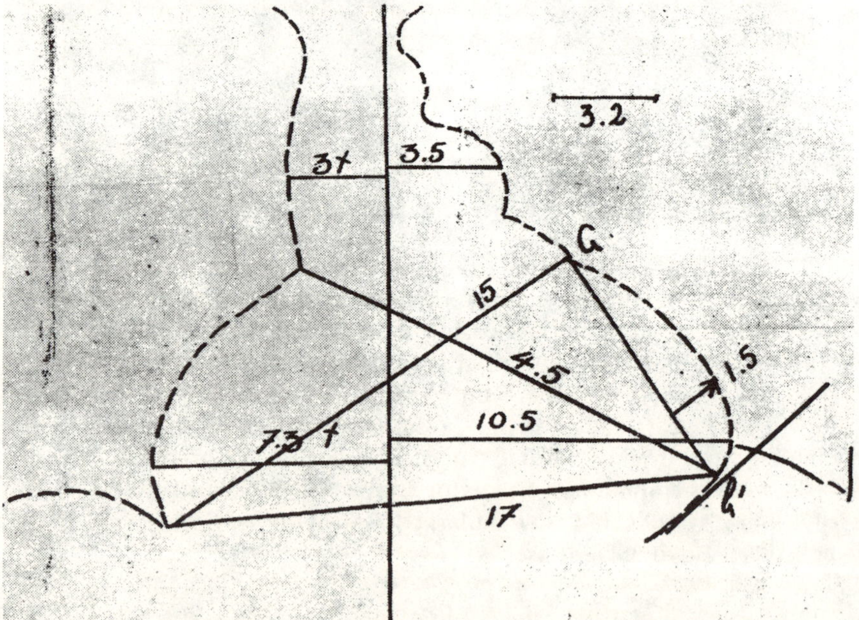

The results of four xenos, two were positive and two negative; perhaps, for a treatment former of tartar emetic.

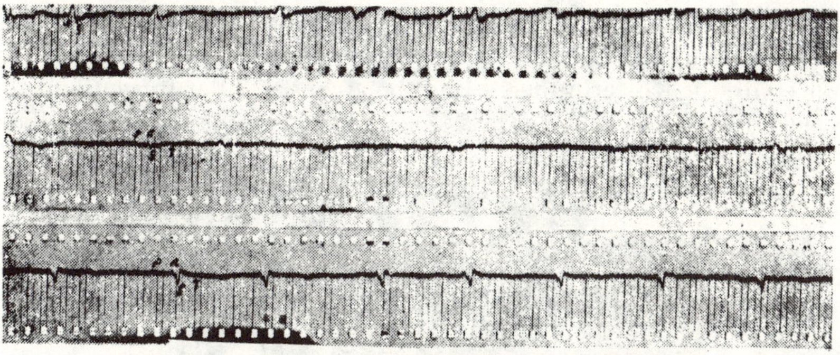

Electro-cardiogram

The result of the autopsy was as follows: pericardium with little overflow; symphisis pericardic; myocardium enlarged, hypertrophy and 600 grammes weight. Total enlargement of the heart, chiefly of the right side. In the right ventricle there is a nodule hard, probably the scar of a infarct; aortic valves well; the pulmonary insufficient to the proof of the water; coronaries well macroscopy.

Conclusions: hypertrophy thyroid; infarct of myocardium; pericardium adherent; cirrhosis hepatic. Probable death for total enlargement of the heart.

The histopathology of the heart of this patient was made in three different places, whose results are following:

Issue 1 - The sample contain several pieces of heart, etc. The piece of heart is covered by epicardium not presenting any change. The pericardium quickly increased and infiltrated, diffuse of numerous cells lymphoid and mononucleares, demonstrating groups around of new vessels. The intima of the coronaries lightly increased. The fibers of the myocardium a few increased and in some sites a light fragmentation. Spreaded nearly all the places groups of cells lymphoid and mononucleares and sometimes eosinophiles. These groups fill often places of the muscular fibres. There is a light fibrosis in focus or around the vessels. *In one of several sections there is a fibre muscular containing in its center a group of leishmani form bodies of the type observed before in the myocarditis produced by the Trypanosoma cruzi in the man. Conclusion: trypanosomiasis cruzi, chronic myocarditis, chronic pericarditis; enlargement of the heart.*

Issue 2 - Myocardium. On observe a total change between the muscular fibres, dissociated, broke and with certain degree of atrophy. The change of the fibers is owned to a double process interstitial of nature infiltrated or proliferating. The infiltrated process is of the type plasmocytaric coexistent with an infiltration of lymphocytes; both are in large focus, not spreaded. The main of this infiltration is represented for a proliferation conjunctive of fibres collagen and reticular tissue; in any places the structure of the myocardium is in total destruction. In certain zones the infiltration is very strong.

The investigation detailed permit to find nodules gigantocellulars with cell in the center, several nucleous, surrounded by a crown infiltrated plasmo-lymphocitic. These characteristics permit us to find any different details with the Koster' tubercle and the gigantocellular formations of the Chagas' disease and brucelliasis and establish identity of syphilitic nodules at initial stages.

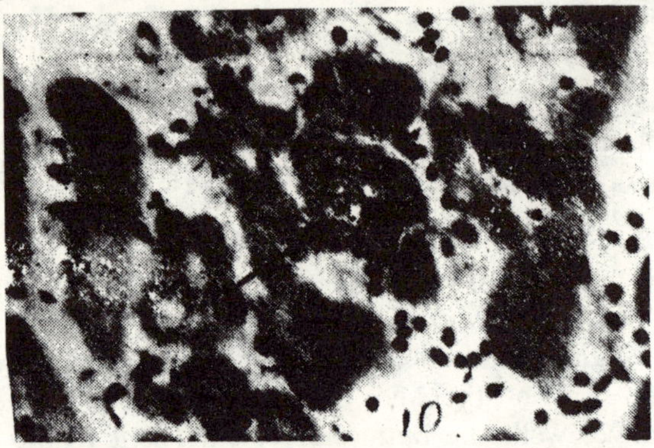

In the center a group of leishmaniform bodies of the type observed in the myocarditis produced by T. cruzi.

By the exposed is possible arrive to the following diagnostic: chronic myocarditis diffuse of syphilitic etiology with formation of gummas, large infiltration interstitial and progressive sclerosis by predominant fibrous proliferation.

Issue 3 - Heart - The sections of heart show deep lesions extended to the cardiac fibres and the tissue around; the vessels also present important lesions.

Call attention in the cardiac fibres a degenerative process and in certain places the fragmentation and the loss of the stration of the fibres and in another one multinucleation and formation of gigantic cells.

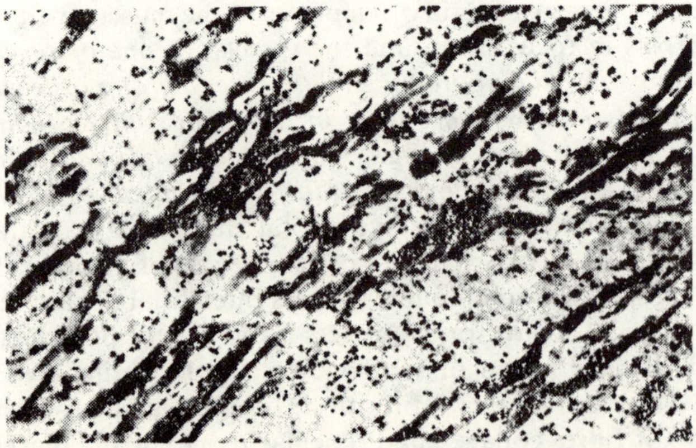

A cellular infiltrate inflammatory and mainly plasmocytic surround almost for all parts many fibres, whose forms and qualities dyeing reveal its poor vitality.

In any points show an infiltrate conjuctive young and scarcely irrigated. There are also necrose points with any frequency without arrive to the caseous stage, seeing groups of cells affected, but conserving yet its structural aspects sufficient recognize it.

Large zones of sclerosis break the noble tissue of the organ, and have the origin in focus of reticular tissue invading around the vessels of medium and small diameter.

The investigation of trypanosomas gave negative result. We could not find elements leishmaniforms.

Neither also histological aspects in order to in Chagas' disease.

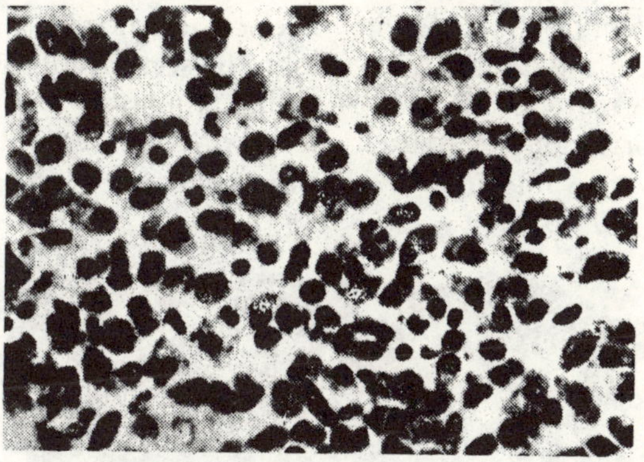

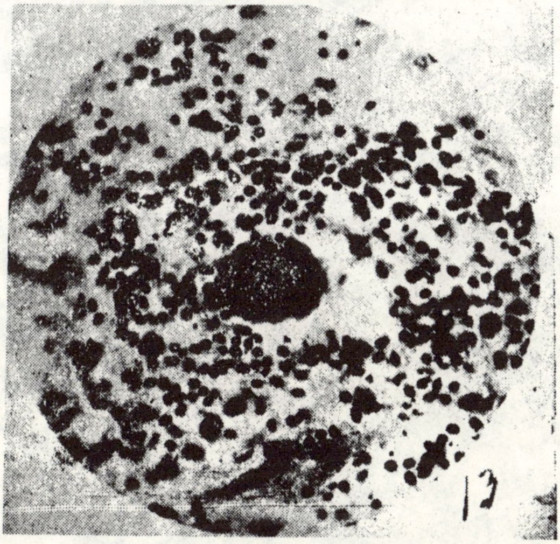

The essential in this patient were whose cardiac lesions, cause of his death, that had given an electro-cardiogram not clear and interrogating. By two of the reports histopathologic and the serology, without doubt the

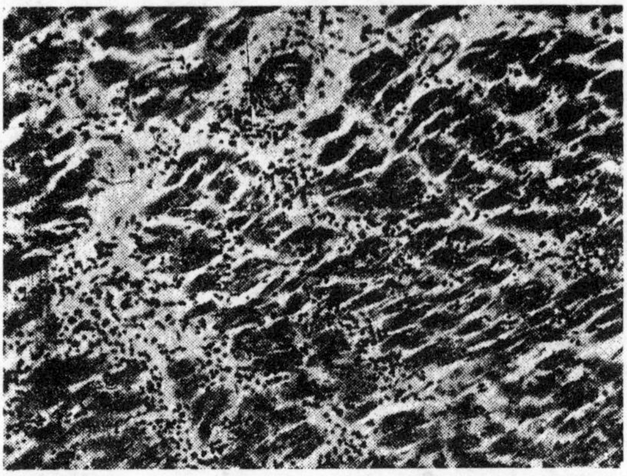

patient was a syphilitic; but also not exist doubt with the posivity of the xenos, the history of the patient, the electrocardiograms and the finding post-mortem of the Leishman' bodies in the sections of the heart, that we are in front a real chronic case of schizotrypanosis. Difficult is find the border line corresponding to each one of both diseases in this cardiopathy. *We remark that is the first chronic case of Chagas verified by the histopathology in our country.*

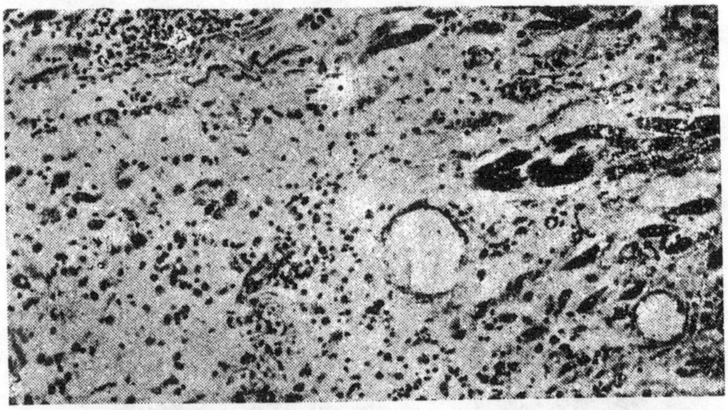

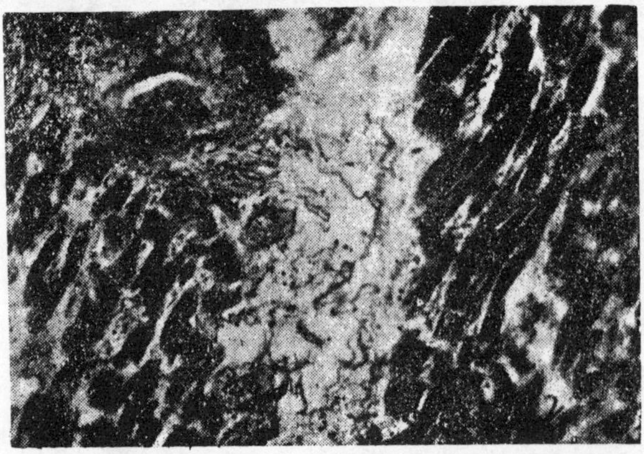

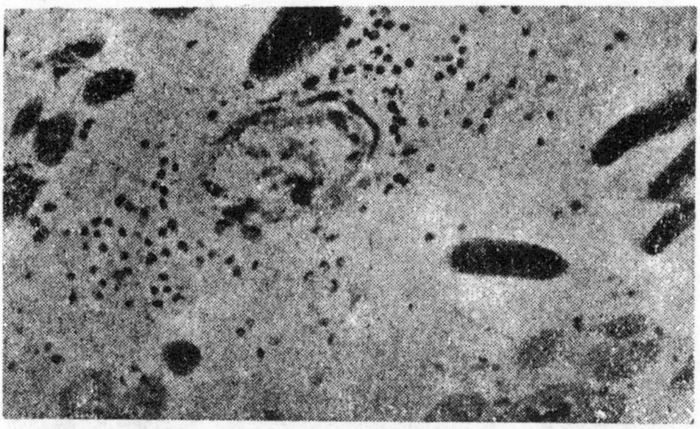

The result of all these investigations bring any meditation, because it is not convenient to think always in front of any cardiac troubles in Chagas' disease.

In one of our investigations taken blood to a patient from zone with reduviidae and advanced cardiopathy, and doing the tests, obtained a Machado-Guerreiro positive and Wassermann the same, having in front of us the equal question. In the State of Minas Geraes, in Brazil, Lacorte has found a positivity united of Wassermann and Machado-Guerreiro of 13%.

CHAPTER IV

Following the histopathological reports of sections of organs of animals infected with S. cruzi coming from human being and from the intestine of R. prolixus infected. In some of these sections in the myocardium of guinea pigs have been found leishmaniforms bodies of the evolving of S. cruzi. *This verify, for the first time between us that the flagellates of the reduviidae infected are Schizotrypanum, and, for the first time, are made sections in organs of animals infected with S. cruzi.*

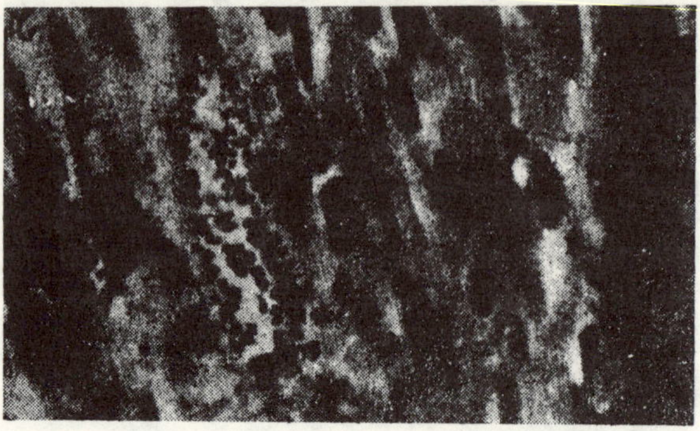

Report of a guinea pig inoculated with S. cruzi from man. Heart - In different points exist small interstitial focus infiltrated for neutrophils, some lymphoid cells and any monocytes of medium size and abundant acidophil cytoplasm and homogeneous. Also recent hemorrhages. Lungs -In any alveolus neutrophils polinucleus, mixed to red cells. Pigment blackish granulate extracellular and the same in the Kuffer's cells.

Report of dog inoculated with intestinal liquid of R. prolixus infected: Heart - A- On see in the epicardium some focus of lymphoid cells. None finding important. B - In different places of the myocardium focus of lymphoids and megacariocytes. These last ones sometimes alone. These focus it seems from hematopoiesis extramedullar.

Report of sections of heart of a guinea pig inoculated with feces of R. prolixus infected: the sections reveal an interstitial myocarditis. Many of the cardiac fibres are full of leishmaniform bodies of S. cruzi.

CHAPTER V

The xeno-diagnostic is a test conceived by Brumpt very useful in diagnostic of the Chagas' disease and extended to another sickness, being as a culture *in vivo*.

We present here four xenos done in patients of the interior, zones with reduviidae, persons accustomed to the stings of these insects, suffering of cardiac troubles, with suspicious of Chagas. In three of them did the control with the reaction of Machado-Guerreiro, utilizing antigen glicero-aqueous of organs of puppies with strong infection.

Today we are more partisan than before of the value of the xeno-diagnosis and of its experimental importance.

In the practice is an inconvenient method needing the ill to wait one month and a half or two months in order to know the result, hard in poor people making expenses in Caracas or staying in a hospital where the beds are scarces. The insects in a laboratory is to maintain, but in the ambient of hospital the lack of discipline of the patients, break the test tubes, the insects escape, the ants doing ravages.

The test of Machado-Guerrerir o has been made, for the first time in Venezuela, by us, and it has served as theme and helped to works of another investigators. We have employed 0.20 for each test tube and 0.40 for verify action anticomplement. The technic is the common of all the test of deviation of the complement.

Reading about this subject we have appreciated that the xeno has gained sphere of action lastly between the brazilian and argentine schools. The Mazza mission has obtained good result with the thick drop and inoculations of blood to the animal for to turn from the trail.

According Brumpt when the xeno is positive, either to ten days is possible to see metacyclic forms in the intestine.

Reports of the xenos:

Patient 1- Woman of Turén, near Acarigua, State Portuguesa, 30 years old. The beginning was with eight larves born in the laboratory lefting three at the end of the proof, being examined 45 days after, with negative results.

Patient 2- Man, fifteen years old, born in State Guárico, white, deep anemia. We did Wassermann with anticomplement results; feces with necator americanus, and urine (twice).

In both albumin; red cells 2,016,000 mm^3; white cells 4.200 and hemoglobin 70%.

This patient was pricked during twenty light days, several times, by twelve larves of R. prolixus born in the laboratory; lefting alives six at the end of the proof, that were examined with negative results. Control with Machado gave the same results.

Patient 3- Man, white, from San José de Tiznados, State Guárico. Test of urine contains albumin, renal cells and granulate cylinders. Wassermann positivity (+); úrea 0.95 by liter; Trichocephallus in the feces; red cells 3.040.000; white cells 6.900 and hemoglobin 72%; differential white count: neutrophils 50; eosinophyles 12.5; basophyles 0; mono large 0.5; mono medium 5; lymphocytes 29.5; transition cells 2.5. Seven larves of R. prolixus born in our laboratory aliving with negative result. The Machado reaction was anticomplement.

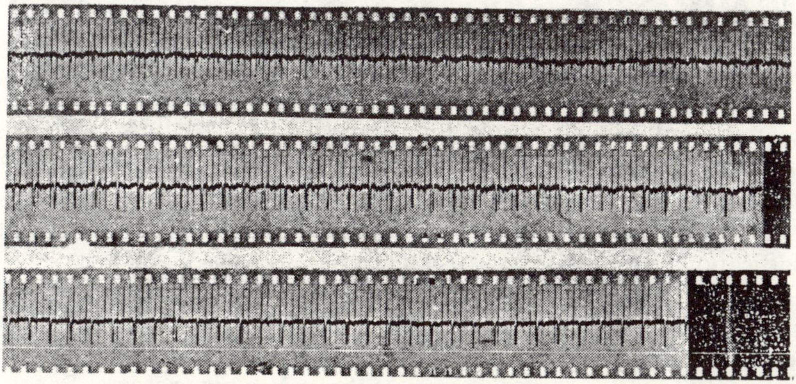

Patien 4 - Woman, 42 years old, from Altagracia de Orituco (State Guárico) and zones with reduviidae, certain cardiac troubles. Ten larves were examined at the end of the proof, one month after, giving negative results. Machado test equally negative.

CHAPTER VI

The electrocardiograms in animals, we believe, are an important matter, being the first made in Venezuela.

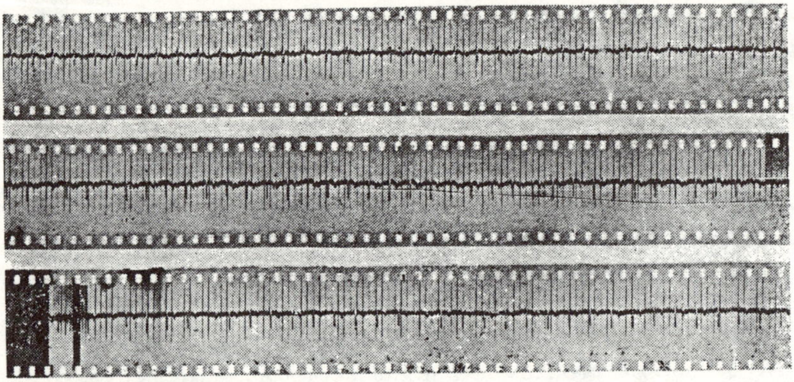

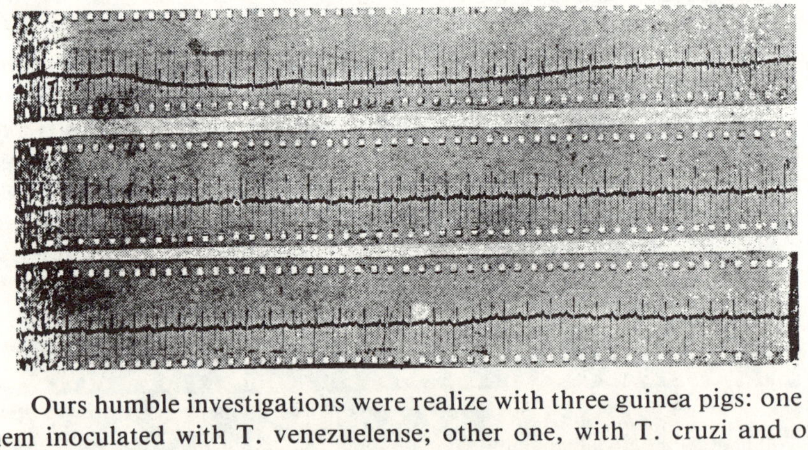

Ours humble investigations were realize with three guinea pigs: one of them inoculated with T. venezuelense; other one, with T. cruzi and one third witness. In the inoculated the trypanosomas had disappeared.

A prime done to the guinea pig with venezuelense, showed none modification respect the witness. It made to the guinea pig inoculated with T. cruzi; three months after, reveales the following:

"The electrocardiograms c II and c III, corresponding to guinea pigs infected with cruzi and venezuelense. There is none modification in comparison with the electrocardiograms of the guinea pigs witness. But, now in the electrocardiogram c IV belonging to guinea pig infected with S. cruzi and that is the same guinea pig c II, but new electrocardiogram long time after, appear anormal signs very interesting. These are: P erased in the first derivation; W Q very remarked in the same and T clearly inverted in the first derivation, without modification of the line S T, which stay to the level of the isoelectric line."

"The inversion of T I indicate suffering of the myocardium and only on find (without modification of S T) and without speak of the T inverted of the patients with angina pectoris in the insufficient hearts; at least, this is the interpretation in human clinic. The P erased indicate hypotony or auricular insufficience; referring the alteration remarkable of Q I, is necessary continue studying it for see if is constant in the experimental infection. It seems, like wise, very important to have in account the beginning of the electric modifications in relation with the date of the infection and try to establish correlation between these alterations and the clinic troubles in the animals infected experimentally."

CHAPTER VII

Inoculations we have made in several animals utilizing the intestinal liquid of reduviidae infected with metacyclic forms. All of the animals have supported well the inoculations, however the great number of germs; only the death of a rat two days after; possibly of peritoneal infection.

The animals more receptive to T. cruzi have been the dogs. The majority have dead few days after with nervious troubles. We inoculate two puppies of one month age intraperitoneal the 1-8-35. The first, not appetite, abundant greenish diarrhea, symptoms of paralysis that is helpless to raise and death 1-16-35.

In the autopsy we find light overflow of the peritoneum and blood of the heart was negative. The other puppy on 1-16-35 is very sad, paralysis of the rear, separation of the front paws trying stability, greenish diarrhea, anxiety, death 1-17-35. It is easy to see the action of the parasite, but it is impossible find it; the same has been observed by others investigators.

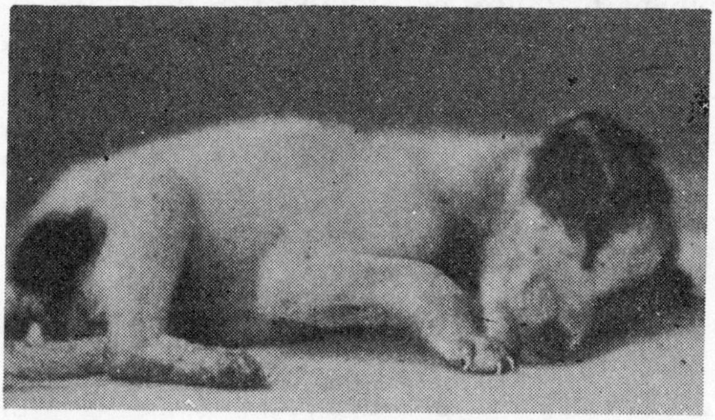

A guinea pig was inoculated intraperitoneal, previous examination of its blood on 1-1-35 and on 1-15-35, fifteen days after, presents scarce parasites in the blood. The little animal, with one month of age, is sad, not appetite, hairy and dead in convulsive stage. With blood of this animal inoculate a new guinea pig presenting this one numerous parasites in the blood one month after.

White rats, with previous examination, avoiding by mistake with T. lewisi, have been inoculating in the peritoneum. There are many important details in the result. One of its; nine days after the inoculation, presents abundant parasites, thing not explained, either, the negative phase, neither, the reproduction in the blood, owning the animal to have presenting the normal curve, that it was not observed. Another one of the rats inoculated with 1 c.c. of the blood of the former animal, four days after presents numerous trypanosomas; it could be accepted, with reserves, as negative phase, or that was a trypanosoma adapted itself to the blood.

These two rats inoculated were male and female and when the male presented strong infection in the female was almost null or on the contrary; phenomenon that we have observed in the T. venezuelense. In this time having to give birth the female rat, the rearings have been negative.

In another inoculations we have seen the negative phase 48 hours after, and the resistance of some animals to the inoculations, between its we remember a small white rat inoculated three times intraperitoneal with trypanosomas from intestine and blood, always with negative results.

A monkey (Callitrix ?) very young and a squirrel have been inoculated and examined during one month, daily, with negative results. The inoculations were made with blood from rat.

Equally, inoculate a picure (P. aguti) and a rabbit, both intraperitoneal, with blood from rat infected. The first, died some days after; the second, was observed during 36 days, date that died, and never we saw flagellates.

Inoculating intraperitoneal an armadillo (Dasypus ?), with blood from rat, fourteen days after presents paralysis of the four paws, greenish diarrhea, lose of weight, epistaxis and death. In this animal the numerous test of blood always negatives. Short time after, we examined a younger armadillo, coming from region El Hatillo, with the same result. Clark, in Panamá, in young armadillos, has found a percentage of 21.4% infected. Lastly, in a armadillo from State Aragua, we have found infection. It has been done the autopsy and the organs studied.

CHAPTER VIII

The insects transmissors of this disease are very abundant in our country. We have travel almost all Venezuela and has permitted us to observe it. We remember that in Barcelona (State Anzoátegui) in the surroundings of the city was easy catch numerous specimens of E. maculata; in Valera (State Trujillo), in the entrance of the village we caught specimens of R. prolixus and here, in Caracas, in Psychiatric hospital, in a house of Los Chorros and in the road called El Atlántico in one of the houses bordering the way, we have caught specimens of P. geniculatus with infection.

Lastly, we had found in all the country four insects of the family Reduviidae, being R. prolixus, E. maculata, Panstrongylus geniculatus, Spiniger rubropictus.

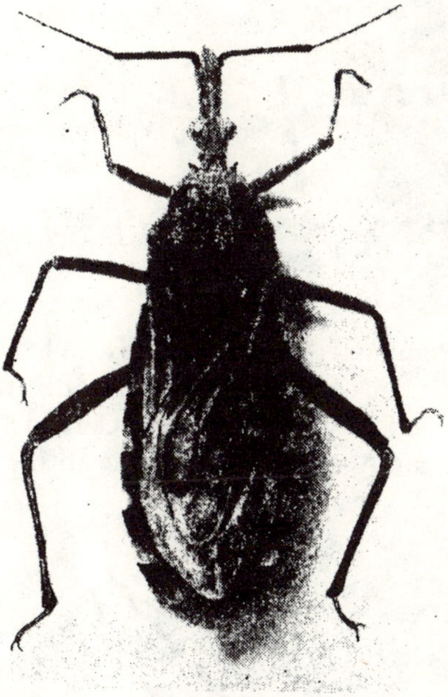

Rhodnius prolixus.

These reduviidae belonging to four genus and four species, the three firsts have been found formely by naturalists abroad, and the fourth has been found, first time, by us. After, we found another two: Psammolestes arthuri and Brontostoma notata Stal. The first has been found between us, but the second, we believe, is found in Venezuela, for the first time, by us, the kindness of Dr. Barber of the Department of Agriculture in Washington (U.S.A.) has been of a great help, in all the details, verifications and classifications of these insects. The classifications of S. rubropictus for the brazilians is yet doubtfull.

The trips to the interior have permitted catch reduviidae in the following States: Bolívar, Cojedes, Portuguesa, Anzoátegui, Guárico, Falcón, Trujillo, Zulia, Barinas and District Federal.

The reduviidae of Bolívar (Ciudad Bolívar), Barinas (farmer two leagues from the town); Anzoátegui (Barcelona) and in some places of the State Guárico (Zaraza) belonging to the genus Eutriatoma, specie maculata Stal.

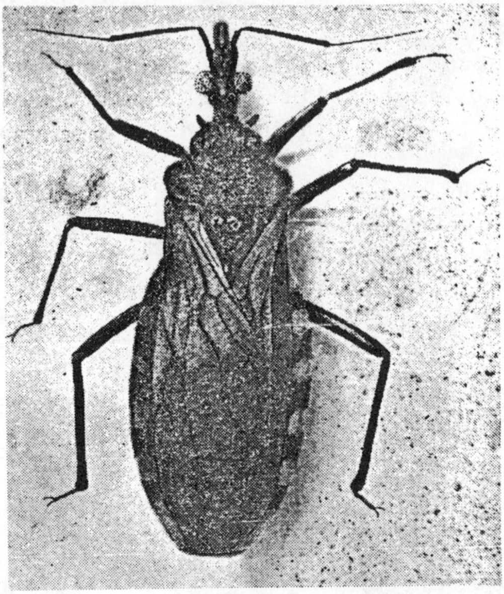

Eutriatoma maculata.

All from Trujillo (Pampán, Valera), almost all from Guárico (Zaraza), a small amount from Anzoátegui (morro de Barcelona); an amount from Cojedes (village Las Vegas, near San Carlos) and from Portuguesa (Durigua, village near Acarigua), belonging to the genus Rhodnius, specie prolixus Stal.

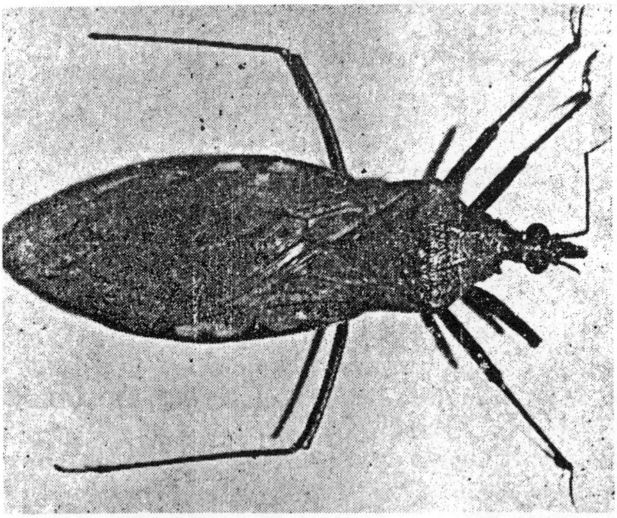

Panstrongylus geniculatus.

An amount from State Zulia, caught in a farmer two leagues from the city Maracaibo, belonging to the genus Spiniger, specie rubropictus H.S.

At last, the capturated in District Federal (El Valle, Los Chorros, Catia) belonging to the genus Panstrongylus and Brontostoma, species geniculatus (Latreille 1811) Pinto 1931 and notata (Stal.).

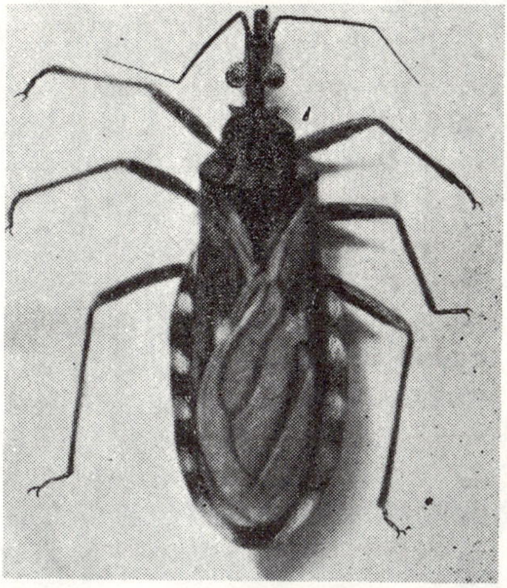

Spiniger rubropictus.

The more interesting of these six reduviidae it seems to be Rhodnius prolixus, because former investigations and the ours verify since the epidemiologycal points that is the true transmissor of the Chagas' disease in Venezuela.

The Eutriatma maculata we thought as told Pinto and by our investigations, that was not infective, either natura, neither in experiences, but last verifications of others investigators have demonstrated opposite opinion.

The Spiniger rubropictus H.S. caught in State Zulia it seems to be reduviidae zoophile (doves, hens); however, we believe can accustom to the human residence and a future transmissor. The specimens caught by us not presented infection, ate blood suctioning guinea pigs and pigeons and the rearings were easy. In that moment, we regret not have had in the laboratory stock of T. cruzi in order to have made some tests. In the center of the town Maracaibo (El Milagro) we found these insects and is called by the people *mamateta*. According the brazilians the genus Spiniger is not hematophagous.

The Panstrongylus found in Caracas, almost 100% have had trypanosomas metacycles in the intestine. One time, the inoculation was positive and the study of the sections were negative, referring leishmanoid bodies in the organs. This detail needs an investigation more wide, because indicate an important fact, either that in the Capital city of the nation, with a high percentage of infection have been caught exemplaries of Panstrongylus geniculatus infected and this specie is a great transmissor of the T. cruzi, as has been demostrated in other places. A light survey done by us with any difficulties, in several huts of the surroundings Las Piñas, between twelve children, near the place we had found the insects, gave negative results.

The Psammolestes was found in big nests of a little bird called *guaiti*, in others sites *cucarachero*, and when leaves the nests come another one called *gonzalito*. In the surroundings of San Carlos, in the place

Chuchango; in the village Manrique and in a small village Las Vegas, from a distance about 8 km. of the town, and in this place, only in one nest found numerous larves, not nymphs and adults.

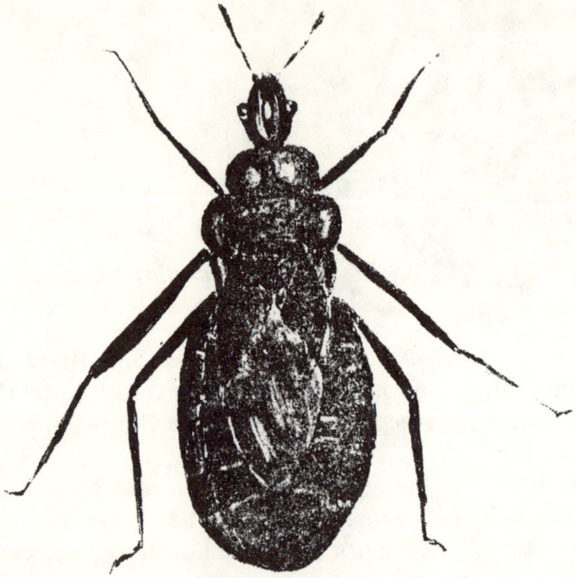

Brontostoma notata.

The examination of the Psammolestes have been negative. In the nests have found also a little blatta with an intestinal spirochaete and a coleopterous; besides, an hyperparasite adhered to the adults specimens, because we have had in test tubes larves and adults and only seek the last ones. We don't know if the hyperparasite lives to expenses of the Psammolestes or if only profit by transportation. We have observed also that the hyperparasite is not attracted for the R. prolixus and when the Psammolestes died is left by the hyperparasite. This hyperparasite is a pseudoscorpion of the family *cheliferidae.*

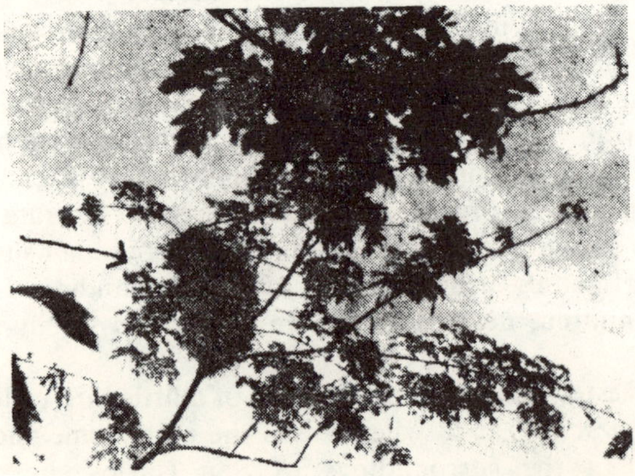

Nest

As not destroy the reatings of this triatomidae, we believe not will be useful in the fight, as we have seen with the ants and rearings of R. prolixus.

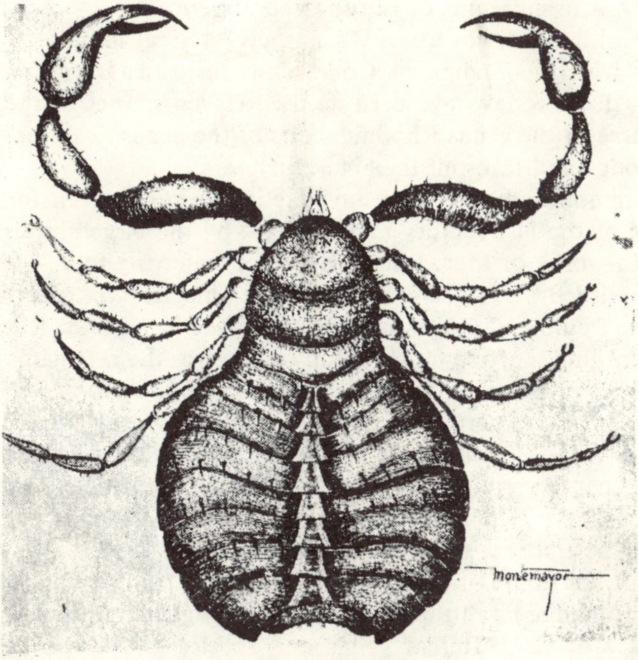

Pseudo-scorpion

Before to begin about the biology of some triatomidae that we have studied widely, will give some details referring the history of these insects.

Pinto (1931) divided this family in nine genus:

Triatoma	Laporte	1832
Eutriatoma	Pinto	1926
Panstrongylus	Berg	1879
Neotriatoma	Pinto	1931
Belminus	Stal	1859
Adricomius	Distant	1859
Rhodnius	Stal	1859
Eratyrus	Stal	1859
Linshcosteus	Distant	1859

According Neiva and Lent, the genus Adricomius has been eliminated and has been created five news: Bolbodera, Cavernicola, Dipetalogaster, Paratriatoma and Triatomaptera, this last one corresponding to Mepraia of the argentineans. To this list on add the genus Psammolestes.

Since the beginning of the last century is known that in North, Center and South America exist big bugs sucking blood, very voracious for the men and animals, and there are the studies of Poepig 1835; Burmeister 1861, Appun 1870-71; Humboldt 1874; Ernst 1877.

The second half of the last century should be called, in accord with Hase "first period of triatomidae exploration", because although in that epoch on found new species of the genus Triatoma, Rhodnius and Eratyrus, had a wide confusion between the finding old and recents, must needs the material was in museums of Europe and America.

The year 1909 with the discovery of Chagas gave a great impulse to this affair, mainly with the finding of Conorhinus megistus Burm. as transmissor. In Brazil till today have been accused eleven species of the genus Triatoma, three of the genus Rhodnius, one of the genus Eratyrus, as capables of to lodge and transmit the Sch. cruzi.

One of the common name of the reduviidae is *vinchucas* given for Poepig to the start of the last century and used yet by the Argentinean school, as is seen in works of Mazza and his school, referring to T. infestans. In accord with Brazilian school Conorhinus megistus Burm. is called *chupao* in Sao Paulo and *fincao* or *bicho de parede* in the State Rio Grande do Sul; according Hoffmann, (1922) in Cuba gives the rare name *chinchorro*. We forgot in Brazil is very used the name of *barbeiro*.

In accord with our notes here the reduviidae have the vulgar names: *pito, chipo, quipito, chipito, chupón, chinche de monte,* being the most used *pito.* We have that in certain regions as Los Llanos, the people only use the name *chupón* and if foreign person gave another word it is not understood. One name embrace different genus and species.

The investigator del Ponte, in 1925, published a map of distribution of the different triatomidae in all the world. Hase, thought more convenient do a summary of the different genus and species in the world; something distinct to del Ponte.

Seeing the square of Hase, on appreciate rapidly that South America is the zone more rich in reduviidae; Center America has abundance in classes; while North America is rich in species.

The T. sanguisuga (Lecomte 1855 -- Neiva 1911) and the P. geniculatus (Latreille 1811 -- Pinto 1931) are species very spreaded for all the American Continent and found in places very far, one of the another, till for 3.500 km. In America are so abundant since American States as Maryland, Illinois, till Patagonia in according Mazza and his school.

The T. rubrofasciata that is a cosmopolitan insect, on believe is the oldest specie that has existed and yet today alives and the initial trunk on bifurcated in two branches: one that is rubrofasciata cosmopolitan, and the other one has continued dividing in numerous American species.

Niño (1926 - 27) has appointed heights for these insects, specially for the infestans, from 0 to 4.000 meters. The colombian Uribe Piedrahita (1927) signed R. prolixus to 1.300 m. in the Andes, and Tejera told to have found E. cuspidatus to 1.200 m. in Boquerón (State Trujillo). The place higher that we can appoint are El Valle, 890 m. and places of Caracas as the road El Atlántico, more or less 900 m.

Around 70 species are known till today; lastly, with the new genus have had an increase of 18 species, of them the following are capables to carry the T. cruzi:

T. chagasi	Brumpt & Gómez	1914
T. brasiliensis	Neiva	1911
T. dimidiata	Latreille 1811	Neiva 1914
T. infestans	Klug 1934	Neiva 1915
T. rubrofasciata	de Geer 1773	Laporte 1832
T. vitticeps	Stal 1859	Neiva 1914
T. rubrovaria	Blanchard 1834	Pinto 1931
T. megistus	Burm 1835	Pinto 1931
R. prolixus	Stal	1859
R. pictipes	Stal	1872
R. domesticus	Neiva & Pinto	1923
R. brethesi	da Matto	1919 ?
E. cuspidatus	Stal	1859

This list is increased today.

Biologycal Notes

We have had the patience of observe during a long time the life of the reduviidae, specially R. prolixus and E. maculata.

The complete evolution of the first is more rapid, being it around of 5 months. So: a larve of R. prolixus born on 1-7-35 did the same day its first meal; on 1-25-35 did its first moulting; second meal on 1-27-35; second moulting 2-10-35; 2-14-35 third moulting; fourth meal 2-28-35; third moulting 3-15-35; fifth meal 3-18-35; sixth meal 3-30-35; fourth moulting 4-28-35; seventh meal 5-17-35; fifth and last moulting 6-19-35. Did 5 moultings, seven meals and a period of five months and thirteen days until the adult stage.

The evolution of E. Maculata is more long and so: larves of E. maculata born on 1-7-35, did its first moulting on 4-20-35, around 3 months and 13 days, doing its second moulting on 6-26-35.

The eggs of R. prolixus are cover of mucilaginous substance that permit the insect to put it on any site, and so, is easy to eggs upper the leaves of gramineous in the plains (Panicum hirsutum S.W. and Panicum maximum Jacq.) and often see specimens of reduviidae on the back of cows and horses sucking blood. That is the reason of the abundance of insects in the straw of roof and walls of the huts, mainly in the news, and many times, the inhabitants left the huts waiting the emigration of the insects by the lack of food.

The eggs of R. prolixus are at the beginning of light pink, color increasing after; ovals, sometimes curving in the end, and in one of the strangled with operculum, that open and go out the larve. When it is empty has appearence wrinkled and white color.

DISTRIBUTION OF THE SPECIES OF TRIATOMIDAE IN THE DIFFERENT PARTS OF THE WORLD

SPECIES	S.A.	C.A.	N.A.	Africa	Asia	Oceania
Triatoma	15	7	12	1	3	1
Eutriatoma	10	2	2	0	0	0
Panstrongylus	9	1	0	2	1	0
Neotriatoma	2	0	0	0	0	0
Belminus	1	1	0	0	0	0
Adricomius	0	0	0	0	0	1
Rhodnius	7	1	0	0	0	0
Eratyrus	3	0	0	0	0	0
Linshcosteus	0	0	0	0	1	0
Conjunto	47	12	14	3	5	2
Psammolestes	2	0	0	0	0	0
Cavernicola	1	1	0	0	0	0
Triatomaptera	1	0	0	0	0	0
Bolbodera	0	1	0	0	0	0
Diperalogaster	0	1	1	0	0	0
Paratriatoma	0	0	1	0	0	0

Picture of Hase completed by us with the last six genus.

Observing to the microscope an egg of R. prolixus we see besides an accented coloration of the operculum, that the surface is drawing by cells and polyhedrical till of seven sides, without relation in the position of these figures.

The middle size of an egg of R. prolixus is: lenght 1 mm 374 microns and half mm of widht; its weight, half milligram.

The eggs of E. maculata are white, changing to the pink; not having mucilaginous substance, compelling the insects to put it on a support, in the fissures of the walls. At the microscope it is not possible to see the strangling, are larger and rounds, the polyhedrical figures are more uniform. The average size is: 1 mm 666 microns lenght and two thirds of mm of widht and weight of one milligrams.

The time of incubation of both species are from 14 to 20 days with an average of two weeks, and coming out larves very different.

The rearings have been made always in test tubes or bottles of wide mouth, using cotton or gauze, because through this last one the animal can do the prinking. It is convenient introduce inside the container filter paper, serving as support and absorb the feces of the insects, because sometimes, gummy, glue it to the wall and dead. This detail is rare in E. maculata, but frequent in the R. prolixus and P. arthuri.

We have seen in the rearings that the insects put the eggs around the cotton plug, like a crown.

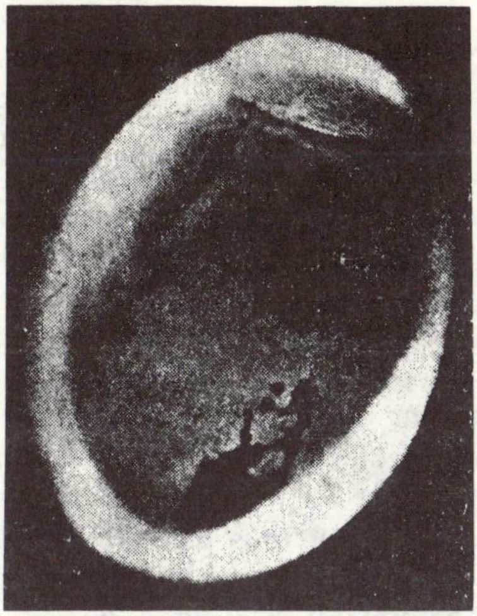

Egg of R. prolixus.

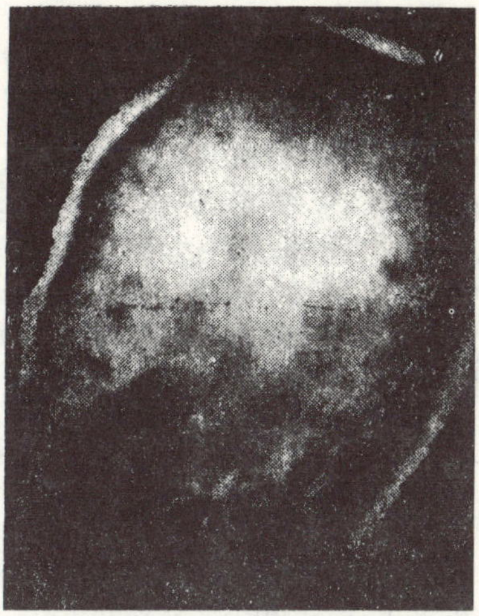

Egg of E. maculata.

The feed seems have not effect about the oviposition. A specimen of R. prolixus in observation since on 12-10-35, had made an oviposition of 15 eggs for 12-31-35; on 3-28-35, one, and on 3-31-35 the total eggs were 32, appreciating an increase of the oviposition at the end of the test. The middle temperature was of 24 c., and observing the influence of the temperature we placed the tube inside an ice-box, more or less, 12 centigrade and leaving it during 8 days, we saw the oviposition stopped, and two days after, being the tube out the oviposition started again.

We feed the insects sucking blood of guinea pigs or pigeons, preferring the last more docile. We have observed that the pigeons are more strong to the sting and sucking of the triatomidae, either for the amount of blood, either for toxins inoculated during the prickling, never seeing the death of the animal, while, one time, utilizing a little guinea pig of 200 grams weight, after a meal to ten insects the animal died. The technic for feeding was: tied the paws, taken the animal for the wings, pull out some feathers and place on the skin the tube or bottle.

In order to appreciate the amount of blood that these insects suck, go the following: a larve of R. prolixus in fasting weighted 0.6 milligrams, weighting after the first meal 1.2 milligrams. A larve of E. maculata in fasting weighted 0.75 milligrams, arriving after the meal to 1.3 milligrams. Morphologically the larve of R. prolixus is long of body and paws, voracious and nimble; the larve of E. maculata, the body is wider and paws shorter.

A larve of E. maculata with weight 6.5 centigrams in fasting, arrived after a meal, done during 23 minutes to 37 centigrams; clairly, the weight increased in 30.5 centigrams, more or less, six times the weight.

This same insect after an evacuation 8 minutes after a meal diminished its weight in 2.5 centigrams. This was made at 10 of the morning and a new weight at 4 of the afternoon, after expelling a gummy liquid, was of

24 centigrams.

The examination to the microscope of the liquid evacuated showed many crystals ronds and any elements, long, as divided, that we consider as the *simbiontes* of Hase, very important in the digestion of the blood.

Working now with adult animals. We take an Eutriatoma with weight of 8 centigrams, arriving with a meal done during 14 minutes, the weight was of 16 centigrams, the double. An expelling made 6 minutes after the meal reduced the weight 1 centigram. Of the same manner a specimen of Rhodnius with weight of 10 centigrams, sucking blood during 18 minutes, arrived to 15 centigrams.

The suction of blood changes according the fasting of the animal, the hour of the meal, the type of the animal, etc., but in general the nymphs and larves are more voracious and suck more blood.

The limpid liquid that expulse the hemipterous after the meal is strongly infective, alkaline reaction, not possible to see crystals noted in the evacuation, gives the reaction of the murexide, as we have appreciate, also positive the Thevenon reaction.

It is very curious to observe the insects in the moment of the meal. Approaching the tube or bottle to the pigeon, the insect by sensations olfactories, visuals, tactiles, thermics, start to move the antennas, approach to the pigeon, stretch the proboscis and with a movement of propulsion do the prickling, put the antennas toward behind and raise the rear of the body.

Some larves after a prolonged meal are full, lift the pigeon, but some minutes after do an evacuation and come again to a new suction; in occasion a larve is sucking, but another larve not stings the pigeon, but prick the full abdomen of the first and so the insect is serving as a duct.

We have noted that to catch the insect expulse by the proboscis a limpid liquid with alkaline reaction, that some one believes has anesthetic properties.

The pricking it seems to be painless for the larves and nymphs, because in adults it seems produce light pain. Taking notes between the rural people it seems to be that the first sting are something painful, later, the person is accustomed or not sensitized. The traces left by the pricking of the reduviidae not exist, and Brumpt it accept; however, one time, in the interior (State Guárico) somebody presented us a child, with numerous marks in all the body and his mother related that a night the boy slept in a hammock hanged inside a hut, was princked for crowd of insects appearing the following all those marks. It is an alone observation heard and pick up by us.

We have found till 60 5 of infection in reduviidae (Rhodnius) and observed that in a lot with this percentage, after some time of cautivity the percentage low to 20%, in according with observations of others investigators, so, the fasting reduces widely the average of infection. On say, about the reduviidae are coprophagous. We think it will be very scarce. Our technic looking for the parasite is removing the rectal blister, dilute with saline solution and examine in the microscope seeing numerous trypanosomas; the crithidies are rare.

It is easy to find eleven parasites for each ten microscopic fields; in others opportunities twenty eight in the same test. Three days after the death of the insect the trypanosomas yet are alives, and so, is very dangerous handle the hemipterous.

CONCLUSIONS

1.- Chagas' disease is as much an endemia in the country as in malaria and hookworm disease; even worse, because in Chagas' disease treatment is unsatisfactory and the profilaxis is very difficult.

2.- It is probable that the condition of a large number of patients suffering from cardiopathies, and that come in from The Llanos, is due to the S. cruzi, since these cases, that are treated through classic methods and are given heart tonics are seldom cured.

3.- The extension and importance of this endemia can better be appreciated if we consider the high percentage of positive reactions obtained by Torrealba (25%). In 24 lots brought in from different parts of the country, we obtained in the rhodnius from Zaraza, a percentage of infection as high as 60%. Seven of the lots were found with infection by Rísquez hijo.

4.- As it is explained in Chapter II, we believe that the Schizotrypanum must subsist and thus consider it best to express S. cruzi and not T. cruzi.

5.- In no one of the twelve boys living in the vicinity of Zaraza, inhabiting straw huts, examined, were we able to get any flagellates. The age of these boys fluctuated between six months and a few years.

6.- We equally examined the blood of a few domestic animals of that same locality and obtained negative results in all. Among the animals examined there were six dogs, almost all of them puppies; seven cats, three of them one month old, and, lastly two pigs.

7.- The little girl which responded positive to Torrealba, was examined anew by us in one of our trips to Zaraza. She was then ten months old. We made the following observations: there was light splenomegaly, skin of the forehead wrinkled, slight edema of the face, polimicroadenopathy and a negative blood examination, made in search for trypanosomas.

8.- The differential count showed increase in mononuclears, a leucocytosis of 38% and 22% of small mononuclear cells. The mononucleosis present has been equally observed by some Argentine investigators.

9.- We obtained a strongly positive Wassermann and Kahn in a patient we brought to Caracas suffering from cardiopathy, with a previous xeno-positive reaction made by Torrealba. Having died, we sent some tissue to the School of Tropical Medicine, Puerto Rico; some to Prof. Salvador Mazza, in Argentine; and some to one of our local pathologist, Dr.

O'Daly Leishmaniform bodies were found in the fibres of the heart and diagnosis of a syphilitic myocarditis was also made, which Mazza assumes to be of congenital origen.

10.- We ignore the role played by the S. cruzi and the T. Schaudinn in the cardiopathy just mentioned and believe that this open new fields to investigation.

11.- The electrocardiograms obtained from inoculated animals tend to show a weakness of the myocardium. We assume that future investigation will make this point clear.

12.- In four suspected cases that came in from The Llanos we tried in each the xeno-diagnosis and obtained a negative in all four. Three were controlled with Machado's reaction.

13.- We have been the first to try Machado-Guerreiro's reaction in the country, using as antigen the extract of spleen obtained from puppies previously inoculated with big infection.

14.- Our findings have demonstrated that the dog is the most susceptible of all the animals inoculated with the S. cruzi; it seems that rats can stand the infection well. We have been unable to find trypanosomas from punctures of the heart, in dying dogs.

15.- We collected four reduvidis bugs in our several trips through the country: Eutriatoma maculata Stal; Rhodnius prolixus Stal, Panstrongylus geniculatus Pinto 1931 and Spiniger rubropictus H.S.

16.- We have been unable to get an infected specimen of the Eutriatoma maculata, nor has it been possible for us to do so experimentally. This bug is very abundant in the country. We have also caught the Panstrongylus geniculatus in gardens from a suburb in Caracas called El Valle, 890 m. above sea level, revealing no infection.*

17.- We have concluded, not only by our own observations, but also by Torrealba's and Tejera's, that in Chagas' disease the chief transmission agent is the Rhodnius prolixus.

18.- By our exposition it is clearly shown that much attention is to be paid to this problem. Far back in 1905 Rangel, referring to Dutton's and Castellani's research work on trypanosomes, assumed as probable the many cases of fever that appeared in The Llanos, not studied then, as having origin in flagellates of this genus.

BIBLIOGRAPHY ADVISED

1.-*Brumpt et González Lugo.*-Bulletin de la Société de Pathologie exotique.-Jun.-1913.

2.-*Brumpt E.*-Précis de Parasitologie.-4 édition 1927.

3.-*Brumpt et Lavier.*-Mode d'action du Bayer 205 sur divers hematozoaires: Trypanosomes, piroplasmes, Theileries, anaplasmes.-Bull. Soc. Path. Exot.-1922.

4.-*Clark Hebert C. and Dunn Lawrence H.*-Experimental studies on Chagas'

* Just we have read in Gaceta Médica de Caracas, that E. Díaz and J. F. Torrealba have obtained success founding this insect infected in nature and experimental.

disease in Panamá.-Reprinted from The American Journal of Tropical Medicina.-January 1932.

5.-*Chaves, Leocadio.*-Processos distroficos na Molestia de Chagas.-M. Ins. Osw.-Cruz.-1915.

6.-*Chagas, Carlos.*-Homenaje.-Revista Medico Cirurgica do Brasil.-1934.

7.-*Chagas, Carlos.*-Nova entidade morbida do homen. (Rezumo geral de estudos etiolojicos e clinicos).- M. Ins. Osw. Cruz.-1911.

8.-*Chagas, Carlos.*-Nova tripanozomiaze humana (estudos sobre a morfolojia e o ciclo evolutivo do Schizotripanum cruzi-n. gen. n. sp., ajente etiolojico de nova entidade morbida do homen.-M. do Ins. Osw.-Cruz.-1909.

9.-*Dias Emmanuel.*-Le tripanosoma cruzi pendent les premières phases de l'infection expérimentale.-Le Trypanosoma cruzi et ses rapports avec le Système réticulo-endothélial.-Sur les déjéctions du Triatoma megista.-Aspects du Trypanosoma cruzi que l'on y rencontre.-Expériences sur la transmission du Trypanosoma cruzi de l'insect au vertébré.-Trabalhos do Ins. Osw.-Cruz.-1932.

10.-*Dias Emmanuel.*-Da presença de formas de evoluçâo do Trypanosoma cruzi Chagas nos tubos de Malphighi do barbeiro.-Reimpresso das Mem. do Ins. Osw.-Cruz.-1930.

11.-*Dias Emmanuel.*-O Trypanosoma cruzi póde evoluir na cavidades geral do triatoma megista.-Reimpresso das Mem. Ins. Osw-Cruz.-1933.

12.-*Dias Emmanuel.*-Trypanosoma cruzi ou Schizotrypanum cruzi.-Reimpresso das Mem. Ins. Osw-Cruz.-1934.

13.-*Dias Emmanuel.*-Sobre un Schizotrypanum de um morcego do Brasil (Nota preliminar).-Reimpresso das Mem. Ins. Osw-Cruz.-1933.

14.-*Dias Emmanuel.*-Estudos sobre o Schizotrypanum cruzi (Tése de coutoramento).-Trabalho do Ins. Osw-Cruz.-1933.

15.-*Dias Ezequiel.*-Molestia de Carlos Chagas.-Estudos hematolojicos.-Mem. do Ins. Osw.-Cruz.-1922.

16.-*Dunn Lawrence H.*-Notes on the reduviid bug, Eratyrus cuspidatus Stal., naturally infected with Trypanosoma cruzi Chagas found in Panamá.-Reprinted from The American Journal of Tropical Medicine.-May.-1934.

17.-*Dunn Lawrence H.*-Attempts to transmit Trypanosoma cruzi Chagas with Ticks of the genus Ornithodoros.-Reprinted from The American Journal of Tropical Medicine.-May. 1934.

18.-*Iriarte, David R.*-Tripanosomiasis cruzi o Enfermedad de Chagas en Venezuela.-Caracas Médico.-1934.

19.-*Iriarte, David R.*-Comentarios al trabajo del Dr. Torrealba sobre Enfermedad de Chagas.-Gaceta Médica de Caracas.-Octubre.-1934.

20.-*Lacorte, Guillermo José.*-A recçao do desvio do complemento na Molestia de Chagas.-Mem. do Ins. Osw-Cruz.-1827.

21.-*Miller, Joh W.*-Chagas' disease in Panamá.-Report of three cases. Reprinted from The Southern Medical Journal.-July.-1931.

22.-*Mazza Salvador, Ruchelli Guillermo y Romaña Cecilio.*-Investigaciones sobre la enfermedad de Chagas. Publicación N°20.-Buenos Aires.-1934.

23.-*Mazza Salvador, Jörg y Romaña.*-Investigaciones sobre la Enfermedad de Chagas.-Buenos Aires.-1934.

24.-*Neiva, Arthur.*-Informaçôes sobre a biolojia da Vinchuca, Triatoma infestans Klug.-Mem. do Ins. Osw-Cruz.-1913.

25.-*Neiva, Arthur.*-Informaçôes sobre a biolojia do Conorhinus megistos. Burm.-Mem. do Ins. Osw-Cruz.-1910.

26.-*Núñez, Tovar.*-Nota sobre dos conorhinus.-Anales Dirección de Sanidad.-1919.

27.-*Pinto, César.*-Rhodnius dunni, n. sp. do Panamá. Revista Medico-Cirurgica do Brasil.-Nov.-1932.

28.-*Pinto, César.*-Tratado de Parasitología.-Tomo I.-Río de Janeiro.-1930.
29.-*Penna de Azevedo, A.*-Histologia pahologica da glandula thyreoide na fórma aguda da Molestia de Chagas (Tripanosome americana).-Mem. do Ins. Osw-Cruz.-1933.
30.-*Pino Pou.*-Enfermedad de Chagas en Barinitas. Gaceta Médica de Caracas.-1927.
31.-*Quintini.*-Nota sobre un conorhinus capturado en Caracas.-Gaceta Médica de Caracas.-1920.
32.-*Romaña, Cecilio.*-Investigaciones sobre la Enfermedad de Chagas.-Buenos Aires.-1934.
33.-*Rodhain, J.*-Trypanosome d'un cheiroptère insectivore Nycteris hispida Schreber au Congo belge.-Bull Soc. Path, Exot. 1923.
34.-*Torrealba, Francisco.*-Pequeñas observaciones sobre Rhodnius prolixus y tripanosomosis en el Distrito Zaraza (Guárico).-Gaceta Médica de Caracas.-1933.
35.-*Torres Magarinos.*-Alguns fatos que interessam á epidemiolojia da molestia de Chagas.-Mem. do Ins. Osw-Cruz.-1915.
36.-*Torres Magarinos.*-Estudo do miocardio na Molestia de Chagas (forma aguda) 1°-Alteraçôes da fibra muscular cardiaca.-Mem. do Ins. Osw-Cruz.-1917.
37.-*Tróes Joao A.C.*-Liçôres & Conferencias.-Doença de Carlos Chagas.-Bahia Médica.-Abril.-1935.
38.-*Tejera.*-La tripanosomosis americana en Venezuela.-Tipografía Americana.-Caracas.-1919.
39.-*Tejera, E.*-Un nouveau flagellé de Rhodnius prolixus.-Trypanosoma (ou crithidia) Rangeli n. sp.-Extrait du Bulletin de la Société de Pathologie Exotique, Julliet.-1920.
40.-*Tejera, E.*-Primer caso de tripanosomosis americana en el Estado Miranda.-Anales de Sanidad Nacional.-1919.
41.-*Uribe Piedrahita, César.*-Notas sobre un tripanosoma de los bovinos de Colombia.-Editorial Minerva. Bogotá.-1931.
42.-*Uribe Piedrahita, César.*-Contribución al estudio de los tripanosomas de los equídeos de Colombia.-Edit. Minerva.-Bogotá.-1929.
43.-*Villela E. y Dias Emmanuel.*-Localisation des formes de multiplication de Schizotrypanum cruzi dans la peau et dans les muqueuses de chiens espérimentalement infectés. Parasitisme de la cellule épithéliale de l'epiderme.-Ext. des comptes rendues des séances de la Société de biologie.-Juillet.-1934.
44.-*Villela E. y Dias Emmanuel.*-Sur la formation d'ulcérations chez les animaux infectés par le Schizotripanum cruzi.-Ext. des comptes rendues des séances de la Soci&t& de biologie.-Juin.-1934.
45.-*Villela E. y Torres Magarinos.*-Estudos histopathologico do systema nervoso central em paralysia experimental determinada pelo Schizotrypanum cruzi.-Mem. do Ins. Osw-Cruz.-1926.
46.-*Villela Eurico y Villela Eudoro.*-Elementos do sistema nervoso central parasitados pelo Trypanosoma cruzi.-Mem. do Ins. Osw-Cruz.-1932.
47.-*Vianna, Gaspar.*-Contribuçâo para o estudo de anatomia patolojica da "Molestia de Carlos Chagas" (esquizotripanoze humana ou tireoidite parazitaria).-Mem. do Ins. Osw-Cruz.-1911.
48.-*Briceño Iragorry, L.*-Contribución al estudio morfológico de los huevos de algunos reduvídeos.-Boletín de la Sociedad de Ciencias Naturales.-Caracas. N°18.
49.-*Chagas, Evandro.*-Forma cardíaca da Trypanosomiase americana.-Mem. do Ins. Osw-Cruz.-1930.
50.-*Dias Emmanuel.*-Estudos sobre o Schizotrypanum cruzi (Tése de doutoramento)-Río de Janeiro. 1933.
51.-*Torrealba, J. Fcco.*-El primer caso de Tripanosomiasis americana diagnosticado en el Estado Guárico por el exámen directo de la sangre.-Gaceta Médica de Caracas.-1934.

52.-*Artículo editorial.*-Figuras de la Ciencia Médica.-Muerte del Profesor Carlos Chagas.-Tomado del Journal do Comercio.-"El Universal".-Caracas.-1934.
53.-*Rafael Sylva (Lino Sutil).*-Entre col y col.-Las Estrellas.-"El Universal".-Caracas.-Abril.-1934.
54.-*Torrealba, J. Fcco.*-Algo más sobre Tripanosomosis.-Xenodiagnóstico.-Gaceta Médica de Caracas.-1934.
55.-*Torrealba, J. Fcco.*-La maladie de Chagas.-Trypanosomose américaine ou Schizotripanose au Vénézuéla.-Tip. Vargas.-Caracas.-1934.
56.-*Rísquez, J.R.*-La Tripanosomiasis de los reduvideos.-Gaceta Médica de Caracas.-1934.
57.-*Le Dantec, A.*-Précis de Pathologie Exotique.-1934.
58.-*Oramas, Luis R.*-Reduvídeos hematófagos de Venezuela.-1934.
59.-*Pittier, H.*-Las Plantas usuales de Venezuela.-Caracas.-Lit. del Comercio.-1926.
60.-*Iriarte, David R.*-La Flageliasis de las Plantas en Venezuela (tesis doctoral).-1928.
61.-*Iturbe, Juan.*-Derrengadera.-The effect of "Bayer 205" on the Trypanosoma Venezuelense.
62.-*González Rincones, R.*-Apuntes hechos en el Laboratorio del Hospital Vargas acerca de dos protozoarios parásitos.-Boletín de los Hospitales.-Caracas.-1906.
63.-*Mazza Salvador.*-Nota sobre tripanosomas de ictéridos del Norte.-Prensa Médica Argentina.-1926.
64.-*Torrealba, J.F.*-Pequeñas notas sobre relaciones biológicas experimentales negativas entre algunos reduvídeos y el Trypanosoma venezuelense o de la Derrengadera de los equídeos de Venezuela.-Gaceta Médica de Caracas.-1935.
65.-*González Rincones, R.*-Revisión del estudio de nuestros tripanosomas.-Tip. Guttemberg.-Caracas.-1914.
66.-*Chagas, Evandro.*-Novos estudos sobre a forma cardiaca da Trypanosomiase americana.-Mem. Ins. Osw-Cruz.-1932.
67.-*Mazza, Romaña y Parma.*-Investigaciones sobre la Enfermedad de Chagas.-Publicación N° 21.-1935.
68.-*Iriarte, David R.*-Presencia del Triatoma maculata en Venezuela.-Medical.-1935.
69.-*Iriarte, David R.*-Ensayos de trasmisión del Trypanosoma venezuelense por insectos de los géneros rhodnius (R. prolixus) y eutriatoma (E. maculata).-Ligero estudio histopatológico de la derrengadera de nuestros equídeos.-Medical.-1935.

LITTLE ASSAYS OF TRANSMISSION OF TRYPANOSOMA VENEZUELENSE*

"With insects of the genus Eutriatoma (E. maculata) and Rhodnius (R. prolixus). Short histo-pathological study of the "Derrengadera" of our equines".

In trip to Zaraza (State Guárico) in december of the last year, in the plain of the farmer Palenque, at side of the way, when going in my car, fallen collapsed a horse of brown color. Asking ahead in the house of the "hato", the animal was sick. We thought in *derrengadera* and tried that animal going up, but only moved the head and the former train because the movement of the rear train was null. It was not thin and had the mouth half opened, ruminating; not edema in the body; the look loose; the anterior train with slight spasticity and tremor; the rear train contracted; ulceration in the penis, going out and viscous urine.

In site we examined the blood taken from the ear showing numerous trypansomas and immediately we inoculated two guinea pigs (8-12-34), intraperitoneal; the inoculation was made with pure blood. To 200 meters ahead of distance we found a female mule in the same conditions, but not so sick as the former horse; perhaps, the mule is more resisting. We had no time to examine the blood of this animal but almost sure was another case of *derrengadera.*

One, of the two guinea pigs inoculated was left as a courtesy to the distinguished colleague Dr. Torrealba and the other one brought to Caracas, being examined for the first time (18-12-34), showing 2 or 3 trypanosomas by field. We inoculated a new guinea pig (22-12-34) and for the first showed abundant parasites, but none the second.

On 25-12-34, we did to sting 3 adults and 7 larves of E. maculata and 10 larves of Rhodnius prolixus (both genus born and rearing in the laboratory) to the animal brought from State Guárico.

One 27-12-34, the first guinea pig showed around 100 trypanosomas by field; the second, more or less, 3 or 4 parasites.

On 3-1-35, the first animal showed a great amount; the second, equally, large abundance. We profit to give the second meal to the invertebrates. Later, 9-1-35, third meal and 13-1-35, fourth meal.

On 14-1-35, died the guinea pig inoculated in Palenque. The autopsy was made 3 hours later. We found little overflow in the peritoneum; bladder full of urine, that examined gave albumin; the test of blood in heart showed numerous trypanosomas alive. We took portions of liver, spleen, kidneys, heart and lungs, fixed in formaldehyde and sent to the School of Tropical Medicine of Puerto Rico, sponsored by the Columbia University, for the histo-pathological study.

On 27-1-35, were killed the hemipterous employed in the research and the result was negative. Referring to trypanosomas in the intestine of the

* Reprinted from "Medical". Año II. N° 14. 1935

insects.

These little assays were made because a disease that is a problem for the country, either is unknown the transmission. Besides, many persons from Los Llanos have seen reduviidae stinging on the body of horses, mules and donkeys, and is easy to think that so as these insects are capable to host in its intestine the T. cruzi, could equally, to do with the Trypanosoma venezuelense coming to be transmissors of the derrengadera.

The report of the School of Tropical Medicine of Puerto Rico is as follows:

"N° 10. 201

Microscopic description - Without description. Microscopic description. HEART - In the epicardium as in the myocardium we see a moderate number of little focus spreaded of lymphoid cells. SPLEEN - The pulp demonstrates a slight congestion and a slight increase of the conjuctive tissue. The cells of the pulp are almost all lymphoids. The follicles are large numerous and protuberant. LIVER - Amount of blackish granular pigment in the Kupffer's cells and extracellular, probably owed to the fixing with formaldehyde. In some places any little focus of necrosis of hepatic tissue. KIDNEYS - Nothing at all interesting. LUNGS - There is a moderate congestion, a little zone of recent hemorrhage, a little of diapedesis in the alveolus and small focus of lymphoid cells in different places of the parenchyma."

We believe it is the first histo-pathological study made in the country about the "Derrengadera" of our Llanos. However, we know that in Panamá there is a similar sickness of the equines widely studies, but we thought that still now it has not been possible demonstrate if Trypanosoma hippicum Darling is equal or different to Trypanosoma venezuelense and then if our endemic is equal or different to the disease of Panamá.

BIBLIOGRAPHY

Torrealba J.F.-Pequeñas notas sobre relaciones biológicas experimentales negativas entre algunos reduvídeos y el Tripanosoma venezuelense o de la Derrengadera de los equídeos de Venezuela.-Gaceta Médica de Caracas.-1933.

Rangel Rafael.-Nota preliminar sobre la Peste Boba y la Derrengadera de los equídeos de los Llanos de Venezuela.-1905.

Uribe César.-Contribución al estudio de los tripanosomas de los equídeos de Colombia.-1929.

Iturbe Juan.-Derrengadera-The effect of Bayer 205 on the Trypanosoma venezuelense.-1924.

EQUINE TRYPANOSOMIASIS*

(Work of Incorporation to the Cuban Society of Biology and Tropical Medicine "Carlos Finlay")

CHAPTER I

The equine trypanosomiasis seems to be an urgent problem for our country. It is not a human endemic, but it is an epizooty destroying the breeding of the horses in Venezuela.

The equine race as the bovine has been diminishing slowly among us. The history speaks of the abundance of horses in the interior of the country. To General Páez the farmers gave a gift of 1,000 white horses during the war of Independence. The families, Pulido and Fernández, also gave presents to the patriot army. Ramón Bescanza also did courtesies, but to royalist troops in Guanare (State Portuguesa).

It was so the scarcity of equines that when we were students we were sent to La Rubiera (1923) by the Direction of Health, order came from Maracay, in order to fight against a strong epizooty among the horses of that region. Notwithstanding, the dictatorial order, the President of the State Guárico, for that time, delayed 24 hours getting two horses to go from Calabozo to El Rastro.

In 1905, Rangel found in the blood of cripple horses of the rear train a trypanosoma; parasite that later (Masnil 1910) called Trypanosoma venezuelense. According to Iturbe this disease began in Apure (1826) and in 1835, spreaded through Los Llanos to the rest of the country (Llanos, Zulia, Lara, Yaracuy, Carabobo, Miranda, Anzoátegui, etc.)

In 1910, Darling in Panamá, mentioned the equine trypanosomiasis in that country, to which called Trypanosoma hippicum. It is not possible yet to say if venezuelense and hippicum are equals. Wenyon believes that they are the same. Possibly the equine trypanosoma of Columbia found by Uribe Piedrahita, will be the same venezuelense.

The seed with which we have worked has been obtained from Los Llanos in the country.

Referring to morphology it is a trypanosoma around 15 to 20 microns length, and of 1.5 to 2 microns width, with rear end sharp. It has a waving membrane with 1 to 5 undulations, often two; nucleus to level of the center of these last waves. The blepharoplaste small or in bacillar form. We have not seen basophiles granulations in the cytoplasme.

As is common, the young animal is more receptive to the inoculation and easily takes the infection. In the old guinea pigs (500 grams or more), many times are very resistant, and so: 4 guinea pigs inoculated on 25-4-40 (N° 1, 340 grams; N° 2, 620 grams; N° 3, 670 grams; N° 4, 490 grams, in-

* Reprinted from the book "Estudios de Patología Tropical." 1942.

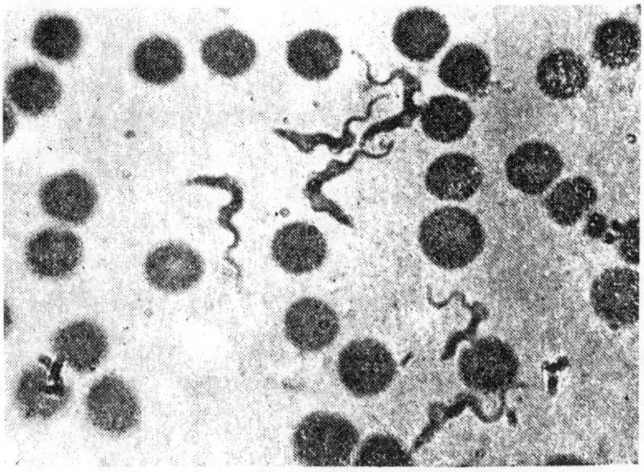
Coloration panoptic Pappenheim.

traperitoneal. On 23-5-40, not presenting infection were re-inoculated and on 6-6-40, only the number 2 showed infection; the others, undamaged.

The periods positive or negative in blood, change very much. In occasions are two or three days positive and negative, and so: a guinea pig positive 11-5-40, on 15-5-40 is negative and on 20-5-40 showed numerous (20 for microscopic field). In other opportunities those periods are of one, two, three or more weeks. When the peripheric blood is negative doing the puncture of the myocardium is also negative.

In these negative periods we have killed guinea pigs or rats in order to see where the parasites are deposited and we have observed the following: in the cephalorachidean liquid we have never found trypanosomas, in opposition to other investigators. We have examined spleen, liver, pancreas, lungs, kidneys, peritoneal serosity. In these organs for smears of apposition and coloration panoptic Pappenheim, we have verified: the spleen as a true depository of trypanosomas; in lungs, kidneys, pancreas, etc., scarce parasites, and in liver almost none. We did the diagnosis by rare nucleus found, because impossible to see complete parasites.

The breeding of guinea pigs infected have been always negative. Referring to temperature it has been completely normal, and so: rats, mice, guinea pigs with high infection, was always 37.5, 37.8, 38.5, 39, taking in account that under 39° it is not abnormal temperature.

We wanted to see the influence of the splenectomy, the negative or positive periods, etc., we did the extirpation of the spleen of a guinea pig weighting 400 grams on 4-7-40, with general anesthesia.

This animal, perfectly of health, was inoculated with 3 c.c. of blood on 13-7-40. On 16-7-40 appeared one trypanosoma for each 5 or 6 fields; on 17-7-40 one parasite for each 3 or 4 fields; the inoculation time seemed to be short. The negative periods increased slowly and on 22-7-40 the animal did not present trypanosomas. On 28-7-40, the guinea pig showed newly scarce parasites, finishing the negative phase. On 31-7-40 the trypanosomas are numerous; on 8-8-40 was negative again; on 18-8-40 was positive and continued presenting parasites till its death. As important details: short inoculation; never, only one time, abundance of trypanosomas; phases positive and negative that are common, and the death very soon. We have seen that the infection with venezuelense can remain several months. Experiences of Meleney with S. recurrentis have demonstrated, that the splenectomy increases the intensity of the infection and the time of the initial attack, facts either mention before in 1911 for Tournade.

Besides the splenectomy we have wanted to observe the action of the pancreotomy of the hydrocarbons metabolism. The pancreotomy has been practiced with general anesthesia and making resection of a great portion of the organ. The animal supported perfectly the intervention. The former glucaemia, the surgical act was of 1 gram and the test after the intervention, gave the same amount or less. The pancreotomy has not changed the course of the infection.

Also, injecting intraperitoneal in rats and mice with abundant parasites, 0.5 or 1 gram of glucose in order to see the effect on the infection, the abundance of the trypanosomas is equal.

The result of the autopsy of a guinea pig with high infection, presenting numerous trypanosomas before the death, is as follows: weight 550 grams, inoculated with T. venezuelense on 20-4-40, and died on 7-6-40. Tests about parasites always positive. Abdomen large, without adiposity in the subcutaneous tissue. The laparotomy revealed the digestive organs in complete normality. Not peritoneal serosity.

Normal peritoneum. Intestinal mucous normal. The liver is increased, double size, not adherences. Surface flat. Hepatic borders congested. In the central region tubercular granulation diffuse yellowish. The biliar vesicle empty.

The spleen enlarged, flat, normal color. The kidneys reveal conjunctive degeneration. The suprarenal enlarged and brown color.

The heart with hemorrhagic overflow peri-auricular hidden the coronaries and extended the pericardium. The intrapleural cavity contains a clear liquid. Good appearance of the respiratory organs.

The cranial trephining did not produce abnormal overflow of

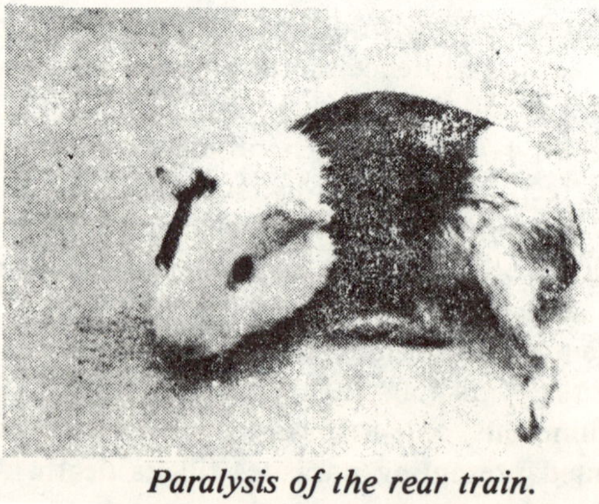

Paralysis of the rear train.

cephalorachidean liquid. The brain and marrow not demonstrating pathologic characteristics. In summary: spleno-hepatomegaly; degeneration of the kidneys and suprarenals. Pericarditis.

* * *

We did inoculations in guinea pigs, white rats, white mice, rabbits, dogs, cats, doves and chickens.

In guinea pigs the inoculation is long, one or two weeks; shorter when the animal is young. The old guinea pigs, of more 500 grams supporting well the infection. They can live a long time without any symptoms. In rare cases presenting paralysis of the rear train, with few sensitiveness. These troubles are durable after the inoculation, never prematurely.

The guinea pig was inoculated on 26-5-40 and the paralysis was observed on 3-9-40. The animal at the beginning dragging along, both paws are impeded and after the paralysis was more appreciable in the left paw. The young guinea pig is not capable to support the disease, dying two, three or four weeks, after the parasites have appeared in the peripheric blood.

The resistance that we have seen in the guinea pig it is not possible in rats and mice. The mouse is more sensitive to the trypanosoma, dying 5 or 6 days after the inoculation, presenting numerous parasites in the blood.

The following day, in rats and mice, after the inoculation, it is easy to find abundant trypanosomas in blood; however, sometimes the test is negative. Often, 24 hours after the inoculation the animal dies, possible the action of the parasites, because of the autopsy the peritoneum is undamaged. In rats is observed the negative phase and so: an animal inoculated on 30-6-40; on 1-7-40, reveal parasites increasing the number till 6-7-40, disappearing, to appear newly on 7-7-40. This animal died the following day, showing parasites in blood from myocardium, agglomerated, unshaken. Never have we found albumin in the urine of infected animals, may be slight quantity, either in the alive animals or dead for punction of the bladder. In infected rats, with treatment sulfanilamide we have found albumin, perhaps owed to the medicine.

In white rats we observed that the animal is sad, walks slowly, there is a slight paralysis of the rear train, but sometimes paralysis of the four paws (quadriplegia). The animal does not move, generalized convulsions, not able to bite, surviving not more than thirteen days. It is so the abundance of trypanosomas that it seems to be more numerous than the red cells.

* * *

A puppy inoculated intraperitoneal on 1-7-40, testing the blood, negative; on 11-7-40 presented the first parasites (5 or 6 by field); on

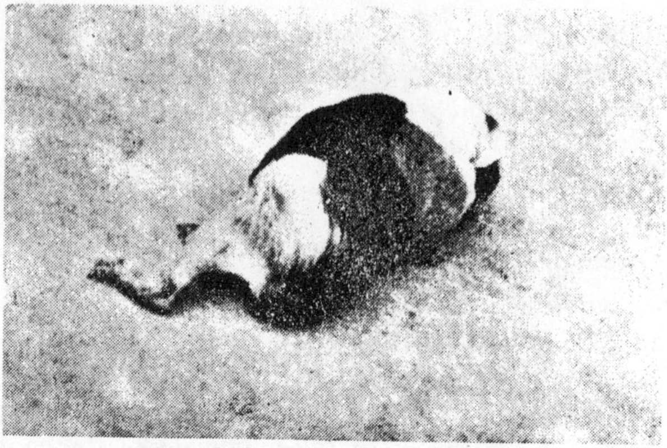

The same former guinea pig.

17-7-40, the number more or less 15 by field, and revealed the first symptoms: sad, no appetite, loss of weight, conjunctivitis monocular (this symptom will be studied carefully in the future). In other animals, as guinea pigs, we have seen the ocular symptoms, sometimes in both eyes, and it seems there is loss of sight.

On 23-7-40, the symptomatology is equal, aggregating troubles for walk and on 24-7-40, the animal died with paralysis of the rear train and convulsions. In the autopsy examined, the blood of the heart was negative, but inoculating this negative blood after the death, appearing parasites in the new animal. Taking ticks of the little dog and examined always negative referring flagellates.

On 16-7-40, we inoculated intraperitoneal two little cats of 250 and 300 grams. On 22-7-40, one of them presents the first parasite. On 27-7-40, the second is positive. On 27-7-40 died the cat that had 250 grams, the first to be positive, and on 31-7-40 died the second. This last one presented paralysis.

On 15-7-40, inoculated intraperitoneal with dilution (3 c.c.) of infectd blood a rabbit of 1.410 grams of weight, presenting parasites on 27-7-40. The following day the blood test was negative to trypanosomas. The animal is sad, loss of weight, drowsiness, deviation of the head to the right, not presenting paralysis of the rear train, but certain instability compeling to the animal to open the former train, continuing this symptomatology till the death.

The inoculations to doves and chickens were negative.

* * *

Doing attempts of transmission we have made the experience of Darling. We took several specimens of domestic fly and put it to suck infected blood; later, we put the insects on the scraping abdomen of a guinea pig. The trypanosomas appeared in the blood of the animal one week after. It is a mechanical transmission, but maybe in the nature will succeed the same. Attempts with Stomoxys sp. has not been possible because the life of these insects in captivity is difficult.

Attempts of cultures we have done in medium modificated of Kast, in medium leptospire of Noguchi, in gelose-blood NNN, in several times, always with negative results. We think that the culture of this trypanosoma is not easy and we do not know any work about this field; perhaps its cycle will be very simple and it is the cause of these failures.

CHAPTER II

It seems the "Derrengadera" of our horses, will be equal to the disease of Columbia and Ecuador. As we have said, before, histopathological has not been studied. Asking to Panamá this affair we have received form Johnson, assistant-director, the following answer: "I received his letter dated 18th of september. I regret not being able to help you in this request about reports related with the histo-pathology of the trypanosomiasis."

"We have made only works about diagnosis, transmission and treatement in the horses."

With this answer from Johnson, from Institute Gorgas, it is very probable, up to date, nothing has been made in this field.

As follows, we give the first histo-pathological reports of the organs of a guinea pig inoculated and died 37 days, later. With the kind help of Koppisch of the School of Tropical Medicine of Puerto Rico, sponsored by Columbia University, New York, U.S.A.

"Macroscopic description, without description. Microscopic description: HEART - In the epicardium as in the myocardium we see a moderate number of little focus spreaded of lymphoid cells. SPLEEN - The pulp demonstrate a slight increase of the conjunctive tissue. The cells of the pulp are almost all lymphoids. The follicles are large numerous and protuberant. LIVER - Amount of blackish pigment granular in the Kupffer' cells and extra-cellular, probably owed to the fixing with formaldehyde. In some places any little focus of necrosis of hepatic tissue. KIDNEYS -Nothing at all interesting. LUNGS - There is a moderate congestion, a little zone of recent hemorrhage, a little of diapedesis in the alveolus and small focus of lymphoids cells in different places of the parenchyma."

CHAPTER III

For two diseases so important Chagas and Equina trypanosomiasis, its germs are very strong, resisting. The T. cruzi, up to date, has no specific treatment; referring T. venezuelense the 205 Bayer, the antimony (Iturbe, Tejera) have effect, but the parasites reappear.

We have attempted with the 7.602, Bayer' product, derived quinolinic used to 3% and handled by Brumpt, Mazza, Torrealba, it seems to have given good results; a second product sulfanilamide and a third derived from the creosol.

The 7.602 has been observed by us in vitro on cruzi of blood and intestinal, putting in contact both drops during 45 minutes for the first and the second two hours. We have not seen no action.

With the venezuelense the same. One drop of infected blood mixed with one drop of the medicament, without observing changes during one hour.

In a test tube mixing saline solution and blood, adding the medicament and making tests to intervals; the effect is null.

A mouse with 25 grams of weight, showing a trypanosoma by field, has been injected with 0.5 c.c. of 7.602, not observing improvement, neither symtoms, nor number of parasites. Injected with 1 c.c. intraperitoneal, no effect and it died some days after. The trypanosomas in blood of the heart are normal and active.

Injecting with 0.5 of 7.602 subcutaneous, a guinea pig with venezuelense weighting 285 grams; one, another, with T. cruzi, seed from triatomidae, infection got with inoculation intraperitoneal, weighting 620 grams, and one, third, guinea pig, strain from triatomidae. In none of the three we have observed any effect.

Two little guinea pigs of 110 grams weight and T. venezuelense positive in peripheric blood, we have injected, intraperitoneal, 0.5 c.c. of 7.602 on 10-6-40. These animals were controlled daily.

The following day of the injection of medicament, no showing trypanosomas in blood, and continues so, till 14-6-40, when newly appeared. Both animals in the moment of the injection presented contractions of the paws and a generalized tremor, during some minutes.

These animals continued in observation, positive always till 21-6-40, that we injected, 1 c.c. of 7.602, intraperitoneal. Both showed nauseas, immovability, for a short time. Tested 3 hours later. The guinea pig of 150 grams was recovered, well, and the blood showed abundant parasites; but the other one, 110 grams, was sad, and numerous trypanosomas in blood. On 23-6-40 not showing trypanosomas and so, till 1-7-40, the smaller died without parasites in blood; the other one on 5-7-40 newly parasites in blood.

In rats and mice with infection venzuelense, we have used a medicament sulfanilamide, called Solfanil. To a rat we have injected 0.2 in 5 c.c. of distilled water, intraperitoneal. Examined daily there was no effect. We thought, two days later, to apply another injection of 0.5, diluted in distilled water. The infection continued equal (clinical and parasitological). In mice we have made the same with equal results. The control has been made two, three or five hours later. We did attempts in-vitro with the same result.

The third medicament to base of creosol, the assays have been null.

SOME OBSERVATIONS ABOUT DISEASES PRODUCED BY PARASITES IN MARACAIBO (STATE ZULIA)*

MALARIA

The Malaria is very abundant in Maracaibo, because in all the districts surrounding the city it is endemial. In the exams of laboratory employing the method panoptic of Pappenheim and thick drop, in many cases we have found P. vivax and only in one case to the care of Dr. Cuenca it was possible to find P. falciparum.

In our visits to the Casa de Beneficencia we saw patients with the common fever and large malaric splenomegalies.

LEISHMANIOSIS

When we started to work in La Beneficencia as adjunt physician, it called our attention a patient of the ward San Jorge, presenting lesions invading both buttoms, humid, painful, bleeding, giving a secretion resembling it produced for the venereal granulome.

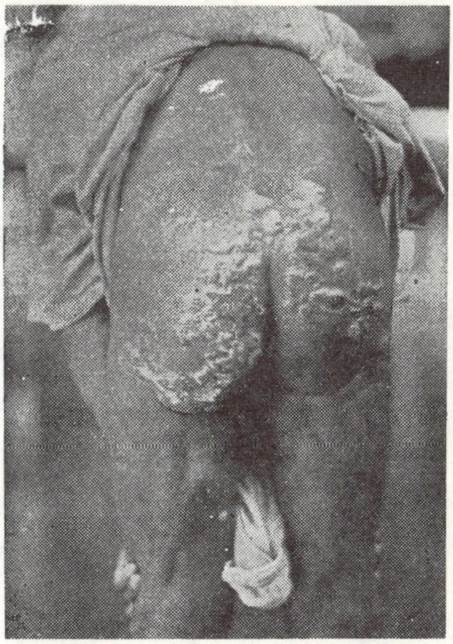

Case of cutaneous leishmaniosis. Observe the aspect and situation of the lesions. Cure with tartar emetic.

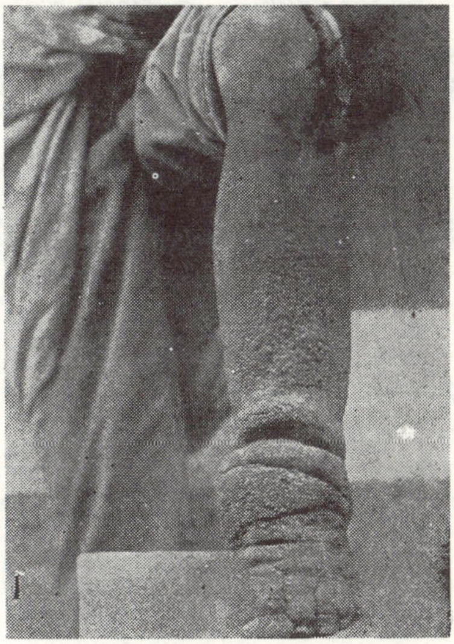

Case probably of it is called "Moosy foot." The skin looks dry, hard, and warty.

* Pamphlet 1929

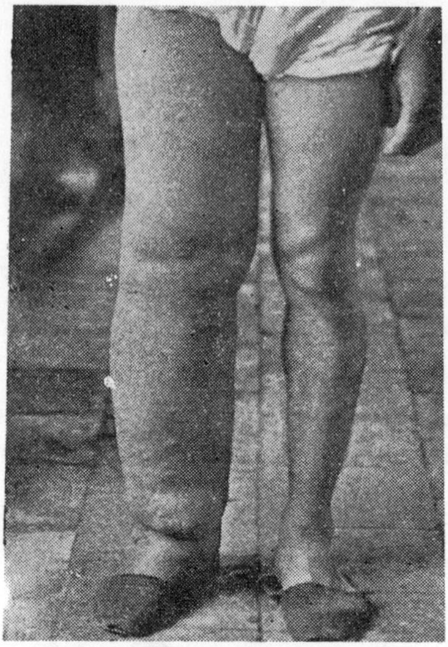

Case, possibly filariosis Bancrofti. Observe the hypertrophy of the leg. Treatment tartar emetic. Improvement.

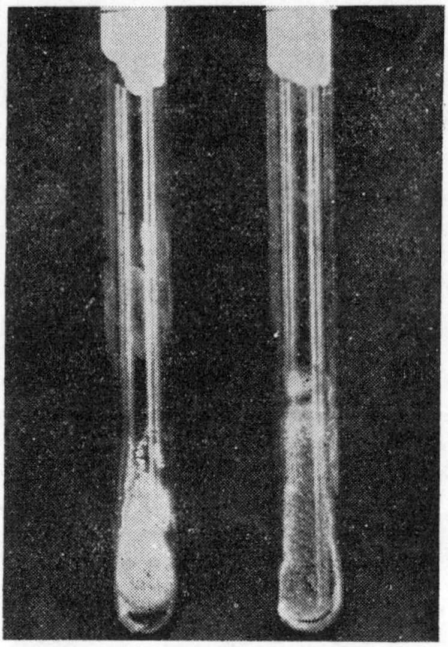

Cultures of Aspergillus in medium of Sabouraud. Material taken from the last two cases.

At the first view we thought in granulome, but after, making smears looking for *kalimatic bacterium gramulomatis,* we had the surprise finding numerous elements ovoids, with nucleus and blepharoplaste very clear, elements that with all security are Leishman' bodies.

This patient, as always, remembered the story of an insect, dark, flat, that had urinated on the place affected, called "pito."

This case is very curious, either for the aspect or for the site of the lesions; not being a region exposed to the sting of the phlebotomus.

Often we saw in the hospital chronic ulcers of the legs, perhaps leishmaniod.

Our patient was cured with the treatment of tartar emetic, but was certain delay.

MOOSY FOOT

Several times we have seen in La Beneficencia patients with large feet, of hard and wrinkled skin, long time of evolution, finishing in surgical treatment.

The photo 3, is an ill person coming from Coro, 38 years old, suffering of this since early age.

To the examination we found a big foot, of corrugated and hard skin, warty, and three thick collars in the anterior face separated by deep furrows. The sensibility to the touch, cold and heat is diminished and the lower part has erysipelatous aspect.

Professor Mühlens in Medical Review of Hamburg (1928), appoint this affection that he saw for the first time in Urama (Venezuela) and later in El Salvador, Guatemala, and Mexico. The warts were studied anatomo-pathological by Rocha Lima and Rísquiz Jr.

According to Cranstom Low could be a type of cutaneous warty tuberculosis.

FILARIOSIS

In Hospital Vargas we often saw cases with suspicious of filariosis; persons born or having lived in Puerto Cabello.

Now, we have had the opportunity to see a patient very interested in Hospital de Chiquinquirá, with an abnormal increase of the right leg.

It is a sick person that lived in the zone of Puerto Cabello, three years ago; later, in Cabimas and Maracaibo, suffering of a crisis of lymphangitis and seeing slowly the increase of the leg.

Tests of blood according to the technician Fülleborn during day and night seeking microfilarias were negative.

Dr. Amado has submited this patient to tartat emetic observing a light improvement.

OTOMYCOSIS

It seems to be that otomycosis is frequent in Maracaibo. We have presented to the Sociedad Médico-Quirúrgica del Zulia three cases with subjective troubles of pain, deafness, hummings, etc.

In these three cases the fungi have been classified in the Department of Agriculture of Washington as belonging to the genus Aspergillus, species niger.

Some of the patients had for a long time the sickness and remembered baths of immersion at the beginning.

All the patients have been cured with enema of the ears and solution of nitrate of silver 1% in instillations, exception of one of the cases, having associated an eczema.

LEISHMANIOSIS*

The American leishmaniosis (cutaneous and mucous) is a disease very frequent among us. We believe that the lapse of time between the works of Iturbe and Tejera and the contributions of Chacín, Pifano, Guerra and Sánchez Covisa, is owed to errors in the diagnosis and in the technic searching the parasites.

One of the few cases published during that period was ours, in a patient of State Zulia, observed in La Beneficencia, with lesions in bottoms, getting his health with a treatment with tartar emetic and we said in that epoch: "often we see in the Hospital chronic ulcers of the legs that probably will be leishmanoid ulcers."

The leishmaniosis was considered only in ulcerations of the pavillion of the ears or in exposed parts of the body, according to photos showed in treaties of Tropical Medicine, never as manifestations of different aspects very good studied by the brazilian researchers appeared in judicious works in the collection of the Memories of Oswaldo Cruz, and besides the investigations of the leishmanias were done for smears in extension and not for apposition.

In our practice in the Service of nose, throat and ears at Hospital Vargas it is common to see the mucous form, chiefly nasal, characterized

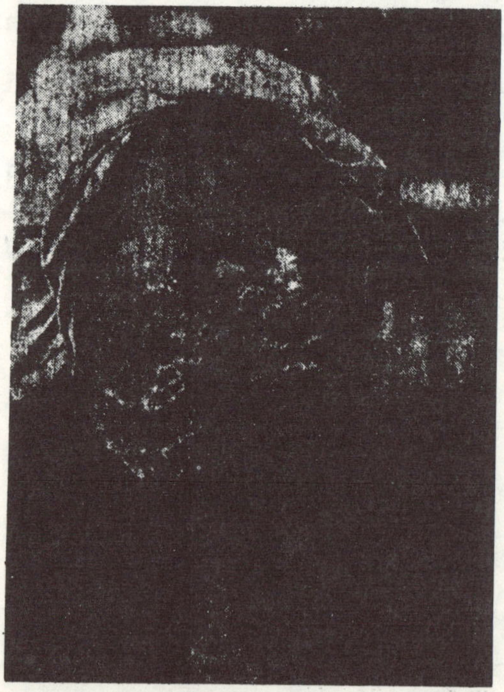

Patient observed by the author, year 1929. Lesions situated in both bottoms. Tartar emetic treatment.

* Reprinted from "Boletín del Laboratorio de la Clínica Luis Razetti" - Año III -Vol. II - Nº 8 - 1942.

for the aspect, slow evolution, destruction of the cartilage of nasal septum, not attacking the osseous portion and this detail helps the differential diagnosis with syphilis.

We expose here a case studied in the mentioned Service. Patient born in Aricagua (State Mérida), 57 years old, with 15 years suffering of a nasal affection causing the enlargement of the nasal pyramid, observing through the rhinoscopy anterior a destruction of the cartilage of the nasal septum with a proliferation of the nasal mucous. R. Kahn negative. Urine normal. Feces: trichocephalus and hookworm. Smears for apposition made with sections of the lesions and panoptic showed leishmanias.

The intradermic reaction with *leishmanin* made in the forearm in National Institute of Hygiene, red 48 and 72 hours after it gave a clear positive result.

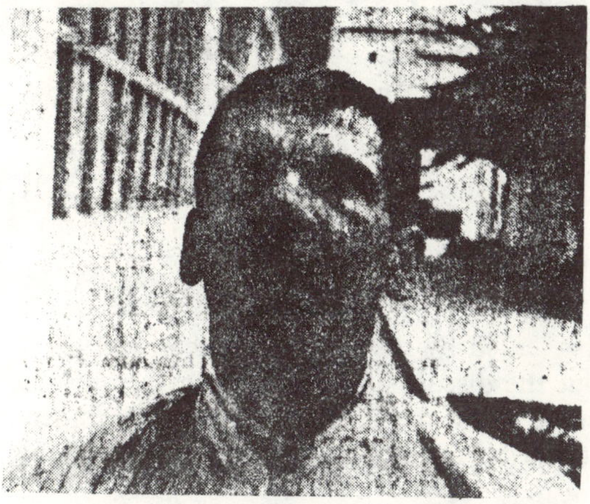

Present case. Leishmaniosis nasal. It is easy appreciate enlargement of the nose.

The patient treated with tartar emetic, received from 15-12-41 to 10-1-42 1 gram 15 centigrams. With this dose was almost a total disappearance of the lesions and a notable increase of the nasal permeability.

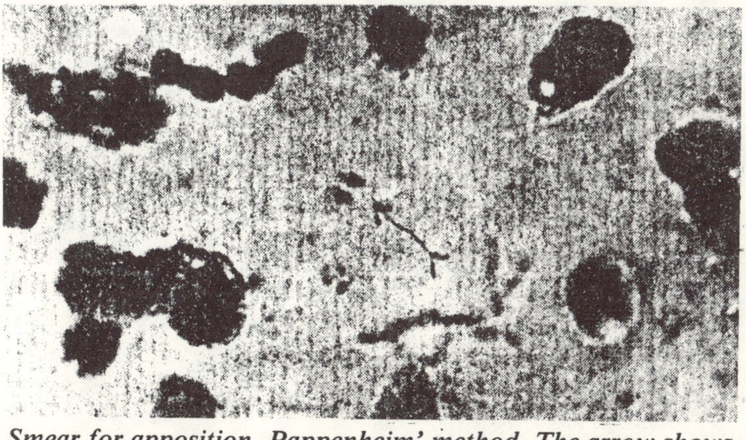

Smear for apposition. Pappenheim' method. The arrow shows two parasites in the center.

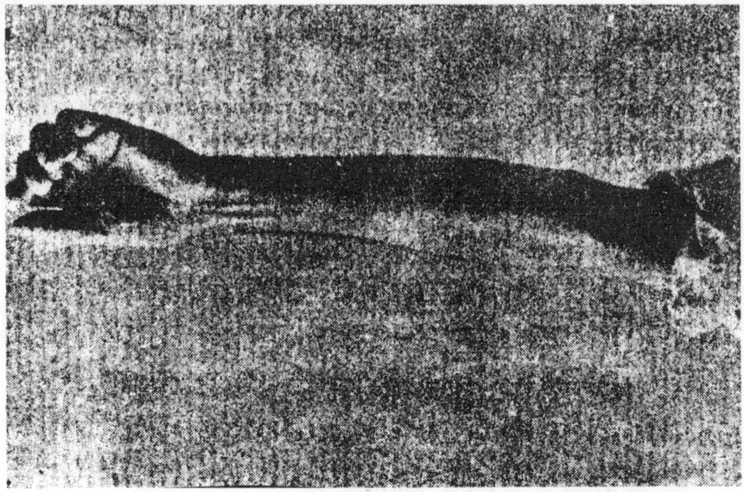

Intradermic reaction to the leishmanin showed strong positivity 72 hours after.

SUMMARY

A case of leishmaniosis presented by the author in the year 1929 is reminded. Commentaries about the disease and why during such a long time was unknown. It is presented a case of nasal leishmaniosis, with finding of leishmanias, positive the test of intradermic reaction and healing with tartar emetic.

OBSERVATIONS TO THE STUDY OF THE LEISHMANIOSIS IN VENEZUELA *

INTRODUCTION

The cutaneous leishmaniosis is an old disease between us. Iturbe and González appointed in the year 1917 the first case in Venezuela; after, Tejera presented a wide monograph, summary of his researches in the State Zulia; scientific work awarded with the prize Vargas and published in 1919.

Since that time the illness was not remarked, owed to two motives: 1°, the investigators only had in mind the descriptions and photos of the teaching books with the known photos of the lesion in the pavillion of the ear, named ulcer of the chewing gum. 2°, that the parasites were not sought for smears of apposition, method very sure according to our experience.

We, in the year 1929, reading the notables contributions of brazilian authors appeared in the Memorias del Instituto Oswaldo Cruz, published a rare case, verified the finding of the parasite, and then in pamphlet "Algunas observaciones sobre enfermedades parasitarias en Maracaibo", wrote: "often, we see in the hospital chronic ulcers of the legs that perhaps, in many cases, will be leishmaniod ulcers."

Later, in the last times, people have had more interest for this affection, and so, there are a communication of Briceño Iragorry, 1935; the doctoral thesis of Chacín; the wide studies of Mayer and Pifano, of Guerra and Sánchez Covisa, and the "Distribución geográfica de la leishmanicosis tegumentaria y algunos datos para el plan de estudios del kalaazar en Venezuela" by Briceño Rossi, works condensing the clinic, parasitology, epidemiology, etc., of this sickness.

CHAPTER I

INVESTIGATION - CULTURES - PARASITOLOGIC CONCEPT

The leishmanias are protozoa, more or less, 2 to 4 microns, round and oval form, scarce or abundant number, often inside the cells, but also out of the cells. With a nucleus, a blepharoplaste long, characteristics helping in its identity. However, we have not been able to obtain clear morphology, maybe to lacks in the technic.

* Reprinted from the book "Estudios Entomológicos y Parasitológicos." 1948.

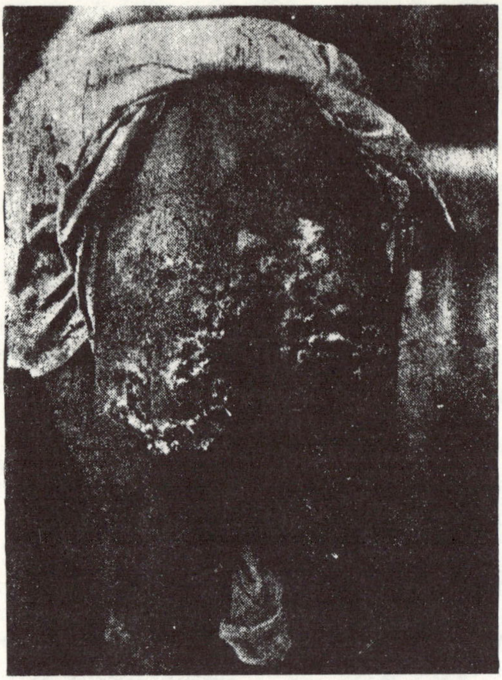

Patient with lesions in the buttoms.

The parasites are very scarce and probable this is the motive of the few positive diagnosis. We do the examination for turns. Many times the clinical diagnosis is clear, but to find parasites it is not possible. In case 1, it was not possible the presence of parasites, not withstanding, in the case N° 11, the leishmanias were very numerous, seeing groups of more than 50 parasites.

In the majority of the patients, almost all with nasal lesions, we take with pincers of the exulceration of the nasal septum or of the edge of the perforation. In the N° 9 we profit to take of the rhino-pharynx and in N° 11,we take form the cutaneous lesions, chiefly, form the edge of the lesions.

The technic that we have used is the panoptic of Pappenheim, also the Giemsa slow (1 drop for each c.c.), during five hours, using before alcohol methylic. The Giemsa has been equally employed in the flagellates forms of the cultures.

We did cultures of the N° 9. In the cultures we have been helped by Professor Pifano, to whom we give our acknowledgement.

Our patients are almost all of nasal leishmaniosis. In them it is very difficult to do cultures, being the nose a part very septic, but in the N° 9, was a type cutaneous-mucous, with a large infiltration of superior lip, we took of this region; and besides, in the patient 11, that had lesions in the left leg and arms, we took material of the leg, place where we had found leishmanias.

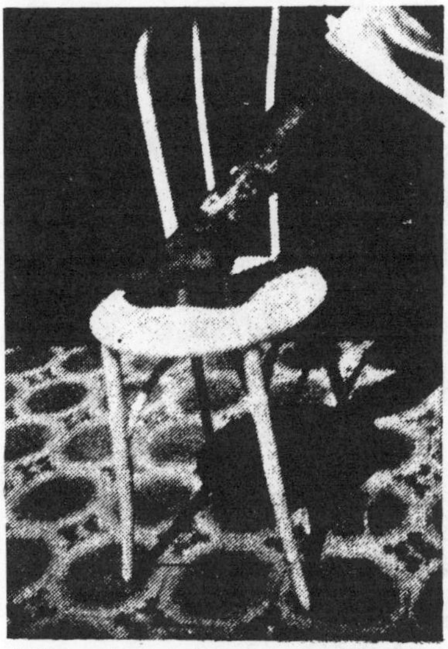

Ulcer leishmaniod verified by us in a patient of Hospital Ruiz of Ciudad Bolívar, born in Tumeremo (State Bolívar).

The cultures have been made in medium NNN, with ph. 7.2. Ten days after one dozen of tubes of the case 9, only one coming infected, and two presented leptomonad forms, positivity in which the motility and the number increasing. Also, we have utilized the medium semisolid of Noguchi, to maintain the cultures with very good success.

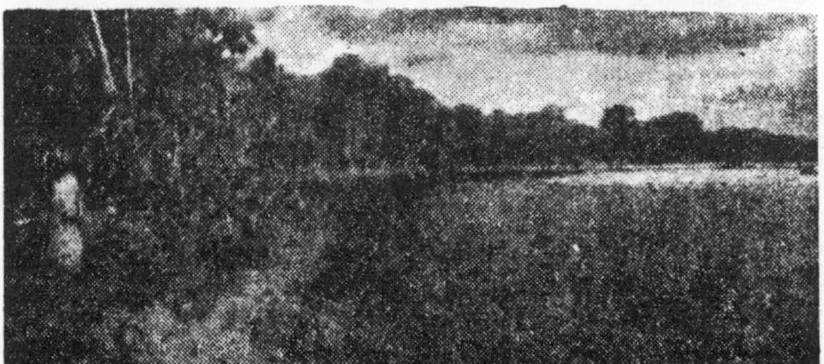

River Canaguá, running around the city of Barinas. In this region very irrigated and bushy, we found a large focus of leishmaniosis, with frequent nasal troubles.

The technic for the culture has been made having a syringe with 1 c.c. of saline solution physiological with acid citrate 3.8%, introducing the needle an little cut the edge of the lesion and moving it; after to inject half c.c., to suck and with this bloody liquid putting 2 or 3 drops in each one of the tubes NNN.

The flagellate forms, as is possible to see in the drawings of the case N° 9, are slender, few wide; some long, others short; alone or in groups with rosy aspect; stages of division and using Giemsa slow, with the water light alkaline; the nucleus, blepharoplaste and flagellum, are seen perfectly.

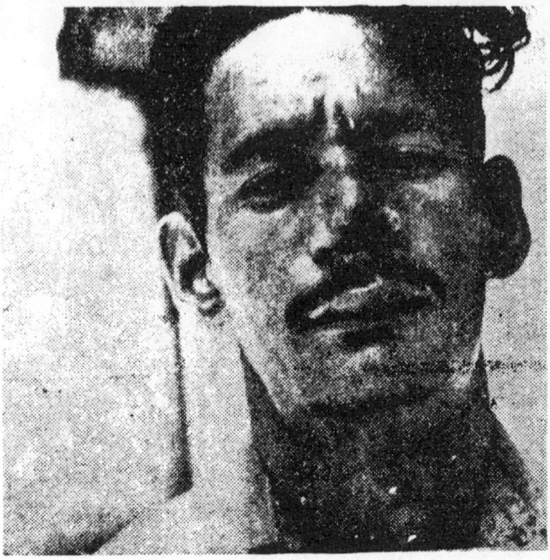

Photo showing the destruction of the lobe, wings, septum and infiltration of the superior lip.

Referring to morphology, it is impossible to separate the Leishmania tropica of the Leishmania americana. In the clinic it is accepted that the Bouton de Oriente is an affection benign, healing easily, very different from the americana that produces cutaneous resisting lesions. However, for the history of our patients we have seen that it is a mild affection, lasting around one year; but, *"the serious are the mucous lesions in nose and pharynx, destructives, mutilators, resisting, for a special tropism, doing it for the ways of blood or lymph, giving malignity to the species. Just, these secondaries mucous lesions are the principal object of this work.*

The course of the disease is a first primary cutaneous lesion and later the nasal secondary lesion; rarely both go together. It seems to be that Christoperson in the Sudan Anglo-Egipcio saw lesions very similar to the espundia of Perú, that will be very probable leishmaniosis cutaneous-mucous.

In our case N° 11, as is seen in photo, was an ulcer primary; after, when it was seen by us, secondary cutaneous lesions and mucous going one at side of the other, and so, the case of Christoperson and other authors, appointing cases of Bouton de Oriente liked to the espundia of Perú or Leishmeniosis American cutaneous-mucous, probably will be a lesion of Bouton de Oriente in the superior lip, invading after the nasal and pharynx mucous and septum. The progress is completely different in both affections.

Laveran, 1917, with material from America, finding large and vacuoleted elements gave the name of Leishmania tropica, American variety; vacuoles have been considered as degenerative shapes. Escomel suggested Leishmania tropica; flagellate variety, and Vianna; pioneer in this sickness, 1911, for the presence of filaments intra-protoplasm, gave the name of Leishmania brasiliensis.

The tests of agglutination handled by Noguchi were accepted, but later, the researchs of Ray revealed: the inmuno-donovani agglutinate equally donovani and tropica var. brasiliensis; anti-brasiliensis agglutinate donovani and tropica from Palestine; anti-Palestine agglutinate brasiliensis, but no donovani; the normal serum of rabbit agglutinate Turkestan, tropica Turkestan and Palestine, donovani and tropica var. brasiliensis. Marques de Cunha sugget that for agglutination it was not possible to separate tropica var. brasiliensis, infamtum, and donovani and thinks L. chagasi is equal to infantum.

Wenyon has suggested not finding differences among tropica and americana the name tropica for both, but possibly will be later, till newer research call the parasite of our American leishmaniosis: L. tropica var. brasiliensis (Wright 1903 - Vianna 1911).

CHAPTER II

CLINICAL CONCEPT

Rabello did a fundamental division among cutaneous leishmaniosis and visceral leishmaniosis. Besides, of the visceral forms from Asia and Europa known. Penna in Brazil 1934, in the Section of Viscerotomy of the Rockefeller, found 41 cases of a new American visceral leishmaniosis, in 47,000 section of liver, giving it the name of L. chagasi.

Pons and Martínez Niochet have found the first case in Venezuela.

The cutaneous leishmaniosis are divided: 1° cutaneous purity; 2° lesions mucous of the nose, pharynx, mouth, beginning for the cutaneous lesions, and 3° mixed forms, cutaneous and mucous lesions.

It is impossible in a picture to include all the clinical forms, because the sites of the lesions, infections, wounds, etc., will change the aspect. To the Bouton of Oriente, Hygoumenakis wrote about its polymorphism, describing 17 varieties. Somebody has told that it is necessary to have in account this polymorphism, before doing the diagnosis.

There is a form simulating a piodermatitis, called piodermoide; other one, cutaneous, with abscess lymphatic, liked for its aspect to the sporotrichosis; there is another one placed in cheeks simulating, as in our case P.C.M., the lupus; other one, with deep lesions, with salient and hard edge, liked syphilitic lesions, and last one, producing increase of the feet, with nodular lesions, salient ulcers, liked the moosy-foot or chromoblastomycosis.

Among this group of appearences there is one typical, that is not other than the old nasal - buccal - pharynx leishmaniosis of Laveran. Just, this form is the motive of this communication, puzzle of the specialist in nose, throat, ears between us.

The common lesions are ulceration in the septum, destroying the cartilage and producing perforation and mainly symptoms of obstruction, expelling crusts and bloody mucosities, sometimes epistaxis, often around the hole where there is the development of a salient edge, easy bleeding.

All these details, a perforation of the septum almost always is related to this affection. Equally, leprosy and tuberculosis also present it, but the leprosy is accompanied for several manifestations and the lupus tubercular is rare in Venezuela.

Characteristics of this affection is the completeness of the bony portion, while the fall for the destruction of the septum.

The tuberculosis does not attack equally the bony parts, but produce atresia and besides the lupus tubercular is not frequent between us.

The leishmaniasis, as other investigators have said (Guerra and Sánchez Covisa) destroy the nasal cartilage and change the nose in a channel that is possible to see the fallen lobe rise; the lupus tubercular try to close both nostrils.

Summary: the syphilitic nose is in riding saddle; the leishmaniod nose in beak of parrot; the leishmaniasis increase the nostrils; the tuberculosis close the nostrils. In a word: the leishmaniasis is ectasis, the tuberculosis is atresia, as opportunely have told the cited authors.

CHAPTER III

HISTO-PATHOLOGY

In almost all of our patients we have made biopsy (our acknowledgment to the Service of histopathology of the Hospital Vargas and Professor Jaffé, chief), sometimes we have obtained more than one report. To make the biopsy we employ special nippers, using Palmer' speculum in order to wider field. We take the biopsy of tissue of the ulcer in septum or the salient edge around the perforation. In the case 11, out the nose, we took another biopsy from other leishmaniod lesion in any part of the body. It is very rare to see leishmaniasis in the sections, said the pathologists, and for that motive only in the case 11 was affirmative.

Among the group of the reports it is easily appreciated, as said Guerra and Sánchez Covisa, the diversity of aspects; however, it is necessary to appoint the proliferation of the epithelium (acantosis) going toward the depth in long files. In the dermis, granular tissue with large infiltrations for ronde cells, plasmocytes and white cells polynuclears.

CHAPTER IV

INSECTS TRANSMISSORS

The researchs of the brothers Sergent and Adler and Theodor referring to the Bouton de Oriente and those of Beaurepaire Aragao in Brazil, with the Ph. intermedius and the American Leishmiasis, have demonstrated the function of the phlebotomus in the transmission of this disease.

We have caught till today, four species of this large family: *evansi, migonei, panamensis,* and *suis* (gomezi?). Classifications done by Rozeboom of John Hopkins, to whom we give our acknowledgment.

Pifano has found in one of our States (Yaracuy) leptomonads in the specie *longipalpis* Lutz and Neiva 1912.

The specie *evansi* was described by Núñez Tovar 1921 and dedicated to Miss Alwen M. Evans of the Liverpool school. In Macuto (Dto.

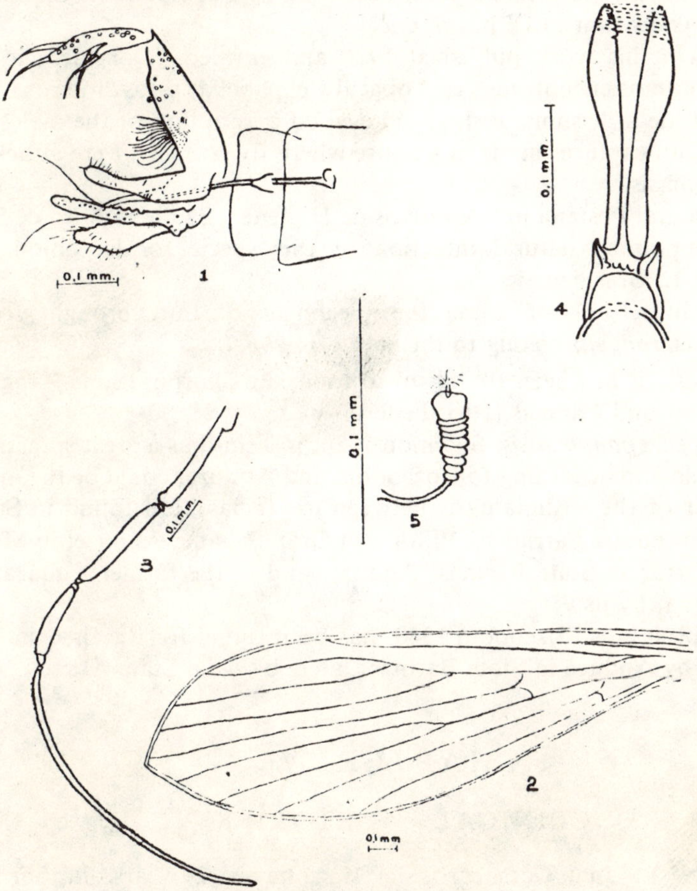

F. suis-Explanation of Plate
Figure 1.- Hypopygium of type male.
Figure 2.- Wing of allotype female.
Figure 3.- Palp of paratype female.
Figure 4.- Buccopharynx of allotype female.
Figure 5.- Spermatheca of allotype female.
All drawings were made with a calibrated camera lucida.
(tomado del trabajo original)

Federal) we have caught it, in the rain season (July and August), doing captures of 30 and 40 specimens.

In 1927-1929 Dyar considered this specie as synonymous of *squamiventris,* but after, have been verified that *evansi* exist, as separated specie.

This specie up to today has been found in four places of the country; Mariara (State Carabobo) Núñez Tovar; Mene Maurea (State Falcón) Ortiz; San Mateo (State Aragua) and Macuto (Dto. Federal) by us.

The specie *migonei* was described by Franca 1920; *Ph. rangeli* Núñez Tovar and Tejera 1924, and *araozi,* described by Patterson and Shannon 1926, are synonymous of Ph. *migonei.*

Mazza in his work published 1926 and entitled "Consideraciones sobre flebotomos encontrados en Tobacal y el papel de estos dípteros en la transmisión de la leishmaniosis", did a good description of the males of this specie, on captures made in a house where five persons were attacked by leishmaniasis.

Pessoa and Pestana in "Arquivos de Higiene y Saúde Pública de Sao Paulo", appointed natural infection of this specie for leptomonads, possibly of L. Brasiliensis.

According to Costa Lima the specimens of Lutz brought from Venezuela as *rangeli,* belong to the specie *migonei.*

In Venezuela, it has been found up to today in Choroní (State Aragua) Núñez Tovar and Caracas (Dto. Federal) by us.

The specie *panamensis,* Shannon 1926, it seems has a great spreading in Venezuela and according to Rozeboom and Anduze, could be the main transmissor of the leishmaniasis between us. It has been found in State Yaracuy, in the site Farriar by Pifano; in Gran Sabana, Anduze; in Mene Mauroa, Ortiz; in State Barinas, Anduze, and in the farmer Aguacatal, State Aragua, by us.

The specie suis Rozeboom 1940, has been found for the first time in Venezuela by Anduze in State Barinas; later, by us in State Aragua.

CHAPTER V

CLINICAL HISTORIES

Case Nº 1 - Juan Camacaro, sick since he was 29 years old, born in Santa Lucía (State Miranda), driver, doing trips often to the interior of the country. Father alive and in complete health. Mother is dead. Three brothers alive and healthy. Eruptives of the infancy. Pneumonie, malaria, blenorrhea. March 1942, test of Kahn + +, submitted Bi and salvarsan.

Eight months started the affection, light troubles and itching in the nose, some bleeding. The disease has gone advancing; total destruction of the nasal septum (cartilage); destruction almost complete of the left wing of nasal pyramid; destruction of the nasal lobe and a part of the right side;

infiltration of the superior lip.

This patient had suffered two intradermic with *leishmanina* in the National Institute of Hygiene, both negative results, and two biopsis in the Institute Anti-Cáncer "Luis Razetti", with the following results: 1° biopsy (20-9-42) acute and chronic inflammation, slight acanthosis of the epithelium. 2° biopsy (13-10-42) exudate inflammatory acute, with remarkable inflammation epithelial, but not qualified as epithelioma.

The intraderma reactions of these patients, exception the case 13 done with antigen prepared by us, were made, kindly, by Professor Mayer, to whom we give our acknowledgment.

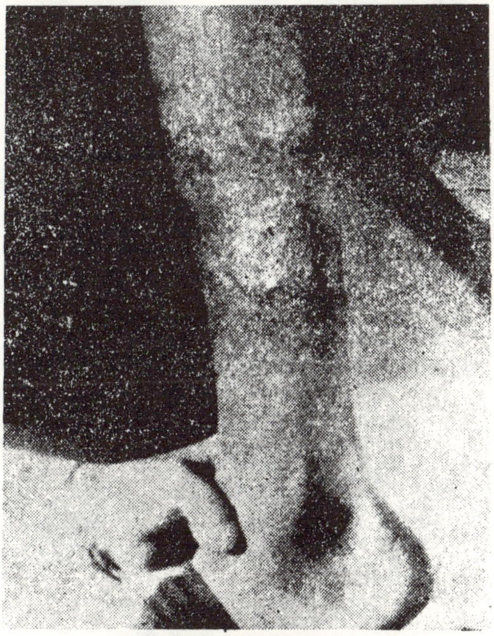

Case - Photo 9 - Scar in the left leg, possibly the beginning of the affection.

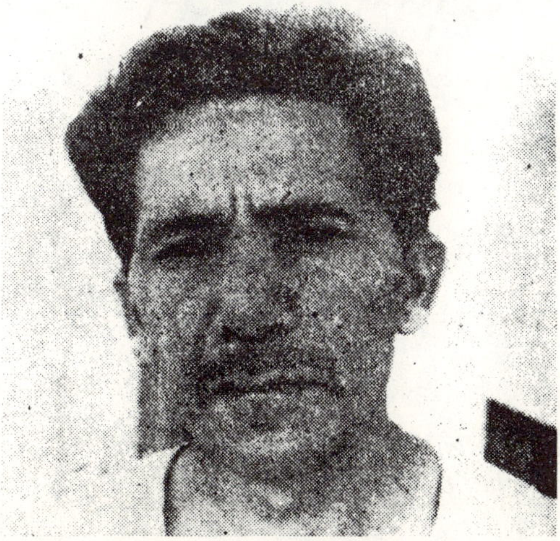

Case - Photo 9 - Show the increase of the nose and the infiltration of the upper lip.

After the entry to the Service in Hospital, we did a new biopsy, studied in the Section of pathologic-anatomy, as follows: notable increase of the epithelial layer in long papillas. Granular tissue with infiltrations of round cells. The aspect it seems to be of leishmaniasis, but without a complete security. It is good apposition smears.

Red cells	4.890.000 mm^3
Hemoglobin	85%
Feces	Necator, trichocephalus and oxyuris
Smears for apposition	ulcers in both legs several times

With the clinical diagnosis and the last report, we submit the patient to treatment with tartar emetic, 20 injections of 0.10, arriving to total dose of 2 grams.

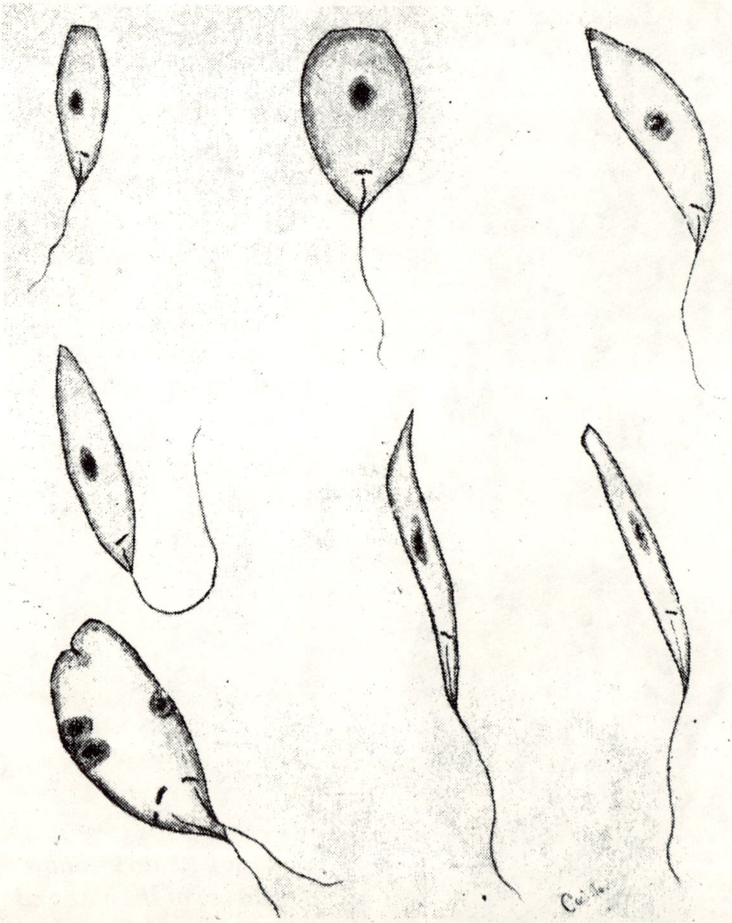

Case Nº 9 - Drawing of the flagellate forms of the cultures. Coloring Giemsa slow. Showing chubby forms, slenders and a division form.

We saw a clear improvement, disappeared the bad smell and the patient left the Hospital.

Case Nº 2 - P.E., 23 years old, born in El Callao (State Bolívar), mechanical.

Two years ago began the affection, with blood secretion and obstruction.

Rhinoscopy: ulcer former part of the septum, some crusts.

R. Kahn	negative
Biopsy	slight acanthosis few gigantic cells
Smears for apposition	leishmanias positive

Submitted to treatment with tartar emetic, rapidly improved and left the hospital owed to his work.

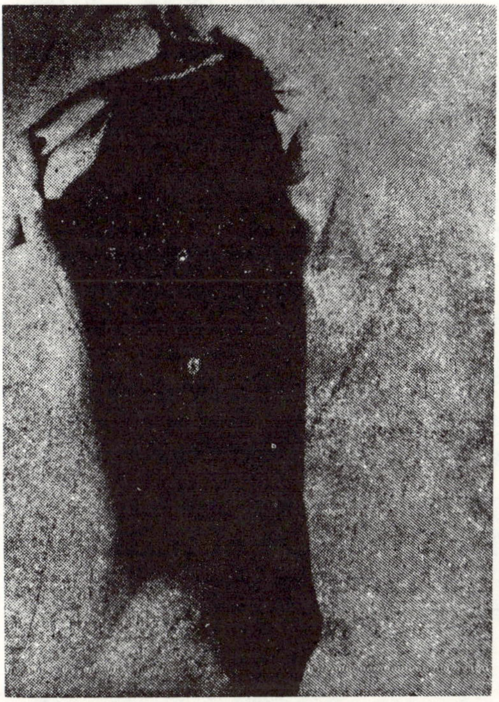

Case Nº 9 - Test of the leishmanina clearly positive.

Case Nº 3 - P.V., 30 years old, born in Maracaibo (State Zulia, agriculturist).

Comes to the Service, because since 4 years stoppage of the nose.

Rhinoscopy: exulceration in both sides of the nose, bloody secretion. Good appearance of the nasal pyramid.

R W. and K.	negatives
Biopsy	was impossible a diagnosis
Smears for apposition	leishmanias positive

Treatment: tartar emetic and nasal pomade. For his work left the town.

Case Nº 4 - R.S., 19 years old, born in El Guayabo (State Yaracuy), agriculturist, comes to the Service on 12-3-43, staying still 14-4-43. Mother alive and has had 14 sons, two miscarriages. Father alive and healthy. Not

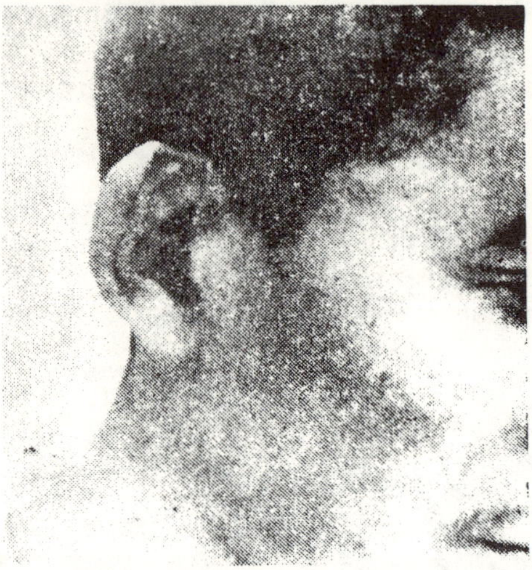

Case N° 10 - Patient, 38 years old, from Albarico (State Yaracuy).

antecedent tuberculosis, cancer, leprosy and mental troubles. Yaws at ten years old. R. Kahn + + + .

The patient says that four years before, during one year, had an exulceration in the chest, resting a white and corrugated scar.

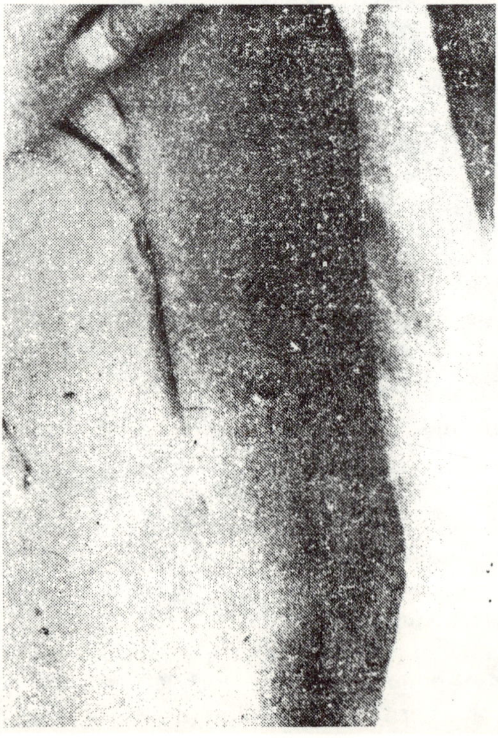

Case N° 10 - The Montenegro' test clearly positive.

One year later cured the ulcer, started bloody secretion from the nostrils. Some time after, increase of the nasal pyramid and obstruction of both sides of the nose.

Rhinoscopy: exulceration on the septum in both sides, easily bleeding.

Biopsy: granular tissue with infiltrations lymphoid and any giant cells type Langhans. Not epitheliums - Probably leishmaniasis.

Smears for apposition leishmanias positive.

Intradermis test to leishmanina: 24 hours clearly positive, 72 hours vesicant aspect. Treatment with tartar emetic. From 12-3-43 to 2-4-43 received 1.25 grams; beginning 0.02, 0.03, 0.04, 0.05, 0.06, 0.07, 0.08, repeating this last dose. It was intolerance. Notable improvement of the lesions.

Case Nº 5 - M.O., 38 years old, born in Pedrazas (State Barinas), agriculturist.

Two years ago began to feel nasal stoppage. Nasal voice.

Rhinoscopy: exulceration of nasal septum in both sides, chiefly in the right.

Biopsy: epithelium increased in long files. Under, a granular tissue with large infiltrations, few giant cells, with different aspect. The diagnosis is possible of leishmaniasis, but it is recommended to send smears for apposition. Smears for apposition: leishmania positive. It was not possible to find the place of the initial lesion.

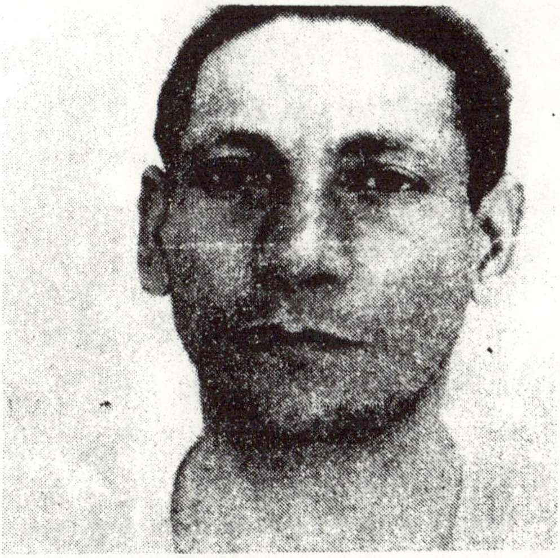

Photo - Case Nº 11 - Patient 39 years old, born in Aroa (State Yaracuy).

He was submitted to antomonial treatment.

Case Nº 6 - R.A., 47 years old, born in Barinas (State Barinas); always rural life.

He has 12 years with troubles in the nose. Rhinoscopy: lesions in both sides of the nasal septum without destruction, crusty. Not defacing of the nasal pyramid.

Biopsy: granular tissue inflammated. The histo-pathological aspect and suspicions of leishmaniasis.

Test Briceño Rossi (blood) negative.

Smears for apposition: leishmanias positive

Scars in right arm and leg, probably sites of the initial lesion.

Tartar emetic treatment.

Case Nº 8 - M.C.V., 15 years old, born in El Limoncito, near Barinitas, State Barinas.

Remember that when he was a child he had an ulcer in the malleolar region in the right foot; after, troubles with the nose.

Rhinoscopy: total destruction of the nasal septum (cartilage). Bony part complete. Perforation, an edge around, crusty, bleeding. Only rest a bridge of skin between the nasal lobe and the upper lip.

Biopsy: miscarried

Smears for apposition: scarce leishmanias

Antimonial treatment

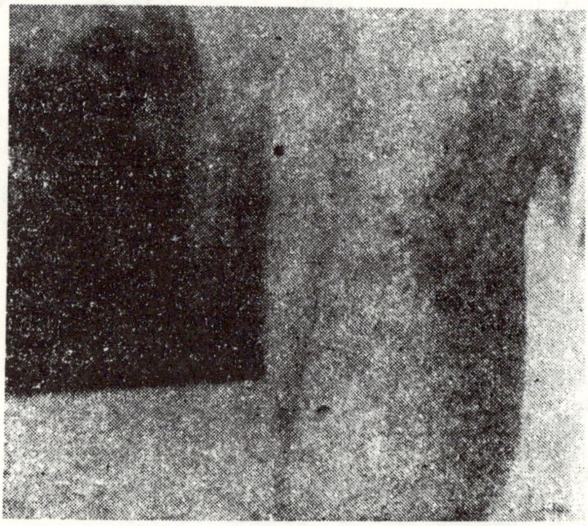

Photo - Case Nº 11 - Lesion situated in the high part of the left leg, where we found leishmanias, going with the nasal lesions.

Case Nº 9 - P.C.M., 35 years old, born in Barcelona (State Anzoátegui), agriculturist; entry to the Service (10-4-43).

Father and mother dead. Eight brothers dead from malaria. Ethylic antecedent in the father. Deny syphilis and yaws. Serology negative.

One year and a half began exulceration in the nose, right side, slight pain. Epistaxis. Bloody secretion. Obstruction in both nostrils. Increase of the nose. Entry to the Service

Case Nº 12 - Rhinoscopy: total destruction of the nasal septum (cartilage). Bony part complete. Nasal lobe down fell with aspect of beak of parrot: Slender bridge of skin between the lobe and the upper lip. Nasal pyramid, upper lip and right cheek redness of the skin. Pharynx infiltrated in the rear part and soft palate.

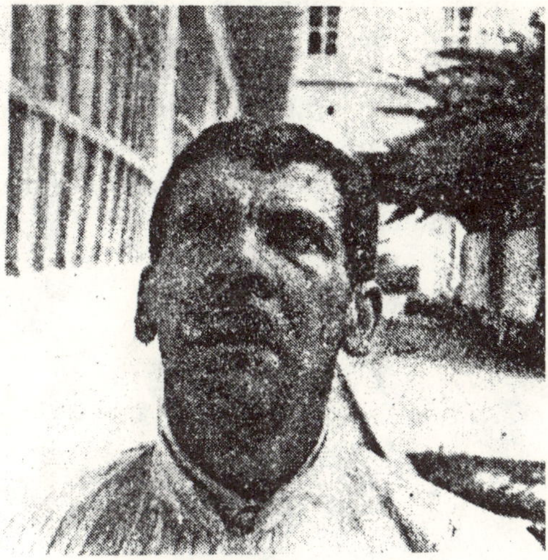

Photo - patient Case N° 12.

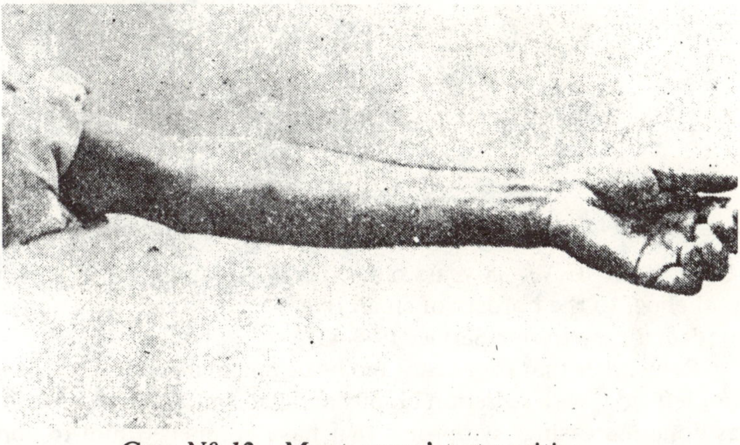

Case N° 12 - Montenegro' test positive.

We took two biopsies.

1° biopsy - (taken from the soft palate) - Chronic infiltration with some giant cells (leishmaniasis?).

2° biopsy - (taken from the uvula) - Shallow epithelium increased and prolonged deeply in files; under, granular tissue with round cells, plasma-cells and some leucocytes polinuclears - Few giant cells - The histo-pathological aspect, suspicious leishmaniasis.

Smears for apposition: leishmanias positive.

Intradermis tests to leishmanina in the left arm (16-4-43) were made two tests with different antigens, prepared in the years 40 and 43. On 19-4-43 the result is clearly positive in both, mainly with the antigen 40, giving vesicle type.

Initial lesion. Living in Cuidad Bolívar had an ulceration in the right leg, ten years ago. It is easy to see a large scar in that place.

Cultures (20-4-43). Were used ten tubes , medium NNN with ph. 7.2, with material taken from the upper lip, for puncture, containing the syringe citrate solution to 3.8 %. Result: one tube infected and the others, two presented flagellate forms.

Treatment with tartar emetic beginning for 0.02, 0.04, 0.06 and 0.08, repeating this dose daily, arriving to the amount of 0.35, and was possible a clear improvement. The patient continued receiving injections with some reposes, till the total dose of 1.48 grams.

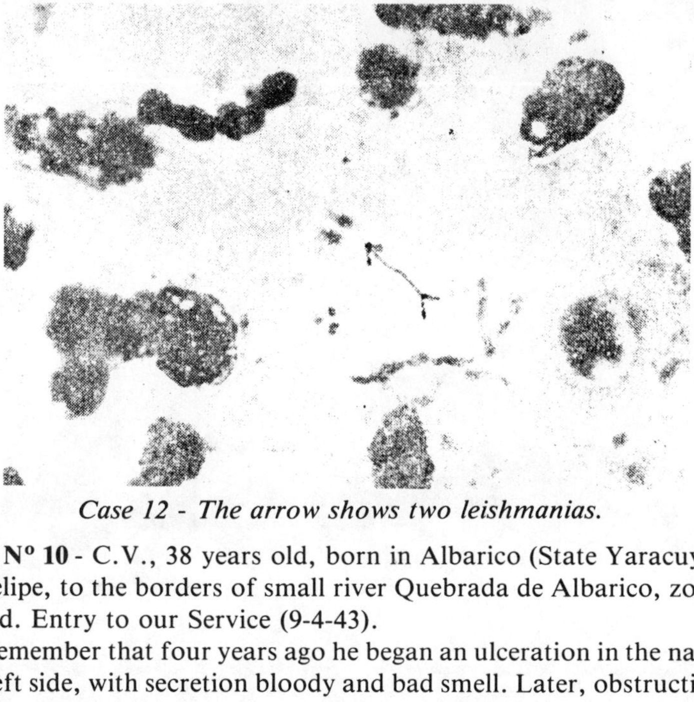

Case 12 - The arrow shows two leishmanias.

Case Nº 10 - C.V., 38 years old, born in Albarico (State Yaracuy), near San Felipe, to the borders of small river Quebrada de Albarico, zone very wooded. Entry to our Service (9-4-43).

Remember that four years ago he began an ulceration in the nasal septum, left side, with secretion bloody and bad smell. Later, obstruction that has gone increasing, symptoms that have compelled him to come to the hospital.

Rhinoscopy: ulceration of the former part of the nasal septum in both sides, chiefly, the left side, presenting a bleeding polyp.

Biopsy: granular tissue with infiltrations denses, but without giant cells; small focus of necrosis. The aspect is not typical of leishmaniasis. It was not possible to find leishmaniod parasites.

Smears for apposition: leishmanias positive.

Intradermis test to the leishmanina done 9-4-43 in the left arm, to 24 hours, clearly positive and 72 hours later, presence of vesicles.

Examination of the eyes: obstruction of the lachrymal channel and recommending to wait for the result of the treatment of the nasal lesions.

Five years ago, ulceration in the upper part of the pavillion right ear. Today, disappearence of part of the pavilion with retractile scar.

Treatment with tartar emetic, receiving a total dose of 2.24 grams.

Case Nº 11 - E.P., 39 years old, born in Arca (State Yaracuy),

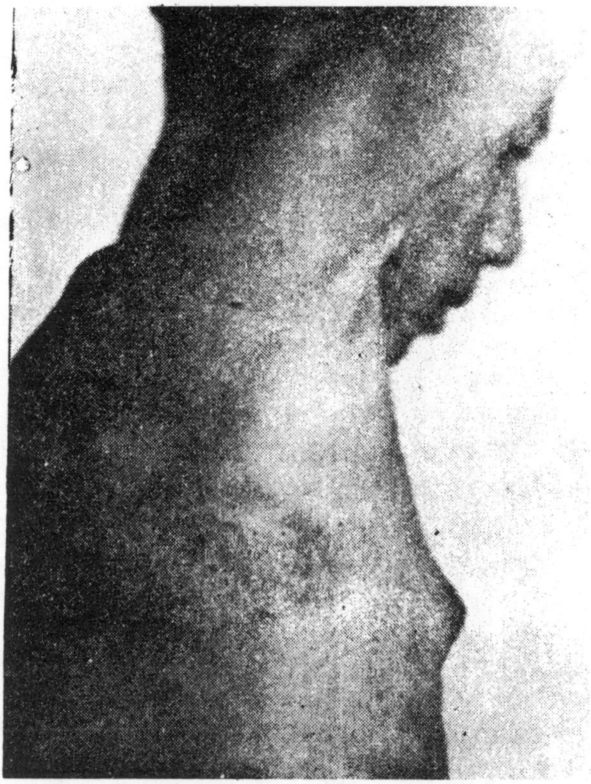

Case Nº 13 - The scar of the possible initial lesion.

mechanic, working in the last years in farmers in Dto. Bolívar (State Yaracuy).

Father and mother dead; nineteen brothers. Ethylic antecedent - Deny syphilis and yaws. Remember an ulcer in left leg, two years ago, that cured after one year and a half of evolution.

Corresponding this lesion, began nasal troubles; obstruction, epistaxis and increase of the nasal pyramid.

This interesting case scraping the scar of the leg, appearance of an ulcer. Some time after, similar lesions appeared in different places of the body. In 1942, R. Kahn + + and lastly new test equally positivity + +. For these results received a treatment with bismuth, without any improvement.

Rhinoscopy: left exulceration nasal septum, infiltration of the nasal pyramid, mainly left side.

Nasal Biopsy: leishmaniasis, with parasites seen in the sections.

Lesion of leg - Biopsy: layer epithelium increased. Among the papillas round cells.

Intradermis test with leishmanina left arm: clearly positive, with node to 72 hours. Another test made in right arm gave a clear positivity.

Treatment with tartar emetic, arriving the quantity of 0.32, with exacerbations of cutaneous lesions. Stop of the injections, started in any day. It was improvement of the nose and also of the cutaneous lesions.

Smears for apposition with nasal material; abundant leishmanias. Thinking the ulceration of the leg should have leishmaniod nature, we did smears for apposition, finding numerous parasites, sometimes, more than 50 elements in a group.

Case N° 12 - X.X., 57 years old, agriculturist, born in Aricagua (State Mérida).

Troubles in the nose last 15 years. Strong obstruction. Rhinoscopy: enlargement of the nasal pyramid; destruction of the nasal cartilage.

Smears for apposition: leishmanias positive.

Test of Montenegro: positive; lecture done 72 hours after.

The site of the initial lesion was not possible to find it.

Treatment: with tartar emetic, receiving the patient since 15-12-41 to 10-1-42 a global dose of 1.15 grams, obtaining a great improvement, referring to the cure of the lesions and the nasal stoppage.

Case N° 13 - M.S., 16 years old, born in San Felipe (State Yaracuy), student. Working in agriculture in the free hours. Parents in complete health. Two brothers dead and two others alive and healthy. Deny syphilis and yaws. R. Kahn + +.

Some time ago he had an ulceration in the trunk, lesion with a size of money piece of five bolívares.

Queloid aspect, starry and dark. After he was cured of this long resistance ulceration, began to feel troubles in the nose, crusts, and stoppage, that compelled him to go to Caracas looking for treatment.

Rhinoscopy: destruction of the cartilage, with a salient edge around the perforation; only rest a cutaneous bridge of the lobe with the upper lip; the nasal pyramid of well appearence.

Biopsy taken of the salient edge of the hole, gave the following report: piece of cartilage. Granular tissue. Ronde cells. Nothing characteristic of leishmaniasis.

Smears for apposition: presence leishmanias.

Test of leishmanina clearly positive, producing necrosis of the skin.

The treatment with tartar emetic has been very well accepted for this patient , arriving at the total dose of 2.00 grams. The nasal lesions are almost cured and the permeability almost normal.

CONCLUSION

1.- A contribution to the study of leishmaniasis cutánea in Venezuela is presented, considering it above all from the otorhinolaryngologic point of view.

2.- A short historical account is given and observations are made about its parasitology and its clinic.

3.- Cultures of one of the cases are presented, obtained in medium NNN and Noguchi.

4.- A brief outline of the histopathology of this disease is given, mentioning the most frequent discoveries.
5.- Treats of transmission by phlebotomus and species (Ph. evansi Nuñez Tovar 1921, Ph. migonei Franca 1920, Ph. panamensis Shannon 1926, Ph. suis Rozeboom 1940, found by the author are reported.
6.- The histories of thirteen observed cases with nasobuccopharyngeal manifestations are given.
7.- The ages of patients ranged from 15 a 57 years. In several of the cases it was possible to determine the place where the initial cutaneous lesion existed. Place of birth according to States were as follows: Anzoátegui 1, Barinas 4, Bolivar 1, Mérida 1, Miranda 1, Yaracuy 4, and Zulia 1.
8.- The characteristic otorhinolaryngologic lesions are exulceration at the septum, destruction of the latter except the bony part, falling of the point, thus, giving the nose the shape of a parrot's beak; ulcerous lesions destructive and mamelonated at the pharynx. The symptom which troubles the patient most is nasal obstruction. The clinical diagnosis is easy to one familiarized with above mentioned lesions.
9.- In all our cases, with the exception of one, the parasitologic diagnosis was made by frotis by apposition and a little patience. Biopsy is very useful but there are no typical anatomico-pathological details and the discovery of the parasites in cuttings is rare.
10.- The intradermic test to the leishmanina or the reaction of Montenegro seems to us very useful for conforming the diagnosis in cases in which it has not been possible to discover the parasites.
11.- The only treatment we have used is the tartar-emetic, obtaining improvement of the lesions but not a total cicatrization, perhaps with 3 or 4 series of emetic at intervals, this may be got. There are patients who have borne 2 grams in doses of 0.10 daily with perfect tolerance, but in general the above dose is too strong for us and should not exceed 0.08. During the treatment, besides the usual nausea and muscular pains, we have observed diarrhea and in one of the cases a generalized rash, accompanied with itching which compelled us to suspend the treatment temporalily.

CHAPTER VII

BIBLIOGRAPHY

1914-*Laveran A.*-Presentation d' un chien inoculé avec succés au moyen de la Leishmania tropica sur souris.-Bull. de la Soc. Path. Exot. Tomo VII. N° 10.

1915-*Dutra e Silva Oscar*-Sobre a Leishmaniose tegumentar seu tratamento. Mem. Ins. Osw. Cruz. Tomo VII. Fasc. II.

1917-*Iturbe Juan i Eudoro González*-First case of Leishmaniosis cutanea in Venezuela. Separata (trabajo presentado al 2° Congreso Venezolano de Medicina) Caracas.

1919-*Tejera Enrique*-La Leishmaniosis americana en Venezuela. Caracas.

1920-*Franca C. i Parrot L.*-Introduction a 1' étude systematique des Dipteres du genre Phlebotomus. Bull. Soc. Path. Exot.

1924-*Núñez Tovar Manuel*-Mosquitos i Flebotomos de Venezuela (trabajo al 4° Congreso Venezolano de Medicina). Caracas.

1926-*Adler S. i Theodor O.*-Further observations on the transmission of cutaneous leishmaniasis to man from Phlebotomus papatasii. Annals of Trop. Medicine and Parasitology. Vol. XX. N° 2.

1926-*Wenyon C.M.*-Protozoology. Vol. 1.

1927-*Beurepaire Aragao Enrique de*-Leishmaniose tegumentar e sua transmissao pelo phlebotomos. Mem. do Ins. Osw. Cruz. Tomo XX. Fasc II.

1929-*Iriarte David R.*-Algunas observaciones sobre enfermedades parasitarias en Venezuela. Taller Gráfico Imp. Caracas.

1929-*Escomel Edmundo.*-La leishmaniose américaine et les leishmanioses en Amerique. Bull. de la Soc. Path. Exot. Tomo XII. N° 1.

1932-*Da Costa Lima A.*-Sobre os phlebotomos americanos (Diptera: Psychodidae) Mem. do Ins. Osw. Cruz. Tomo XXVI. Fasc. I.

1935-*Briceño Iragorry L.*-Un caso de leishmaniosis americana. Rev. de la Policlínica Caracas. N° 20.

1936-*Weinman David*-Factors affecting the morphology of Leishmania tropica. The production of leishmania forms in cultures. Parasitology. Vol. XXXI. N° 2.

1938-*Southwell T. i Kirshner A.*-On the transmission of leishmaniasis. Ann. of Trop. Med. and Paras. Vol. 32. N° 1.

1939-*Adler S. i Theodor O.*-The behaviour of Leishmania chagasi in Phlebotomus papatasii. Ann. of Trop. Med. and Paras. Vol. 33. N° 1.

1940-*Pifano Félix*-Sobre el desarrollo de Leishmania tropica brasiliensis en flebotomos de Venezuela. Gaceta Médica de Caracas. N° 2.

1940-*Sánchez Covisa José i Guerra Pablo*-Las leishmaniosis tegumentarias en Venezuela. Rev. de la Policlínica Caracas. N° 54.

1940-*Pifano Félix*-La leishmaniosis tegumentaria en el Estado Yaracuy. Rev. de la Policlínica Caracas. N° 55.

1940-*Pestana Bruno R., Pessoa S.B. i Correa Aniceto*-Notas sóbre a leishmaniose no municipio de Marinia. Arquivos de Higiene e Saúde Pública. Año V. N° 8.

1940-*Villela Francisco*-Dados estatisticos sóbre a leishmanioses das mucosas em Aracatuba. Arquivos de Higiene e Saúde Pùblica. Año V. N° 8.

1940-*Pestana Bruno R. i Pessoa S.B.*-Leishmaniose tegumentar autóctone no municipio de S. Paulo. Arquivos de Higiene e Sáude Pública. Año V. N° 8.

1940-*Pessoa S.B. i Rangel Pestana B.*-Sóbre a disseminacao da leishmaniose tegumentar no Estado de S. Paulo. Arquivos de Higiene e Saúde Pública. Año V. N° 8.

1940-*Pessoa S.B. i Pestana Bruno R.*-Leishmaniose tegumentar urbana. Arquivos de Higiene e Saúde Pública. Año V. N° 8.

1940-*Pessoa S.B. i Pestana Bruno Rangel*-Lesoes iniciaes na leishmaniose tegumentar americana. Arquivos de Higiene e Saúde Pública. Año V. N° 9.

1940-*Villela F., Pestana Bruno R. i Pessoa S.B.*-Presenca da "Leishmania brasiliensis" na mucosa sem lesao aparente, em casos recentes de leishmaniose cutanea. Arquivos de Higiene e Saúde Pública. Año V. N° 9.

1940-*Francia Martins A.*-Do diagnóstico serológico das leishmaniose. Arquivos de Higiene e Saúde Pública. Año V. N° 9.

1940-*Ayrosa Galvao A.L. i Coutinho J.O.*-Contribuicao ao estudo dos flebótomos do Est. de S. Paulo. Arquivos de Higiene e Saúde Pública. Año V. N° 9.

1940-*Coutinho J.O.*-Observacoes sóbre algunas espécies de flebótomos com a descricao do macho de Phlebotomus lloydi antunes. 1937. Arquivos de Higiene e Saúde Pública. Año V. N° 9.

1940-*Pessoa S.B. i Pestana Bruno Rangel*-Infeccao do Phlebotomus migonei por formas de leptomonas provavelmente da Leishmania brasiliensis. Arquivos de Higiene e Saúde Pública. Año V. N° 9.

1941-*Mayer Martin i Pifano Félix*-Sobre el cultivo de Leishmania tropica en Venezuela e intra-reacciones con leishmania-antígeno. Rev. de Sanidad i Asist. Social. N° 3.

1941-*Pessoa S.B.*-Dados sobre a epidemiología de leishmaniose tegumentar em Sao Paulo. Arquivos de Higiene e Saúde Pública. Año V. N° 11.

1941-*Franco do Amaral, Antonio Dacio.*-Contribuicao para o estudo da inoculacao experimental da leishmania brasiliensis. Ann. da Facultad. de Med. da Univ. de S. Paulo. Vol.XVII. Tomo I.

1942-*Iriarte David R.*-Leishmaniosis. Bol. del Lab. de la Clínica Razetti, N° 8.

1942-*Briceño Rossi A.L.*-Distribución geográfica de la Leishmaniosis tegumentaria i algunos datos para el plan de estudios del Kala-azar en Venezuela. Tip. Garrido. Caracas.

1943-*Senekji Harry A.*-Hematologic and inmunologic studies on natural and induced leishmaniasis in paretics. Amer. Jour. of Trop. Med. Vol.XXIII. N° 1.

THE FLAGELLIASE OF THE PLANTS IN VENEZUELA*

The discoveries of Lafont (1) referring to the finding of a flagellate in the euphorbiae, had a great importance, because for the first time it was possible to see protozoons living in the latex of the plants.

The fact of why the leishmaniasis cutaneous is observed commonly among the people living or working in the forest, came to the attention to several investigators that any lactiferous plants, the same as any insects living on it, could be deposits of leishmaniod parasites.

Just, Strong (2) says to have found a leptomonad, morphological equally in the latex of an euphorbia, in the intestinal containt of an insect (Chariesterus cuspidatus) and the intestinal containt of a small lizard (Cnemidophorus lemniscatus) hosts of it.

Inoculations subcutaneous and intraperitoneum to monkeys, dogs, guinea pigs, mice, gave a negative result. Exception of the inoculation to a monkey in the abdominal region, giving a papule and exulceration sixteen days after. Smears and cuttings of this lesion revealed to Strong the presence of leishmanias.

As in the inoculations with the latex and intestinal containt of the insect were null, somebody thought that the flagellates had been capable to attack the skin of the monkey for having had a modification in the intestine of the lizard.

Franchini (3) infected mice with phytotripanosomas verified it for examination in fresh of the blood and cultures of it. Besides, this same author has obtained hepatic abscess in mice for inoculations of phytoamoebas.

All these studies show the importance of the protozoons of the plants; However, the last works of Noguchi (4) destroyed completely the relation among the flagellate of the plants and the leishmaniosis.

Noguchi worked with immune serums anti-brasiliensis, anti-tropica, anti-infantum and anti-donovani referring the action on the leptomonads. Observed that form and motility continued equals; it was only possible to see a light agglomeration that is produced also for the normal serum of rabbit and finish: "the flagellates of the latex of Asclepias curassavica, Asclepias syriaca and intestine of the Oncopeltus are immunologicaly different of the four strains of human leishmanias."

Another important question is the future problem with the

* These doctoral. 1928.

(1) C. R. Soc. Biol. 1909 and Ann. Ins. Past. 1910.

(2) Am. Journal Trop. Med. 1924.

(3) Bull. Soc. Path. Exot. 1923 and Ann. Inst. Past. 1922.

(4) Proc, Internat. Conf. on Health Prob. in Trop. Med. 1924.

agriculture, because the spreading of the phyto-proptozoons are increasing. It is not the presence of a leptomanad in the little euphorbiae, but of its presence in several families of plants. So, the Professor Petri of the School of Florence, found in a disease of the vineyard protozoons like trypanosomidos. Ray Nelson (5) speaks of protozoons, flagellates or not, in the mosaic of the tomato, string beans and trefoil. Frank P.M. Worther (6) discovered a protozoon, like an amoeba in a disease (agalla de Fiji) of the sugar cane.*

FIRST PART

CHAPTER I

FLAGELLIASE OF THE PLANTS (7)

Some years ago (1909) David and Lafont in the island of Mauricio, discovered in the latex of some euphorbiae (Euphorbia pilulifera, Euphorbia hypericifolia, Euphorbia thymifolia) a flagellate with characteristic of leptomonad, giving it the name of Leptomonas davidi (Lafont).

In this one, his first work, Lafont thought in a disease of the plants and described the parasite.

After, appeared the works of Donovan (8) in Madrás, and Carougeau and Le Fers (9) in Madagascar. Immediately it is possible to see a spreading in all of the tropical zone, according to the research of Rhodain and Bequaert (10) in the Congo Belga; Bouet and Roubaud (11) in Dahoney; Leger (12) in Senegal; Noc and Stevenel (13) in Martinique, and Leboeuf and Tavelly (14) in Nueva Caledonia.

It is in 1911 when Franca (15) discovered for the first time the infection in Portugal, out the tropic, in the Euphorbia peplus and E. segetalis.

Findings similar to Monti and Vicentini (16) and Laveran and Franchini (17), in Italy, Sicily and Sardinia. In 1921, Galli-Valario found infected the Euphorbia gerardiana to a height of 1.300 m. in the Canton Valais in Switzerland. In the same year Sergent (18) appointed the

(5) Technical Bulletin, 1922.
(6) The Phillippine Agriculturist, 1922.
(x) Our deep acknowledgement to wise Professor H. Pittier, for the classification of the plants and sending the insects to the United States.
(7) Name given by Galli-Valerio.
(8) The Lancet, 1909.
(9) Bull. Soc. Pathol. Exot. 1911.
(10) Bull. Soc. Path. Exot. 1911.
(11) C. R. Soc. Path. Exot. 1911.
(12) Bull. Soc. Path. Exot. 1911.
(13) Bull. Soc. Path. Exot. 1911.
(14) F. Mesnil. Ann. Soc. Sc. Nat. 1921.
(15) Bull. Soc. Path. Exot. 1911.
(16) Academia del Lincei. 1924.
(17) Mesnil Ann. Soc. Nat. 1921.
(18) Schw. Med. Woche. 1921.

flagelliase in Algerie; in 1923, Aubertot (20) found infected the Euphorbia cyparissias in Alsace.

The flagelliase had been found only in Euphorbia, but Migone, 1917, (21) said to find a phytomonas in an Asclepiadacea (Arauja Angustifolia) (Funastrum bonneariensis) in Paraguay and callet it Leptomonas elmasiani.
boneariensis) in Paraguay and called it Leptomonas elmasiani.

Franca (22) found a leptomonas in a new asclepiadacea. Called the flagellate Leptomonas bordasi and the plant Morreira odorata. Holmes (23) appointed infected the Asclepia syriaca in Central America. Noguchi, 1924, speaks about the infection in Asclepia curassavica and Euphorbia brasiliensis in Honduras. Fantham (24), in 1926, signalized in the Africa of Sud infected an urticacea (Ficus edulis) and gave to the parasite the name of Herpetomonas ficuum.

Lastly, the Italian Franchini (25) has published several works, appointing infection for leptomonads and other protozoons (amoebas, spirochetes, crithidias, trypanosomas) in different families; euphorbiacea (E. calyculata, E. nereifolia, E. virosa); asclepiadacea (Chlorocodon whitei and Cryptostegia grandiflora); apocinacea (Cerbera odollam, Caudrania javanensis); urticacea (Ficus tholloni, Ficus carica); artocarpea (Antiaris toxicaria, Lakoocha artocarpus); sapotacea (Sideraxylon inerme, Chrysophyllium glabrum).

CHAPTER II

GENERAL CHARACTERISTICS OF THE PHYTOMONAS

To avoid confusions among leptomonads, herpetomonas and phytomonas, look at the following picture.

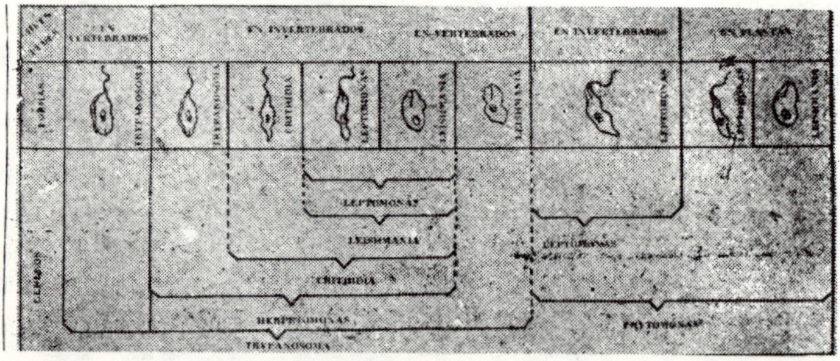

Taken from Wenyon, Prozoology, Tome I, to which Dr. Arnoldo Gabaldón, aggregated the genus phytomonas.

(19) Arch. Ins. Past. Afrique du Nord. 1921.
(20) C. R. Soc. Path. Exot. 1916.
(21) Bull. Soc. Path. Exot. 1916.
(22) Ann. Soc. Belge Med. Trop. 1921.
(23) Biology and Anatomy. 1924.
(24) Trans. of the Roy. Soc. Trop. Med. 1926.
(25) Bull. Soc. Path. Exot. 1919-1923.
(26) Name adopted by Galli-Valerio.

The Phytomonas davidi has all the characteristics of a leptomonad. The lenght of the body between 16 and 20 microns and the width 1 to 2 microns; the length of the flagellum 10 to 16 microns. Often it is possible to see a light twist of the rear portion of the body around the longitudinal axis, arriving to 2 or 3 spiral turns.

It seems to be the influence of the medium, because researches of Shortt, 1923, inoculating the Leptomonad ctenocephali of the flea of the dog in small fissures practiced in the stems of euphorbiae, it can live for about six days showing longer a certain twist similar to phytomonas.

The nucleus is situated between the anterior third part and the middle third part of the body; the blepharoplaste before the nucleus and gives birth to the flagellum. The multiplication is made by longitudinal division. Also are seen flagellate and leishmaniod forms.

The motility of the parasite changes with the climate it seems. In the moderate zones the parasites are of rapid movement, and in the hot zones are slow moving, probably owed to a higher concentration of the latex.

The authors are not in accord with the pathogenicity of the leptomonads. Lafont spook of a true disease of the plant: "la plante parasitée est de mauvaise venue." Franca thought the same.

The histo-pathological studies of this last one, it seems demonstrate that it is a disease of nutrition, because in cutting the healthy leaves full of abundant latex, including particles of starch; while in the sick plants, in cutting of an ill leaf, the lactiferous tubes are empty, full of embolies of phytomonas, having then the plant a poor nourishing, succumbing.

Franca arrives to find flagellates in the cover of the fruit and in the proper fruit believed to find elements suspicious in relation with flagellates capable to infect the seeds, doing possible the hereditary transmission.

The majority of the researchers that deny the disease in the plants, have worked in the tropic, and perhaps will have a stronger resistance; maybe, as said Gaschen (28), the climate conditions have any action increasing the resistance of the plants.

We can not give opinions, because the exemplairs of E. pilulifera infected showed to be in not good appearence, in change, the specimens of E. hypericifolia had complete health.

CHAPTER III

NATURAL TRANSMISSION OF THE INFECTION

Lafont was the first to suspect the spreading of the infection through insects and accused the *Nysius euphorbiae* Herv.; Bouet and Roubaud appointed the *Dieuches humilis.* Franca in Portugal accused two insects of

(28) Contri. a l étude la Flag. des Euphorb. en Suisse. Thesis. 1926.

nocturnal life as transmissors, the *Stenocephalus agilis* Scop. and *Brachipelta aterrima* Forst, and described the evolutive cycle of the parasite. Noc and Stevenel in Martinique said about an hemipterous *Pamera bilobata* Say. Carougeau and Le Fers in Madagascar accused the same insect of Lafont. Galli-Valerio in Suisse appointed the *Steno cephalus agilis.* Strong, in Central America the *Chariesterus cuspidatus.* Franchini (30) a muscid *Anthomyia maculata.* Holmes in Baltimore, the *Oncopeltus fasciatus* Dall., and ending, Noguchi in Honduras *Oncopeltus cingulifer* classified for Barber.

CHAPTER IV

EXPERIMENTAL TRANSMISSION

Noc and Stevensel were the first (31) transmitting infection from plant to plant, utilizing pipette Pasteur. Franca utilized capillary tubes introduced inside the stems. The other investigators have not obtained success, showing the importance of the insects. Franchini has verified infection of the plants with Herpetomonas muscae domesticae and Herpetomonas Ctenocephali.

CHAPTER V

CULTURES

The cultures of the leptomonads of plants has been very difficult. Noguchi has done assays in medium leptospira with a ph similar to ph of latex, in milk of coconut fresh and hot, whose ph is similar to the acidity of latex and in medium NNN., always with negative results. Only, he obtained to maintain alive during twelve days the leptomonads in the medium leptospira, but without reproduction. (33).

Franchini has done many tests in order to obtain cultures of phyto-amoebas and phyto-trypanosomas in medium Noller. The cultures were of a protozoon flagellate in the latex and flagellate in the cultures, from *Euphorbia cereiformis* in medium of latex + simple broth in equal parts; in simple broth + blood and gelose + human broth.

Migone cultivated the Leptomonas elmassiani in gelose + human blood.

Franca said: "the culture of leptomonads of euphorbia is very difficult and we believe the cause is the impossibility to obtain latex pure."

(29) Arch. Für Bratisterkunde. 1941.
(30) Bull. Soc. Path. Exot. 1922.
(31) Bull. Soc. Path. Exot. 1922.
(32) Bull. Soc. Path. Exot. 1922.
(33) In accord with verbal communication of Dr. Iturbe, it seems to be, Noguchi in his last cultures could cultivate, inconstantly, the Leptomonas davidi.

Gaschen told: "the adaptation of the flagellate to a so special medium as the latex is the reason for which the culture in any medium is very difficult."

SECOND PART

CHAPTER I

FLAGELLIASE IN VENEZUELA

The study of the flagelliase of the plants in Venezuela began with the research of Dr. Juan Iturbe (34), who found infected the Euphorbia hypericifolia; after, the investigations of Dr. E. Tejera found the infection of the E. pilulífera (35), the E. tymifolia and E. segetalis and our researchs consigned in a communication to the Academy of Medicine (36 - Algo sobre la flagelosis de las euforbráceas (Gaceta Médica de Caracas - 5 de mayo 1927).

Up till today, the plants that we have found infected, are: E. hypericifolia and E. pilulífera. Many specimens so in plants of the same family, as belonging to another, have been always negative.

We have made excursions to Los Chorros, La Vega, El Paraíso, Los Teques, Maiquetía, finding two zones of infection: Los Chorros and El Paraíso.

Our center of research has been the gardens of the Hospital Vargas, where the presentation in this work has been made.

In Los Teques we have found a scarce number of plant lactiferous; it seems to be, more abundant in the hot places.

200 specimens of E. pilulífera, 150 of E. hypericifolia and 80 of E. thymifolia have been examined. This last one has not been found infected and possible for its small size and skimming the ground will not host of insects, but in it we could capture ants (hymenopterous) that will be classified.

The E. pilulífera infected has a sick appearence (the leaves are few, hard and yellowish, the latex is scarce); however, E. pilulífera is an annual plant and thc disease is present to the end of its life, when the plant is faded, not with the E. hypericifolia infected it always has a good aspect and complete health.

In many of these euphorbias, sick or healthy, we have seen little stains, dark, in stems or leaves and that Franca called "prime lesion", because it should be the site of the sting.

Very curious, in these sick plants the infection was very abundant in a

(34) Presencia del Leptomonas davidi Lafont en la savia de la Euphorbia hypericifolia. Ext. de "Actualidades" N° 17 de 38 abril de 1918. El Dr. Iturbe encontró, además, infectada la Jatropha manihot.

(35) La leishmaniosis americana en Venezuela. 1919.

(36) Algo sobre la flageliasis de las Euforbiáceas. Gaceta Médica de Caracas. Mayo 1927.

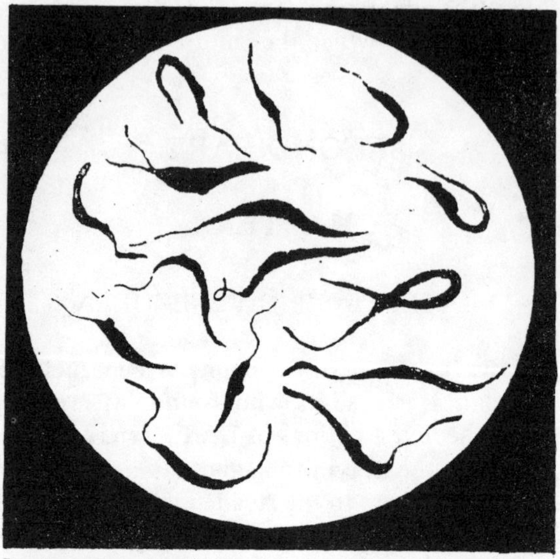

Leptomonads of the Euphorbia pilulífera; seeing a form of division. Coloration panoptic Pappenheim. Oc. 3. Ob. imm. 1-12 Leitz.

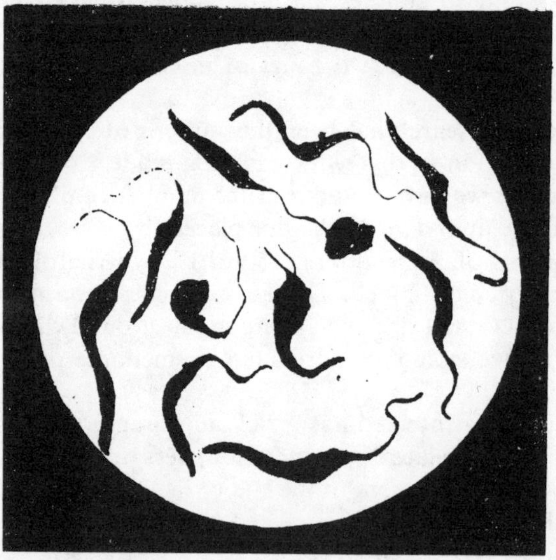

Lepromonads of the E. hypericifolia, showing a division and a leishmanoid form. Coloration panoptic Pappenheim. Oc. 3. Ob. imm. 1-12 Leitz.

branch today, tomorrow it will be null or very rare and the amount of leptomonads has relation with the hour of the test. When it is made in the early morning, the result is negative and when it is made at noon or afternoon it is always positive. May be solar influence?

In any moment the infection verified in several branches of the plant; suddenly has been null and then testing the trunk, it almost always is positive for leptomonads.

We have photos of E. hypericifolia with several branches where in a group of eight, five presented parasites and the others negative. In occasions in a dicotomy, one is positive and the other one negative.

CHAPTER II

MORPHOLOGY OF THE FLAGELLATES OF THE EUPHORBIAS

The examination of the latex is very easy, only to put a little drop between lamina and lamel and to see with an ob. 6. Surprise is the quantity of leptomonads by field. At the beginning they have a rapid movement, being very difficult to see the flagellum; little by little it is slow, permitting to do the test with preciseness; with dark field the motility is appreciated perfectly.

In the E. hypericifolia the late is very heavy and the abundance of granulations with brownian movement, do the examination difficult, having as guide the movement of the crystals impelled by the flagellums.

After the coloration with Leishmann or panoptic Pappenheim, body and flagellum are seen very clearly. The body is lenghtened, wide in the former end and slender in the rear part. Nucleus in the middle body, round or elongated. Blepharoplast toward the anterior end, very clear and perpendicular to the nucleus. The flagellum undulated, sometimes undulated in the base and straight in the rest.

CHAPTER III

NATURAL TRANSMISSION OF THE INFECTION

Many insects (hemipterous, coleopterous, etc.) we have found living on the E. pilulífera and hypericifolia.

In this last one, chiefly, and in the gardens of the Hospital Vargas, we have caught two hemipterous classified in Washington as Corizus sidae Fabr. and Orthaea bilobata Say. The first of these two insects is more abundant and in the 50 % of them we have found a flagellate with all the characteristics of a leptomonad. In the E. pilulífera the presence of these is rare.

The leptomonad of the insect is very similar to the leptomonad of the euphorbias; however, the body is larger and wider. Are very numerous. The flagellum are very easy to see, in fact difficult in the latex. The

MEASURES OF THE LEPTOMONADS OF THE E. PILULIFERA

	Long Cuerpo	Ext-ant a Blefaroplasto	Blefaroplasto a. núcleo	Núcleo	Núcleo a ext. post.	Anchura	Long Flagelo
	20	2	2	2	16	2	10
	20	2	2.2	1.5	16	2	9
	21	2	2	2	14	2	5
	20	2.5	2	2	16	3	10
	22	2	2	2	18	2.5	8
	20	2	2	1.5	15	2	8
	21	1.5	2	2	16	2	5
	19	2	2	2	15	2	5
	20	1.5	2	2	16	2.5	10
	20	2	1.5	2	16	2	5
Promed.	20.3	1.95	1.93	1.90	18	2.2	7.5
Diferen.	19-22	1.5-2.5	1.5-2.2	1.5-2	14-18	2-3	5-10

movements are rapid and sometimes as a snake or shaking as Noguchi said. One hour after, the movement continues equal.

Very good coloration using the panoptic of Pappenheim. The body does not appear so clear as in the euphorbias, but presenting any vacuoles. The nucleus large, round, sometimes in kidney shaped, situated in the middle of the body. Blepharoplast is bacillar, placed in the middle between the nucleus and former end; this end is round and the rear is sharp; for its fragility many are seen without flagellum and deformed.

In last investigation in State Zulia it was not possible to find Corizus sidae Fabr. but catching numerous specimens of Orthaea bilobata Say., without infection.

MEASURES OF THE LEPTOMONADS OF THE E. HYPERICIFOLIA

	Long Cuerpo	Ext-ant a Blefaroplasto	Blefaroplasto a. núcleo	Núcleo	Núcleo a ext. post.	Anchura	Flagelo
	26	2	2	3	21	2	9
	26	2	2	2	20	3	8
	25	2	2	2	20	2.5	5
	20	2	2	2	20	2	10
	25	2.2	2	3	16	3	10
	26	2	2	3	18	3	5
	25	2	2	3	15	3	8
	22	1.5	1.5	2	15	3	5
	25	3	2	3	18	2.5	10
	24	2	2	2	20	3	5
Promed.	24.4	2.07	1.95	2.5	18.3	2.75	7.5
Diferen.	20-26	1.5-3	1.5-2	2-3	15-20	2.5-3	5-10

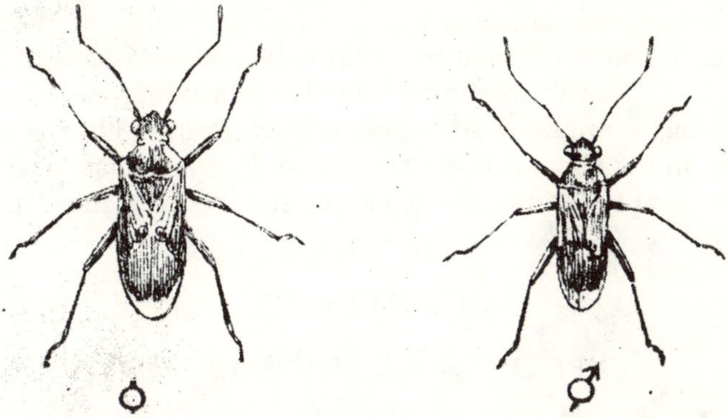

Corizus sidae Fabr. Insect transmissor of the Flagelliase of the Euphorbiaceae in Venezuela. The male size 5mm. and 8 mm. the female.

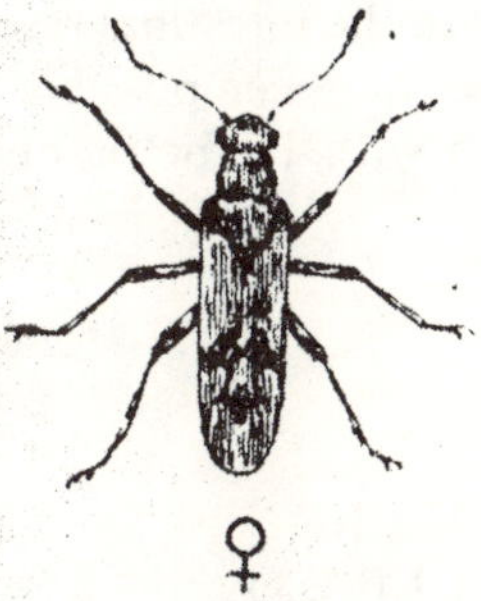

Orthaea bilobata Say. Insect inseparable of the Corizus, accused by Noc and Stevenel as the transmissor of the flagelliase of the euphorbiaceae in Marthinique, but, we could never find infected, nor obtain it experimentally.

The Corizus sidae Fabr. is an insect that the male has around 5mm. and the female has 8mm., pretty colors, dark in the thorax, brown in the hemelitres and a triangle nacreus in the rear parts of the wings; joining often; very restless; always jumping among the groups of E. hypericifolia, putting on the leaves its graceful clusters of reddish eggs.

The incubation of the eggs is of 10 to 12 days, going out a tranverse larve of black and red. This one suffering several moulting, arriving the adult stage in a few days. When they are captured, there is the expulsion of an aromatic liquid.

Easily we have obtained larves of Orthaea bilobata and Corizus sidae in the laboratory, introduced inside test tubes, specimens with inflourescences as food, and the following days are covered with eggs.

Placing larves on E. pilulifera and E. hypericifolia they seek the flowers, but sometimes stay on leaves and stems sucking latex. Insects submitted daily two hours and a half living on sick plants we have found a leptomonad similar to the leptomonad of the plants. Taking specimens of Corizus that have lived several days on sick euphorbias and placing them on healthy E. pilulifera and E. hypericifolia, we have got the transmission of the infection.

The Orthaea bilobata being always a close fellow of the Corizus, never has been found infected by us. However, in accord with Noc and Stevenel it is the transmissor in the island of Marthinique.

Employing exemplaires of Nezara stictica Dallas (37) that had been found by us in the zone of Los Chorros, with an intestinal flagellate, we could not transmit the infection from one euphorbia to the other.

CHAPTER IV

EXPERIMENTAL TRANSMISSION

Lastly we have made attempts to transmit experimentally the infection, utilizing pippetes Pasteur with negative results.

Not withstanding, in our first research (1925) was obtained a 10%. We thought, as said Gaschen: "for producing the infection are necessary the infectant forms of the salivary glands."

E. pilulifera and E. hypericifolia inocoluated with the intestinal reservoir of Corizus sidae with leptomonads positive, it has not been possible to obtain infection. The same result with inoculations with Herpetomonas muscae domesticae.

CHAPTER V

ACTION OF THE DIFFERENT LATEX. ACTION OF THE LATEX OF E. PILULIFERA AND E. HYPERICIFOLIA ABOUT THE TRYPANOSOMA VENEZUELENSE

Placing in the microscope a drop of infected latex and adding a new drop, either of E. pilulifera or E. hypericifolia healthy latex, the leptomonad absolutely does not change and the motility continues equal. Now, adding latex of another plant the leptomonad disappeared immediatly, probably owed to autolysis, influenced by the ph., density, refraction' index.

Reading the experiences of Franchini (38) and Drbohlav (39) about the action of the latex of different plants on several flagellates (Trypanosoma cruzi, lewisi, equinum, etc.), we wished to see the action of the latex of E. pilulifera and E. hypericifolia on the Trypanosoma venezuelense to which adds 2 or 3 drops of latex of these plants, putting paraffin around the lamel, and then the trypanosomas are capable to live several hours, with morphology and motility equal.

(37) Classified by James Zetek.
(38) Bull. Soc. Path. Exot. 1923.
(39) American Journ. of Hyg. 1925.

CHAPTER VI

INVESTIGATION OF THE FLAGELLIASE IN OTHER PLANTS

Many specimens of the following plants have been examined without finding leptomonads, neither none of the protozoons (trypanosomas, crthidias, spirochetes, amoeba), appointed by Franchini:

Croton rhamnifolius (barredero)	euphorbiaceae
Jatropha gossypifolia (túa-túa)	,,
Euphorbia graminea	,,
Euphorbia pulcherrima (papagallo)	,,
Jatropha manihot (yuca)	,,
Euphorbia caracacasana (lechero)	,,
Jatropha curcas (piñón)	,,
Plumeria alba(anapola)	apocinaceae
Tabernaemontana (nardo)	,,
Allamanda cathartica (jazmín falcón)	,,
Callotropis procera (algodón de seda)	asclepiadaceae
Ficus prinoides (sio)	urticaceae
Lactuca scariola (lechuga)	compuesta

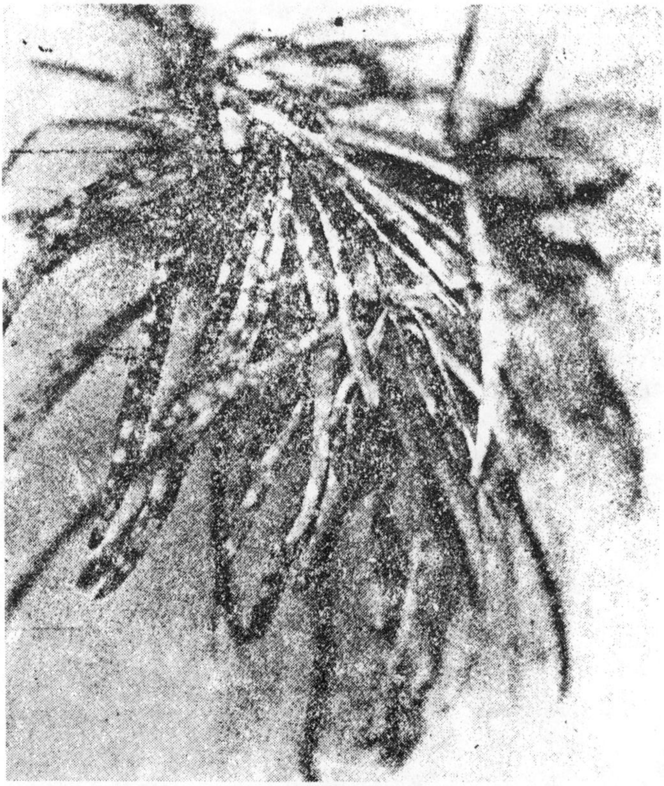

Codiaeum variegatum Blume.

Lastly, we have examined, with the same motive, a great number of plants (convolvulaceae, apocinaceae, etc.,) always with negative results, exception of an euporbiaceae (Codiaeum variegatum Blume) where we have found an amoeba.

It is the first time that is appointed in Venezuela another protozoon, besides of the leptomonad davidi, living in plants. Franchini, who has worked enough in this field, has demonstrated the patogenicity of these amoebas, verifying to produce abscess in the liver of mice.

The Codiaeum variegatum Blume, is a plant very cultivated in the gardens of Caracas, commonly called "lluvia de oro" in some places of Venezuela, and it is not native of America. It is a plant imported from Oceania, islands of Java and Sumatra.

Formerly, we had examined: Ipomea calonyction bonanox (convolvulaceae), Rauwolfia lamarkii (apocináceae), Hippomane mancinella (euphorbiaceac), Croton fragilis H.B.K. (euphorbiaceae).

CHAPTER VII

CULTURES

Our assays in this field have been the following:
Simple broth: negative.
Simple broth with latex euphorbia: negative.
Gelose-blood NNN: (24 hours later all the parasites died).
Zotta' medium: (with this medium, Gaschen could be maintain alives, during 15 days, the leptomonads and obtain the passage to a second tube of culture. Our attempts have been null with this medium).
Latex E. pilulifera and E. hypericifolia: (placing latex of these plants in small test tubes and rearing it in latex of the same extracted from infected plants, the leptomonads have disappeared completely 48 hours after).

THE PLANTS AS RESERVATION OF VIRUS *

(Dedicated to Professor Paz Soldán Carlos)

Many years ago, David and Lafont (1) in the island of Mauricio found a flagellate (leptomonad) in the latex of some euphorbiaceae, discovering that had a great importance, because was the first time that knew a protozoom living in the latex of plants. This flagellate was named Leptomonad davidi Lafont.

At the same time was observed that the leishmaniasis cutaneous existed frequently in the persons working or staying in the forest, and then, some scientific men thought that those plants lactiferous and the insects living on it could be reservoirs of leishmaniasis.

In effect, Strong (2) found a leptomonad morphologically similar in the latex of an euphorbia, in the intestinal containt of an insect (Chariesterus cuspidatus) and the intestinal containt of a small lizard (Cnemidophorus lemniscatus) living on that plant.

Inoculations made by Strong, subcutaneous and intra-peritoneal in monkeys, guinea pigs, dogs, mice, gave negative results. Exception of one, done in a monkey in the abdominal region with intestinal containt of lizard, giving a papule eight days later, taking ulcerative aspect two weeks after. Smears and cuttings of this lesion revealed to Strong the presence of leishmanias.

As the inoculations with the latex and the intestinal containt of the insect were negative, was accepted that the flagellates were capable to infect the skin of the monkey as result of a change in the intestine of the lizard. It is unknown if the intestinal containt of the insect is equal to the intestinal containt of the lizard.

Franchini (3), from Italy, has obtained hepatic abscess in mice for inoculations of phyto-amoebae. Besides, he could infected mice with phytotrypanosomas verified by examination in fresh blood and cultures.

The flagelliase had been found only in euphorbiaceae and in the tropic, when, Franca, in 1911, in Portugal, appointed for the first time (4) the flagelliase, finding infected the E. peplus and E. segetalis. In 1921, Professor Galli-Valerio (5) in the Canton Valais, in Switzerland, to a height of 1.300 m., found infected the E. ferardiana, and Aubertot (6), in Alsace, the E. cyparissias.

Lastly, the Italian Franchini (7) appointed the infection not only for phytomonas, also for different protozoons (amoeba, spirochete, crthidia, trypanosoma) in several families: euphorbiae (*E. calyculata, E. nereifolia, E. virosa*); asclepiadae (*Chlorocodon whitei, Cryptostegia grandiflora*); apocinaceae *(Cervera odollam, Caudiana javanensis*); urticaceae (*Ficus tolloni, Ficus carica*); artocarpeae (*Artiaris toxicaria, Lacoocha artocar-*

* Read in the Academy of Medicine of Lima (Perú). Published in "La Reforma Médica" of Lima (Perú) N° 185. "Gaceta Muskus" Año V. N° 57. 1934. Caracas.

pus); Sapotaceae (*Sideroxylon inerme, Chrysophylium glabrum*).

According to us, it seems to be that it is better the name of phytomonas for the flagellate (leptomonad) of the plants, because in accord the picture of Wenyon (8), to which we add something, the leptomonad is only of the invertebrates and the phytomonas is for invertebrates and plants.

Our contribution almost ready "Contribución al Estudio de la Flageliasis de las Plantas en Venezuela" (9), we read the research of Noguchi (10) in this field. The wise japanese did investigations with inmuneserums: antibrasiliensis, antitropica, antiinfantum and antidonovani, referring the action about the leptomonad, observing that the form and motility continue equal, only a little agglutination produced by the normal serum of rabbit, and conclude: "the flagellates of the latex of *Asclepias curassavica, Asclepias syriaca* and intestine of the *Oncopeltus cingulifer* are inmunological different to the four types of human leishmanias."

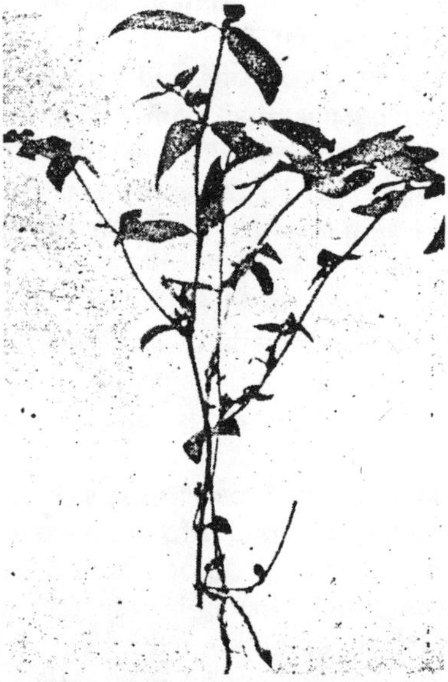

Euphorbia pilulifera healthy.

For that time we tried to demonstrate the future problem referring the agriculture, because it was not only a host protozoon in the latex of small euphorbiae, either Pietri, from Florence, "find in a disease of the vineyard, protozoons liked to trypanosomas"; Ray Nelson (11) says of protozoons, flagellates in the mosaic of the tomatoes, of the string beans and trefoil; and Frank M. Worther (12), discovered a protozoon, similar an amoeba, in a sickness of the sugar cane (agalla de Fiji).

Our research here in Venezuela, about 200 specimens of E. pilulifera, 150 of E. hypericifolia, 80 of E. thymifolia. The infection was seen in the two first, because in the third never was possible to find infection.

The sick plants have a sad aspect, the leaves are hard and pale, scarce latex. However, the E. pilulifera is an annual plant and the infection is

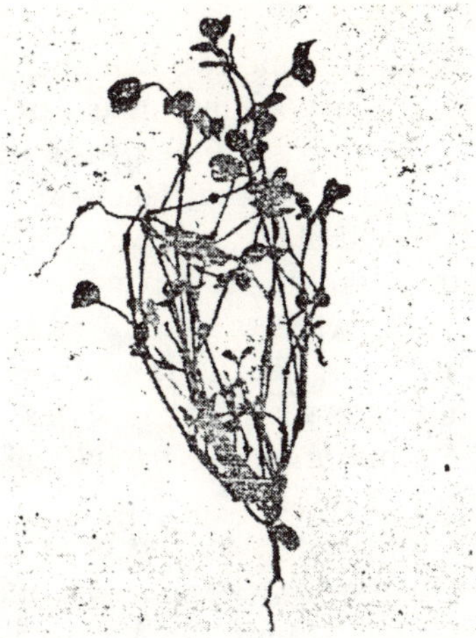

Euphorbia thymifolia healthy.

almost always in the adult stage; the E. hypericifolia, in change, the sickness has not relation with the freshness of the plant.

Curious detail that we observed is that in the parasitic plant, the infection in a branch is very abundant today and tomorrow, the same branch is negative or light. It seems to be the influence of the sun has action about the presence of the phytomonas; because, when the test is practiced early in the morning the result is null, but, when the test is done at noon or afternoon is positive. The infection in the trunk is always positive. Sometimes in a dicotomy, one side is positive and the other one negative.

The size of our phytomonas are as following:

Phytomonas E. pilulifera (average)	
Lenght of the body	20.3 microns
Ext. ant. to blepharoplast	1.95 "
Blepharoplast to nucleus	1.93 "
Nucleus	1.90 "
Nucleus to rear end	15.80 "
Width	2.20 "
Long flagellum	7.50 "

Phytomonas E. hypericifolia (average)	
Lenght of the body	24.40 "
Former end to blepharoplast	2.07 "
Blepharoplast to nucleus	1.93 "
Nucleus	2.50 "
Nucleus to rear end	18.30 "
Width	2.75 "
Long flagellum	7.50 "

* * *

Seeking the insect transmissor we have found two hemipterous, common hosts, of the euphorbiaea, classified in Washington as Corizus sidae Fabr. and Orthaea bilobata, Say. In the digestive tube of the first, only, we have found a flagellate, exactly similar, to the flagellate of plants. Besides, through them to infect undamaged plants and we obtained to infected specimens born in the laboratory, sucking sick plants.

The Corizus sidae Fabr. is an insect whose female 8 m.m. and the male 5 m.m., with attractive colors: dark in thorax, brown in the hemelitres, and a triangle nacreous in the rear part of the wings. Restless, jumper. When are caught there is the expulsion of an aromatic liquid and the incubation of the eggs are of 10 to 12 days.

The other insect named is a fellow of Corizus and has been accused by Noc and Stevenel as the transmissor of the flagelliase in Martinique, but we have never found infection and we could not infected it experimentally. The same result with specimens of Nezara stictica Dallas.

All this researchs were made in surroundings of Caracas. Now, in our stay in Maracaibo, State Zulia, found the mentioned euphorbiae and also the two hemipterous named, but always, without infection.

Up till today only we have found the flagelliase in euphorbiae, not withstanding, we have investigated in other families cited as infected in several countries: asclepiadacea, urticaceae, apocinacea, etc.

The experimental infection utilizing pippetes Pasteur has been rare and only 10%. The cultures employing different mediums, were negative and for that epoch, we did the following conclusions:

1st - The flagelliase of the plants in Venezuela has been found up till today in the family of euphorbiae.
2nd - The infected plants are the following: E. pilulifera, E. hypericifolia, E. thymifolia, E. secretalis (segetalis?) and Jatropha manihot.
3rd - It has been appointed in State Zulia and District Federal.
4th - The transmissor insect is the Corizus sidae Fabr.
5th - Another hemipterous, Orthaea bilobata Say, accused by Noc and Stevenel as the transmissor in Martinique, never has been possible to find infected, nor experimentally.
6th - The experimental infection using pippetes Pasteur has been possible, only, in a percentage of 10%.
7th - The assays of cultures have been negative always.
8th - The Trypanosoma venezuelense can lives during some hours in the latex of E. pilulifera and E. hypericifolia.

* * *

The researchs of Noguchi and his authority (13), destroyed completely any relation between those flagellates of the plants and the cutaneous leishmaniasis and for extension with human pathology, but knowing now the important investigations made in our brother country Perú, by Professor Daniel Mackehenie (14) and his adjunct Coronado have brought newly the attention, the interesting of the phyto-pathology and the plants as deposit of virus.

Formerly, Dr. Maldonado had appointed that the focus of *verruga peruana* had coincidence with the flora lactiferous. The focus of the Coast, for example, are included in the xerophilus flora, specially with lactiferous plants (huanarpo male and female, huancoy, mito, brincamoza, pate) among a height of 700 m. to 1.200 m. over sea level.

The Professor Mackehenie fortunately has cultivated the elements of the Jatropha basiacantha and also the elements containt in the intestinal of those insects living on those plants, very important for the agglutination.

The tests of agglutination with serum of Carrion' disease, serum of guinea pigs inoculated with *Bartonella baciliformis*, serum of guinea pig inoculated with elements of latex of Jatropha and with human serums coming from other sickness, with the following results: Bartonella baciliformis, eight patients positive 1 x 4.000 to 1 x 3.200; serum of warty not agglutination Bartonella muris; serum of inoculation Jatropha basiacantha, was agglutinated in two cases, percentage, 1 x 6.000, and the serum obtained for inoculation of the insect, gave the same percentage. The microscopic agglutination test was negative clearly from 1 x 50 to 1 x 1.600 with serum typhus, paratyphus and melitococcus.

All these researchs of the Peruvian medicine shows the attachment between Bartonellas and Rickettsias, mainly for the phenomenon of Mataro and Mooser and that the diagnosis of the Carrion' disease could be practiced: hemo culture, histological test of the skin, Mataro's phenomenon and Mooser's phenomenon and two sure signs: one clinical, the verruga peruana and the other one, hematologic, the presence of bartonellas.

We wait the definitive conclusions, to praise the Peruvian school, and to regret not presenting a personal opinion about the Verruga peruana, because, everyone knows, is a sickness limited to the brother country.

BIBLIOGRAPHY

1st - C. R. Biol. 1909 and Ann. I. Past 1910.
2nd - Am. Journ. Trop. Med. 1924.
3rd - Bull. Soc. Path. Exot. 1923 and Ann. I. Past. 1922.
4th - Bull. Soc. Path. Exot. 1911.
5th - Schw. Med. Woche. 1921.
6th - C. R. Soc. Biol. 1923.
7th - Bull. Soc. Path. Exot. 1919 - 1923.
8th - Wenyon. Protozoology. Tome I.
9th - Cont. al Est. de la Flag. de las Plan. in Venezuela. 1928.
10th - Proc. Inter. Conf. on Health Trop. Am. 1924.
11th - Tech. Bull. 1922.
12th - Phillip. Agricult. 1922.
13th - Journ. Exp. Medicine 1926 - 1927.
14th - Ref. Médica. 1933. Bull. Of. San. Panam. 1933.
15th - Path. Exot. Le Dantec. 1929.

THE PLANTS. THE PHYTO-PATHOGENESIS AND ITS RELATIONS WITH THE HUMAN PATHOLOGY *

We want to say four words more about the plants, the phyto-pathogenesis and its relations with human pathology. Short time ago we presented to the Academy of Medicine of Perú a little work about the same subject and now we wish to expose the results obtained in some light investigations made here, among us, in the same way.

The discovery of Mackehenie and his research about the theme of this Conference, it seems to be, one of the landmark done in the world in Tropical Pathology. The trajectory of Mackehenie has been wonderful. After his magnificent discovery, the Academy of Medicine of Lima has open the doors for him and when we have read his interesting work of entrance, making ostentation of erudition, we have appreciated in him a prepared and cultivated spirit, capable to give to his country and the world the key of the phyto-pathogenesis of the *Verruga peruana*. As said Paz Soldán: "in Mackehenie are united the wise and the technician, and of the fight of these two imponderables has born that work of Science and Art, that it is of Incorporation mentioned."

Recently understood to the colleague Dr. Mir says that the interesting part of his trip to those brother countries was to see nearly that group of diseases of Rickettsiosis and Bartonellosis, or clearly, the tifus de Santiago and the Verruga peruana. Our fellow spoke of a great difference among one and another, but resulted that both groups tried to attack each other, progressively.

The Rickettsias and Bartonellas during its evolutive cycle for a stage of two chromatic mass united by a slender filament and it is necessary to distinguish the involutive forms, as are seen in the Decement's membrane, after the Mataro's phenomenon, and probably are the origins of the monococoides forms of Japonese Sato. The differences are more biologic than morphologic, not withstanding, the Rickettsias attack chiefly the nervous system, the Bartonellas seems to attack more the blood and hematopoietic organs. However, the case of a patient of Professor Monge cited by Mackehenie with nervous troubles, presenting a scarce Bartonellas in the blood, but very abundant in the cephalo-rachidean liquid. The autopsy of this patient revealed a strong congestion of the meningeal vessels; besides, thrombosis of the longitudinal sinus. In the cerebellum and bulb were found Bartonellas.

Time after, Dr. Mir published some Commentaries about our work in the review of Policlínica Caracas.

The germs found by Mackehenie in the intestinal containt of the insects living on the Huanarpo and cultivated being inoculated to guinea

* Reprinted from "Trabajos Científicos" (book 1937)

pigs, produced nervous troubles, as instability, convulsions and paralysis of the rear train.

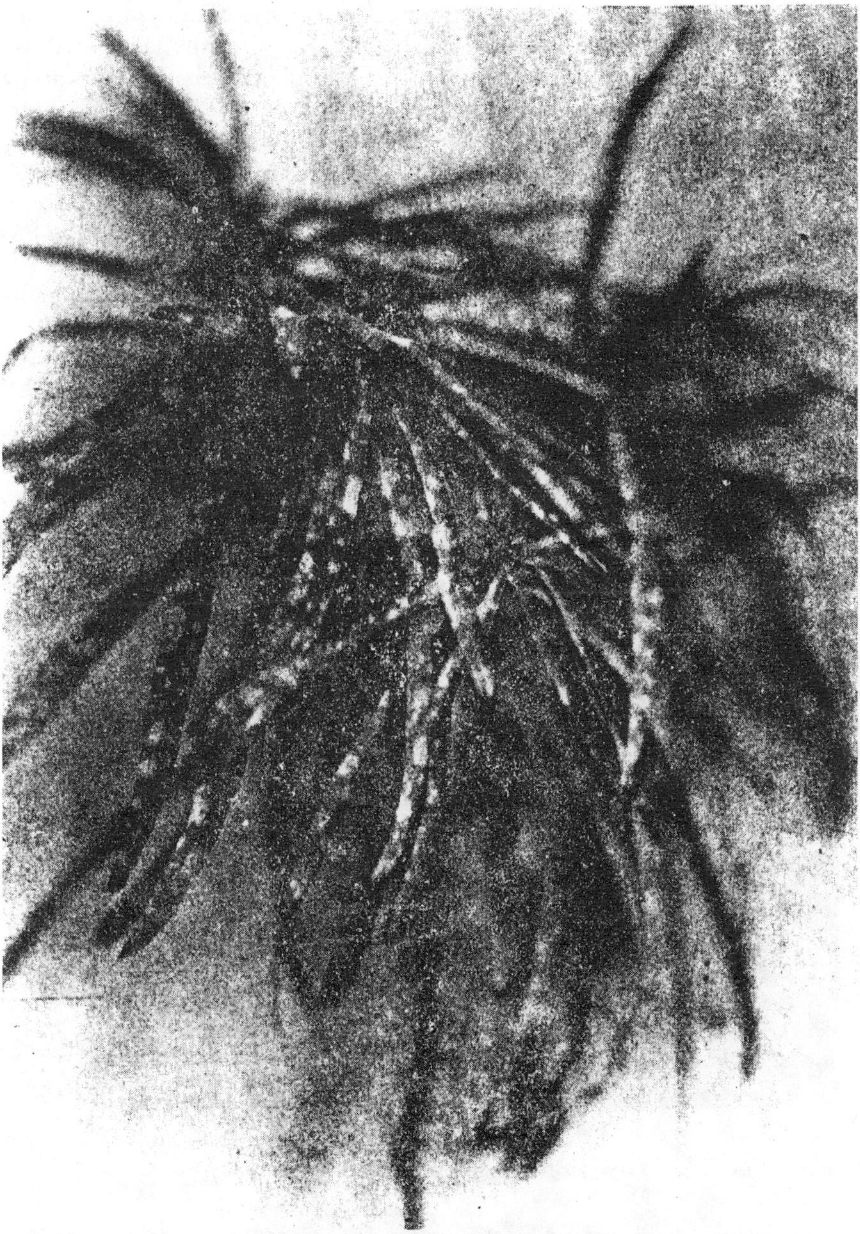

Codiaeum variegatum Blume, where we have found an amoeba.

The Mooser's phenomenon (edema scrotumtesticle) and iridocyclitis of the Japanese Mataro and Nagayo, attack still more the Rickettsias and

Bartonellas and in the Mooser's phenomenon there are more bartonellas in the cells of connective tissue than in the brain and spleen. The reticular system, it seemed to be, the deposit of bartonellas, as said Mackehenie.

The Professor Angel Maldonado for his studies about the flora of the xerophilus regions, and Pedro Weiss having found in the latex of those plants bartonelloid elements, opened the path of Mackehenie, who doing the test of the latex of an aciculate euphorbia called *Huanarpo male* (Jatrpha basiacantha), found bartonelloid element and that latex inoculated to guinea pigs, 48 hours later died. Another species, called Huanarpo female, not aciculate, produced also the death of the animal; the same results with the latex of another species Jatropha macrantha.

Mackehenie has obtained cultures of the bartonelloid forms of the latex, rearing in broth simple, agar-agar and agar-blood. These germs of

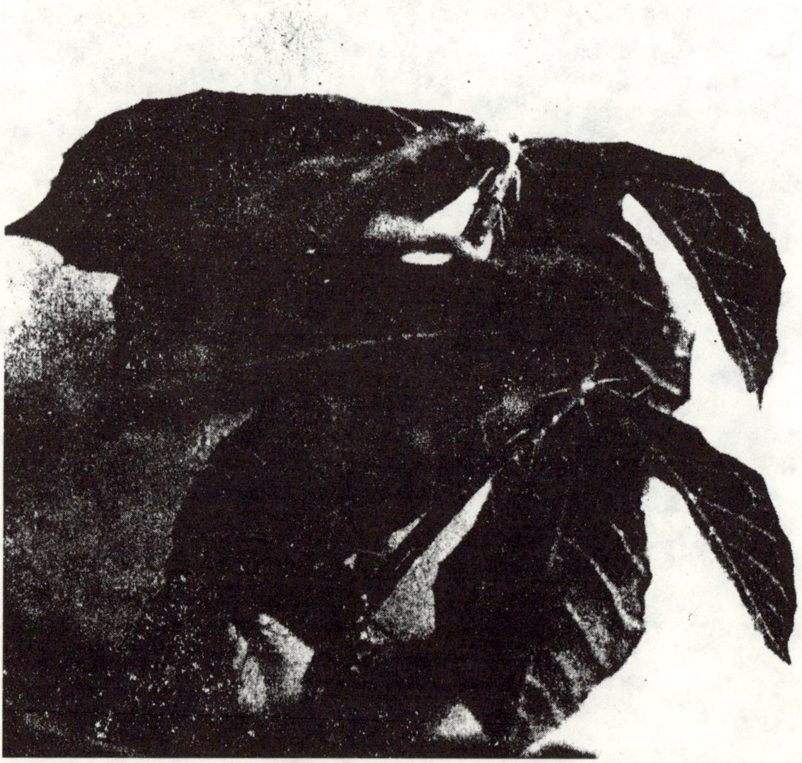

Jatropha urens L. of the xerophytic region of Maiquetiía, D.F., in whose latex we have not seen bartonellas.

the culture are agglutinated by the serum of patients with verruga peruana till 1 x 3.200. The Bartonella muris ratti is not agglutinated. Comparing with serums of typhus, para typhus and melitococcus have been negative referring the agglutination.

Will be an human germ the elements found by Mackehenie in those jatrophas? It is probable. It is an element that biological and morphological is equal to the B. bacilliformis. Afranio do Amaral and Lemos Monteiro, believe that in the evolution of the typhus was an epoch living in plants and after attacked the man.

It lacked only to Mackehenie produce warts in inoculated animals and he has found a very receptive animal, the hen of race Leghorn. This fowl inoculated in the comb, 20 days later, presents warts in the site of the inoculation. Placing these warts in normal saline solution and injecting in new animal, this one presented Bartonellas in his blood and spreading of the warts in the comb, in the chin and in the tarses.

Among us it does not exist either the Jatropha basiacantha, nor the Jatropha macrantha. These are plants limited to those region of Perú and Brazil; but we have two plants, with urticating poils, sisters of the J. basiacantha: the Jatropha urens L. and the Jatropha kurthiana, small plants, abundant in the dry zones of Maiquetía, called *guaritoto*, but in some places of Maracaibo is named *pringamoza*.

Continuing the advices of Mackehenie we have examined in fresh and with coloration the latex of these plants, but we have only found crystals and moving particles, but not germs. After, we have inoculated this latex to guinea pigs without producing any trouble and the examination of blood negative. Rearing this latex in broth and agar-agar, none colonies. These reaserch are good for Mackehenie, but should be convenient practice investigations of control in countries around Perú, as Ecuador, Brazil, Bolivia. Curious things in the nature: the germ of the Verruga Peruana, having its bed in any small plants, uglies, with a latex highly caustic and full of urticating poils!

We have examined other plants, that have not been searched before: Ipomea calonyction bona nox (convolvulácea), Rawwolfia Lamarkii A.D.C. (apocynaceae), Hippomane mancinella L. (euphorbiaceae), Croton fragilis H.B.K.(euphorbiaceae).

We are going to do mention of the finding in a plant from Barinas, for examination in fresh, of an amoeba, small, similar to Amoeba nana, scarce in the sap of the plant, not moving too much, lazy, slender form, central nucleus. Is the first time, we think, that it is found, among us, another protozoon, besides the Leptomonad davidi, living in plants. Franchini, one of the first in this field has demonstrated the pathogenesis of these amoebae producing hepatic abscess. The plant where we have found this amoeba is an euphorbia and is called "lluvia de oro", in some parts of the country. It is not a Venezuelan plant, it is imported from the islands of Java and Sumatra.

The problem of phyto-pathology and phyto-pathogenesis is very important, because Franchini has found amoebae, crithidias, trypanosomas, etc., in plants; the mosaic has been considered as result of protozoons. Today is accepted definitive a virus filtrable, and in a disease of the sugar cane (agalla de Fiji) has been found amoebae.

Before finishing, our acknowledgement, for his kind help in the botanic classifications to Professor Henry Pittier and also congratulations to the School of Medicine of Perú for have given to his country and the world the key of the phyto-pathogenesis of the Verruga peruana.

(This work was realized in the Laboratory of the Clínica Luis Razetti)

LITTLE NOTE ABOUT THE FLAGELLIASE OF THE PLANTS IN THE STATE ZULIA *

In several excursions to the surroundings of the town of Maracaibo and some near Districts, we have had the agreable task to do research about the flagelliase of the plants in these regions.

Before, in our doctoral thesis of the last year we exposed our investigations in this field.

The drought of our lands has disable our research, because we walked long extensions without finding the plants that we seeked. In Caracas it was different, we found in any place, euphorbiaceae, that were often infected.

Up till today only we have found with infection the Euphorbia pilulifera in a farmer called Urrutia, from an hour of distance of the city. This plant has been found infected in Caracas.

The plants infected are all a sad aspect as we have seen before.

The Euphorbia hypericifolia and the Euphorbia tymifolia were also common in these zones, but did not show infection.

Living on the sock plants we have caught insects whose intestinal liquid has been negative, referring to leptomonads. Among them we captured some exemplairies of Orthaea bilobata Say, insect that we could not accuse as transmissor in Caracas. According to Noc and Stevenel it should be the transmissor of the flagelliase in Martinique.

We have investigated several plants belonging to different families. Have been classified the following:

Croton rhamnifolius (barredero)
Jatropha gossypifolia (túa-túa)
Jatropha manihot (yuca)
Plumeria alba (amapola)
Ipomea cairica (bejuquillo)
Calotropis procera (algodón de seda)
Ricinus communis L. (tártaro)
Fragia volubilis L. (pringa-moza)

* Reprinted from Revista de la Sociedad Médico-Quirúrgica de Zulia - 1929.

SOMETHING ABOUT AN INTESTINAL FLAGELLATE OF THE DYSDERCUS MAURUS DISTANT.

Read in the meeting of the Clínica Luis Razetti (July 17th 1935) Published in "Medical".

In Acarigua (State Portuguesa) we found in a tree called *camoruco* (Sterculla carthogenensis) and under its shadows sucking, voraceously, the fruits fallen, numerous specimens of an insect called by the people *candelilla,* attracted our attention, like the hemipterous appointed by us, for the first time, as the transmissor of flagelliase of plants in Venezuela.

The insect has pretty colors, having the male 5 m.m. and the female 8m.m., moving nimbly trying to join often and very sensitive to the cautivity.

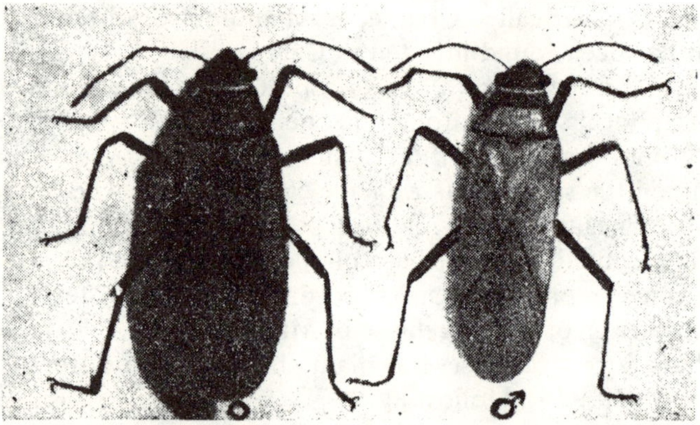

Dysdercus maurus Dist. The male has 5 m.m. and the female has 8 m.m.

The examination of the intestinal containt in fresh and coloration to the panoptic of Pappenheim, we have found in several specimens, abundant leptomonads, having around 18 microns of lenght and 2.5 microns width, with a form shorter than the leptomonad davidi Lafont, living in the intestine of Corizus sidae Fabr., found by us.

Searching the sap of the mentioned tree, and also the sap of some bushes around it, have been negative for flagellates.

Our fellow in the laboratory Dr. Briceño Iragorry brought to us any exemplairies caught in the gardens of the Hospital Vargas, and its intestinal containt revealed, equaly, the presence of a leptomonad.

Specimens of the insect sent to the Department of Agriculture in Washington have been classified as belonging to the family Phyrrhocoridae and under the name Dysdercus maurus Dist. The classification was made by H.G. Barber, to whom we give our acknowledgement.

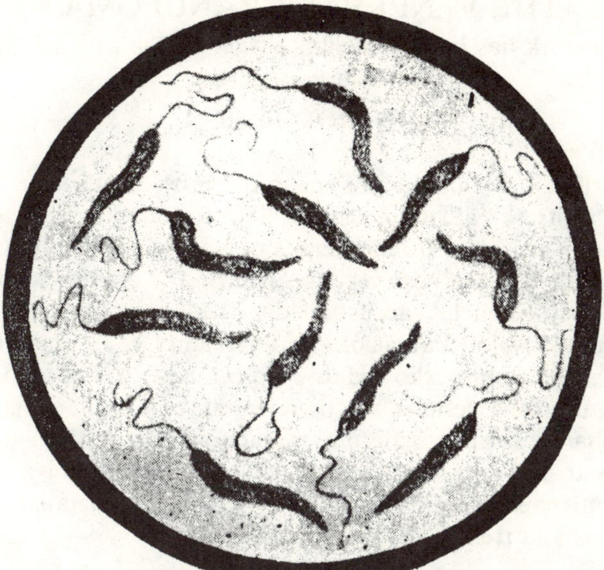

Leptomonad found in the intestine of Dysdercus maurus Dist. Length 18 microns; width 2.5 microns. Panoptic Pappenheim.

BIBLIOGRAPHY

1.-*Iriarte David R.:* La flageliasis de las plantas en Venezuela (Tesis doctoral)-1928.

2.-*Iriarte David R.:* Algo sobre la flageliasis de las euforbiáceas-Gaceta Médica de Caracas-1926.

3.-*Iriarte David R.:* Las plantas como reservorios de virus. La Reforma Médica. Lima, Perú, 1934.

4.-*Gabaldón Arnoldo:* Estudio sobre Herpetomonas muscarum-1928.

5.-*Noguchi Hideyo*-Plant Flagellates and Leishmania. International Conference on Health Problems in Tropical América-1924.

6.-*Gaschen Hans L.*-Contribution a l'étude de la Flagelliase des Euphorbiacées en Suisse-1926.

7.-*Franchini G.*-Serie de trabajos. Bull Soc. Path. Exot.-1922-23-24.

8.-*Iturbe Juan*-Presencia del leptomonas davidi (Lafont), en la savia de la Euphorbia hypericifolia.-Actualidades-1918.

9.-*Tejera Enrique:* La *leishmaniosis americana en Venezuela-1919.*

10.-*Pittier H.*-Plantas usuales de Venezuela, 1926.

11.-*Beaurepaire Aragao H.*-Pesquizas sobre Phytomonas francai.-Memorias do Ins. Osw. Cruz-1931

THE VENEREAL GRANULOMA *

This work has had the collaboration of Dr. Luis M. Salas

INTRODUCTION

The brief study that we present to the Fifth Venezuelan Congress of Medicine, waits to call the attention about a common disease, but not much taken in account in Venezuela. The Venereal Granuloma or Granuloma Inguinale is a sickness very frequent in the country, chiefly among persons of low social class accustomed to the lack of hygiene. We and our fellows in the Hospital Vargas often found, and Dr. Tejera in his cathedra of Tropical Medicine, showed us typical cases. It is confound with numerous ulcerous lesions of the genital parts: ulcerous papilloma, ulcerous chancres, phagolytic ulcers, tuberculosis of the vulva, etc. We believe it is an affection very current between us, and doing a deep study in all the antivenereal centers, should give lights details on etiology, pathogenesis and treatment, yet in controversy.

SYNONYMY

Who described for the first time this disease was the Colonel McLeod in the India (1892) seeing a specific granulomatous process. C. Donovan in 1905, say intracellular bodies, found in the smears taken from the ulcerations and that the authors of the english language call yet "Donovan's bodies".

The rich synonymy that this disease has; up to this day it is difficult to know in what nosological site must be placed. The same referring to the suspicious causative agent; everything this, do arduous the correlation among the numerous studies made in many parts of the world.

There is variety of names: Venereal granuloma inguinale, Granuloma inguinale, Lymphogranuloma inguinale, Ulcerating granuloma of the pudenda, Granuloma pudendi, Granuloma ulcereux des parties genitaux, etc. We believe, that the name of Venereal granuloma is not justified, because the illness not always is venereal as the syphilis and the blemorrhea; neither, Granuloma inguinale is not correct, because the process can invade other regions out the inguinal. The name more appropriated according to us should be: *Ulcerating granuloma.*

HISTORY

It was after the interesting work of Aragao and Vianna in 1913, that related the etiologycal effect of the Donovan's bodies with the illness and did to know the good results with the treatment with tartar emetic, that medical literature of this affair comes to be very abundant, and a list, not

* Reprinted from the book "Estudios de Patología Tropical. 1942.

complete, will be given at the end in the bibliography. It is necessary to rebound the recent communications of Foster M. Johns who made attempts to cultivate the Donovan's bodies without success (29) and other one of J.A. McIntosh, who said he obtained positive cultures and produced specific lesions (41). Unfortunately for us our assays in this field were always negative. Referring to Venezuela the bibliography about this question is very poor, and only we know the case studied by Juan Iturbe and Eudoro González (28).

DESCRIPTION OF THE LESION

In the field of dermatology the exact description is very difficult. The affection begins often for one or more vesicles or small papules, some itching, opening some days after, giving a clear liquid, not purulent. Later, little erosion, bordering it slight inflammation, invading slowly, seeming to heal, but newly, start to extend through out the border, arriving to the former size rapidly.

The aspect of the lesions when the patients enter the hospital, is the following:

Region - The ulceration almost always is situated in the genital organs and perineal and genital regions, but this place as has been demonstrated by Johns (29) and photo taken of his study, it is not exclusive. In the man is seen in penis, glands, prepuce, inguinal region, perineum and perineal region. In the woman, all the vulve, low part of the vagina, peri-anal region.

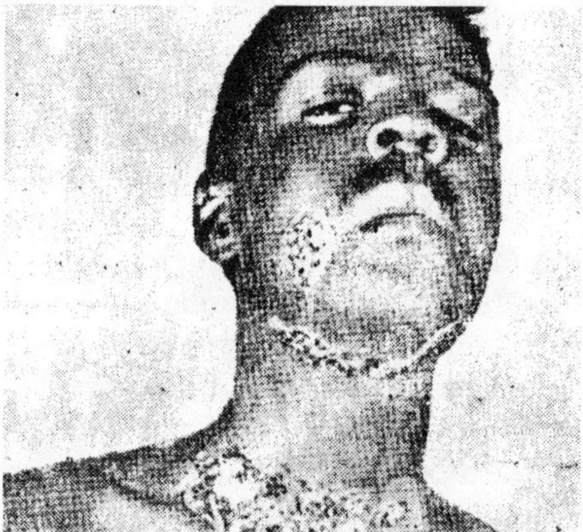

Photo taken from John's work (lesions on face and neck).

Size - The ulcers are of different sizes, arriving to large dimensions, as is seen in the photos of this work.

Aspect - The ulcerations have salient edges, with small protuberances covert for granular tissue; the bottom, never deep, covert also for granulation. In the patients without no treatment and with secondary infection, the lesions are covert with an exudate, giving a smell not fetid, but characteristic. The lesions are painful and bleeding easily. The peripheric ganglions are not presenting infarction. The main details, are: the process is slow; not peripheric inflammation; good appearance of the ill; and many times there are cases with several years in evolution, doing to discard a cancer. The disease is auto-contaminant by scraping or excoriation.

Frequency - The sickness is frequent in persons of low social class, it is common in the patients of hospital.

Sex - We have not seen no difference.

The venereal granuloma is accompanied often for syphilis, bubos, chancres infected, bringing inconvenients for the diagnosis and the treatment.

ETIOLOGY

This is a point very discussed in the field of this disease. Since the discovery of Donovan inside the cells mononucleares, have been considered as the cause of the sickness for many investigators, and the majority are in accord giving it a pathogenical activity. Donovan thought it was a protozoon; Siebert, classified it as a diplococcus capsulary (47); Martini said to have verified positive the cultures with material from the ulceration (38); Wise (56). Maitland (35), McLennon (33) and other researchers have found spirochetes, type treponema and to approach to syphilis. Noguchi also found spirochetes type Tryponema genitalis (29). In smears done with the exudate of the lesions exist a rich bacterial flora. In these smears it is frequent to find a certain amount of spirochetes, employing the methods of Giemsa or Leishmann; not having the characteristics of the Treponema pallidum.

Aragao and Vianna in their interesting work found often the intracellular organism and, according to them, obtained cultures in Sabouraud's medium. Taking in account the morphology and its reproduction, founded the genus "kalimmato-bacterium" and called this species "Kalimmato-bacterium granulomatis". The english authors continue with the name "Donovan's bodies". The Brazilian authors verified positive intraperitoneal inoculations in cats, guinea pigs and rats.

Many communications have appeared after the study of Aragao and Vianna. Some deny that it is a bacterium, may be a protozoon; others, have doubts about the cultures and the inoculations and believe it is simply a banal bacillum capsulat type "Friedlander".

In that epoch appeared the work of Johns (29) who did large attempts for the cultivation and inoculation in the animals. We reprinted here the conclusions: "Many times we have tried to inject or transplant material scraping the ulcerations, pieces of sick tissues, do grafts in dogs, guinea pigs, rabbits and rats, utilizing all the ways, intradermic, subcutaneous, intraperitoneal, intra-testicle, in vesicles produced by cautery or in old lesions with protuberances granular; never, have we obtained reproduction of the disease, neither, death of the inoculated animals."

"Besides, of the usual mediums we have assaid with different degrees of ionic concentration, with or without sugar, aerobic and anaerobic, with atmospheres of hydrogen of nitrogen. Pieces of tissues containing abundant organisms mixed with citrated blood, gelose blood, liquid of hydrocele. The rearings tests have been always negative."

After this affirmation coming of a known researcher, who accompanied by Bass, cultivated for the first time the plasmodium of the malaria, came to our hands, a study of the American J.A. McIntosh (41) telling that the kalimmato-bacterium was easily cultivated and the inoculations were positive. We have tried to do experiences in both fields, with numerous assays, always with negative results.

It lacks to know if, really, it is the producer germ, because it must fill the biological cycle of Koch.

Seeking the kalimmato it is better not to wash the lesion two or three days before, nor treat with tartar emetic the patient. Not to do the smears with the exudate, it is necessary to scrap deeply the ulceration profiting the bloody lymph; the smears must be thick; coloration with the methods of Giemsa or Leishmann. Referring to morphology, the germ has aspect of little coccus., of 2 to 3 tenth of micron, around a capsule; other times in form bacillar with the end round shaped, in accord with the division stage, that is binary. It is Gram negative.

The organism is intracellular, showing groups near the nucleus; the cells enlarged, later break, giving liberty to the germs. The organism must be found in any part of the lesion, but it is more sure to seek it in the salient edges.

PATHOGENY

According to the present *status* is difficult to speak about the pathogeny of this disease. It is necessary to know which is the way of introduction. Probably will be the sexual relations, helping this assert the name venereal and the situation, chiefly in the majority of the cases in the genital region; however, McIntosh (41) says that the sexual contact between two persons, healthy and sick, not transmitting the disease; should be necessary an excoriation of the skin. The slow development of the illness, its slight on the human organism, not presence of ganglionar reaction, do think that the effect of the germ are simply local. These facts try to approach the granuloma to the cutaneous leishmaniosis and both reply to the antimonial treatment.

HISTO-PATHOLOGY

The photo 104, taken from the work of McIntosh gives an idea of the histo-pathological lesions.

The micro-organisms are abundant intracellulares, chiefly, inside the macrophages and Johns (29) is astonished with the quantity inside one cell, without destroy its chemical composition, revealed by the coloration.

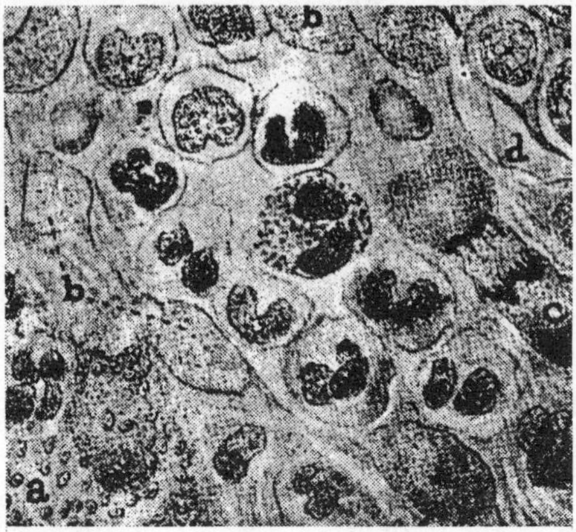

Section - Numerous Donovan's bodies inside the macrophages.

Schochet (48) told the following: "It is an hyperplasia of epithelial and conjunctives cells, with the formation of sclerotic bands of conjunctive tissue. There is also an infiltration diffuse perivascular of rond cells and proliferation of new vessels, giving origin to the granulations. Never, giant cells or elements in process of caseation."

TREATMENT

Were Aragao and Vianna the firsts to use the tartar emetic for treating the granuloma; may be thinking in the good results treating the leishmaniosis. The technic are intravenous injections of solution of emetic to 1% in saline solution, 2 or 3 times a week. These injections are caustics and toxics. The injections must be made with special care, avoiding spread the liquid out the vein. It is convenient to begin for 1 c.c., increasing till arrive to the best dose, almost always of 5 or 6 c.c. To the minor sign of intoxication is necessary to stop the treatment. The global dose elevated produces troubles in the liver, kidneys, etc. After the first injection the parasite disappeared from the ulcerations, and if the patient had not received before none antimonial treatment, at the starting, the lesions it seems suffer a recrudescence: painful, bleeding, but all these symptoms return slowly. Up today there is a tendence to high doses avoiding emetic resistance.

RELAPSES AFTER THE TREATMENT

This is possible in some cases. The relapses appeared after the total epithelization of the ulceration and often the new ulceration begins in some of the edges of the former lesion, either appear one focus, or may be several.

SURGICAL TREATMENT

This treatment is a downfall in the extirpation of the sick parts. The lesions increase, try to extend. A colleague says that has obtained good results with the cautery on the small granulomas.

DIFFERENTIAL DIAGNOSIS

The venereal granuloma can be confounded with the common lesions of the affection situated in genital organs or inguinal region.

Le Dantec (30) consider it of tuberculosis nature; but, should be interesting to get the *kalimmato.* An ulceration with the characteristics mentioned, not improving with anti-syphilitic drugs and not finding the kalimmato, could be a possible case of veneral *granuloma* and a assay with tartar emetic is indicated.

TEST OF THE FORMALDEHYDE

This test has been devised by McIntosh (41) who it called "formol gel test", or in other words: test of gelatification of sanguineous serum for the formaldehyde. The technic is the following: to x 1 c.c. of serum of the patient, to add 1 drop of formaldehyde diluted to 37% and to mix; wait 24 hours. If the test is positive the serum is opaque and gelatinous; many times, 10 minutes after add the drop of formaldehyde, McIntosh said the test was positive in 14 cases and negative in 1 case.

We have employed this test twice. In one case was completely negative and in the other new after 4 hours a slight opacity, but not, gelatification of the American researchers.

Besides, with serum of persons that never have had lesions of granuloma, with Wassermann negative, we have observed positive results; on the contrary, with syphilitic serums, in accord to Calmette (57), are gel for formaldehyde in high percentage; in our hands have been always negative.

RELATION AMONG THE VENEREAL GRANULOMA AND THE INGUINAL PORADENITIS

Lastly, we knew a communication signed by Robert Clement (58) that we have left astonished. This author wrote that the venereal granuloma and the inguinal poradenitis or lymphogranulomatosis are the same disease. Before, we have never seen that kind of information. Are till today two different illness: the first, is an affection with an ulceration without glands infarcted; the other one, is a suppuration of the inguinal glands, very studied between us by E.P. de Bellard in communication to the IV Venezuelan Medical Congress and others. This publication of Clement without scientific basis, will bring only confusion, because are two sickness completely different. The similitude is only in the name.

CONCLUSIONS

1 - The venereal granuloma is a chronic disease it seems very spreaded in Venezuela; possibly, often, confounded with ulcerations of the genital parts.

2 - The etiology, yet is not clear.

3 - The best treatment till today is the tartar emetic, not either

definitive.

4 - In order to obtain food effect of the antimonial treatment it is necessary high doses, continued and prolonged.

5 - The disease relapses frequently.

6 - The gelatification of the serum for the formaldehyde it seems to be a reaction not specific of the disease.

EXPOSITION OF THE CASES

CASE A - R. S., single, 18 years old.

Father died. Mother alive. Six brothers, healthy. In 1925 came to Hospital Vargas for papillomas ano-perineal, that began six months before, that were treated for cautery; without cicatrization left the hospital.

Comes back again to the hospital in 1926, with ulcerations in perineal region, superior parts of thighs and vulve. These ulcerations are reddish, with salient edges, painful and feels itchy. R. Wasseramnn negative.

Smears, coloration panoptico Pappenheim, was possible to see numerous ''kalimmato-bacterium granulomatis'' inside the cells, similar the photos from Aragao and Vianna (1). In these smears saw another similar germ, like the pneumococcus. Besides, the smears showed spirochetes, diplococcus and diplo-bacillum.

He was treated with arsenic, bismuth and tartar emetic.

On 2-11-26, with exudate of the lesions was inoculated a guinea pig in the inguinal region. The result was negative. Also we did cultures with material for scraping, giving only development of colonies of staphylococcus.

The biopsy was examined by Rísquez Jr., giving: ''epithelial granulations surrounded of inflammation tissue; cuttings of capillary vessels wiht endothellium hypertrophic.''

This patient received a global dose of emetic and showed a notable improvement when left the hospital.

CASE B - This case is the most characteristic and it had been studied before by Martín Vegas, who did the diagnosis.

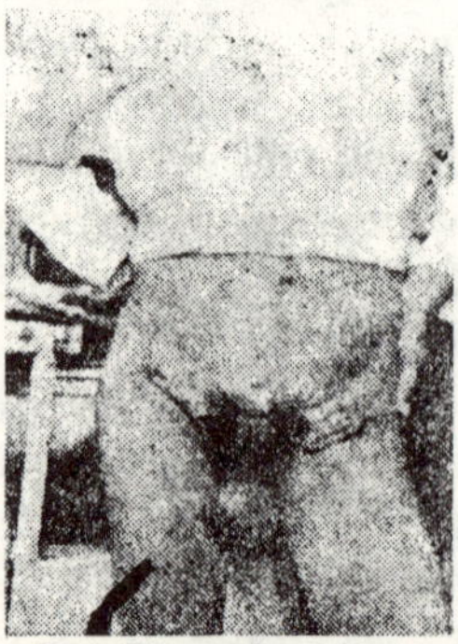

Dr. Vegas' patient seen by us.

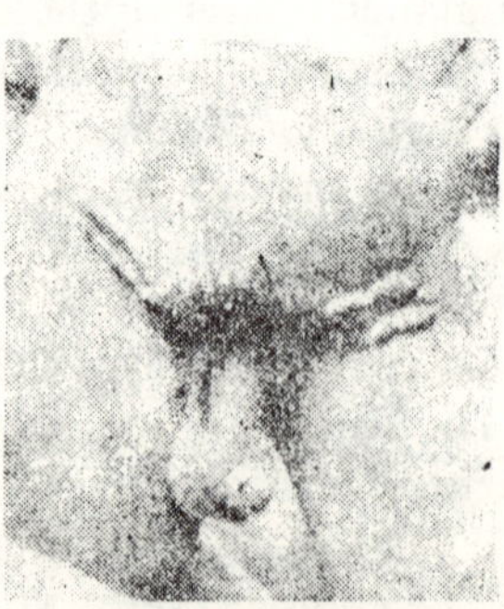

The former case.

The patient said that one month after sexual relations, appeared a little ulceration in glands (frenum) of the penis, that some days after disappeared. Some time later, showed up, similar lesions that invaded all the glands and prepuce with abundant suppuration; 15 days afterward began a small lesion in left groin, with surface of raspberry and 1 month later, a similar lesion in the right groin.

Dr. Vegas did smears of the exudate finding numerous Donovan's bodies.

The treatment was with emetic and the patient received from 16 of June until the 17 of July (1926) 1 gram 39 c.g. with notable improvement. From 29 of July to 12 of August received 0.90 c.g. more of emetic. The healing was complete.

On 13-11-26 had a relapse with presence of inguinal lesions. New treatment with tartar emetic with rapid betterment. Please see the photos showing the aspect when looked for treatment and when the relapse.

In the smears of the relapse, abundant Donovan's bodies inside the mononuclears; we also found bacillus type Ducrey.

Cultures with exudate from these lesions in the Sabouraud's medium, gelose, broth, giving negative results. Then we made attempts with gelose-blood, gelose-starch-blood, gelose-milk-glycerine.

The cultures in these last mediums have been null; only, in the tubes gelose-blood there are brown colonies of a large germ, type coccus, perhaps, may be, kalimmato-bacterium, but we have no security.

Inoculations to guinea pigs have been negative. Histo-pathological cuttings nothing special.

CASE C - 29 years old. Worker. History of waws, venereal diseases. In July 1926 began two ulcerations in the inguinal region: the higher irregular borders and the lower like a deep fissure. Both have salient and hard edges. The tissues around are normal. There is a third ulceration to the right side upper an old scar in the inguinal fold. The aspect of the lesions gave way to thinking of venereal granuloma.

On 11-9-26 the patient had received a global dose of emetic of 1.35 grams. The cicatrization was complete and the ill could be operated of an inguinal hernia.

The bacteriological investigation referring to kalimmato-bacterium was negative.

CASE D - 15 years old, domestic worker. On July 1926 started the lesions in the vulva. These ulcerations extended to the perineum and anal region.

When admitted in the Service presented reddish ulceration of the vulva, something hard and painful.

The treatment with emetic was during one month and a half, receiving 2.20 grams. The daily dose has been changeable and with days of repose. The lesions have been a little rebellious to tartar emetic.

* * *

Lastly, we presented in one of the weekly scientific meetings of the Clínica Luis Razetti a new case, accompanied by photos and a microphoto with finding of the Donovan's bodies, reaction of the formaldehyde positive and treatment with *fuadina,* obtaining very good results. This Communication was published in ''Caracas Médico''. Año II. N° 6. 1935.

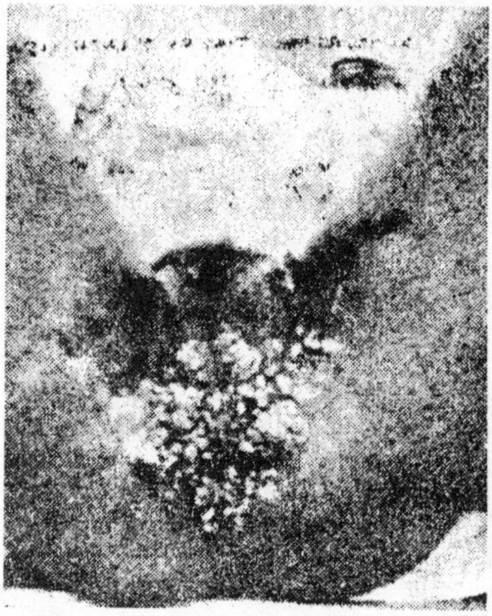

Lesions vulva-perineals papillomatous.

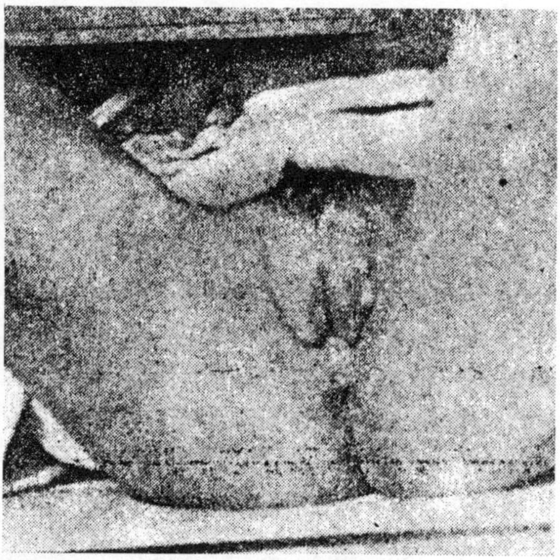

The former patient improved.

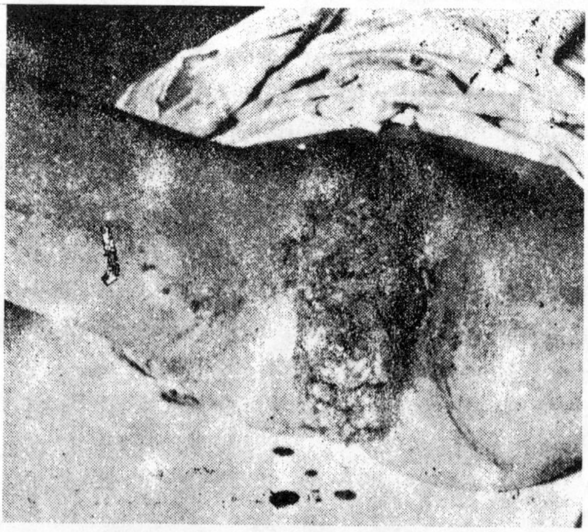

Case with Donovan's bodies and formaldehyde gel test positives. Notable improvement with fuadina. Studied lastly.

BIBLIOGRAPHY

(1) *Aragao, H.D.B. y Vianna, G.* -"Pesquizas sobre Granuloma Venéro", Mem. do Instituto Oswaldo Cruz, 1913, 11, 211-238.

(2) *Aragao, H.D.B.* -"Notes on Granuloma Venereum", New Orleans Med. and Surg. Journ., 1917, XX, 369-374.

(3) *Beeson, B.B.* -"Granuloma inguinale with a lesion on the lower lip", Arch. Dermat. and Syph., 1922, n.s. VI, 342.

(4) *Cornwall, L.H. and Peck, S.M.* -"Etiology of Granuloma Inguinale etc., Arch. Dermat., and Syph, 12, 613, 1925.

(5) *Clément, Robert.* -"L'Etiology du Granuloma Vénérien, Adenopathie Inguinale Subaigue simple a suppuration intro-ganglionaire, Presse Médicale, N° 91, Nov. 13,1926.

(6) *Campbell, J.* -"Granuloma Inguinale", Journ. Americ. Med. Assoc. 1921, XXVI, 648.

(7) *Carter, M.R.* -"Ulcerative Granuloma of the Pudenda", The Lancet, London, 1910, 11, 1128.

(8) *Castellani A. y Chalmers.* -Tropical Medicine.

(9) *Castellani A.* -"Granuloma Inguinale", Nelson's Loose Leaf Living Medicine, Vol. 11, p.347.

(10) *Claasen U.L.* -"Granuloma Inguinale", Ohio Med. Journ. 1922, XVIII, 685-689.

(11) *Cleland, J. and Huckinbothan.* -"On the etiology of ulcerative granuloma of the pudenda", Journ. Trop. Med. and Hyg., 1909, XII, 10, 142-151.

(12) *Conyers, J.H. and Daniels, C.W.* -"The lupoid form of the so-called grain ulceration of this colony", British Guaina Med. Assoc. 1896, VIII, 13.

(13) *Driscoll, F.L.* -Erosive Vulvitis, Arch. Dermat. and Syph., 1920, XXXVIII, 170.

(14) *Donovan.* -"Piroplasma" and "Medical Cases from Madras General Hospital", Indian Med. Gaz., 40:414, 1905, vol. 39. -Also 1004, X, 321.

(15) *Daniels, Abutt and Rollestan's.* -"System of Medicine", vol. II, part II, 70, 1906.

(16) *Ehrich, W.S.* -"Granuloma Inguinale", Surg Gynnec. and Obstetrics, 40:107, 1925.

(17) *Fraser, A.A.* -"Granuloma Inguinale", British Jour. Dermat., 37:14, 1925. -Also in Journal of Urology, 13:227, 1925.

(18) *Flu, P.C.* -"Die Etiologie des Granulom Venereum", Arch. f. Schiffs, und Tropen Hyg., 1911, IX, 87. -También Centralb. f. Bak., 1912.

(19) *Fox, Howard.* -Granuloma Inguinale". Journ. Americ. Med. Assoc., Vol. 87, Nov. 27, 1926.

(20) *Frai W.* -"Eine neue Hautreacktion bei Lym, Phogranuloma inguinale". -Klinic. 4:2148.

(21) *Gougerot, H.* -"La Dermatologie en Clientéle", 1922. pg. 603.

(22) *Gage, I.M.* -"Granuloma Inguinale", Arch. Dermat. and Syph. n.s. VII, 303-325, March, 1923.

(23) *Golloway, James.* -"Ulcerating Granuloma of the Pudenda". British Journ., 1927, IX, 133, April.

(24) *Goodman, M.* -Ulcerative Granuloma", Journ. Americ. Med. Assoc., 1922, XXIX, 86-92.

(25) *Idem.* -"Ulcerative Granuloma", Urolog. and Cutaneous Review, St. Louis, 1923, XXVII, 86-92.

(26) *Grindon.* -"Granuloma Inguinale, with report of three cases". Journ. Cutaneous Diseases, 1913, XXXI, 236.

(27) *Hoffmann, W.H.* -"Das Venerische Granulom". Muenchen Med. Wchnschr., 1920, XVII, 159.

(28) *Iturbe, Juan y González, Eudoro.* -"Contrib. del Lab. Iturbe en el 3er. Congreso Venezolano de Medicina, 1921, pág. 21.

(29) *Johns, F.M.* -"Some observations on Granuloma Inguinale and cultural studies of the Donovan bodies", Proc. International Conference on Health Problems in Tropical America, 1924, page 440. United Fruit Company.

(30) *Le Dantec, A.* -"Précis de Pathologie Exotique", 1924, Tomo II, 817.

(31) *Litterer W.* -"Granuloma Inguinale", Nashville City Hospital, Journ. Americ. Med. Assoc. 1922, XXIX, 819.

(32) *Low, C.C. and Newham, D.* -"Ulcerative Granuloma", British Med. Journal. 1916, 11, 387.

(33) *Linch.* -"Granuloma Inguinale", Journal of Americ. Med. Assoc. 77, 925, Sept. 17, 1901.

(34) *Mac Lennon, A.* -"Memorandum on the observation of spirachaetoe in yaws and granuloma pudenda", British Med. Journal, 1906, II, 995.

(35) *Mac Roe, J.C.* -"Granuloma Inguinale and Syphilis", Jour. Americ. Med. Assoc., 84, 512, 1925.

(36) *Maitiand.* -"Etiology of Granuloma pudenda", British Med. Journ., 1906, I, 1463.

(37) *Manson-Bahr.* -"Manson Tropical Diseases", ed. S. London, 1925, pág. 478.

(38) *Martini E.* -"Ueber ein Fall von Granuloma venereum und seine ursache", Arch. f. Schiffs und Tropen Hyg., 1913, V. 160.

(39) *Idem.* -"Reinkultur des Erragos von Granuloma Venereum", Münch. Med. Woch.

(40) *Mc Leod K.* -"Precis of operations performed in the wards of the first surgeon Medical College Hospital during the year 1881". indian Med. Gaz., 1882, XVII, 121.

(41) *Morrisey P.G.* -"Granuloma Inguinale", Journal Tennessee Med. Assoc. Nashville, 1922-1923, XV, 106-107.

(42) *Mc Intosh, J.A.* -"The Etiology of Granuloma Inguinale", Journ. of the American Medical Association", Vol. 87, N° 13, September 25, 1926.

(43) *Randall, Small and Belk.* -"Granuloma Inguinale", Surg. Gynec. and Obstetrics. 1922, XXXIV, 717.

(44) *Raed and Walf.* -"Preliminary report on treatment of granuloma inguinale with exhibit of cases", New Orleans Med. and Surg. Journ. 1921, XXIV, 25.

(45) *Ross, C.F.* -"Granuloma Inguinale", Virginia Med. Semi-Month., Richmond, 1921-1922, XVIII, 579-582.

(46) *Rabello, E.* -"Pesquizas sobre o *Granuloma* Venéreo", Comunicacao a Sociedade Brazileira de Dermatologia, 1912.

(47) *Siebert, W.* -"Zur Aetiologie des Venerische Granulom", Arch. f. Schiffs und Tropen Hygiene. Vol. 16, N° 8.

(48) *Siebert, W.* -"Zur Aetiology des infectiesen oder Venerischen Granulome", Arch. fur Schiffs und Tropen Hyg. Vol. II, N° 12, 1912.

(49) *Schochet, S.S.* -"Granuloma Inguinale", Surgery, Gynecology and Obstetrics, 1914. XXXVIII, 759-767.

(50) *Shattuck, G.C.* -"Granuloma Inguinale in Boston". Boston Med. and Surg. Jul., 1923, XVIII, 530-532.

(51) *Steele, D.* -"An investigation into ulcerative granuloma of the pudenda, etc." The Lancet, 1912, XXXVII, 225.

(52) *Symmers, D. and Frost Albert D.* -"Granuloma Inguinale in the United States", Journ. Americ. Med. Assoc., 74, 1304, May 8, 1920.

(53) *Sabella, P.* -"Due casi di Granuloma Ucerosi delli pudendi guariti col Neo-salvarsani a Tripoli". Malaria (ital.), 1913, anno 4, N° 2.

(54) *Walker, E.L.* -"Etiology of Granuloma Inguinale", Journ. Med. Research, 1918, XXXVII, 427.

(55) *Weinberg, Milton.* -"Granuloma Inguinale", Journ. Urol. 1923, IX, 505-507.

(56) *Winfield, J.M.* -"A report of cases of so-called tropical granuloma observed in Kings Country Hospital", Medic. Record. New York, 1922, 57-60.

(57) *Wise, K.S.* -"A note on the etiology of Granuloma Pudenda", British Medical Journal, 1916, 1 y 11, 1274.

(58) *Calmette.* -"Manuel de Microbiologie et Sérologie".

YAWS IN VENEZUELA *

ETIOLOGY AND GEOGRAPHICAL DISTRIBUTION

The buba o bubas, pian, framboesia or yaws, is a chronic disease, produced by an organism (T. of Castellani) almost indistinguishable of the producer of the syphilis. With this sickness has clinical resemblance attacking the skin and the mucous in the recent stages and destructive bucco-pharingeal lesions in the last stages, giving a positive serology.

The buba has been also called *coko* in the Fiji islands; *Parangi* in Ceylan (this word means foreigner and is used for the natives to sign the European); *Dube* in Gold Coast; *Purru* in Malaya; *Boubas* in Brazil.

The producer organism was found by Castellani in Ceylan in 1906, in the spleen and lymphatic glands, very slender and subtile, and denominated T. *pertenue.* It is easy to see it by scrapping of buboes tissues, to the dark field or colorations as the Giemsa or silver nitrate as Fontana. It is a germ of 5 to 14 microns lenght, with regular spirals of one micros and sharp ends. Resembling organisms, not pathologic, are : in the mouth (Sp. dentium), in the throat (Sp. vincenti), in the intestine (Sp. eurygyratum), in ulcers (Sp. schaudinni), ubicuitous (Sp. refringens).

A strain of treponemas from Haiti and maintained in rabbits in John Hopkins Medical School during three years, showed differences of a strain of syphilis, isolated and maintained equally. 4 strains of T. pertenue and 7 of pallidum have been studied in order to see the lesions produced in the first generations, and in each culture, and observations have been made as characteristic of yaws or syphilis. Of 12 attempts to transmit human yaws to rabbits, only 4 had success; while of 7 to transmit syphilis, all had success. The T. pertenue is more malignant than pallidum in rabbits.

The yaws is spreaded between the tropics Cancer and Capricornio; it is very common in the West Indies: Jamaica, Haiti, Santo Domingo, Trinidad and a little in Puerto Rico; almost has disappeared in Barbados. In Cuba, with the entrance of people from Haiti and Jamaica for working in the sugar cane has had some cases in Cayo Manibí and later in Sagua (Oriental province) and so Pardo Castelló found 500 patients in december 1938.

In Central America it is a common disease in Nicaragua, Panamá, Costa Rica. There are details about the other countries. In Mexico, it seems not to exist. On speaks of cases in the United States and France, but the infection has been taken in the tropics.

In South America the yaws is common in the Guiennes, chiefly the english part; in the Amazon (Brazil); in Venezuela, where according data, are infected the District Federal and 15 States, as follows: Miranda, Aragua, Guárico, Carabobo, Cojedes, Yaracuy, Portuguesa, Zulia, Tru-

* Reprinted from the book "Estudios de Patología Tropical" 1942.

jillo, Mérida, Táchira, Anzoátegui, Sucre, Nueva Esparta and Bolívar. (We have seen it in the States Zulia, Barinas, Cojedes, Guárico, Miranda and Portuguesa); Western part of Columbia. It has been appointed in Perú. According to Rebagliati, the yaws is very extended in wild regions, calling it *cuchipe*. In 1935, only in the Loreto Department were found 2.105 cases, and possibly exist in other South American countries, perhaps undamaged the South-end.

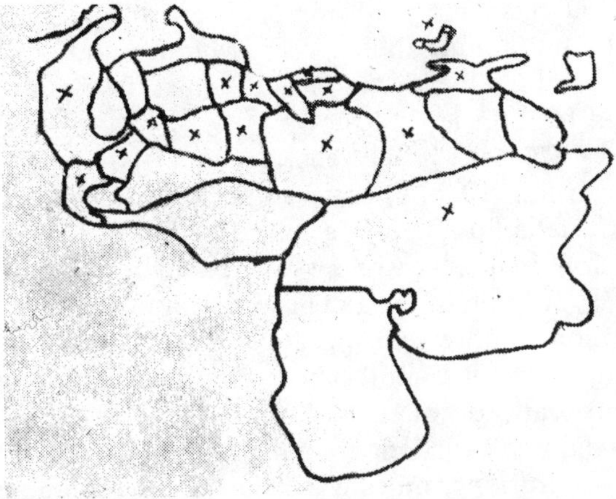

Map of Venezuela showing the probable distribution of the yaws in the country (District Federal and the States, including State Barinas). We have seen it in trips to those regions. It is almost sure that there must exist focus in other States and the two Federal Territories, coming to be and endemic spreaded in all Venezuela.

Africa is the Continent more affected, mainly the intertropical zone extended from the Atlantic Coast to the East - Indian Ocean. It is very frequent in Senegal, very common in Sierra Leona and Liberia. It exist in Ivory Coast, Gold Coast, Togo, Nigeria, Camerum, Africa Equatorial French, Rhodesia, Kenia, Belgian Congo, Tanganyka, Uganda, High region of Nile, Sudan anglo-egyptian, Madagascar. In Tripoli, twelve cases were reported in 1935.

Castellani said of cases in the italian Somaliland, in Bas-Uebi-Scebeli and Boulo-Burti, reporting 1.000 cases in 1936 and 1.502 in 1937 and more in 1938. In Eritrea, appointed 12 cases in 1936 and 9 in 1937. In Ethiopia, in the provinces of Amhara, Harrar and Choa, has not been found and the same in Libya.

Asia: in India: Assam, Burna and part of Bengala, Madras, Hyderabad. Very frequent, according Spitel, in Ceylan, Indochina, Siam, Malay Península, Dutch Indies, Philippines.

Some cases in Formosa. Frequent in the North and Central Australia. It seems to exist in the islands of South Pacific, including Melanesia and Polynesia.

PATHOGENY

The conditions of life in the endemic areas aid the direct contagion: lack of hygiene; promiscuity among numerous families; children mixed with cases of secundary yaws; wet nurses taking care of bubous children; boys that play with sick people or use the same utensils.

Bancroft, in 1769, said: "secretion there is always on wound covert of flies, that these insects later go to stop on ulcers or ripping, commonly not in white people, but among the negroes, whipped and often naked."

In 1770, Schilling believed that the yaws in South America was possibly carried for a little fly "the yaws fly."

Wilson in 1870, cited the general belief that in West Indies the sickness was transmited from person to person through flies.

In 1907, Castellani referring to this affection in Ceylan, told that: in accord his opinion, in many cases the yaws could be transmitted for insects and that was easy for him to see it in hospitals, inmediately that the patient with bubous lesions, undressed, was coverted for abundant flies trying to suck the secretion, and it is almost sure that later will go to do the same procedure on ulcerations not buboes of another person.

Castellani did two experiences: in the first took the exudate for scraping of buboes ulcerations, putting it inside sterile containers. After, introduced specimens of domestic fly and other species, during half hour. Examining the proboscis and paws, in two of them found spirochetes. In the second assay, several groups of flies were tested, during two hours on buboes ulcerations with positive treponema; smears made with the proboscis, two of them revealed treponemas.

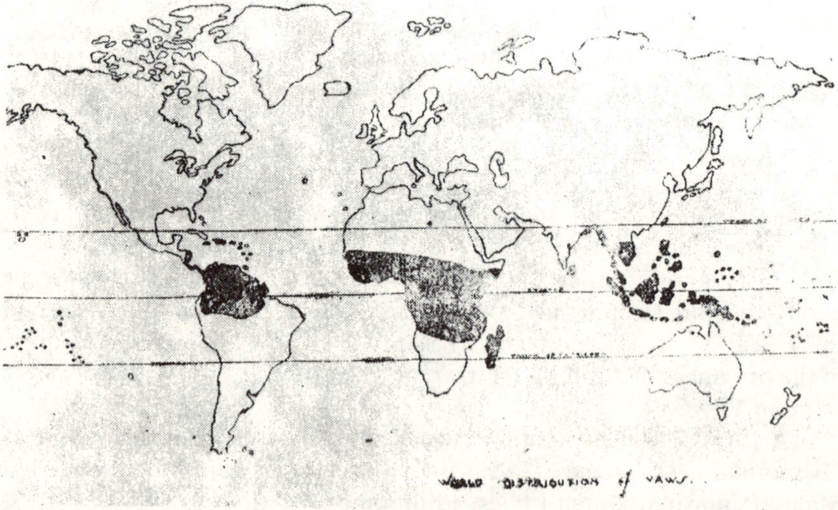

Map demonstrating the world distribution of the yaws. Four Continents, exception Europe, are attacked with this disease. It is an intertropical sickness.

In the Gibert's islands of the Polynesia, in 1908, Robertson took 200 specimens of flies caught sucking on buboes lesions and did a crush with distilled water and put it to centrifugate. In four of twelve smears found treponemas.

In 1910, Austen for observations in Dominica accused the fly Sarcophaga plinthopygia Wied., and Nicholls with an abundant material in Saint Lucy, said: "I believe that the majority of the cases of yaws are transmitted for the fly Oscinia pallipes." He mentioned that a fly abundant not in the town Castries, but in the rural zones of the island seeking the ulcerations of the arms and legs trying to suck any secretion. In 1930, Wilson and Mathis thought that the same fly Hippelates pallipes = Oscina pallipes was the transmissor in Hawaii.

In 1934, Thomson and Lamborn fed specimens of Mosca sorbons Wied. on buboes ulcerations, verifying treponemas in the dejections and that the protozons pass through the intestinal walls. Transmission will be done for the dejections or regurgitations.

The interesting research about the transmission for insects have been made by Kumm in Jamaica in 1934; .1.218 specimens of Hippelates were caught on the leg of a man in Cherry Garden in 15 minutes, or to be about 4. 872 in one hour. In another opportunity, on the ulceration of the leg of a monkey, in 15 minutes, caught 1. 395 Hippelates. Kumm wrote that in a fly has found 304 T. pertenue, one minute after the eating on a buboes lesion.

Seven to eight species of the genus Hippelates have been found in Jamaica, but the more frequent is the pallipes, and here is a picture of Kumm's work.

Sitios de captura	Número total de moscas Hippelates	Porcentaje del total representado por H. pallipes	Porcentaje del total representado por otras especies de Hip. no especie pallipes
Mount pleasant	31.071	97.13%	2.87%
16 otras localidades donde la buba es endémica.	10.748	93.99%	6.01%
Papine	70.474	80.01%	19.99%
Kingston	783	2.43%	97.57%
Capturas hechas en trampas de moscas en Papine y Mount pleasant.	1.654	1.65%	98.95%

Kumm's work

The factor seems to be very important. On human ulcerations, monkeys or dogs, the common specie is Hippelates pallipes; while placing traps with pieces of liver in decomposition, pallipes is scarce. Then, being the specie pallipes the most frequent on ulcerations, probably, will be the true transmissor from lesion to lesion. In 1933, in a total of 667 seizures were captured 117.476 flies of the genus Hippelates and of these, 98.580, or a percentage of 83.92%, were species pallipes. The male of this species, rarely feeds on the ulcerations. Of 2.266 killed and studied by Kumm in 1934, only 40 specimens, or to be a percentage of 10.13% were males that had sucked blood, and in two of them was found one T. pertenue, not moving.

The Hippelates introduced under the crusts, may be seeking to feed on more flesh, and it is not rare to find them under the crusts.

Researchers of Kumm have showed the size and situation of the esophageal diverticulum in order to appreciate the regurgitation or "vomit drops", fact possibly very interesting in the spreading of this disease. Have been found T. pertenue in these vomiting and in the stains of the regurgitations glued to the walls of the containers used. An Hippelates deposited 55 vomitings in the following 24 hours, after the eating on the ulceration.

The majority of T. pertenue sucked by an Hippelates remain active, more or less, 7 hours in the esophageal diverticulum; in the stomach lose the mobility; in the proboscis scarce specimens with little mobility.

To the following day of an infective eating, less than half of the insects presenting treponemas, and no spirochetes, two days later.

Hippelates were dissected daily until 14 days after the infected meal, and yet 21 and 28 days after, but in none of these tests were found treponemas; these results it seems verify that the T. pertenue has no development extrinsic, cyclical, in the fly.

In the inoculations in animals it has been verified that none has resulted positive. Monkeys and rabbits have been utilized and the intratesticular inoculation in this last one, according to Kumm, produced

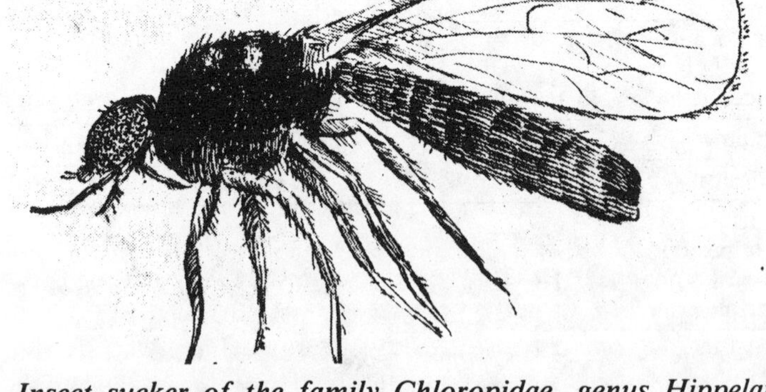

Insect sucker of the family Chloropidae, genus Hippelates, without to arrive to the species, found by us in the zone of Guarenas (State Miranda). Specimens of this same genus we have caught in Macuto (District Federal).

yaws in the rabbits, but it is necessary that the strain has been inoculated formerly to several rabbits. Sixty-five rabbits inoculated with material taken directly from the lesions have been successful; attempts with Hippelates from fly to fly were negative.

The genus Hippelates have demonstrated a clear helio and phototropism, but only to diurnal light not to the artificial, because never have been seen sucking during the night, always to diurnal hours; being very voracious.

The hours in which the Hippelates are very abundant are from 9 to 10 a.m.; before 6 a.m. and after 6 p.m. are very scarce. This, has been verified for seizures done for Kumm in three groups, to different hours and continued during ten weeks, in dry and humid stations. The same author demonstrated the influence of the wind, utilizing an anemometer, one minute before and one minute after the seizure, verifying that the abundance of the capture was on the inverse to the speed of the wind.

It has been important to take in account the temperature, observing that to higher temperature, higher captures, but it seems to be that the importance is the daylight. Referring to the rain, observations of Kumm in Jamaica (Mount Pleasant and Papine) demonstrated that in Paine in rainy season the number of sucking insects was greater.

The Hippelates never or rarely has been found inside the houses, they prefer to rest under the leaves of the bushes and frequently in Jamaica, in the tree Maranga maculata. These flies could maintained alives in boxes of Petri with sugar; few specimens have been rearing on humid soil and the larves could be fed on dung of dog mixed. Eggs have been obtained from females, fed with water and sugar.

We have caught exemplaires of the genus Hippelates in the region of Guarenas, to the borders of the river, accompanied for Simulium exiguum; also, we have done seizures in Macuto. In both times on arrived to the genus, but without to know the species, even helped by North American specialists.

SYMPTOMATOLOGY

The primary lesion, mother's pian or frambuesoma, often is adquired in the infancy and rarely is genital; however, it is seen in penis, groin, scrotal region, appearing inguinal glands, but not characteristic as in syphilis. The chosen sites are the discovered places, chiefly the low parts of the legs and feet. Spittel, in 32 cases, gives the following places: Buttocks, 2; thighs, 1; knees 2; high part of the leg, 2; low part of the leg, including ankles, 11; feet, 7; heels, 3; toes, 2; elbow, 1; forearm 1. Also are frequent places: the breasts of wet nurses, the mouth of the newborns nourished on breasts with lesions; the hips of women carrying the children to astride.

The incubation of the primary lesion is of 2 to 4 weeks, beginning for an itching papule and later vesicle. This one, for the scraping changes in a

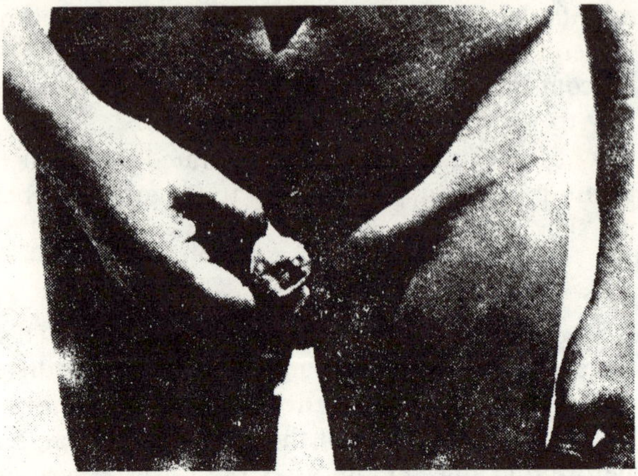

Frambesoma of the penis with positive treponemas. Boy of 10 years old, born in State Yaracuy. This localization is very scarce. Cured rapidly with bismuth (observation and photo given gently by Dr. Briceño Rossi).

granular, small lesion, exudative, crusty, that continues increasing, adquiring of a typical lesion of yaws, receiving the name of frambesia, similar to the raspberry.

The sickness continues slowly and this primary lesion remains six months or one year, and is called first period.

The secondary period is characterized for generalized eruption of several aspects: papular miliary as head of pins, diseminated or in groups; in form of lentil seeds; papule-scaly, papule-crusty, or also, as is frequent, numerous frambesiform lesions; equally, will be possible to see lesions in the commissure of the lips, in the vulva, nostrils, around the anus.

Sometimes, two or three frambueses can constitute all the secondary period and this brings confusion in the diagnosis or to appear tertiary manifestations after a long time, without to have appreciate secondary lesions.

In the negroes (color people) the secondary period of the syphilis is few ostensible, while the secondary period of the yaws is terrible, stage that they never forget and help in the history of the diagnosis between syphilis and yaws.

A group of frambesiform papules can appear in the place of the primary lesion, as has been seen in Ceylan. The cicatrization of the frambesia may appear from the center to the periphery or inverted appering in circle of dark pigmentation.

Slowly, the sickness pass to tertiary period, very similar to syphilis, and has two characteristic lesions: gummas and fibrous indurations. Among the variety of clinical manifestations, there are: gummany infiltration localized on the bones or ulcerations of the skin and subcutaneous tissues.

The yaws attack commonly the bones more than the syphilis and

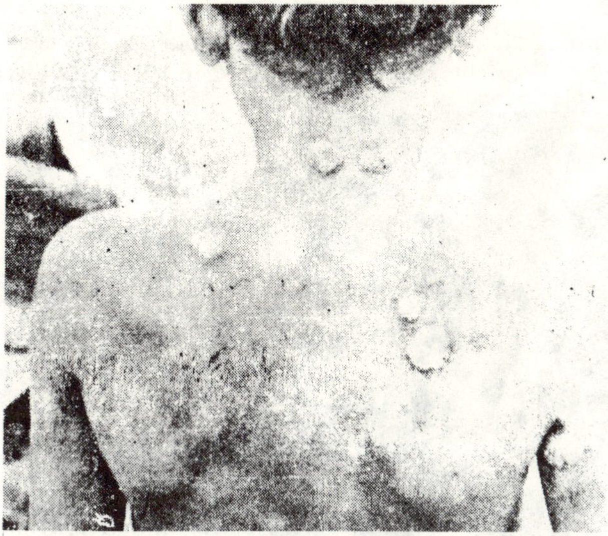

Photo done by us in the surroundings of San Carlos (State Cojedes). Boy, 12 years old, secondary period. Very net the frambesiform lesions.

chiefly those near the cutaneous surface, as tibia, malleolus, humerus, ulna, radius and places of insertion of the muscles, and so, probably, traumas and tractions are prejudice.

In the nodules and infiltrations appear ulcerations with granular tissue. Necrosis could happen with expelling of osseous fragments, coming later very ugly cicatrizations.

In the diffuse infiltration under the periosteum, there are increase, alteration of the Harver's conducts. The tibias take the aspect of a saber, called in Australia "boomerang legs", enlarging ahead to behind. In 17 cases of boomerang legs, 88% had negative Wassermann.

In the nose and palate there are communication between mouth and nose. The lesions extending lips and cheeks. Sometimes, through this cavity, it is possible to see the tongue, the pharyngeal wall, the hole of the trumpets, the sphenoidal sinus. This picture is called in some regions "gangosa."

The nodes yuxta-articulars appear in knees, ankles, elbows. It seems to be characteristic of the yaws. Ferrer Viera, if we are not mistaked was the pioneer to signed these nodes between us. This patient was seen by us.

The frambeside is another characteristic of the tertiary bubous period. The scars are cheloid in yaws, while in the syphilis wrinkled. Are situated in any site, but frequently on buttocks, back, etc., increasing slowly, employing one or several years.

Other important troubles are the lesions on the nervous system and the circulatory aparatus. In Jamaica, among 12.500 persons examined, 13 were found with neurological troubles.

According Nicholls, in the asylum for buboes of the island of Saint Lucy, of 2.353 patients admitted from 1882 to 1910, 1.444 were males and

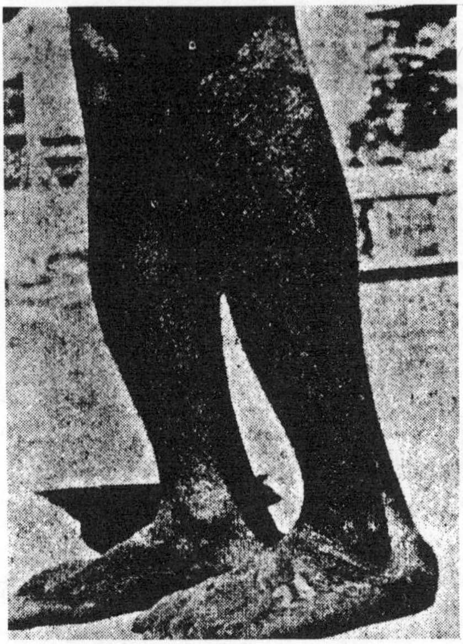

Boomerang legs or legs in saber of the tertiary period. Photo of an Australian native. It has been taken from the Hackett's work. This type of legs are easy to find in Venezuela.

909 females. The population of the island in that time was of 20.839 males and 22.919 females. The percentage referring the age was the following:

0 - 10	11 - 20	21 - 30	31 - 40	41 - 50	51 - 60
43.6	26.1	12.9	11.5	4.5	1.1

Infected zones: Castries 3.4%; Villegas 33.2%; Rural completely 63.2%.

In the Philippines in 26 cases (15 males and 11 females), the youngest was 17 years and the oldest 48 years. Seventeen patients (65.4%) had ages under 25 years, from several provinces; 23 cases presented renal lesions; 20 cases ulcerations and scars in pharinx; 3 with lesions in larinx. The test of Wassermann gave 8 positive + + + +, 8 positive + + + and 10 weakly positive. The Wassermann in cephalorachidean liquid was always negative.

In these patients it is very difficult to distinguish between syphilis and yaws. Besides, we have diseases with similar lesions, as the leishmaniosis and paracoccidiosis. Cases of these sickness we have seen often with the finding of the parasites.

Spittel tested the cephalorachidean liquid in 9 cases of secondary period and 5 of tertiary period. In the first group, exception one weakly positive, were negative. In the second group, 2 gave result weakly positive. It was not an increase of cytological elements, not globulines, concluding that it seems that the nervous system is not attacked by the yaws.

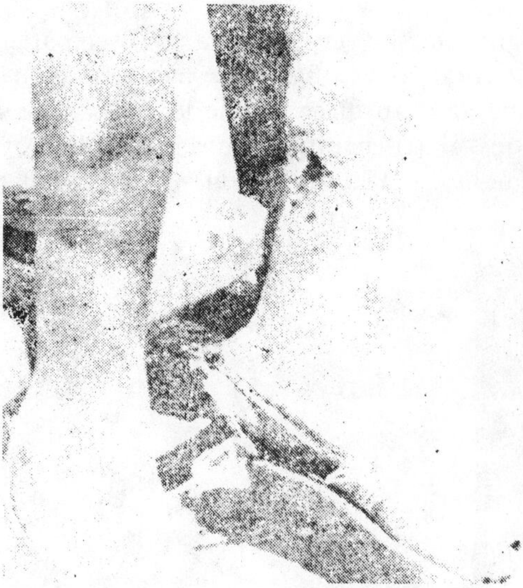

Photo made by us in the surroundings of Pedrazas (State Barinas), showing the osseous lesions and the scars characteristics of the yaws, different from the syphilitic scars. Boy of 10 years old.

Chamber in 1.000 autopsies done in Haiti, said: ''there is no histopathological differentiation, either in aorta, nor in other organs, in order to distinguish syphilis and yaws. Concluding that in 5.4% of those autopsies found aortic changes owed to syphilis or yaws.

Fernando and Ocampo, from the Philippines, thought that the test of cephalo-rachidean liquid could be very useful in the diagnosis of tertiary lesions of nose and throat of syphilis and yaws; being positive in the first and negative in the second, because yaws does not attack the nervous system.

These authors also remark that syphilis and yaws could be different in the primary and second stages, because in the third it is very difficult. The Wassermann, the histo-pathological cuttings does not have a definitive value. The same treatment. Many times the yaws improve rapidly to arsenic, in other cases are very resisting.

The yaws are not hereditary. Maxwell (1893), Baermann and Hollenberger (1916), Mass and Bigelow (1922), Rogers and Megow (1930), Hermans (1931), Martlett (1933), Stannus (1935). In 6.500 histories and examinations made in Jamaica of patients with yaws, in none was congenital lesions or birthmark.

DIAGNOSIS

The principal differentiation is with its sister the syphilis. The history and the clinical signs must be very important. If the patient explains that he comes from the rural zones, that never has suffered of genital lesion, that had, long time ago, an ulcer on the leg, and after an eruption of frambesiform lesions. Later, painful lesions in the plant of the feet, tibias enlarged, scars of nodes sticked to the bones. All these manifestations are in favor of yaws.

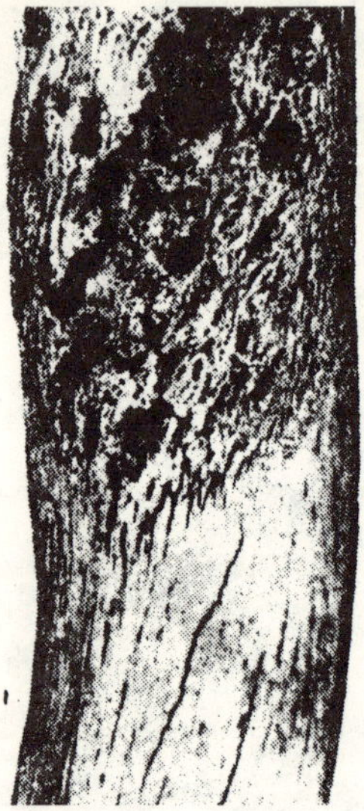

Section of bone showing the lesions (tibia).

Some affections of the skin, perhaps, can produce a certain confusion; as the same manner, the appearance of an epithelioma in the site of the scar.

YAWS	SYPHILIS
Not congenital	Hereditary
Not reciprocal immunity	Mucous membranes often attacked. Rare itching
Primary lesion extra-genital	Alopecia and iritis
	Cirrhosis
Characteristic frambesiform lesions	Gumma of the liver, kidneys, testicles
Itching. Desquamation furfur	Nervous system attacked: myelitis, nervous cranial paralysis. Gumma in brain and marrow. Tabes. General paralysis. Endo-arteritis obstructive. Trombosis vessels of the brain. Arteriosclerosis. Aneurisms
Lesions in the plant of the feet	
Scarcely attacks the muccous	
Not alopecia	
No lesions of the eyes	

Visceral lesions very scarce	The attack on the human being is stronger
Nervous system rarely attacked	General damage on the organism
Histo-pathology: infiltration peri-vascular and proliferation endothelial	Attack vital structures, the yaws attack the conjunctive tissue
It is better supported than the syphilis	
Slight general attack	
Eruption more exuberance	
Cheloideal scars	
Often lesions in legs	

PROPHYLAXIS

The prophylaxis may be individual or general:
1 - To cover the lesions.
2 - Desinfection or destruction burning the material employed in the dressing.
3 - Isolation and to avoid the direct contagion.
4 - To submit the ill to treatment promptly.

GENERAL

1 - Hygienic measures in the infected zones.
2 - To fight against the flies.
3 - To avoid passing suspicious cases to undamaged zones.
4 - When an undamaged country is to return the person attacked, notify the Sanitary office.
5 - Any way the physicians or persons advice the cases to the chief of Sanitary Services or Commission for yaws if there is a campaign against the yaws.

TREATMENT

The yaws, as the syphilis, are cured with arsenic and bismuth, because the mercury is slow; however, Spittel is partisan of the use of KY and Hg in the tertiary period.

Spittel prepared a solution, as follows: iodide of mercury 3.24 grams; iodide of sodium 28.42 grams; solution of phenolphthaleina 0.5% 1 c.c.; Na OH (sol. 25%) 2 dracmas; distilled water 100 c.c. The solution prepared is acid, but the Na OH changes it to alkaline. The treatment with this solution should be one injection weekly of 6 to 8 c.c., arriving 6.

It is not rare to observe diarrhea, fever, gingivitis, chills, malaise.

While the eradication of syphilis is difficult, in yaws it is different, and Spittel, said: "If the eradication of the syphilis it seemed a task of Sisifo; referring yaws we thought different". Pardo Castelló said that it was completely mistaken to believe that the yaws is cured with 2 or 3 injections of arsenic. This illness is so difficult to treat as the syphilis; the patient improve, but it is necessary a long treatment, because, often the lesions relapse and the ill person is infected again.

This author in the campaign against the yaws in Cuba brought two patterns of treatment, for children and adults, using arsenic and bismuth, alternating with periods of repose; checking with tests of urine and blood; to practice annually serology.

One or two injections of arsenic disappear all the signs and symptoms of the secondary period, leaving in the places of the lesion a slight pigmentation. Gumma and tertiary lesions also cure with only one injection. The osseous lesions are more resisting, but disappear the strong pains.

In Nigeria, Wilson recommended the acetylarsan, employed in both stages. In the cases of "gangosa" is very good. The serology comes to be negative, result not obtained with the bismuth.

In Nigeria and Tanganyika, Dale has used arsamilato de bismuth in injections with very good results (Bi 2 03 53% and arsenic 17%).

The best campaign about the study and treatment of the yaws has been done in the years 1932, 33, 34, 35 and 36, for the Jamaica Yaws Commission. The serology demonstrated almost 100% of positivity.

Recaídas o lesiones persistentes en pacientes bubosos tratados

Número de tratamientos	Tratados con neoarsfenamina				Tratados con salicilato de bismuto			
	Lesiones a los 5 meses		Lesiones a los 11 meses		Lesiones a los 5 meses		Lesiones a los 11 meses	
	Número de casos seguidos	Porcentaje con lesiones	Número de casos seguidos	Porcentaje con lesiones	Número de casos seguidos	Porcentaje con lesiones	Número de casos seguidos	Porcentaje con lesiones
1	51	19.6%	39	30.7%	46	6.6%	28	10.7%
2	107	14.9%	83	30.1%	115	15.6%	93	23.7%
3	181	9.7%	142	14.8%	147	10.9%	126	13.5%
4	441	12.2%	315	20.3%	293	6.5%	221	14.5%
5	177	9.0%	75	25.3%	139	5.7%	70	8.8%
6	288	5.9%	102	12.8%	270	7.4%	111	16.2%
Total	1.245	10.5%	816	20.3%	1.010	8.3%	649	15.3%

In 1933, the plan consisted in eradication of all the infected cases, control and discovery of the relapses, checking to intervals the area, in order to appreciate the work and the progress of the treatment. The Commission tried to see the effect of the arsenic and the bismuth and had two unities: inspection and treatment. The first, for one or two inspectors preceded the second, doing a visit to each house. The unit treatment had medical chief, major official and inspectors. The areas Castleton, Rock River, Belfield, Clommel and Red Wood, were submitted to the arsenic and controlled in different times. Redcood was not checked.

The areas Richmond, Brainard, Broad gate and Troya were submitted to the action of bismuth and controlled later, several times.

The following tables taken of the cited work, showed more relapses in the patients treated with arsenic than in those treated with bismuth. At the end of one year the results were not satisfactory in 20 % of the cases treated with arsenic and 15% in the cases treated with bismuth.

CAMPAIGN IN VENEZUELA

The Ministry of Health started in the country in the beginning of the year 1930 a campaign in order to eradicate this disease, commencing for the Department Vargas del Distrito Federal and the States Miranda, Yaracuy and Carabobo. The plan was similar to the campaign of Turner and Saunders in Jamaica. The medicament used was bismuth in 6 injections, and sometimes 9.

In certain cases were used 10 or more injections. Bismuth was the choice, because it is easily handled, less dangerous and the price is lower. Turner and Saunders obtained a percentage of success of 92%, using the arsenic and 85% using the bismuth. A 7% of difference.

It was an organization of 3 commissions, each one of physician chief, an inspector and two assistants; without technical of laboratory. The patients were divided in patients of prophylaxis and patients of assistance. The first were subdivided in two groups: some ones presenting lesions in evolution, and the other ones, without evident lesions, only had 5 years with the sickness. Are patients in latency and just Turner and Saunders observed that the relapses (85%) appeared in that type of sickness. The patients of attendance are those that have suffered with the illness for a long time, not contagious, are human beings not apt to work and cause a problem to the economy. In this group were included those suffering of the two late accidents of the yaws.

The Commission of the Departamento Vargas found that the parish Macuto was undamaged; Caraballeda, with 26 patients; Naiguatá, with 107; Caruao, with 307; Maiquetía, with 6; Carayaca, divided in three sections: Carayaca, with 32 of prophylaxis, Chichiriviche, 129 of prophylaxis and 89 of assistance, and El Limón with 139. In total, 835 ills in the Departamento Vargas. Controls done for the Commission 6 months and 1 year after the treatment in the parishs: Caraballeda, Carayaca, Naiguatá and Caruao, gave the following results: the two first, free of new cases; Naiguatá, 4 new cases in the village of La Hondonada on a total of 35 patients seen and treated formerly, and in the small village Los Caracas, 2 cases on 33. In Caruao, was 14 new cases on 307 seen before and treated, distributed, so: small village La Sabana none; in this site had been treated 86 patients, 27 contagious; small village Caruao none; when this settlement was treated had 44, 13 contagious; small village Todasana, two cases, having been treated 6 sick, 2 contagious; settlement Uritapo 3, having attended 57 sick, 18 contagious; settlement Chuspa 9, formerly were treated 114 patients, 63 contagious.

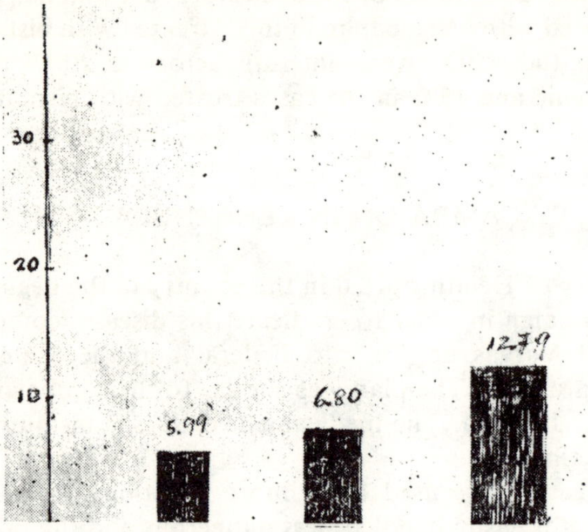

State Yaracuy

The campaign in State Miranda was divided in two sections: Tuy section and Barlovento section.

In the first arrived to the amount of 915 patients, distributed in the Districts Sucre (La Carlina, La Mata, Requena and San José) and Paz Castillo (small villages Quintana, Turgua, Cedralito, Playa Grande, La Caiba, El Manguito, La Secreta, La Vega, Tun Tun, Mamonal, El Volcán, El Milagro, La Vigilia, Las Plazas, Las Adjuntas, Santa Rita, El Loro, San Vicente, Urapal Arriba, Urapal Abajo, Boca de Siquire, Palmar del Siquire, El Placer del Siquire).

The Barlovento's Commission for december 1939 had treated 1947 sick, of them 729 of assistance and 1.213 of prophylaxis and had in treatment 1.437 patients more. This campaign include the villages and settlements, following: Guayabal, Aricagua, Chirimena, Carenero, Higuerote, Sotillo, Las Colonias, Curiepe, Birongo, Ganga, Tacarigua, Maturín, La Fundición, Los González, Los Martínez, Los Araminas (including Aramina La Maravilla, Aramina Los Toros, and Aramina Los Serranos), El Colorado, La Trinidad, Velázquez, Mayoral, etc., Rosalía, Belén, El

Toro, Santa Teresa (village and surroundings), Sauce, El Negro, Quebrada de Agua, Agua Amarilla, Casupo El Medio, Los Dos Caminos, Morocopo Arriba, Casupo Hurtado, Banqueo, Los Flores, Los Mermales, Morocopo Abajo, Las Marías and Trinidad.

STATE YARACUY

Were studied three districts: Nirgua, Urachiche and Yaritagua, including the 40% of the global population. It was found a percentage of infection of 12.79%. The ends for all the villages were 1 to 37%. Referring to the districts amounts were: Nirgua 15.34%, Urachiche 8.34% and Yaritagua 6.65%.

Taking totally the area studied, patients of prophylaxis and assitance were, more or less, of 50%, with very few predominance in prophylaxis.

Almost all the sick were treated, having obtained 91.87% of healings.

Absolute numbers and percentage of infection for yaws, distributed for Districts in the States Yaracuy and Carabobo (1939 to 1941).

DISTRITOS	Población censada	Total de enfermos	Enfermos por 100 habitantes
Nirgua	17.580	2.698	15.34
Yaritagua	5.007	333	6.65
Urachiche	3.222	269	8.34
Estado Yaracuy	*25.809*	*3.300*	*12.78*
Bejuma	4.513	425	941
Montalbán	3.623	250	6.90
Valencia	346	108	31.21
Estado Carabobo	*8.482*	*783*	*9.23*

STATE CARABOBO

Were studied the districts Bejuma, Montalban and Valencia (only the rural part of this one); besides, the district Falcón of the State Cojedes. The census included a 15% of the total population.

The percentage of infection was of 10%, being the ends of 2 to 37% in all the area. In the districts separated the amounts were: Bejuma 9.41%, Montalbán 6.90%, Valencia (rural zones) 31.31%. The 77.42% of the patients found were treated.

CONCLUSIONS

1 - The yaws is very probable, a disease spreaded to all the country. It is appointed in District Federal and 16 States. We have seen it in 6 States: Zulia, Barinas, Cojedes, Guárico, Miranda and Portuguesa.

2 - It is almost demonstrated and accepted that the indirect contagion of this disease is made through insects of the genus Hippelates. Specimens of this genus, not arriving to the species, have been caught by us in Guarenas (State Miranda) and Macuto (District Federal).

3 - We presented a case of frambesoma of the penis (patient of Dr. Briceño Rossi) and photos of cases with lesions of the secondary and tertiary stages. We exposed to have seen nodes yuxta-articulares, legs in saber, destructive rhino-pharhngeal lesions, etc.

4 - We did a good and large exposition about the treatment employed in different countries and wrote the campaign done in Venezuela in the Departamento Vargas of the District Federal and States Miranda, Yaracuy and Carabobo.

5 - The bismuth has been the medicament used in this campaign and currently for the low toxicity, easy handling and low price. In Jamaica, Turner and Saunders employed the arsenic and the bismuth, seeing only a difference of 7% among the effectiveness of both. The standard treatment in Venezuela has been of 6 injections of bismuth (bivatol, insol-bi and others) of 2 c.c., arriving sometimes to 10, 12 or more injections, obtaining the whitening of the patient.

6 - In the Departamento Vargas, exception Macuto, all the parishs were infected, finding the number of 835 sick. In the State Miranda, the campaign was divided in two zones: Tuy and Barlovento. In the first, were found 915 patients, and in the second, december 1939, had been treated 729 sick of assistance and 1.218 of prophylaxis; 1.437 more of prophylaxis were in treatment.

7 - We showed tables giving account of the works in the State Yaracuy and Carabobo. In the first were studied 3 districts, arriving around the 40% of the population and finding an average of infection of 12.79%. The ends

were of 1 to 37%. The percentage for the districts was: Nirgua 15.24%, Urachiche 8.34%, and Yaritagua 6.65%. It was obtained a 91.87% of healings.

8 - In the State Carabobo were studied the districts Bejuma, Montalbán and Valencia (rural part) and the District Falcón of the State Cojedes, arriving around 15% of the total population. The average of infection was of 10%. The ends of 2 to 37%. The infection for districts, was the following: Bejuma 9.41%, Montalbán 6.90%, Valencia (rural part) 31.21%. 77.42% of the patients found were submitted to treatment.

Our acknowledgement to Drs. Curiel and Mejía, chiefs of the Division of Epidemiology and Venereal Diseases by their help and advices.

BIBLIOGRAPHY

Reports of the Jamaica Yaws Commission.-Government Printing Office.-Kingston, Jamaica, 1932-1933-1934-1935-1936.

R.L. Spittel.-Framboesia trópica.-Bailliere, Tindall and Cox-Londres. 1923.

D.B. Blacklock.-Yaws and Siphilis.-Annals of Tropical Medicine and Parasitology.-October 1932.

Philip Manson Bahr.-Manson Tropical Disease.-1935.

Fco. Alfonzo Rivas.-Contribución al estudio del agente patógeno de la buba. Tesis doctoral.-1906.

W.A. Lamborn.-The experimental trasmission to man of Treponema pertenue by the fly Musca sorbens Wied.-The Journal of Trop. Med. and Hyg. Oct.1936.

L. Nicholls.-Framboesia Trópica.-A short review of a colonia report concerning statistics and Hippelates flavipes. Ann. of Trop. Med. and Paras.-Liverpool, Oct. 1936.

V. Pardo Castelló.-Frambesia.-Imprenta Librería Nueva.-Habana. 1938.

Frambesia.-Estado actual de esta enfermedad en Cuba.-Vida Nueva.-Feb. 1939.

Cecil J. Hackett.-Boomerang legs and yaws in australian aborigines.-Transactions of the Royal Society of Trop. Med. and Hyg. July 1936.

H. Chambers.-Review of the pathology observed in 1.018 post mortem examinations in Haití. U.S. Navy Med. Bull.-1936.

Antonio S. Fernando y Geminiano de Ocampo.-Wassermann's reaction of the cerebrospinal fluid in the diagnosis of yaws of the nose and throat.-The Journal of the Philippine Islands Med. Assoc. June 1938.

C. Wilson.-The treatment of yaws with acetylarsan.-The West African Medical Journal.-June 1937.

H.D. Chambers.-Further light on the "yaws-syphilis" problem.-Transactions of the Royal Soc. of Trop. Med. and Hyg.-June 1937.

Aldo Castellani.-Le pian dans les colonies italiennes.-Office international d'hygiene publique.-Bulletin Mensuel.-Feb. 1939.

Ildemaro Lovera.-Contribución a los estudios clinico, serológico y sanitario de la buba. Tesis doctoral.-1938.

Leonard Rogers and John W.D. Megan.-Tropical Medicine.-1939.

OBSERVATIONS ABOUT THE CARATE IN THE DISTRICT PERIJA OF THE STATA ZULIA *

The carate is a dermatomycosis very frequent in the District Perijá of the State Zulia. The borders of this District, are: North, line going from the mouth of the river San Juan, to the site known Paso de la Candelaria on the river Palmar; South, rivers Lara and Santa Ana; West, Republic of Colombia, and East, lake of Maracaibo.

Doctor Madina Jiménez in his interesting work entitled "Las Afecciones Micósicas en Venezuela", published in 1925, referring to the geographical distribution, spoke about a large focus in the plains of Zamora extending toward South to the rivers Apure, Arauca and Meta; by the North, toward a little portion of the States Mérida and Trujillo; West, State Táchira, and East, the State Portuguesa.

Besides of this principal focus do mention of four secondaries focus: one, in the District Perijá of the State Zulia; another one in the State Lara; one third, in the District Buchivacoa of the State Falcón, arriving to the Lake of Maracaibo, through the Districts Miranda and Bolívar, and a fourth focus, small, in the State Miranda.

He says in one of his paragraphs: "De modo que si se exceptúa el pequeño foco mirandino, puede decirse que los carates son afecciones del Occidente i del Sur de Occidente de Venezuela, pues en las regiones centrales i orientales son casi desconocidas".

The disease seems to have been introduced, long time ago, by colombian people through the frontier. Colombia is a country with many caratosos and in the zones infected, the percentage is of 4%, according Montoya.

Machiques, capital of the District, is the cradle of the carate, because all the caratosos seen by us, the 100% were born in that village. Others small villages as Las Piedras, San José, La Villa, presented some cases, but rarely. A decrease of this affection is appreciable in last years; seeing only around twenty cases. Before, on spoak with afraid of Perijá. We knew the wife of a Governor that was drinking mineral water, avoiding to be infected, during seven months. In this diminution of the sickness has had influence the use of the arsenic.

Between the population of Perijá are several versions about the transmission: for ingestion, scrapping the scales; taking bath in places named *pozos,* with the stagmant water, and the sting of some insects, abundant to the rivers Apon, belonging to the family Simuliidae. Lutz in his book "Estudios de Zoología i Parasitología Venezolanas" determina 8 species.

* Published in the book "Trabajos Científicos" 1936

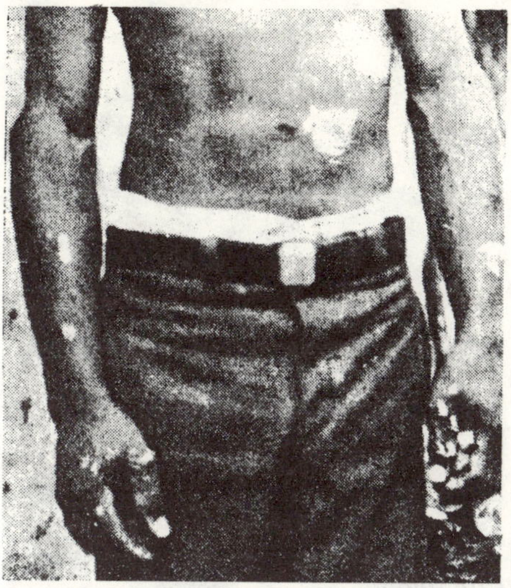

Fig. 1

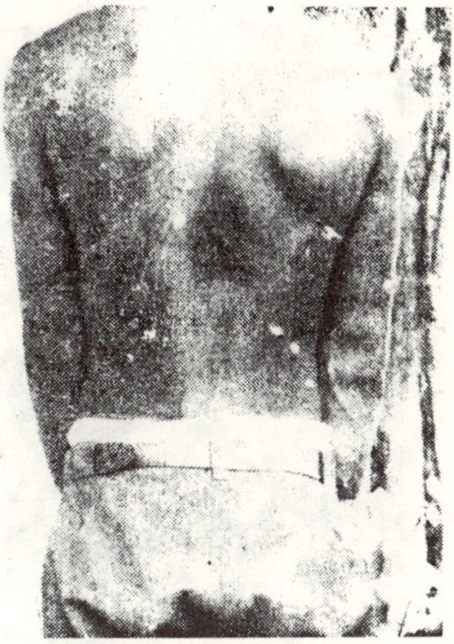

Fig. 2

We met the case of a man, 61 years old, infected long time ago, variety white, married three times and had fifteen sons, and none of the family ever presented carate.

In farmers as Yasa in a total of thirty persons only three had carate; Now then, nevertheless the promiscuity of their lives there is not transmission. Between them the percentage is of 100%; the disease starts in early age and in both sexes. All our patients were men.

The disease seems to start for a large lesion in any place, salient, itching; after continue coming out smaller lesions simultaneously.

The general aspect of the patient is of good appearance; some of them speak of fever, but it is zone of malaria. The examination of the fresh blood and smears are normal. The differential white blood count is normal with light eosinophylia.

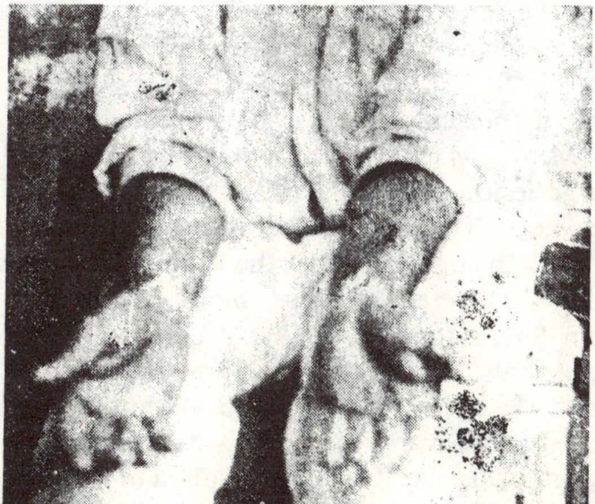

Fig. 3

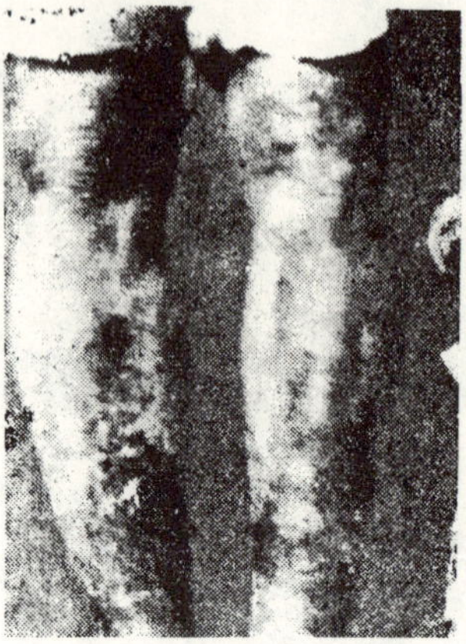

Fig. 4

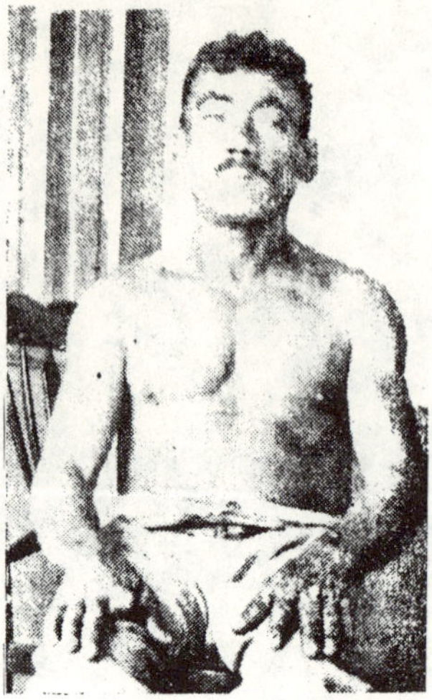

Fig. 5-Case of blue carate-
Notice the lesions on the hands.

The lesions continue presenting desquamation, itch and taking different colors. In accord with patients the lesion suffer a lot of colors. We did not see troubles in the nails and mucous membranes. According to González Urueña the blue variety is very frequent in México and the variety white is doubtful.

Frequently the lesions are more abundant in the sites more exposed to the sun, and in the hands are common in the joints, called "picadura". All the patients were from low social class. Two of them were white.

We took scales and seeding in Sabouraud' medium. The inoculation we did in the back of guinea pigs, scraping the skin. Fifteen days later the skin appeared dry and bright. Taking scales and putting them in Sabouraud gave the same fungi inoculated. The scales were taken of an incipient case and a case of blue carate since was a child. When taking the scales around the lesions the hair falls easily. Montoya said about a folliculitis. The inoculations disappeared spontaneously, after forty five days.

Summary of four cases that we have studied:

Case N° 1 - M.M., Machiques, 30 years old. Two months started the carate for large lesion in abdomen, very itching; after, new outbreaks. General aspect good. He has a brother caratoso. Living with the brother it is correct to think in contagion, but the fungi are different in both. Fresh blood negative - Differential white blood count: Lymphocytes 26%; Mono-medium 9%; Mono-large 1%; Neutrophiles 60%; Eosinophiles 4%; Basophiles 0%.

Cultures of the scales in Sabouraud, 48 hours after development of colonies greenish, increasing the color with the time. Test with hidrate sodium only epithelial cells. The fungi resulted to be: Aspergillus nidulans. The classification of these fungi has been made by Ch.W. Emmons of Columbia University. Our acknowledgment.

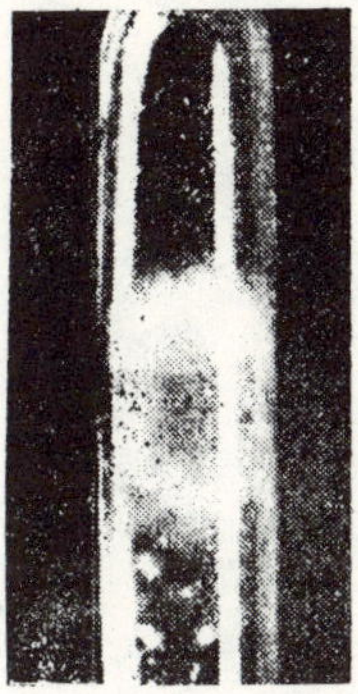

Culture of case 1 - Aspergillus nidulans. Sabouraud medium.

Fig. 6

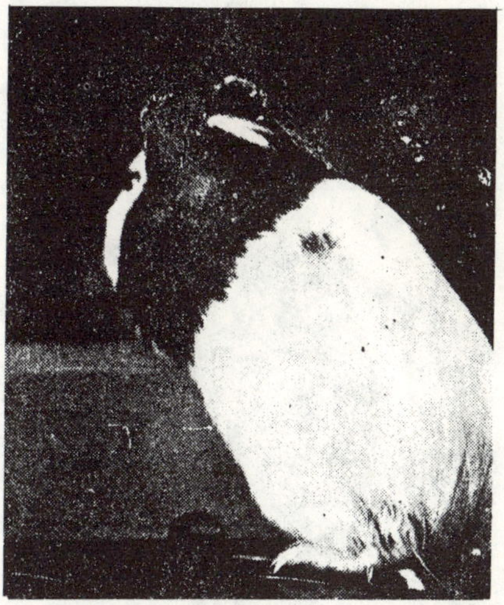

Fig. 7

Lesion in the back of a guinea pig, 15 days after the inoculation.

Case 2 - H.M., 72 years old, born in Machiques, husband epileptic, promiscuity in the faminly, brother of the former case 1. The culture of the fungus likes cotton on over the surface of the medium. Classified, resulted to be: Fusarium sanguineum.

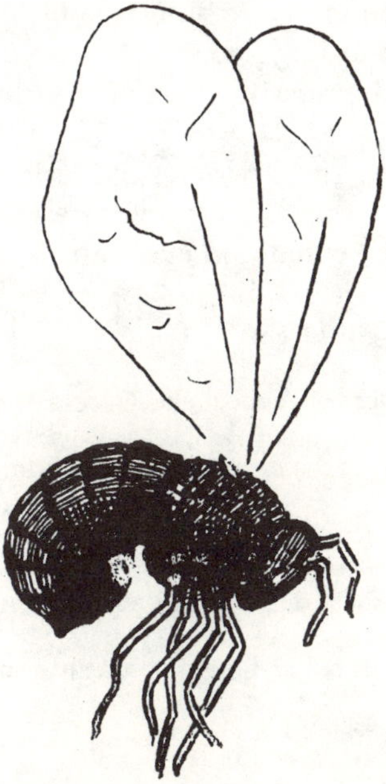

Fig. 8 - Simulium sp. very abundant in the borders of the river Apón. Accused by the people as transmissor of the carate.

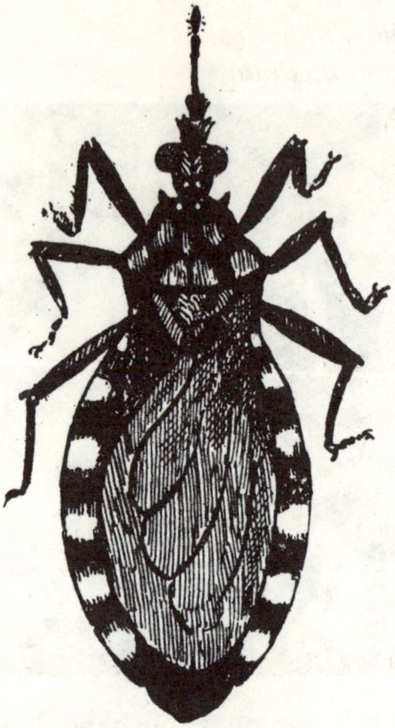

Fig. 9 - Spiniger rubropictus H.S.

Case 3 - L.R.N. born in Machiques, 35 years old, husband suffering of blue carate in different parts of the body.

The color of the culture at the beginning is white, but after blackish. Test in fresh blood negative. differential white blood count: Lymphocytes 26%, Mono-medium 12%, Mono-large 5%, Neutrophiles 55%, Eosinophiles 2%, Basophiles 0%. The classification of the fungus resulted to be: Cephalosporium curtipes.

Case 4 - N.N., 55 years, Machiques, rural people, old lesions caratosas. Two other caratosos in the same farmer. In the cultures there are two fungi: Penicillium matris meae and Penicillium cyaneum.

BIBLIOGRAPHY

Medina Jiménez.-Las afecciones micósicas en Venezuela.-Gaceta Médica de Caracas.-1926.

J.B. Jiménez.-Nota clínica acerca de tres casos de actinomicosis humana.-IV Congreso Venezolano de Medicina.

Castellani & Chalmers.-Manual of Tropical Medicine.

Escomel.-La blastomicosis humana en el Perú y Bolivia.

Martín Vegas.-Los carates o carares.-Revista del Centro de Estudiantes de Medicina.-1918.

Eudoro González.-Algunas observaciones sobre hongos parásitos encontrados en Venezuela.-1922.

Brumpt.-Précis de Parasitologie.-4° edition.

Varios.-Geografía Médica del Zulia.

R.P. Strong.-Harvard African Expedition.-1926-1927.

VOYAGE A MENE MAUROA
CONTIBUTION A L'ETUDE DU CARATE DANS L'AMERIQUE TROPICALE

Published in Paris, France - Year 1932 - Jouve and Co.

On peut définir le carate, selon Peña Chavarria et Shipley (1) "une dermatose tenace, cliniquement caractérisée par prurit, desquamation et troubles pigmentaires de la peau".

L'année dernière nous avons publié un petit travail sur cette question (2). Comme nous l'avons dit, le carate de Perijá est seulement un petit foyer secondaire, et nous répétions une fois de plus, ce qu'a écrit le Dr. Medina Jiménez (3) quand il se réfère á la situation géographique, en signalant un grand foyer dans les plaines de l'Etat de Zamora, en s'étendant vers le Sud jusqu'aux fleuves Apure, Arauca et Meta; au Nord vers une petite partie des Etats de Mérida et de Trujillo; à l'Est dans l'Etat de Portuguesa et à l'Ouest dans l'Etat de Tachira.

En plus de ce foyer principal, il signale quatre foyers secondaires: un foyer dans le district de Perijá de l'Etat de Zulia; un autre dans l'Etat de Lara; un troisième dans le district de Buchivacoa de l'Etat de Falcon, envahissant jusqu'au lac de Maracaibo, à travers des districts de Miranda et de Bolívar, et dernièrement un quatreième foyer de petite extension dans l'Etat de Miranda (4).

Ce troisième foyer secondaire qui en partie se trouve dans l'Etate de Zulia est celui que nous avons étudié dernièrement et duquel nous apportons ici quelques observations.

Nos idées sur cette maladie ont changé depuis, et nous commençons notre étude en disant que le carate est une dermatomicose. Par les études faites dernièrement, surtout au Mexique, et par ce que nous avons observé, le rôle que jouent les champignons dans le carate est un rôle tout à fait secondaire et beaucoup des investigateurs (5) les ont cherchés en vain chez beaucoup de malades.

Nous ne croyons pas que ce soient les champignons les producteurs du carate:

1° Parce que ces champignous n'ont aucune spécificité; depuis Montoya jusqu'à nos jours les variétés de champignons sont trés nombreuses, et parmi ceux que nous avons trouvés, nous n'avons pas encore vu qu'on peut considérer, comme nous dit le Dr. Emmons, qu'ils soient capables de

(1)-Contribución al estudio de los carates de América Tropical.-Rev. Med. Latino-Americana.-1925.

(2)-Observaciones sobre el carate en el distrito Perijá del Estado Zulia.

(3)-Las afecciones micósicas en Venezuela.

(4)-Selon une communication verbale du Dr. A. J. Fernández, il y a un autre foyer sur les rives du fleuve Orinoco, surtout dans les tribus Piaroas et Goahibos.

(5)-Folkes, Med. Rev. Mississippi.-Castellani, Observations on some diseases of Central America.-J. Trop. Med. Hyg., 1925; Arch. Dermat. y Syph., 1928.

produire des lésions comme celles du carate.

Les inoculations que nous avons pratiquées antérieurement et que nous faisons constater dans notre travail, et que nous avons considérées comme positives, aujourd'hui avec un peu plus d'expérience, nous savons que nos cultures en Sabouraud, pratiquées 15 jours aprés avoir inoculé le cobaye par scarification de la peau, avec du matériel pris par grattage du lieu de l'inoculation, ont très peu de valeur, parce que certainement les champignons qui ont germé et que nous avons trouvés étant égaux aux innoculés, ne seront autres que ceux que nous avons mis sur la peau du cobaye, et qui seront restés saprophitiques sur la peau de l'animal.

2° Depuis quelques années les habitants du Perijá prenaient des pilules mercurielles pour se guérir du carate; on faisait de même au Mexique, (6) et à l'ingestion de mercure on ajouta des frictions du même médicament. Dans l'autre travail, nous avons fait constater que le nombre des malades au Perijá a diminué d'une façon remarquable, puisque le natif sait qu'au commencement, deux ou trois piqûres de neo-salvarsan suffisent pour le guérir. (7) Même dans les anciens cas, dans lesquels n'existe qu la tache acromique finale, où on trouve des vestiges de prurit et de desquamation, ces deux symptômes disparaissent, l'acromie persistant, qui est inguérissable; cependant au Mexique on a observé, dans certains cas, de faibles pigmentations ces taches après le traitement arsenical (8). Les Mexicains ont employé le bismuth avec succès. Jusqu'à présent pour le traitement par ces médicaments, nous ne croyons pas qu'ils agissent sur les champignons. Cependant en acceptant pour l'arsenic une certaine efficacité, quoique dans quelques affections de la peau il ait réussi, comment s'expliquer l'action du mercure et du bismuth? Si on guérissait avec de l'iode, avec des sels d'argent, spécifiques pour les champignons, on le comprendrait. Pourtant l'épreuve thérapeutique est une raison de plus qui, nous le croyons, vient détruire la théorie micosique.

Le carate, paraît-il, est une infection générale (9), et probablement d'origine spécifique, et peut-être c'est la cause de la grande quantité de Wassermann positifs chez les malades et la grande action du traitement mercure-bismuth-arsenical, et encoré on peut croire que ce soit un germe en spirale de nature inconnue avec des manifestations de prédominance cutanée. Les inoculations qu'on a pratiquées au Mexique en se servant du sang et des dilutions de biopsies prises des lésion, n'ont pas réussi.

Il y a une théorie sympathique défendue par González Guzmán et

(6)-Según González Urueña (Primer Censo del Mal del Pinto en la República Mexicana.-1929-1931.-Departamento de Salubridad Pública.-1934) en el Estado de Guerrero que es el más infectado, en 554.570 censados, halló el 23.67% de infección, y en 15 Entidades Federativas (Michoacán. Oaxaca, Puebla, etc.), en una población de 2.496.808 censados encontró un porcentaje de enfermos de 10.84%.

(7)-En trabajo último, Pardo-Castelló ha obtenido magníficos resultados con arsénico y bismuto en Cuba (Revista de Medicina Tropical y Parasitología, Bacteriología Clínica y Laboratorio) 1936.

(8)-Communication verbale du Dr. Galo Soberon y Parra.

(9)-Voir le travail: Is carate (pinta) a dermatomycosis. Annual Report. United Fruit Company, 1930.

González Herrejon y Pallares (10) dans laquelle le principe du carate serait une auto-intoxication particulière des tropiques et probablement d'origine intestinale, de telle manière que le carate serait finalement la manifestation cutanée d'un système sympathique malade. Cette théorie nerveuse ferait ressembler le carate au vitiligo.

* * *

Nous sommes sorti de Maracaibo un matin du mois de mars et une heure après nous arrivâmes à Puertos de Altagracia; nous continuons à La Estacada, Bureau de la British Controlled Oilfields. La gentillesse de M. Rapapport, gérant de la dite compagnie, nous offrit un troley, et nous arrivâmes à Mene Mauroa, qui se trouve à une distance par voie ferrée de 54 kilomètres.

La végétation dans ce parcours n'est pas trop exubérante, surtout dans la première vingtaine de kilomètres; mais à cause des abondantes pluies les arbres sont fraichement verts.

Durant le parcours nous avons pu voir le sibucara (Bombax Carabobense) Pittier, le curieux indio desnudo-indien nu-(Bursera simaruba) L., la maya (Bromelia chrysantha Jacq), le barredero (Croton rhamnifolius), l'abondant aritibar (Ipomea abutiloidea) H.B.K. avec ses nombreuses fleurs blanches qui enchantent le paysage, le araña-gato (Fagata pterota) L., le pendare avec une floraison jaune qui attire le regard du voyageur, el zorrocloco (Morisonia) L., le dividive (Caesalpinia coriara) Wild et le cuji (Piptadenia flava) Benth.

Mene Mauroa, est un village de l'Etat de Falcon divisé en deux parties: une de ces parties appartient à la British, située sur une colline, et c'est la plus saine; l'autre partie qu'on appele El Pueblo, sa fondation est une conséquence des travaux pétrolifères. La population du village est actuellement de 2.500 habitants environ et de 600 maisons toutes avec le toit en zinc.

La British avait à notre disposition une automobile avec laquelle nous sommes allé au village El Consejo, centre de ce foyer secondaire de carate du district de Buchivacoa de l'Etat de Falcon et des dictricts Miranda et de Bolívar de l'Etat de Zulia. La distance est de 25 km. environ à travers un mauvais chemin. A mi-chemin nous traversons une rivière et nous sommes sur le territoire de l'Etat de Zulia.

La végétation est exubérante parfois dans ce chemin et nous trouvons le caudero (Mimosa cabrera) Karst qui est très abondant, et on dit qu'il guérit les morsures du tigre; la guadua (Guadua latifolia) Kunth, le cabimo (Copaifera Langsdorfii) Desf, le tártago (Ricinus communis) L., et les cactacées, parmi lesquelles le Cactus caesius Wendl, le gigantesque caracaro (Enterolobium cyclocarpum) Griseb, la pringamoza (Jatropha Kumthiana Müll et Jatropha urens L), el algodón de seda (Calotropis procera) Ait.

(10)-González Guzmán. Algunas ideas acerca de la fisiología del mal del pinto.-Rev. de Biol.

Dans certains lieux la végétation devient rare et nous trouvons des petites plaines qu'on appelle Sabanas del Consejo, oú nous avons trouvé un palmier d'une hauteur de 2 à 3 mètres appelé Palmiche et dont les natifs utilisent les feuilles pour construire la toiture de leurs maisons, et le mastranto (Hyptis suaveolens) Poit, dont on brule les tiges pour chasser les moustiques.

El Consejo est un petit village de l'Etat de Zulia avec une population de 600 habitants, comprenant les environs.

Le carate n'est pas très abondant dans cette région, il paraît qu'on exagère un peu, et nous n'avons vu que 8 cas. Le carate chez eux est plus honteux que chez ceux de Perijá; ceux-ci ont de la maladie une conception plus nette. Le malade de El Consejo ingnore d'où provient la maladie, comment s'effectue la contagion et comment on peut la traiter (11). Tous ces cas avient des taches noirâtres, sauf un qui les avait de couleur bleue, et que nous avons rencontré pendant le trajet de Mene à El Consejo. Les jambes ont le même aspect que chez les habitants du Perijá, la peau devient sèche, crevassée et avec de grosses écailles.

Quelques-uns des malades ont de la fièvre, mais la cause peut être le paludisme, et l'etat général ne s'altère point. Il n'y a pas chez eux l'idée de la transmission par les insectes. Un autre des villages infectés est Rio Chiquito près de El Consejo.

Les examens en frais et les frottements avec coloration panoptique ont eu des résultats négatifs. Les formules leucocitaires normales.

Dans quatre cas on a pris des écailles de la peau et elles ont été semées au milieu de la preuve de Sabouraud, elles ont donné des colonies de champignons vingt-six heures après. Les colonies du tube n° 1 sont rondes, plates et pendant la fructification prennent une couleur verte. Au microscope c'est un champignon cliosonné de petites spores rondes et de couleur faiblement verte. La culture du tube n° 2 est au commencement de couleur blanchàtre et après d'une couleur rouge. La culture n° 3 est d'une couleur blanche. Celle du n° 4 est un penicillium des spores grandes, rondes et vérdâtres.

On a pratiqué des inoculations par scarificaitons de la peau chez deux cobayes et un singe. Celle de celui-ci fut complètement négative, de même que l'inoculation chez un des deux cobayes. L'inoculaton de l'autre produisit dans la peau de l'animal, quelques jours après, une légére desquamation, avec un aspect luisant de la plaque et la chute facile des poils environnants quand on les tire. Le grattage de cette plaque, vingt jour après, et en semant les écailles en Sabouraud nous avons obtenu les mêmes champignons que nous avons inoculé sur la peau. Un mois après, la desquamation cessa, les poils poussèrent et la peau revint à son état normal. Antérieurement nous avons dit comment nous apprécions les résultats de

(11)-Dans notre travail antérieur, nous avons cité un moustique que nous avons rencontré à Perijá, classifié aux Etats-Unis comme étant du genre simulido. Des moustiques de ce même genre ont été cités par Montoya en 1898. Actuellement on espérimente au Mexique avec des tiques et des punaises.

ces inoculations.

Actuellement M. le professeur Langeron (12) qui nous a reçu avec amabilité est en train de classifier ces champignons et nous l'en remercions beaucoup.

Enfin le carate est une infection qui mérite d'être étudiée, puisque la Colombie a 400.000 malades environ, et le Mexique 300.000. Nous admirons l'école mexicaine pour les importantes études qu'elle a faites dernièrement sur cette question.

(12)-Hasta ahora no hemos tenido noticias sobre la clasificación de estos hongos.

"CARATE" OR "CARARE" IS TODAY ONE OF THE MOST CURABLE DISEASES. VENEZUELA MAY HAVE ABOUT 50,000 PEOPLE WITH THIS DISEASE. A CAMPAIGN AGAINST IT IS NECESSARY. *

Caracas-March, 1936. There is a disease which is very odd, very rare and very interesting because no one knows its cause or how it is transmitted; but, fortunately, and I want to emphasize this, today there is a cure for it. This ailment to which I am referring is called Carate or Carare.

This disease is a problem for many countries such as Columbia which has about 400,000 people with the disease in a population of 9 million; Mexico has 300,000 in a population of 18 million, and in Venezuela, if a count were taken, we would probably find about 50,000.

Venezuela has a great source of Carate located in the state of Zamora, and five small sources located as follows: one in the district of Perijá, state of Zulia; another in the state of Lara; a third in the district of Buchivacoa, state of Falcón; a fourth source of small range in the state of Miranda; and lastly, a fifth among the tribes of Gohaibos and Piaroas on the shores of the Orinoco river in the state of Bolívar.

Judging from the geographical distribution of this disease in our country, it seems to have come to us from Colombia, since the great source is in Zamora; and from the data we obtained from the source at Perijá, one of the districts of the state of Zulia, we clearly saw that it has been brought over the Colombian immigrants.

A person with Carate is an outcast. Since it is an ostensible disease as leprosy, everyone feels disgust for a person with Carate.

In Maracaibo, many years ago. people spoke of Perijá with horror because of its Carate; and to think of going to that place was like a nightmare. We know of a woman from Maracaibo, wife of an ex-governor of Perijá, who, during seven months that she spent in that region, ate only eggs and soda water for fear of being infected. When we were in Mene Mauroa, a bordering town between the states of Falcón and Zulia, as soon as we arrived at the Carate center of that region called El Consejo and asked for the assistance of the Commissioner for whom we had a letter from his superior, he told me: "Doctor, I can assist you in anything, except in gathering up the people with Carate," since this man was afraid that if he insisted in having them do something, these would retaliate by infecting him with the disease.

The cause of Carate is unknown, since the theory of the fungi which were always considered as its producer, was destroyed by our two strong objections. The first objection is that fungi have no specificity, and many

* Published in the book "Trabajos Científicos"-1937-Editorial Elite-Caracas.

times we find in a person with Carate, two or three different fungi which, when inoculated or ingested, do not produce the disease; the second is even more decisive: Carate is cured with the same three medicaments with which syphilis is cured. Until now. these medicaments are not known to produce any effect on the fungi.

The transmission of this disease is unknown. In Perijá I met a patriarchal gentleman of about sixty years of age who had married three times and had twenty children, and who had never shown, nor his wives or children, any manifestation of Carate. During the same journey, I came across a plantation with thirty laborers among which two were infected, and despite the promiscuity in which these people lived, sleeping in the same hammocks and eating with the same utensils, etc., the disease had not become contagious.

An honorable gentleman from the state of Barinas was telling me that he once saw a man with Carate wounds on his foot. The bleeding was contained with rags as is usually done among the poor. During the incident, a pig and a donkey approached the area and ate the blood-filled rags. Twenty days later, both animales showed signs of Carate on their bodies. What we thought to be mere hearsay, lately we find, by reading some Mexican publications, that Carate is transmissible to animals.

In Perijá, and not too long ago in the state of Zamora, on the shores of the Socopó river, we have gathered mosquitos which the inhabitants of those regions claim to transmit the disease. Strangely enough, these same mosquitos were accused thirty-eight years ago by a Colombian gentleman by the name of Montoya y Flores, of being the ones to transmit the disease.

Through the publication of this article, I want the people of Venezuela to know that Carate is curable. (1) With a hygienic campaign, we will be able to see in several years the almost total elimination of ths disease from our country.

Today, a person with Carate, just as the leper, has realized that his illness is curable and he no longer sees the doctor and society as his enemies. In Quebrada Seca, a town in the state of Zamora, it was enough to have someone say that a doctor was coming to do a study on Carate, for me to have in a matter of minutes between thirty and forty patients ready for any type of examination or treatment. During that same occasion, I was able to see a poor woman to whom I had offered a box of bismuth injections as treatment, walk several kilometers to Barinas to pick up my small present, all in the interest of being cured.

Carate is curable with arsenic, with bismuth and with mercury. Arsenic is the most active, being enough six injections of Neosalvarsán to see the disease disappear; however, we have noticed that the people in the

(1) According to R. Sanguinetti Rangel-living in Santa Bárbara, state of Zamora-he has treated ninety cases (ages: ten to seventy years old; sex: 62 M. and 28 F.) withing a period of nine years. All patients have been submitted to a bismuthic cure (Muthanol), needing only a box each (10 injections), with the exception of two cases which have needed two boxes each. Among the ninety cases, he mentions a case of relapse and another of resistance of failure.

infected areas use Neosalvarsán very little because of its high price and the lack of people in those places capable of applying intra-venous injections, using then Sulfarsenol, Acetilarsán, etc., injections which are applied intra-muscularly.

Bismuth is used the most, and among the various compounds, the most renowned is Muthanol. One box is sufficient to see a patient cured.

Nowadays, mercury has been the first medicine which has successfully cured the disease. Years ago, witch doctors exploited this business. In Zamora, I learned of a woman witch doctor who charged a hundred "pesos", as we used to say it then, for curing a person, a treatment which was discovered later, and turned out, to be with mercury applied as much internally as externally. This medicament has had the difficulty that these people have used it ad-libitum, and this has caused illness of the mouth, kidneys, etc.

Carate is curable in any of its colorations "with the exception of the white spotting which has no cure." (2)

We wish that this small publication arrive at all the infected areas of the country, any may we have eradicated in a few years this depressing and repulsive disease.

(2) In the state of Zamora, according to popular belief, very good results are obtained on these achromic spots using gum-resin from Tampaco or Isfuque (Clusia rosaeflora - Gutiferous).

THE "CARATE" IN VENEZUELA *

(With the collaboration of Dr. A. L. Briceño Rossi)

CHAPTER I

DEFINITION - HISTORY - ORIGIN GEOGRAPHICAL DISTRIBUTION

The carate, carare or cute, as is called in Los Andes, is an odd and curious disease. The study of it attracts because its origin has had many stages; its transmission is still unknown, but fortunately for the persons that suffer of it, the healing can be obtained, mainly at the beginning.

It is a chronic dyscromasia, adquired after the age of 3 or 4 years in accord with our observations, invading almost all the body, without fever, existing at determinated places of México, Columbia, Venezuela, as also in Center-America countries and islands of the Caribbean: Cuba (Fox, Pardo Castelló, Sáenz and his school); Haiti; in South American countries: Ecuador, Perú (Escomel), Bolivia, Brazil (Ramos E. Silva), and probably in the Philippines and Africa.

Perhaps, with the name of Carate have been catalogued different illness. We have seen patients sent of the interior of the country or of surrounding countries, listed carate, and later, being examined, have resulted cases of pityriasis, vitiligo, leukodermias post pityriasis. Colleagues have sent us descriptions of some patients and it is easy to see confusions in the diagnostic.

The carate has several names in the different nations and so the carate or venezuelan cute may be the quirica from Panama; the kcaras of the valleys of Arequipa and Vitor that have been cited by Escomal in Peru; the Mal-azul in Bolivia; the Puru-puru in Brazil; la guasarola of the Dominican Republic; the cative of Central America; la busarola of Haiti; the picuití of Guadalupe; el mal del pinto of Mexico; the lota of Guayana; the carate of Colombia. Not withstanding, it will be not rare another one affection in the large field of the dermatology.

Still now, there are doubts about the origin of the Carate: american or african. Peña Chavarría and Shipley in noteworthy monograph bring to explain the american origin, the book "Historia de Indias" of Oviedo, where referring about the transportation of the notable caribes for the slaves indian carates, says: "al indio que naturalmente tiene toda persona o la mayor parte de ellas, como descostrada, levantados los cueros a manera de empeynes. Ellos parescen feos, mas comunmente son recios e de mejores fuerzas é parescen frisados, é aquella frisa es dolencia que se acaba cuando ha acabado de les andar todo el cuerpo toda aquella comecon o en-

* Published in the book "Estudios de Patología Tropical"-Caracas-1942.

fermedad é han mudado todo el cuero de la persona''.

The Oviedo' description does not seem to be in accord with the general symtoms of the carate and besides, this is a disease that does not disappear spontaneously. In that time, the promiscuity and uncleanliness for those indians, helped the development of multitude of diseases of the skin.

On tell it was a letter of Hernán Cortés sent to the Emperor Charles V, where in a paragraph, told: ''en este país de ventura existen rarezas en el color de sus habitantes, presentando variedades''.

José Casani, missionary preacher, wrote the ''Historia de los Jesuitas en el Reino de Nueva Granada'', did mention about the spots in the Tunebos, signs of beauty and necessaries to get marriage between them.

Some of the mexican authors sympathizing with the american origin bring to critical comparison the indian word *tzalzayanalixtli* meaning carate; and Dr. Francisco Fernández, physician of Felipe II, told in a book that he left, referring to the qualities of the plant *ixtenexti:* ''que su raiz machacada i puesta sobre lienzos deshace i limpia la lepra lo mismo que el zarpullido i también cura la enfermedad llamada: *tzalzayanalixtli''*.

Relating to the african origin, it is unknown yet, we believe that this illness may exist in that continent, because the descriptions of european authors have been made through references.

It is possible that the negro slaves, so they brought the pigmentation and plagues, as the hookworm and yellow fever, also brought the carate. In recent days we see scourges imported from Africa to America, as the importation of the Anopheles gambiae, transmissor of the malaria carried by the traffic between Natal and Costa de Oro.

Relating our opinion we are partisan of the american origin of this disease, as we think about syphilis, her sister, because we have observed virgin tribes of virgin indians: maquiritares, piaroas, goahibos, places unknown for negros, where the carate is an ancient disease, transmitted from fathers to sons, with paternal spirit loving, of beauty for the progeny and tribe.

The first in the study in Venezuela of the carate it seems to be J. J. Freites, Freites Pineda and Antonio M. Pineda, perhaps ought for living near the secondary focus of Sarare in the State Lara.

After, Dr. Medina Jiménez, in several scientific works about mycosis, published in the Gaceta Médica de Caracas (1913-1916); later, in ''Afecciones Micósicas en Venezuela'', 1926, speak about his investigations in this field, thinking in a fungus genus Malassezia, as cause of the stains.

Martín Vegas, being student, observed some cases of the region of Guatire, finding fungi, searchs published in the Revista del Centro de Estudiantes de Medicina, 1918.

The doctoral thesis of Padilla, 1907, being made long time ago, when there was difficulty and scarce the bibliography, is very interesting.

He says that the carate is a disease known in America before the discovery in 1492, being the etymology probably of tamanaco or caribbean origin. It is known that the caribes, in accord with Rojas and Jahn, in their conquest from South to North, impose, between another thing, their language, and it seems to be, the word *carate* or *carare,* word compounds of *gua,* that means spot; *ra,* sprinkled, and *are,* river or rivulet, that together should be: stain sprinkled of the river. Truly, in Mexico and referring to our observations, all the focus of carate are to the borders of the rivers, giving origin to the hydric theory very accepted some time ago.

In the vocabulary of several indians tribes there are many words like the word carare, designating things with any similitude of the skin of a patient with carate, and so, we see that the morrocoyo is called *ahará* or *huarará;* some trees named *carapa* and *carateo* have different spots in leaves and stems; the word *caraire,* stamps the tiger by his stains in the body.

The word *Sarare,* name of a village in the State Barinas, center of a secondary focus, it seems to be that some years ago was called *Carare.* The refreshment very known, called *carato,* perhaps its name comes that exist the belief that was used perversely for transmitting the disease profiting the heterogeneous aspect of beverage.

The caratoso is a person with moral decayed, faded the spirit like the leprous. We make memory, sadly, of the history of a Governors wife of Perijá that related us that in the period of seven months living there, ate only eggs and acidolous water of fear of becoming infected.

We make also memory that traveling to El Consejo, village between the States Zulia and Falcón, center of a secondary focus of this illness, begging to the police chief to help us to gather some caratosos for some investigations, answered: "doctor, I can help you in everything, but less in to meet the caratosos". It was the fear of becoming infected by revenge.

The slow progress of the country, the roads and paths, the influence of the oil companies, our preachments since the year 1931, have going modifying that complex of the caratoso, and so, four years ago in a trip to Barinas, in Quebrada Seca, region which almost all of the inhabitants have the disease, doing the offering to treat and cure the patients, some time after, we were surrounded by a hundred of ills disposed to suffer any kind of tests. In the same region we could see the interest of the caratoso in his healing, because with the offer, a box of ampoules of bismuth, some of them walked several kilometers, distance between Pedrazas and Barinas.

This disease, Panneus carateus of Alibert or Karataflek of the Germans, it is a problem for some countries. So, we see that in the census of Mal del Pinto in Mexico, published the year 1934, made under the direction of González Urueña, found in some States, as Guerrero, that it is the most infected: in 554.570 persons, 131.315 sicks or a percentage of 22.67%. In the State of Mexico of 93.763 persons, 32.570 displayed the infection or 34.67%, and in a whole of 15 States with 2.496.000 persons there, was 270.585 or a total percentage of 10.84%. In Columbia, since the monograph of Montoya, knew that in the infected regions the percentage arrives to 4% of the population.

In Cuba, for the works that we have in hands is scarce, the same in Brazil, in the areas central and coast, because in the Amazonic zone it is frequent in indians. In Central America, in accord with the studies of Castellani in Honduras and Panama, it seems to be very common in certain regions; in Peru, in accord with Escomel, it is not frequent.

In Venezuela, about our opinion, the carate is an illness that must be had and regarded with attention; we believe that with good sanitary campaigns it will be possible to erradicate it.

The carate is an endemic for Venezuela, as it is for Colombia and Mexico. Recently, we found that the infection in the municipalities of Pedrazas and Quebrada Seca, in State of Barinas arrives more than 50%, and the whole State 10%. In census verified in municipality of Pedrazas or Ciudad Bolivia we have found in 600 inhabitants distributed in the small villages: Mijaguas 113; La Caldereña 15; Las Monjas 28; Palmasola 26; Anime 43 and Curbatí 36; in total 261 caratosos being an alarmant figure. In other near settlement to Pedrazas, in 136 residents there was 59%.

Today it is not an aesthetic problem affecting deeply the psychology of whom has it, but, it seems to be a general sickness with positive serology and attack the lymphoid organs and aorta.

The carate, we think goes invading our nation. At present exist a main focus in the State of Barinas, that invade toward the South till the rivers Apure, Arauca, and Meta; to the North toward a small portion of the States Mérida and Trujillo, to the East encroaching upon the State Portuguesa, and the West, the State Táchira. Besides this central and pricipal focus there are five secondary focus: one, in the District Perijá of the State Zulia; another one, in the State Lara, in the region of Sarare, extending in accord Padilla and Pérez Carreño to the State Yaracuy and Carabobo; one third, in the District Buchivacoa of the State Falcón, region called Mene Mauroa, arriving till the Lake of Maracaibo, through the districts Miranda and Bolívar of the State Zulia; a fourth focus, in the region of Guarenas, Guatire and Caucagua, in the places Naranjal, Oruza, Copure and Canare, in the State Miranda, and another one fifth focus between the indians maquiritares, piaroas, goahibos, tamanacos, etc., focus that in accord with Alvarado arrives through Meta i Casanare to the bordering Colombian focus, and through the region Rio Negro, till Brazil.

In summary, seeing the joined may the Carate is an endemic from West and South-West of our country. We have infected the States Barinas, Apure, Mérida, Táchira, Trujillo, Lara, Zulia, Carabobo and the territories Delta Amacuro and Amazonas. Total; 12 States of the 20 that the Republic has and the 2 territories.

The largest distribution toward the West think that the carate came from Colombia and could be the first Perijá, and comes in affirmation of this idea that the focus of Perijá by its antiquity try to disappear, as is observed in epidemiology. In Machiques, capital of the District, speaking with old people, told us that many years ago, arrived from Colombia exiled politics, between them the Zeledon Family showing all the signs of the sickness.

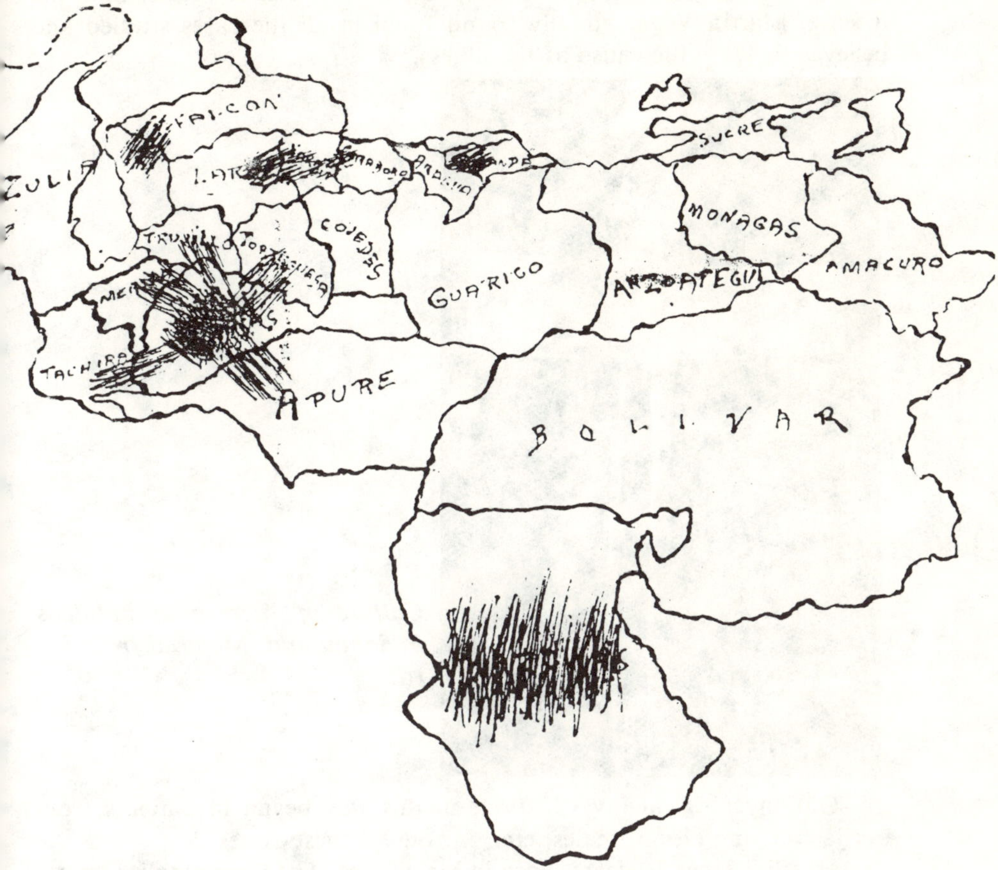

Map showing the geographical distribution of Carate in Venezuela.

CHAPTER II

ETIOLOGY OF THE CARATE

We consider two stages in this CHAPTER: the montóyica and the post-montóyica, rather, the mycological stage and the spirochetal stage.

The first started at the end of the last century (1898) when the Colombian Montoya i Flores published his thesis "Recherches sur les caratés de Colombia", that possibly acquired celebrity to be made and published in Paris and written in french.

After this work, the investigators of all parts of the world, found and saw fungi in any lesion and Mexican, Colombians and Venezuelan finish accepting this origin. Medina Jiménez says that in the skin there are many saprophytic fungi, but conclude accepting a Malassezia as the origin of the disease. Martín Vegas equally found fungi in all the cases studied and believes they are the cause of the illness.

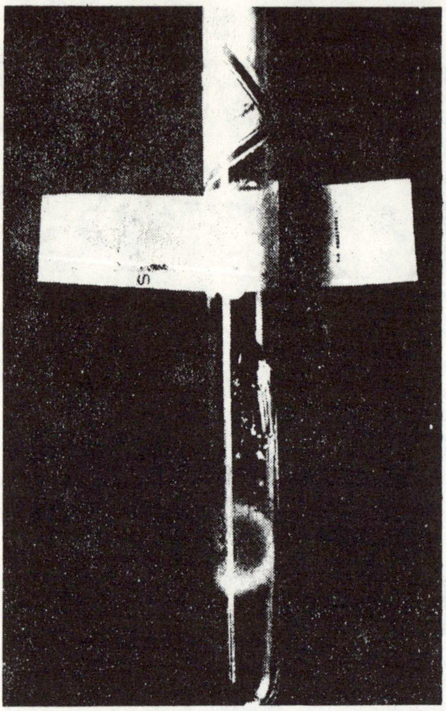

Culture of Aspergillus nidulans in Sabouraud. Material from Perijá.

Our mycological investigations in this way began in patients from Perijá studying blood, scales, etc., in four of these zones.

1° - Sick since 30 years, born in Machiques. The beginning is very recent. In the family there is a brother infected. Taking scales of the lesions in different parts of the body by scraping and cultivating it in Sabouraud, two days after, development of a fungus not raised of the surface of the colony, green color, increasing with the time the coloring. New cultures positive 24 hours later. Direct examination with sodium hydrate did not discover any fungus. Classified, the result was Aspergillus nidulans.

2° - Second case born also in Machiques, 32 years old, several years sick, brother of N° 1, agriculturist. Scrapings of the spots and cultures of the scales in Sabouraud, development after 48 hours of an exuberant fungus at the beginning white, but later reddish. Classified to come out Fusarium sanguineum. Direct examination of the scales was negative.

3° - Another patient from Machiques, 35 years old, stains blue-slated colored. Scrapings and cultures in Sabouraud gave colonies white, that after change to blackish. Classified, to come out Cephalosporium curtipes.

4° - A fourth case, born in same village, 55 years old, since young has had the disease. The cultures of the scales in Sabouraud gave colonies

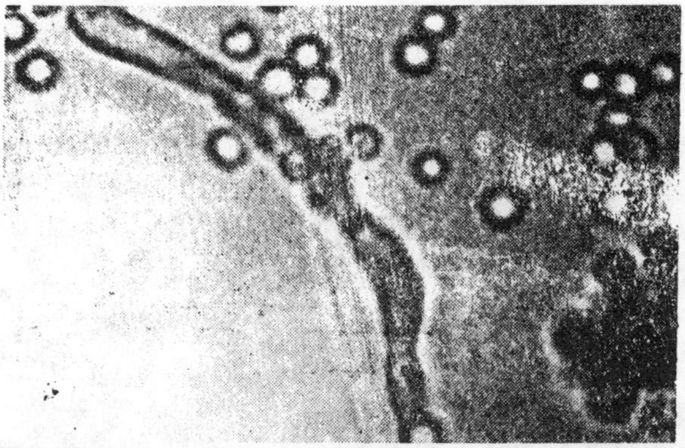

Myceliums and spores of the fungus found in the skin of caratosos.

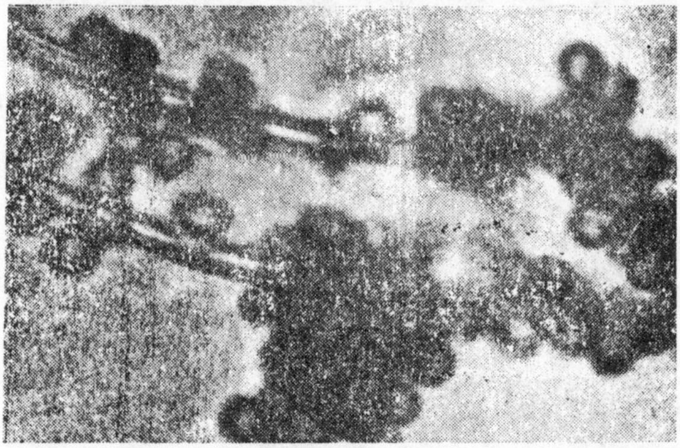

Myceliums and spores of the fungus found in the skin of caratosos.

greenish. Classified the fungis to come out Penicillium matrae meae and Penicillium cyaneum.

Later, in Mene Mauroa, thinking always in fungi, we examined another four cases, finding in all the patients different kinds of fungi.

The searchers in Barinas in 100% of the ills had the presence of fungi. In one of them, we found the appearance of a yeast in culture medium of acid Raulin with small development and not veil.

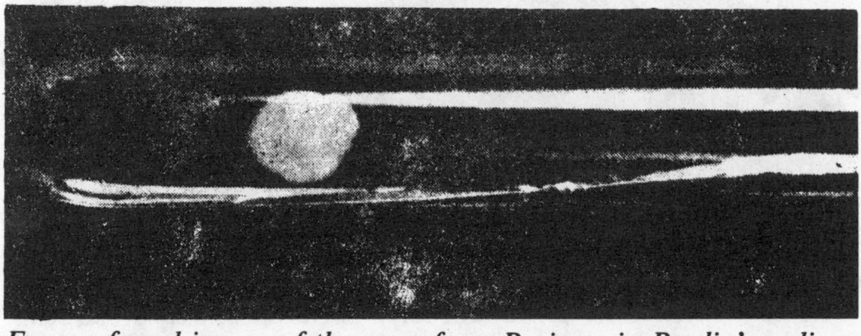

Fungus found in one of the cases from Barinas, in Raulin' medium.

With the fungi obtained in Perijá and El Consejo, we made by scrapings, inoculations in back of guinea pigs and thinking in the infections p er os put clots of fungi in the water for the animals to drink.

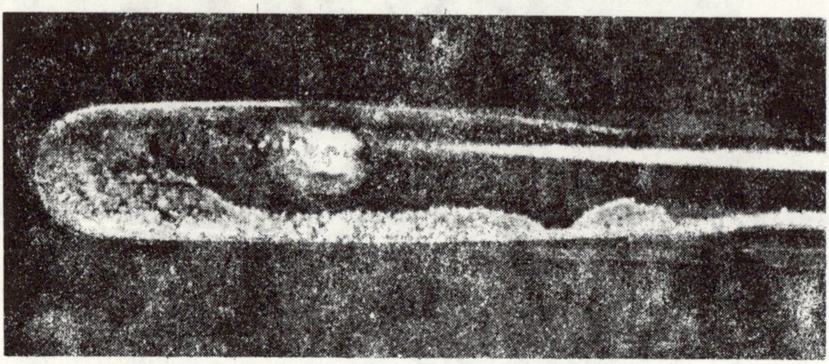

The same fungus in Sabouraud' medium.

In the sites of the inoculations 10 or 15 days after appeared light desquamation looking dry and rough. In the cultures appeared the same fungi that we have cultivated. The pseudo-lesions disappear 45 days later. We inoculated also a monkey, with negative result.

The cure of this endemic with the anti-syphilitics and the serologic tests clearly positive in high percentage and other details, did think that this disease had a spirochaetal origin, like the syphilis.

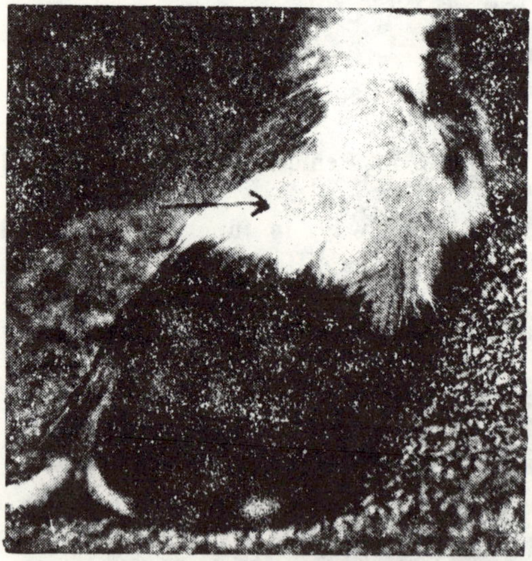

Inoculations made in the back of guinea pigs with fungi obtained of caratosos from Perijá, 30 days after the scraping.

Just, González Herrejón in 1927, gave the alarm, suspicions corroborated when Sáenz, Grau Triana and Alfonzo Armenteros, the last year 1938, seeing in dark field the lymph taken from the border of lesions of the skin situated in hands and feet, by surprise, saw a spirochaetal germ, treponema type, similar to the germ of the syphilis, details published in a preliminary report: "Demostración de un espiroqueta en el borde activo de un caso de Pinta de las manos i pies i en la linfa de ganglios superficiales. Reporte preliminar".

Francisco León i Blanco, attached to the Service of Professor Saénz, went to Mexico, where moreover to be common the illness it will be easy the verification of the Cuban finding. In effect, Blanco in almost the 100% of the caratosos examined in that country found the germ, patients some of them done the dignostic by Professor González Herrejón, who is very able in this field, researches published in "Medicina".

Between us, here in Venezuela, we feel pride to be the third nation in America, finding the spirochaetal agent, before than Brazil, more advanced, and Colombia, more infected. This finding prove that the Cuba discovery is true, than tha Mexican suspicions had good reason and that the carate, carare of cute, from Venezuela, is similar to Mal del Pinto of Mexico or the Pinta of Cuba, and so, is very possible the unity of this disease in America.

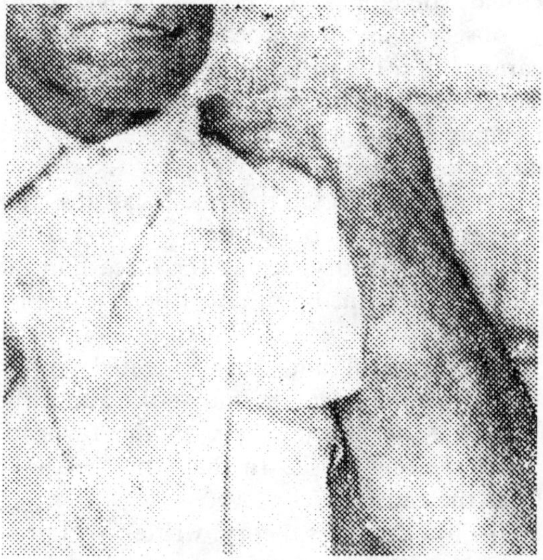

Case of Carate of the zone of Guatire. In lesions of the arms, how is appreciated in the photo, and more over in the lesions of the legs, we have found spirochetes.

In ten patients, the examination of a drop of lymph taken from the border of any lesion; in one, only, we obtained positive result. In the other cases, very probable, we had not practice in the taking of the material, the presence of the protozoan is scarce; sometimes, one or two hours in order to see an element. Notwithstanding, certain time later, accompanying Professor Brumpt in a trip, it was very easy to find the spirochete.

Frequently, in dark field, it is easy to see a protozoan with spiral form, one, two or three spires; seven or eight microns of length.

The technic for the seizure of the lymph is the following: pinch with a nipper the center or the border of a lesion, and scrape it, until the lymph comes out, or better, thrust it with a needle waiting the lymph-bloody, where there is large probabilities to find the spiral germ. It is an author modification to the Cuban technic.

We have not in accord with the aseverations of the Mexican school. For us, the spirochete then is considered belonging to the genus Treponema of Noguchi, calling it, Treponema carateum, is very rare, scarce, on need of big patience to see it; only one time could we see two in a field. It seems, that in Mexico it is easily found. The coloring for us, considering the scarcety, is difficult. The spirochete never has been seen for dyeing with silver nitrate. With Giemsa, rarely nevertheless, we have seen smears made in Mexico, sent kindly by León i Blanco, where easily it is possible to see numerous samples.

The features of the protozoan found by us is as follow: thin body; 15 to 18 microns, sometimes more; 12 to 16 stiff spires; ends a little slender; active mobility in rotation on his axis, and finding an obstacle the action is like a whip. His propulsion is slow; presenting forms of circle, hook, walking cane, coming again to the spiral aspect.

The observation in dark field, sometimes, has been prolonged more than three hours and we have observed as the spirochete goes losing his mobility and taking the appearance of a file of refringent points. Details of these are in accord with the Cuban descriptions.

The investigation in the glands of the groin was negative; the same than it was made in the axillar region, with difficulty.

Finishing this Chapter it is convenient to tell that the Mexicans have produced the bibliography more serious and abundant.

So, the priest Alzate, in the XVII century, seeing the disease in the hills of the volcano Jorullo, thought in divine punishment or volcanic influence.

In the XVIII century Ruiz Sandoval and Iris presented to the Academy of Medicine of Mexico a communication and spoke about the fungi, but it is good to say that it was Montoya, with the favor of Sabouraud, who published an interesting thesis. In that time he spoke about the water and the corn, as the causes.

González Guzmán emited the intoxications theory, written: "el principio del padecimiento puede ser una auto-intoxicación propia de los apises cálidos i probablemente de origen intestinal, quizás, orginada por protozoarios o protofitos".

CHAPTER III

TRANSMISSION OF THE CARATE

In this disease exists yet two large problems: 1° the transmission.

2° to explain if the spirochete of the carate is the same of the syphilis and the yaws.

The contagion possible is made of two ways: direct and indirect; but having many contradictions between one and another, the situation is embarrassing.

Our inquiries in this way reveal that the caratoso, says always: "por que otra persona se la echó"; or, because there are some gnats that sting and are the cause of the spread of it.

The caratoso believes that perversily other person has tried to infect himself, well with the scales or blood throw in the coffee, "chicha", fruits. When we have been in our investigations, one time, going from Barinas to San Cristóbal, a trip of two days, avoided meals and beverages.

In Perijá, we have visited farms as Yasa, with 30 day laborers, only two caratosos between them. Living in promiscuity and the illness did not spread.

In Machiques, we met a man with a certain social position, married three times and had 15 sons, and no-one in the family had adquired the disease.

Some, incriminate the bath; el caratoso bathing in the dead water of the river, leaf in the surface of the water, a greasy mantle, that should be infected.

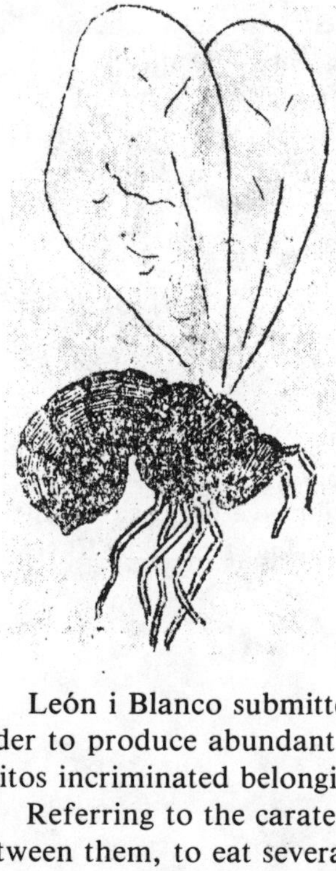

Simulium sp. captured by us on the border of the river Apón (Perijá) and cited by the perijaneros as transmissor of the Carate.

León i Blanco submitted a group of caratosos to strong exercises in order to produce abundant sweating, finding in it spirochetes. The mosquitos incriminated belonging to the family Simuliidae.

Referring to the carate it is an endemic not inherited. It is common, between them, to eat several in the same container, cold meals, with hot sauce, not admitting the children, and believe that simuliums after sting, filled of blood, fall in the vessel, spreading the disease by ingestion. Simuliums, we have seen many in the State Barinas, to the border of the river Socopó and they are incriminated also as transmissors of the carate.

In region Guarenas, Guatire, the patient thinks equally in the transmission by simuliums, classified as Simulium exiguum.

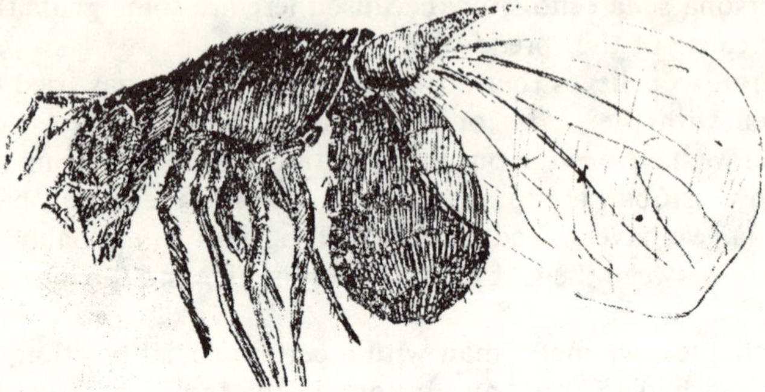

Simulium exiguum captured by us in the zone of Guarenas (State Miranda).

The Mexicans say to have found spirochetes in the simuliums of the caratosas zones. In the mycologic epoch we put simuliidae in culture tubes trying to find fungi. With simuliidae from Guarenas, we have examined in dark field seeking spirochetes, always with negative results. Carrying simuliidae from the caratosas zones, the rearings are very difficult; the gnats in cautivity not eat and the survival is only of three days. The Colombian Montoya i Flores, since 1898, signaled the simuliidae as transmissors.

CHAPTER IV

SYMPTOMATOLOGY OF CARATE

The carate is adquired in the first years of life; it is not inherited. In Mexico, where it is very common probably will have confusions in the diagnostic. Referring to Mexicans bring the following: from 0 to 10 years,

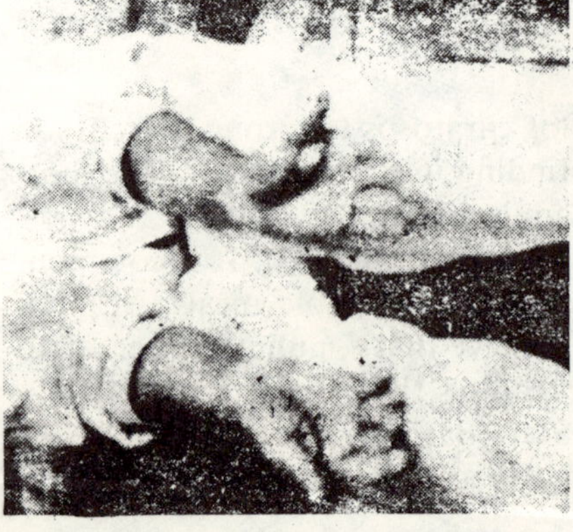

Carate white from Perijá. Symmetrical spots in both hands.

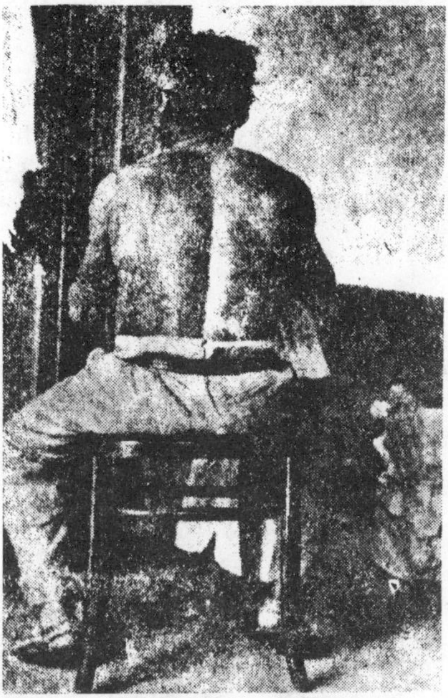

Carate blue-slate from Perijá. Stains in all the body. Region on back.

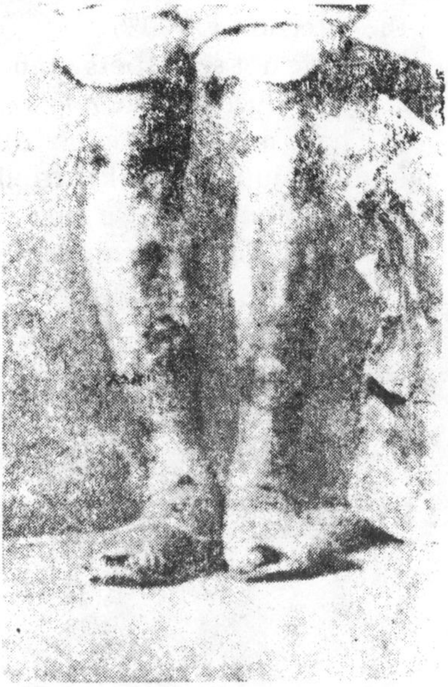

Photo of a caratoso in Perijá. Skin is crusty, scaly and bright.

started the disease in 638 cases; from 11 to 20, in 471 cases; from 31 to 40, in 61 cases; from 41 to 50, in 19 cases, and from 51 to 60, 11 cases.

Between us, it seems to be more frequent from 15 to 40 years old, and the percentage is increasing after 6 years old. Under this age it is very rare and almost exceptional.

About our inquiry in State Barinas in 281 patients the results is the following:

From	0 to 1	1 case
,,	2 to 5	12 ,,
,,	6 to 9	32 ,,
,,	10 to 14	53 ,,
,,	15 to 25	74 ,,
,,	26 to 40	67 ,,
,,	41 to 69	41 ,,
,,	70	1 ,,
,,	80	1 ,,

Observe the figure between 15 to 25 and 26 to 40 they are the double of the figures between 6 to 9 and 10 to 14.

Relating to sex it seems to be that the male is more attacked than the female, and about our inquiry (census) in 281 patients, there were 118 males and 163 females and we have noted referring to the work are the boatman, because they are obliged to be always on the border of the river, and the infection is 100%.

We have not seen spots in the buccal mucous and sometimes are very frequent, produced in the *mulatos*.

We have not seen trophic troubles in nails, as gryposis, leukonychia, longitudinal flutings, neither troubles in the pilous system as say the Mexicans and Colombians; we have not found modifications in sensibility to the pain, cold, hot and contact.

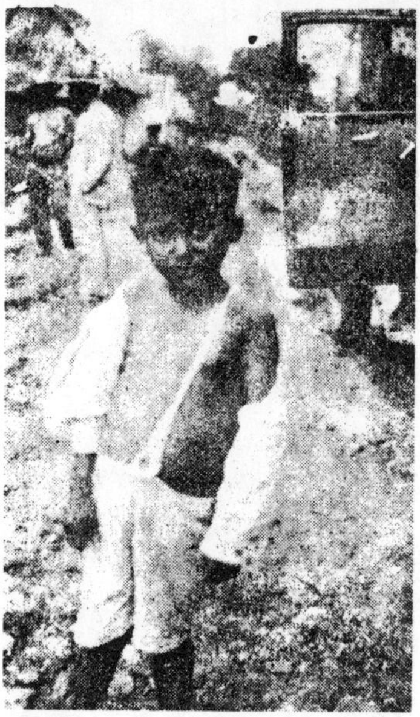

Photo of a boy from Quebrada Seca (S. Barinas). Carate blue. Is one of the cases with lowest age in which we have seen the disease.

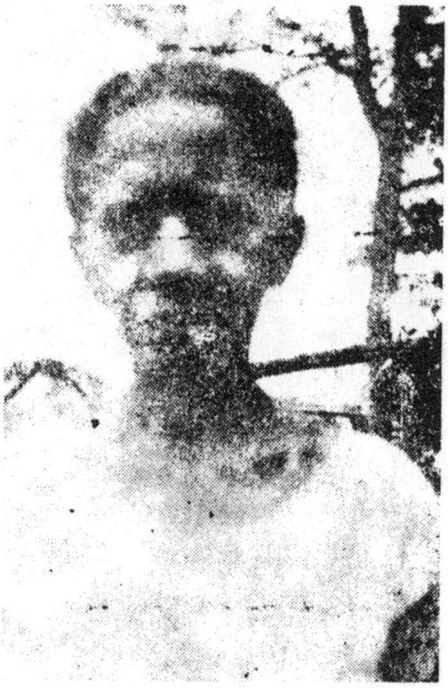

Photo of a patient of the region of Barinas. Is one of the few cases in which we have observed the blackish coloring of the skin that almost disfigures the face and are the patients more attacked morally.

The symptomatology is very difficult, exactly is necessary to stay for a long time where is endemic the illness, and besides the authors change often the clinical pictures.

By our own observations the sickness start always by a large lesion inany part of the body, projecting, itching; after, with intervals monthly continuing coming out new lesions smaller. It is astonishing when we see a patient in this stage, the diagnostic is made by the rural people that since the infancy are seeing the same pictures.

The health of the caratoso is good, only in the lapse of time of the appearance of the lesions they suffer of fever. Many observers believe to be malaria and we think they are in reason.

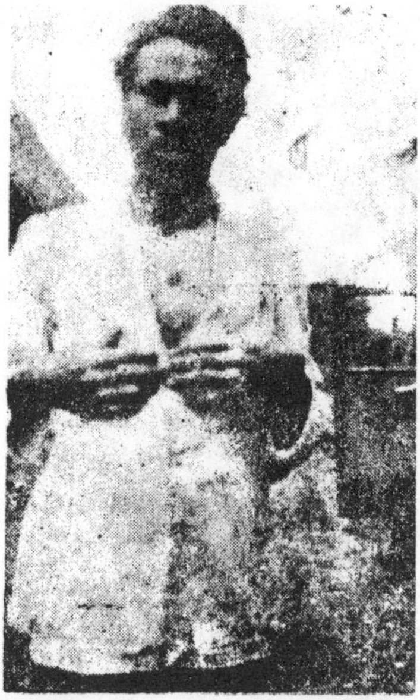

Caratoso from Barinas. Stains in the hands.

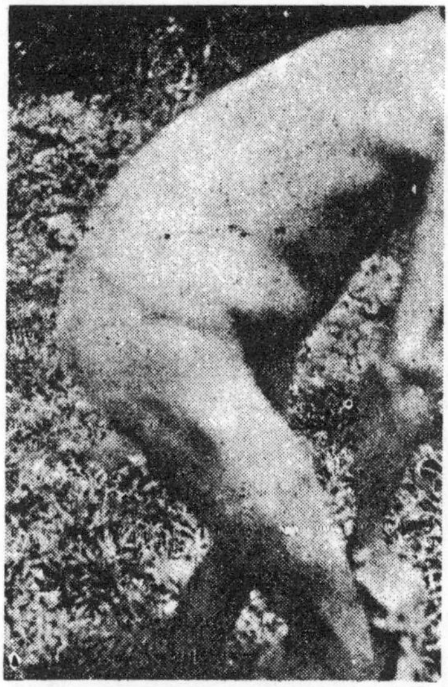

Case of carate white from Barinas. Stains in back and legs.

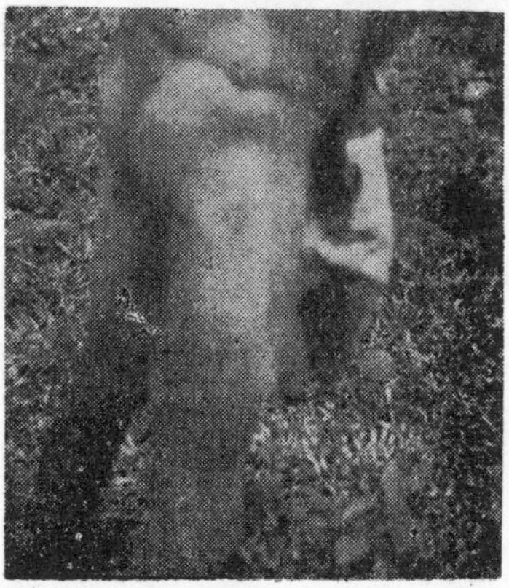

The same anterior case. Observe the spots in the legs and the buttocks.

The lesions continue growing, are scales, itching, dry, bright, contrasting with the rest of the skin, healthy, soft, humid, thin. The white color yet is doubtful if it is the definitive spot or it is a variety of the sickness.

The coloration more frequent is the white and the blue-slaty; the dark-blue, we believe has relation with our racial types, and so, in the mulatto is common to see it. In these lesions we are in accord with the Mexicans, observing that the spots are more dark in the center, and in periphery there is an achromic strip.

We have not seen stains in the palm of the hands and sole of the feet as it seems to be frequent in the Pinta of Cuba.

The place of the spots is very common in the face often in the forehead, nose, cheeks, in the chest, very frequent; in the back, buttocks. In the arms, forearms, hands, chiefly in the joints.

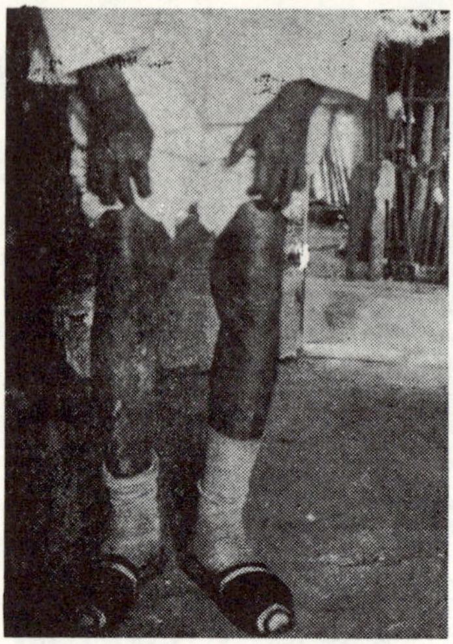

Caratoso from Quebrada Seca (S. Barinas). Lesion scales, dry and bright.

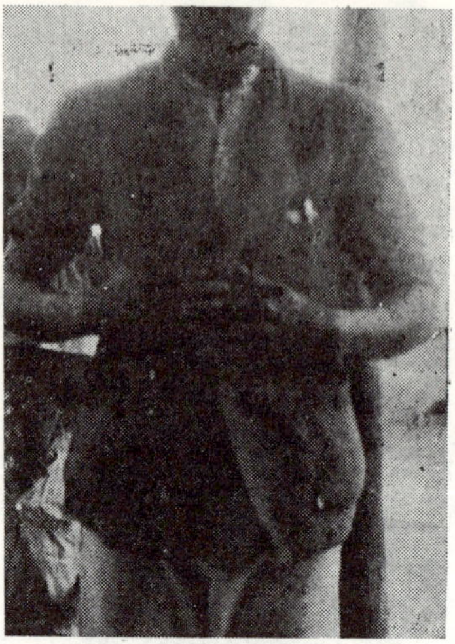

Caratoso from Barinas. Achromic lesions in both hands, chiefly in the joints, called "picadura".

In the thighs, knees, legs, feet. It seems to be more frequent in some places like the knees, malleolus and scarce in others, as the inguinal regions, popliteal regions, between the fingers.

For the crossed topography of the stains, sometimes unilateral distributions, called hemi-pinto; sometimes, same aspect in both sides, do believe in the action of nervous system.

CHAPTER V

SEROLOGY AND HEMATOLOGY OF THE CARATE

In the year 1926, Dr. Menck published in one of the Reports (N° 15) annuals of the bananera' company United Fruit, a work made in the Hospital of Santa Marta (Colombia), entitled: "The percentage of positive Wassermann reactions found associated with various diseases", where he made known that practicing the Wassermann in 67 caratosos, in 69.5% of them the test was clearly positive.

The Commission for the study of Mal del Pinto in Mexico, found in 130 reactions of Wassermann made in caratosos in different times of the evolution, in the town of Iguala, in the State of Guerrero, 125 clearly positive, 3 negative and 2 anti-complementaries. Making control taken blood of persons not infected in the same town, obtaining 86% of negative results and 14% of positive results.

Pérez Rodríguez, equally in México and in the same State of Guerrero in 109 tests of blood taken to caratosos, found 104 with positive results, 1 with light positive result, 3 anti-complementaries and 1 negative.

Referring to us we have made 111 reactions of Kahn between 161 patients that we have had in treatment in the District of Pedrazas of the State Barinas, seeing that the 78% of those patient treated and cured gave Kahn positive and the patients in evolution of the illness, without treatment, the positive result was of 100%. In Quebrada Seca, near Barinitas, in collaboration with Sanguinetti, we have found equally 100% for not treated and 77% for those treated and cured

Observe with brightness that the carate as the yaws, continue giving a positive result being a potential sign in the sickness.

We did not use Wassermann in Barinas, because the technic is very complicated in those far regions.

It is comprobated that the carate gave a serology yet more positive than the syphilis and yaws and is convenient to have all these results in mind, either that the carate and yaws are national endemics and not think obstinately in syphilis.

Referring to hematology, the amount of red cells, white cells, hemoglobin is necessary to have in account that all these people are infected by malaria, intestinal worms, etc., and so many times you see an increase of the eosinophiles, lymphocytes.

The white blood count made by us in Perijá, Mene Mauroa, Barinas have been normal.

Here, two from Perijá:

Nº 1

Lymphocytes	26%
Monocytes	10%
Neutrophyles	60%
Eosinophyles	4%
Basophyles	0%

Nº 2

Lymphocytes	26%
Monocytes	17%
Neutrophyles	55%
Eosinophyles	2%
Basophyles	0%

CHAPTER VI

THE CARDIO-AORTIC LESIONS IN THE CARATE

In the interesting work that we have in hands, published in the 19th Annual Report, the year 1930, entitled: "Is carate (Pinta) a dermatomycosis?" by Thonnard Neumann, Camacho Moya and Bruster, explains that in 75 cases studied from the region Santa Marta (Colombia), 90% presented Wassermann and Kahn positives; 80%, exposed to the X-rays, enlargement of the aorta; 55, cardiac enlargement; 50%, pathologic troubles of cardiac rumors, and in 20 of 34 cases under thirty years old, troubles of their circulatory system, arriving to consider that the carate as a general disease to treponema, as the syphilis.

The Mexican Commission for the study of the carate made investigations about neuro-vegetative unbalanced condition in caratosos with troubles in cardiac rumors, finding frequently hipo-enfotonismo hypo-sympathetic and hypo-vago.

Grau Triana thinks that the 75% of the caratosos studied by him presented clinical and screen increase of the heart by dilatation of the left ventricle and enlargement of the aorta.

In 10 caratosos of the focus of Guatire studied lastly by us we have found clinical signs of troubles cardiac-aortics and two of them brought to Caracas, our suspicions have been comprobated. In that sense 40%; believing that the carate as trepanomatosis, is capable to attack the heart and vessels. We know that the syphilis is responsible for 91% of the cardiac-aortics lesions.

In these ills the age was between 14 to 70 years, but chiefly 30 to 40. In some of them it was very old, and sometimes arrived to 38 years of evolution. Referring race: 7 were niggers, 1 mulatto, 2 whites.

The clinical examination of these sick people has demonstrated the following:

E. B., nigger, 48, stains blue-slaty, 38 years suffering the disease; nine sane sons; his wife never miscarried; no increase of the spleen or ganglions; gets tired when walks; pulse 70; metalic rumor in the second time.

P.A., mulatto, 29, spots blue-slaty; increase of lymphatic nodes in neck and groins; normal spleen; pulse 92.

J.E., nigger, spots blue-slaty; age 76; normal spleen; increased lymphatic nodes.

J.D., blue-slaty; 28; ganglions and spleen normal.

B.D., blue-slaty; 34; increased lymphatic nodes; normal spleen.

R.R., red stains; age 56.

A.D., blue-slaty; age 12.

J.R., blue-slaty; age 40.

I.V., red spots; normal spleen. Increased lymphatic nodes; age 66.

Tests of laboratory and electric-cardiographics of the two patients treated by us:

R.R. - Wassermann positive (+ + + + +)
Kahn positive (+ + + +)
Malaria (smears and thick drop) negative
Red cells 4.616.000 mm^3
Leukocytes 10.800 mm^3

Hemoglobin	80%
Globular value	0.82

White blood count:

Lymphocytes	18%
Monocytes	11%
Neutrophyles	54%
Walking cane	6%
Metamielocytes	5%
Basophyles	0%
Eosinophyles	6%
Mielocytes	0%

Uraemia	0.279
Glucaemia	0. 75
Basal metabolism	- 10%

Urine

Albumin	negative
Glucose	negative
Urobiline	positive (+ + +)
Bile pigments	positive (+ +)

Feces

Eggs of worms	negative

Eyes

N o r m a l

Blood pressure	Mx 12.5	Mn 7
Arteriosclerosis		
Aortic focus		second rumor metallic
Tricuspid focus		second rumor metallic
Balance		normal
Standardization	1mv:	10 mm

Electrocardiogram of R.R. - positive case Treponemas in the different sites of the body.

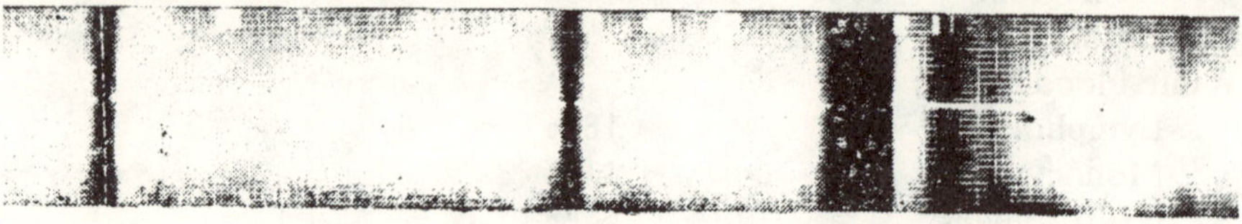

Electro cardiogram of the patient J.R.

Voltage		R II	8mm
Conduction		atrio-ventricular (P.R.):	0.20 in II
Interval		Q R S:	0.08 seconds in II
Electric			axis- - 42° to the left
Rhythm	sinusoidal		
		frequency	
		auricular	60
		venticular	60

Conclusion: Slow pulse, normal cycle. Sinusoidal heart block.

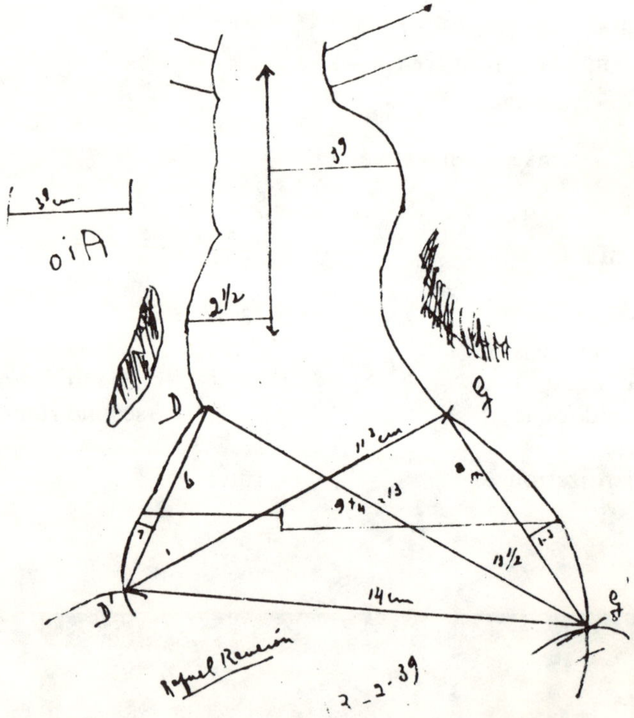

Ortodiagram of R.R. (positive case)

Diameter of the left heart normal

Diameter of the right heart: auricle normal; ventricle increased lightly, with tendency traingular for dilatation (D'G' - 14 cm)

Ascending aorta with tendency to take form of walking cane of 3.9 and dyeing as III.

In O.T.A. 3.9 cm.

Visible pulmonary artery

Consclusions: aortitis and light right dilatation.

J.R. normal eyes

Radioscopy: aortitis and left enlargement

Electrocardiogram:

P-R O.20 seconds

Interval Q.R.S.: 0.08 seconds

Electric axis: 120° to the left

Voltage‘ 10mm in R II

Rhythm sinusoidal: ventricular 90 in D I and D II

auricular 100 in D I and D II

80 in D III

Observations:

Wave P presents in D I, D II, D III R of 3 mm lack S.

Interval S.T. presents in D I, D II, lack S in D III.

Wave T D I diphasic, D III diphasic, D III iso-electric.

Summary:

Electric axis devious to left to 120°

R small of 3mm

S negative in D III

T diphasic in D I and D II. Iso-electric in D III

Consclusions:

Probable degeneration of the heart.

The preceding papers demonstrate that the carate must be had in account in cardio-aortic lesions. We know something about the bilharziosis in this sense; wait till the surprise of the future.

CHAPTER VII

HISTOPATHOLOGY OF THE CARATE

The histopathologic study of this disease is related to the names of Pallares, Martínez Báez, Ochoterena, Fox and others.

The majority of the authors, excepting Ochoterena, that we know, found a thinness of the skin, as we could see in our cuttings and the number of files of cells, often is of eight.

The typical in the carate blue-slaty is the abundance of pigment, either in the epidermis as in dermis. The corneus layer, not taking in account the color of the spots is always very thin, as it has been verified by us.

In summary: we have found atrophy of the epidermis, the superficial layers of cells very narrow. The papillas are visible, but short and scarce. Thinness diffuse of the corneus layer. In the red carate we have not found an increase of the pigment. In the layer sub-epidermic many conjunctival fibres hyalines.

Infiltration of round cells and plamacells chiefly in the conjunctival, superficial layers, but also continuing with the vessels till more deeper layers.

In the cutting of red carate we have not verified an increase of dilatation of the vessels and cells as say the Mexican authors.

CHAPTER VIII

DIFFERENTIAL DIAGNOSIS

About this Chapter there are many things to tell, because in these endemic regions any lesions in the skin is called carate, but it is necessary to tell that, as any disease, useful to have seen many cases and to have lived between them, in order to make a sure and rapid diagnosis.

The chloasma is characterized by its localization in the face, common in the woman, always hepatic troubles, pregnancy, lack of itching and scales.

The pityriasis versicolor tropical or tiña flava of the list of Castellani is very easy to know for the situation, the coloring coffee and milk, the preesence of the fungi in the cultures. The residual achromia, uniformly achromic leaf, sometimes a small evolutionary focus that help to do the diagnosis.

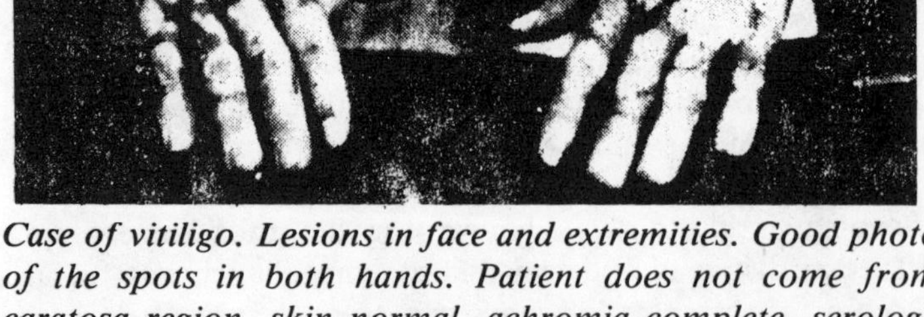

Case of vitiligo. Lesions in face and extremities. Good photo of the spots in both hands. Patient does not come from caratosa region, skin normal, achromia complete, serology negative and the prolonged treatment gave negative result.

The keratosis nigricans palmaris or tiña negra, is located on the hands and material taken of these lesions give fungi Cladosporium and Wernecki. This keratosis must be interesting in Cuba, where the Pinta has similar lesions in hands and feet.

The necklace of Venus or pigmentary syphilide is a lesion localized on the neck, more frequent in woman than in men. The specific previous helping to do the diagnosis.

The variety white of the carate and the nervious leprosy, but the stains can present another coloring, there is no trouble in the sensibility, there is no atrophy, no swelling of the cubital nerve, no rhinitis, no other symptoms that the leprosy shows. It is possible to look for the bacillus, because the serology is highly positive in both diseases.

Some authors exaggerating, believe confound it to the Addison disease. Referring us to the carate in Venezuela is very confounded with the vitiligo, lucky, both have characteristic symptoms:

WHITE PINTO	VITILIGO
Spots always hypochromics. Achromia increased in some sites, as knees, malleolus, joints metacarpal, elbows, wrists.	Spots uniformly achromics. Rarely hypochromics.
The lesions are dry, chiefly scaly.	The skin always with normal aspect, there is no xerodermis, no scales.
The spots are rare in the genital organs, scalp, back medium, folds of flexure.	The spots are very frequent in all those sites. In the head and genital region observe the whiteness of the hair.
The patients coming from endemic zones.	The patient is from any region.
The serology tests are positive in 100%, clearly and durable.	The serologic tests are often negative, at least it is associated to syphilis.
The disease disappears with bismuth, mercury and arsenic, excepting the residual white spots, incurable.	The disease commonly is incurable. Bismuth, mercury and arsenic have no action upon it.

CHAPTER IX

PROGNOSTIC - REACTIVATION - RELAPSE RE-INFECTION - INMUNITY

The prognosis of the carate before this epoch spirochetosic was very benign. The caratoso could be buried in life morally bearing this stigma of malediction, making its transmission, involuntarily, generation to generation, as a destroyer and malign inheritance, but the material ravages were of no account. On believed, that were the aspergillus and penicilliums, accused by Montoya, living on the skin producing that series of dischromatosis.

The prognosis has changed deeply since 1927 when González Herrejón considered the cause of this disease was a spirochete, suspicion verified years later by the Cubans, observing lympho-adenopathies, enlarge of the spleen and aortic lesions, findings about we have referred before.

During the treatment we have observed reactivation of the spots, either with the arsenic as the bismuth, after an improvement appreciable and the body was invaded for new stains.

In some of the patients we have seen re-infections, explainable, because are persons to stay in the same life: promiscuity, accumulation, stings of the same entomological fauna.

The child in the photo, from Quebrada Seca, possibly, is a case of re-infection, because had been cured with bismuth one year before.

About the inmunity in the carate, we do not accept it, and besides the treponemosis in common does not produce inmunity.

CHAPTER X

PROPHYLAXIS OF THE CARATE

Today we think the prophylaxis of the carate is simple. Knowing the origen and treatment, disregarding the transmission, we believe have large advancements in the study of this sickness.

Sympathiser of a transmitting host unknowed yet, the campaign will be difficult. As in similar events: houses with walls and zinc in the roof, in order to avoid the development of insects; metallic webs in doors and windows; mosquito net; forbidding the construction of houses near the border of the rivers, avoiding the stings of the numerous insects, between them, the simuliidae.

With a campaign well organized it will be possible the erradication of this scourge; placing dispensaries for the treatment and to profit researchs as the commissions in Mexico, that will not be very expensive. Our positive case, with 14 injections of Bivatol, 2 cc, had an advanced improvement and the spirochetes had disappeared. We have been helped in the treatment of the patients of State Miranda by laboratories Bayer and Ponce and Benzo.

CHAPTER XI

TREATMENT OF THE CARATE

This Chapter is one of the most interesting of this disease.

The treatment is very ancient, perhaps since the last century. Galo Soberón i Parra an able mexican physician in question of Hygiene and Tropical Medicine to whom we met in Paris, was the first who gave me details in this way, for that when coming back to Venezuela, we published in the main journal of that time, an article about the treatment of this disease and we were so ignorant in this field that few times after we were receiving letter of many colleagues from different regions of the country asking us about this problem and physicians of Caracas inquired referring to this question.

The secret treatment had been in hands of the empiricits or quacks. We knew that the "piaches" of the native tribes used the mercury with good results; but handle by these ignorants *adlibitum* produced intestinal troubles, gingivitis and general poisoning. Referring that a famous empiricist had the ill in a room without light several days giving him rubbings and pills daily. Both things, probably, was mercury.

Little by little with the influence of the Mexicans that have been the first in these investigations, we knew that the carate was curable.

We have seen in our trips to Perijá, Mene Mauroa and Barinas that the medicament more used was the bismuth for the easiness to inject and the low cost, because the neosalvarsan, of rapid and surprising results, its price is higher and needs intravenous application.

The cure of the carate with these three medicaments had made to think that the carate was not a local affection, but a general disease likes the syphilis produced by a spirochete. Just, we went the pioneer divulger in our country and at the same time the first to lessen the value of the mycologic theory of Montoya, that have been published in Paris and Written in french arrived praise.

The medicaments more used by us, with the useful collaboration of Sanguinetti, were arsenic: neo and solusalvarsan, novarsan, acetilarsan and bismuth: muthanol, biazan, bivatol and lipo-bi.

The average of c.c. employed in the treatment, was of 24 to 30 c.c. Relating to bivatol that was the most used and each c.c. correspond to 7 centigrams of bi-metal; we have a total dose of more or less of 200 centigrams of bi-metal for obtaining a curation.

It is so rapid the action of these medicines that in the case with spirochetes positive, after 182 centigrams of bi-metal the lesions were almost disappeared and negative the spirochetes.

At the beginning in observe the disappearance of the itching and light hyperesthesia that presents the caratoso. A symptom very frequent in the caratosos are the rheumatismal nocturnal pains as in syphilis, that disappear gast with the treatment.

There are patients that have been cured with 56 c.c. of bi-metal or 42 centigrams of bi-metal. The age, it seems, does not have relation with the dose, because patients of 21 to 28 years old cured with 6 c.c. of bismuth (Bivatol), and others of the same age needed 24 and 36 c.c., and others of minor age (14 years old) needed 36 c.c.

We believe that the standard treatment must be started with arsenic (neo-salvarsan 0.15, 0.30 and 0.45) and to continue with bismuth until complete healthy. With the previous arsenic the treatment is more swift and patient increase his faith.

The population in the State Barinas believe that the gum-resin of a gutífera called "tampaco or isfuque" (Clusia rosaeflora) applied on the spots gives good results. Is a case where *voz del pueblo, voz de Dios* is mistaken.

In present, we have in treatment several cases in the region of Guatire, with the help of P.P.L. using solu-salvarsan, neolesal and paroxil, medicaments given kindly by laboratories Bayer and we are very satisfied for the campaign started and the results obtained.

THE INITIAL LESIONS OF THE CARATE *

(Píntides de León i Blanco - Carampanchos of the Venezuelan people - Empeines or Jiotes of the Mexican people)

In different trips that we have made (sometimes alone, others, accompanied by Briceño Rossi) to the big caratosa zone or main focus in the nation (State Barinas), both had observed in more than an opportunity, in children as in adults, lesions of the skin mycotic type, light redness, scaly, psoriasiform, syphiloid, trichophytic, redness-pigment-pigmentary, without the characteristic coloring of the carate.

During those trips, neither Briceño Rossi nor me, arrived to have suspicions that were of caratoso origin, but, for the aspect were of mycotic nature, and for those persons, we prescribed pomade with salicylic acid (5%) or iodic's alcohol (1%).

For that time not one of the people gave us any suggestion about the nature caratosa of these lesions.

If this there was happening, it was not written until two Venezuelans described these lesions for the first time, because the spirochete of the sickness was unknown. It was later, the discovery of the germ, that a Cuban, León i Blanco, studying and seeing the lymph of these stains found the Treponema herrejoni or carateum. But there must always be a reason of pride for the Venezuelan medical school, that so as two Venezuelan (Brinceño Rossi and I) discovered for the second time in the world the spirochete, so equally, for the second time verified the spirochetic nature of these lesions that our people call "carampancho" and the Mexicans "empeines or jiotes", verigying the findings of the distinguished Cuban caratologist.

León i Blanco could, innoculated himself with the lymph of positive patients, seeing and observing the development of the beginning.

However, nihil novum sub sole, the knowledge of the empeines mexicans and the details of the lesions have had the following chronologic order: Fernández de Oviedo, 1506 to 1516; Sahagun, 1529; F. Jimérez, 1615; Corona, 1811; Yryz, 1879; Ruiz Sandoval, 1881; Flores, 1886; Téllez, 1889; Terrés, 1907.

Aguirre Pequeño, commented a work presented by Latapí and León i Blanco to the Academy of Medicine of Mexico on August 13, 1930, entitled "Las lesiones del principio del Mal del Pinto. Una nueva dermatosis" refer that the authors say: "que revisando la literatura nacional y extranjera solo encontramos que Iriarte en 1937 en Venezuela y Ruiz Sandoval en

* Published in the book "Estudios Entomológicos i Parasitológicos" Caracas-1948.

1881 se refirieron en unos cuantos renglones a las lesiones de principio del mal''

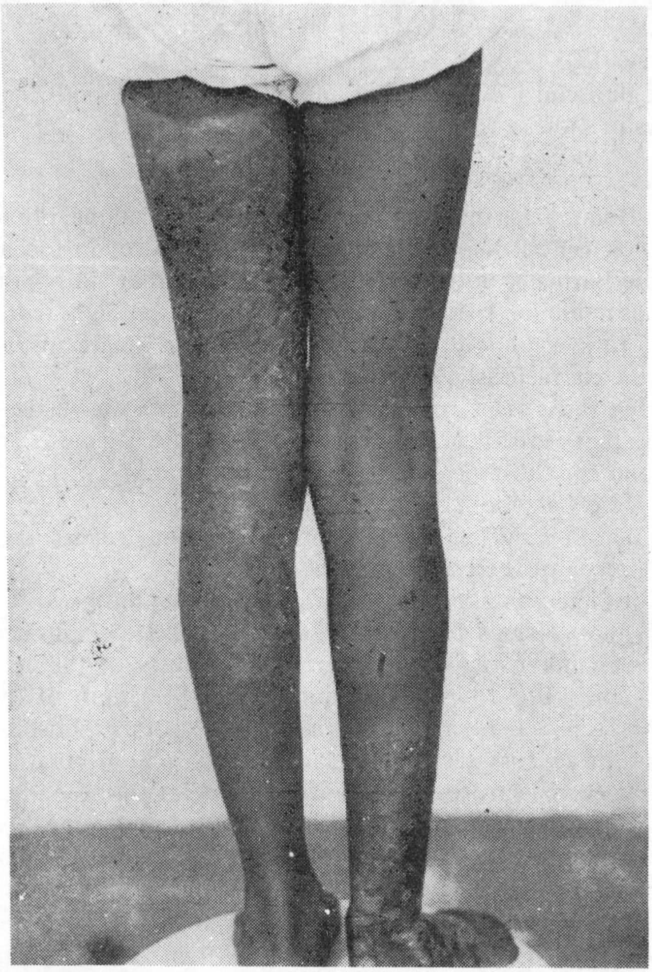

Píntide, empeine, jiote or carampancho, type redness-pigmentary.

León i Blanco years after, with a better documentation referring the work of Corona published 1881, wrote the following: ''en ninguna publicación posterior a ésta hemos leido una descripción más exacta que ésta de la marcha evolutiva de la enfermedad desde su inicio. Ciento veintiocho años después, la experimentación y la observación de un amplio material clínico condujeron al autor (León i Blanco) a las mismas conclusiones''.

It is true, for us that the report of Corona in 1881, explains clearly that the carate begins by the empeines and that the disease is cured with mercury. Successively, one paragraph of the most interesting: ''Los rápidos progresos que ha hecho esta enfermedad los ha causado principalmente la pobreza, la desidia. Yo fuí sub-delegado de Tuxtla y observé con bastante cuidado, lo muy fácil que es su curación. Nunca se manifiestan las manchas desde su principio, primero le salen unos empeines con los cuales se mantienen mucho tiempo, éstos se van extendiendo a proporción que en el centro va desapareciendo el empeine, dejando la mancha negra, blanca,

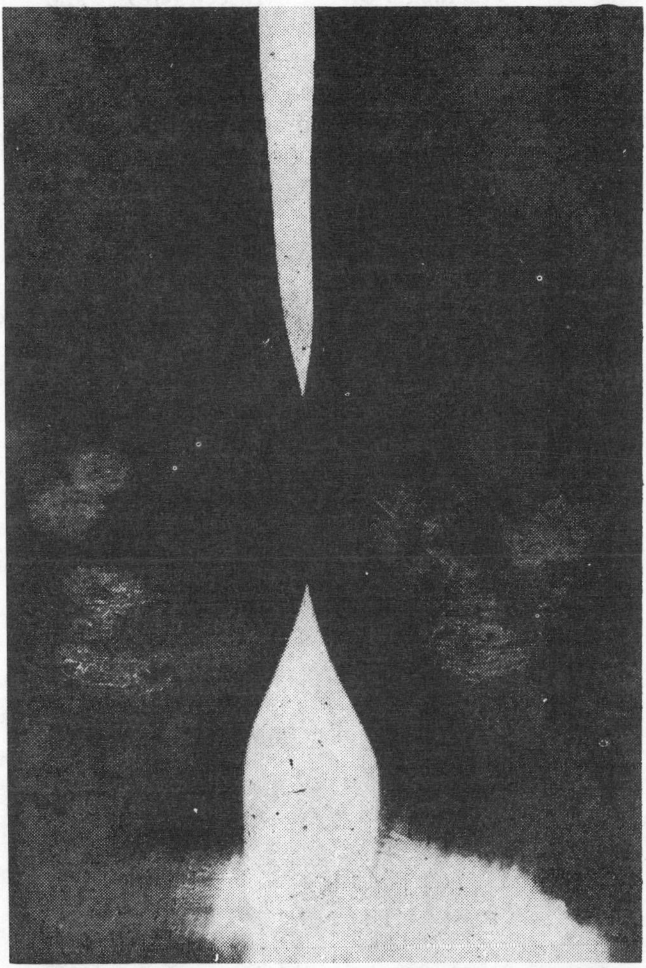

Pintide, empeine, jiote, carampancho, type psoriasiform.

azul o encarnada y así se van cundiendo hasta que se ponen como pintados. Si en el principio se cura aquel con la simple untura de sebo y azogue desaparece dentro de breve en aquel lugar. Yo conozco muchas familias de Tuxtla que con sólo este preservativo han logrado conservarse limpias con toda su familia, a pesar de estar tratando diariamente con los tiñosos''.

In our last investigations accompanied by Briceño Rossi (december 1942) about the carate in Barinas, both had in mind as an important matter of the program, although a little incredulous, the verification of the pintides. The first case was in the forearm of a boy from Pedrazas, living on the border of the river Canaguá.

This skepticism probably existed in the mind of the former researchers preceding us: Padilla, Freites Pineda, Medina Jiménez, Martín Vegas and others.

Perhaps the preachments of both (Briceño Rossi and us) since the year 1933, our trips making investigations in all those zones, the sanitary campaigns, did consciousness in all those people, and so in our last investigation in the zone of Pedrazas, on the border of the river Pagüey, in Quebrada Seca and in the surroundings of Barinitas, asking for the empeines or carampanchos, the majority of the people knew perfectly how the disease started.

The carampanchos, pintides, jiotes or empeines, in opinion of both, prefer the exposed sites, and so, in 12 cases of carampanchos positive, and also in dischromic patients that make history of the beginning lesion, we can verify this belief. In the 12 cases mentioned, in 10 of them are there are exposed places: legs 5, arms and forearms 3, faces 2; the others in trunk and buttocks.

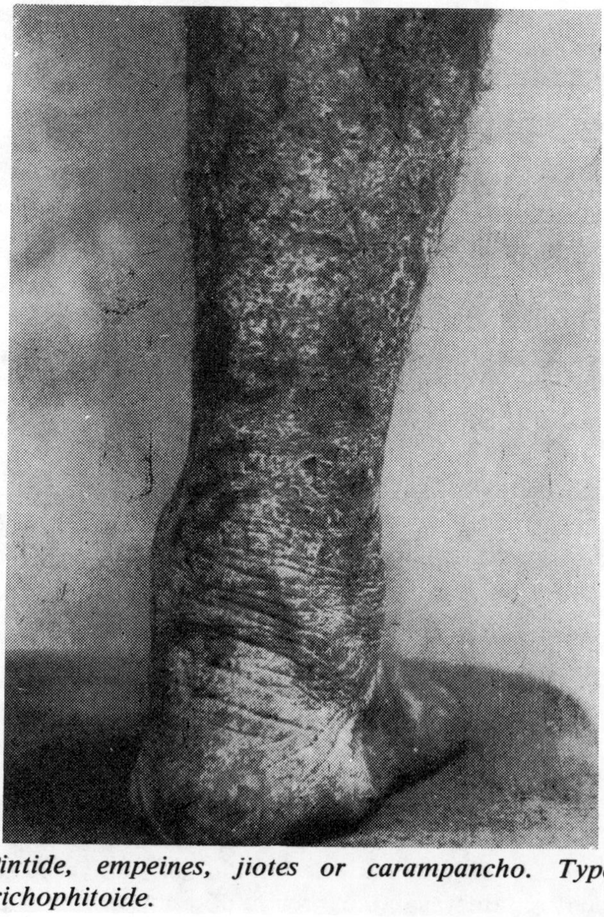

Pintide, empeines, jiotes or carampancho. Type trichophitoide.

The carampanchos have different sizes. We have seen large, in sheet or reduced. The aspect is variable, similar lesions of psoriasis, impétigo, syphilis. The number is variable also; sometimes, one only, and others, several, distributed in different sites of the body as a child living on the border of the river Pagüey, where we count around 20.

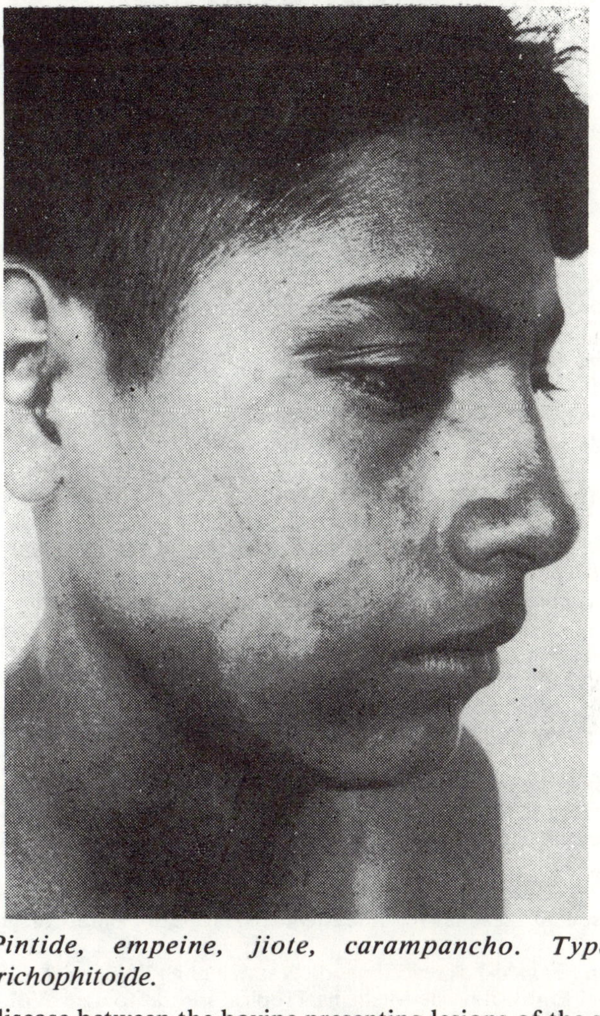

Pintide, empeine, jiote, carampancho. Type trichophitoide.

There is a disease between the bovine presenting lesions of the skin in different sites of the body, alopecia, variable size; that the farmers call *carare* and the animals that suffer of it, *cararosas*. By advices of Professor Brumpt we examined in several opportunities the lymph of these lesions and never found spirochetes.

Finishing, we recommend the following conclusions:

1° - the carate starts between us for lesions that the people in Barinas call carampanchos, that are equal to the pintides of León i Blanco; called also by the people of Mexico jiotes or empeines.

2° - it is necessary in order to be sure of the diagnosis, do the examination in dark field of the lymph taken of the carampanchos.
3° - the positive carampanchos that according to us are the majority (95% at least), must be treated with arsenic, bismuth or mercury.
4° - the carampanchos of other nature (mycotic, etc., will be treated with pomade of salicylic acid (5%) or iodic alcohol (1%).
5° - at the beginning of the carampancho, the serology is always negative, but a short time later, with the evolution, it changes to positive.
6° - is convenient seeing resistence with the iodine and the salicylic acid, although not finding spirochetes, use medicaments anti-syphilis.

BIBLIOGRAPHY

Consulted Foreign

1-*Fcco. León i Blanco*-Estudios sobre la etiología del Mal del Pinto. Medicina-Tomo XIX. No. 334.

2-*Fcco. León i Blanco*-El Treponema herrejoni. Rev. de Medicina Tropical i Parasitología. Vol. VI No. 1.

3-*Fcco León i Blanco*-La presencia de Treponema herrejoni en la serosidad de las grietas, fisuras i rasguños. Rev. de Medicina Tropical i Parasitología. Vol. VI. No. 1.

4-*Fcco. León i Blanco*-Presencia de treponemas en la superficie no erosionada de lesiones discrómicas. Medicina. Tomo XIX. No. 333.

5-*Fcco. León i Blanco*-Presencia constante de Treponemas herrejoni en las lesiones cutáneas del período discrómico del Mal del Pinto i en las pintides. Ausencia de los mismos en la piel de las personas sanas que conviven con los pintos. Rev. Medicina.

6-*Fcco. León i Blanco*-La lesión inicial en el Mal del Pinto. Rev. de Medicina Tropical i Parasitología. Vol. No. 1.

7-*Fcco. León i Blanco*-Histología patológica de las lesiones cutáneas i de los ganglios linfáticos en el Mal del Pinto. Rev. de Medicina Tropical i Parasitología. Vol. V. No. 6.

8-*Fcco. León i Blanco i Fernando Latapi*-Las lesiones de principio del Mal del Pinto (Una nueva dermatosis) Medicina, Tomo XX, No. 367.

9-*Fcco. León i Blanco*-La noción del contagio i la idea del vector en el Mal del Pinto. Medicina.

10-*Fcco. León i Blanco*-Cuarta nota sobre la trasmisión experimental del Mal del Pinto de persona a persona. Rev. de Medicina Tropical i Parasitología. Vol. VI. No. 1.

11-*Fcco. León i Blanco*-Las reacciones de Wassermann i Kahn en el período primario del Mal del Pinto. Rev. de Medicina Tropical i Parasitología. Vol. VI. No. 1.

12-*Fcco. León i Blanco*-Las reacciones de Bordet-Wassermann i Kahn en el período secundario del Mal del Pinto. Rev. de Medicina Tropical i Parasitología Vol. VI. No. 4.

13-*Fcco. León i Blanco*-Las queratosis palmares i plantares en el Mal del Pinto. Rev. de Medicina Tropical i Parasitología.

14-*Fcco. León i Blanco*-Estudio epidemiológico del Mal del Pinto en una pequeña aldea del Estado de Guerrero (México). Rev. de Medicina Tropical i Parasitología. Vol. VI. No. 4.

15-*Fcco. León i Blanco*-Tercera nota sobre la trasmisión experimental del Mal del Pinto de persona a persona-Revista Médica Militar-Tomo II No. 10.

16-*Fcco. León i Blanco*-Treponema del Mal del Pinto. Rev. Médica Militar. Tomo II. No. 8.
17-*Fcco. León i Blanco*-Las lesiones de principio del Mal del Pinto. Rev. Médica Militar. Tomo II. No. 8.
18-*Fcco. León i Blanco*-Histología patológica de las lesiones cutáneas de los ganglios linfáticos en el Mal del Pinto. Rev. Médica Militar. Tomo II. No. 10.
19-*Fcco. León i Blanco*-El Mal del Pinto. Obra. 1942.
20-*Guillermo González Peris*-Bosquejo histórico sobre la etiología de la pinta o carate. Villa Clara Médica. Vol VI. No. 10.
21-*Ignacio González Guzmán*-Contribución para la serología del Mal del Pinto. Gaceta Médica de México. Tomo LXXI. No. 4.
22-*Ignacio González Guzmán*-Acción de la dilución sobre la capacidad reactora de los sueros de pintos. Gaceta Médica de México. Tomo LXXI. No. 4.
23-*Ignacio González Guzmán*-Estudio serológico de los enfermos portadores de pintides. Gaceta Médica de México. Tomo LXXI. No. 4.
24-*R.L. Kahn*-False positive reactions in serology of syphilis. University Hospital Bulletin. University of Michigan, Ann. Arbor. Vol. VI.
25-*E.J. Thonnard Neumann, Moya Camacho i K.C. Brewster*-Is carate (pinta) a desmatomycois?. Report United Fruit Co. Vol. IXX.
26-*Howard Fox*-Mal de Pinto as observed in Mexico its relation to carate. Proc. of 8th International Congress of Derm. and Syph.
27-*Howard Fox*-Discovery of the causative organism of pinta. Arch. of Dermat. and Syphilis. 1939.
28-*A.L. Carrión, R. Nazario i F. Hernández Morales*-Mal del Pinto en Puerto Rico. Bol. de la Soc. Méd. de Pto. Rico. 1941.
29-*E. Brumpt*-Un nouveau troponema parasite de l'homme Treponema Agent des carates ou Mal de Pinto. C.R. Soc. Biol. 1939.
30-*E. Brumpt*-Concernant l'agent et l'epidemiologie du carate ou Mal de Pinto. Ann. de Paras. Humm. et comparee. 1939.
31-*A. Peña Chavarria i P. Shipley*-Contribución al estudio de los carates de la América Tropical. Rev. Médica Latino-americana. 1925.
32-*J. Grau i Triana*-Contribución al estudio de la pinta o carate en Cuba. Arch. de Medicina Int. 1937.
33-*J. Grau i Triana*-La pinta en Cuba. Rev. de Med. i Cir. de La Habana. 1933.
34-*Salvador González Herrejón*-El Mal del Pinto. Ed. de la Rev. Int. Terapéutica. 1938.
35-*S. González Herrejón i H. Pallares*-Nuevas orientaciones para el estudio del Mal del Pinto. Revista del Hospital General. 1927.
36-*J.I. Escobar*-La enfermedad azul de los indios Chillos (Ecuador). Bol. Cli. Fac. de Med. de Antioquía. 1940.
37-*Braulio Saénz, J. Grau i Triana i José A. Armenteros*-Aspectos clínicos de la pinta o carate en Cuba. Su agente etiológico. El Día Médico. 1941.
38-*Luis A. León*-El mal del pinto en el Ecuador. Previsión Social. Bol. del Minis. de Prev. Soc. 1941.
39-*Luis A. León*-Ojeada histórica sobre el carate o mal del pinto en los países de la Gran Colombia. Rev. Médica. IV año 1942.
40-*Helia Bravo Hollis*-Bibliografía del Mal del Pinto i de algunas dermatosis cromógenas afines. Rev. Mex. de Biología. Tomo X. No. 3.
41-*Pardo Castello e Ismael Ferrer*-Pinta, mal del pinto, carate. Arch. of Derm. and Syph. Vol 45. 1942.
42-*Eddo. Aguirre Pequeño*-Empeines o jiotes. Lesiones de principio. Ensayo crítico. Medicina. Tomo XXII. Año XXIII. No. 424.
43-*Rodolfo Gómez Farías*-El Mal del Pinto. Revista Médica Militar. Tomo II. No. 8.

44-*Rodolfo Gómez Farías*-Investigaciones del Treponema en las lesiones de 500 casos de Mal del Pinto. Revista Médica Militar. Tomo II. No. 8.

BIBLIOGRAPHY

Consulted Venezuelan

45-*Briceño Rossi Antonio*-El valor del verification test en la serología del carate o mal del pinnto i buba. Rev. de Sanidad i Asistencia Social. Vol. VIII. No. 1.
46-*Antonio Briceño Rossi*-Carate or Mal del Pinto. Proc. of the Sixth Pacific Science Congress. Vol V. 1939.
47-*Antonio Briceño Rossi i David R. Iriarte*-Consideraciones sobre el estado actual del carate i su distribución geográfica en Venezuela. Folleto. 1939.
48-*Antonio Briceño Rossi i David R. Iriarte*-Breves notas sobre últimas investigaciones verificadas en las zonas pintógenas de Venezuela en relación al estado actual del conocimiento del carate o mal del pinto. Rev. de Sanidad i Asistencia Social. 1943.
49-*David R. Iriarte*-Trabajos Científicos. Obra 1937.
50-*David R. Iriarte*-El carate en Venezuela. Bol. del Lab. de la Clínica Razetti 1940.
51-*David R. Iriarte*-Estudios de Patología Tropical. Obra. 1942.
52-*J. Medina Jiménez*-Las afecciones micósicas en Venezuela-Gaceta Médica de Caracas. 1926.
53-*Alberto Fernández, Brumpt, Pifano, Mayer, Briceño Iragorry, Iriarte, Vegas, etc.*-Carate. Bol. Of. Sanitaria Panamericana-1940.
54-*Martín Vegas*-Los carates o carares. Rev. Centro Est. Medicina. 1918.
55-*Fernando Padilla*-Tesis Fac. de Medicina de Caracas. 1907.

THE CARATE - THE PINTA OF CUBA IS NOT CARATE *

The carate, always it has been, a sickness suggestive and mysterious, its etiology and treatment had several stops.

Since the author was a boy in his place of birth (Maracaibo, State Zulia) had heard speak with afraid of the region of Perijá and its focus of carate. Until few time ago the caratoso was a pariah as the leprous. Remember that in 1942 in the "Revista de Medicina Tropical i Parasitología de La Habana". Vol. VIII, No 6, we wrote: "el caratoso es una persona moralmente aplanada, acabado el espíritu como pasa en el leproso". Remind with horror the history of a woman, ex-wife of a governor that described the disease and did mention that was during seven months with a diet of eggs and spring water fearing the infection. Remember that in a trip to El Consejo, village bordering the States Falcón and Zulia, center of a secondary focus of carate, begging to the police commissioner help in order to gather a group of ills, trying to obtain material for the study, answered: "doctor, I can aid you in everything, less in gathering them". It was the fear that the chief had.

"The slow civilization of the country, the roads and paths constructed, the power and influence of the oil companies, our preachments since 1931, have gone modifying the mind of the caratosos, and so, four years ago in trip to Barinas, in Quebrada Seca, where almost all the population are infected, inmediately knew the arrival of a physician studying the disease, few minutes later had around us a hundred of persons ready to suffer any test. In this visit we offered to a sick, one box of bismuth, and the followed day walks 20 km. looking for the medicament.

The carate in Venezuela is called also carare, but the word cute that we had as synonymous, today, we believe they used it for designate other affections of the skin.

We did our first investigations about this illness in the year 1931, in communication published in Gaceta Médica de Caracas, page 173, entitled "Observaciones sobre el Carate en el Distrito Perijá del Estado Zulia". In 1932, we published in Paris, printed Jouve & Co., something about the same subject, entitled: "Voyage a Mene Mauroa. Contribution a l'etude du Carate dans l' Amerique Tropicale"; after, an article spreading abroad, in 1933, in the newspaper "El Nuevo Diario", entitled: "El carate o carare es una de las enfermedades más curables hoy. Venezuela puede tener alrededor de 50.000 caratosos", reproduced in the "Boletín Clínico de Medellín", Colombia, Año V, No. 12 pages 591-600.

The following paragraph has been taken of the Revista de Medicina Tropical i Parasitología of Havana (Cuba) either mentioned: "El carate es una endemia alarmante para Venezuela, como lo es, por las cifras que ha-

* Read in the National Academy of Venezuelan Medicine (7-11-1966)

blan, para nuestras hermanas Colombia i México. Acabamos de encontrar que en los Municipios Pedrazas i Quebrada Seca del Estado Barinas la infección llega a más del 50% i para todo el Estado a un 10% , cifras parecidas a las anteriores de las estadísticas mejicanas. En censo hecho en el Municipio Pedrazas o Ciudad Bolivia hemos hallado que para 600 habitantes, distribuidos en los caserios: Mijaguas, 133; La Caldereña, 15; Las Monjas, 28; Palmasola, 26; Anime i Cubatí, 43; Población, 36. Existen 281 caratosos, lo cual es una cifra alarmante. En otra aldea cercana a Pedrazas, en 136 habitantes hay 59 caratosos.

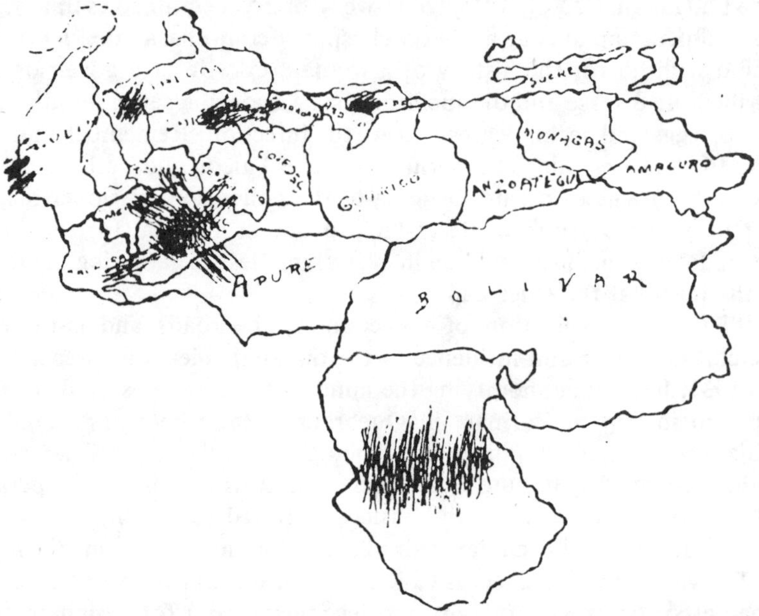

Map showing the geographical distribution of the carate in Venezuela.

We continue speaking about the distribution accompanied of a map: "El carate nos da la impresión se va extendiendo en nuestro país. Actualmente tenemos un foco principal situado en el Estado Barinas, que emite prolongamientos hacia el Sur hasta los ríos Arauca, Apure y Meta; al Norte hacia una pequeña parte de los Estados Mérida y Trujillo; al Este en el Estado Portuguesa y hacia el Oeste al Estado Táchira. Fuera de este gran foco central y principal, tenemos cinco focos secundarios: un foco en el Distrito Perijá del Estado Zulia; otro, en el Estado Lara, en la región de Sarare, que es posible se extienda a Yaracuy y Carabobo, según Padilla y Pérez Carreño (citados por Medina Jiménez); un tercero, en el Distrito Buchivacoa del Estado Falcón, región llamada Mene de Mauroa, llegando hasta el Lago de Maracaibo a través de los Distritos Miranda y Bolívar del Estado Zulia; un cuarto foco en el Estado Miranda, región de Guarenas,

Guatire y Caucagua en los vecindarios Naranjal, Oruza, Copure y Sanare; un quinto foco en el Territorio Amazonas, entre los indios maquiritares, goahibos, tamanacos, etc., foco que, según Alvarado, va por las regiones del Meta y Casanare hasta continuarse con los focos limítrofes colombianos, y por Río Negro hasta el Brasil".

En resumen, se ve por el mapa adjunto, que el carate es sobre todo una endemia de Occidente y del Sur de Occidente de nuestro país. Tenemos infectados los Estados Barinas, Apure, Mérida, Táchira, Trujillo, Lara, Zulia, Portuguesa, Falcón, Bolívar, Yaracuy, Carabobo y los dos Territorios Federales.

"La distribución geográfica hacia el Occidente da la idea que el carate nuestro viene de Colombia y nos hace pensar que el primer foco pudo ser el de Perijá, yendo en aserto de esto, como sucede en epidemiología, que el foco de Perijá trata de desaparecer, posiblemente por su antigüedad. En Machiques, capital de este Distrito, logramos recoger datos entre la gente vieja, de cierta cultura, y nos contaban que con motivo de las revolucioes de otros tiempos en el país vecino, llegaban a través de la Sierra de Perijá, que nos sirve de límite, muchos exiliados inmigrantes, recordando una familia Zeledón que presentaba la enfermedad y que probablemente fuera la semilla en esa comarca."

Rafael Medina in "Dermatología Venezolana", Vol. III, No. 3 y 4, 160-230, in "El carate en Venezuela" (Estudio de la enfermedad en el medio natural y resultados de los ensayos de inoculación experimental), br-

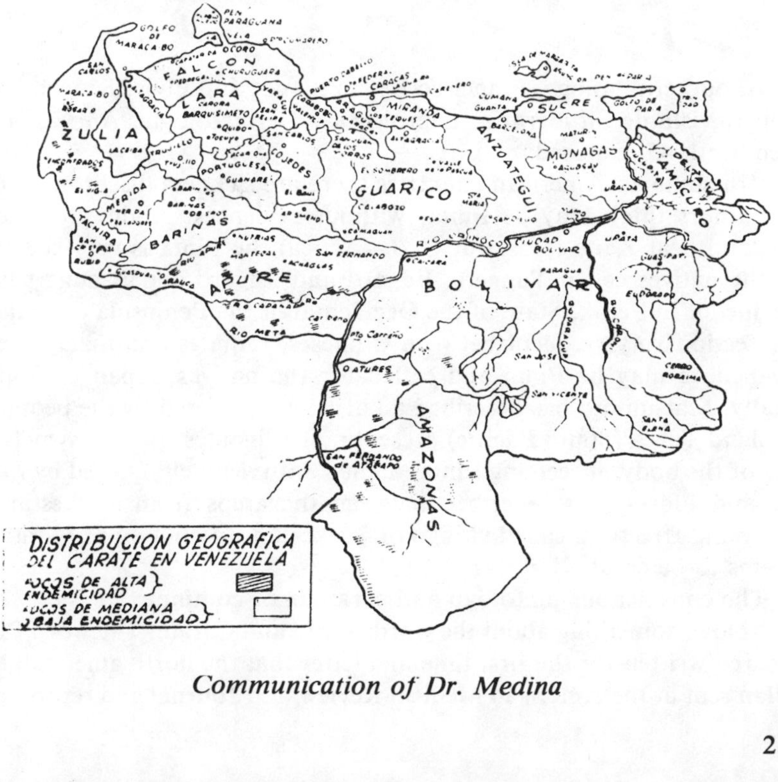

Communication of Dr. Medina

ings in the Chapter of Epidemiology large details about geographycal distribution with a map and wrote: "Today the greographycal distribution of the carate in Venezuela, is as follow:

1° - Focus of high infection situated in the Territorio Federal Amazonas, South of the State Apure and Sierra de Perijá in the State Zulia".

2° - Focus of medium and low infection, in the States Barinas, Miranda, Aragua, Carabobo, Bolívar, Lara, Portuguesa, Cojedes, Trujillo, Falcón, Monagas, Mérida and the Territorio Amacuro".

"Zone of Perijá, situated at the West of the State Zulia and with aspects bioclimatics and physiographics that remember the zones para-equatorials".

"The groups more infected of carate are integrate for indians belonging to the tribes japrería and pariries, living in villages near Tucuco, and others living to the borders the rivers Negro, Apón, Tucuco and Aaraguisa, toward the Sierra de Perijá in the borders with Colombia, and some of them are unknown".

"State Barinas, 20 years ago the zone of Barinas was the most infected in all the country. In that epoch the disease spreaded to The Andes and also to the plains toward the South, invading the araucans and focus of Colombia. Today is possible to find little focus Pedrazas, San Silvestre, Libertad, Mijagual and villages near to Suripá, Santa Lucía and rivers Santo Domingo, Masparro and Caparro".

* * *

About terminology, Francisco León i Blanco and Elvira Sánchez García in Revista de Sifilografía, Leprología y Dermatología, Año 2, N° 4, december 1945, exposed:

"In some no American countries there are sickness dischromics that any authors think may be Pinta, without evidences. About Browne in Hausland near Kano (Costa de Oro - Africa) the Pinta is very common and the natives call it Tungere. Edgard and Edgard and Beddaert have described it in Perak, State of the Occidental of the Peninsula of Malaca, an affection very frequent between Chineses, tamules and malayos that they believe may be Pinta and called for the natives Sopah or Sopak. Equally, Matsumoto has described an affection suffered by the people of the island Turca (South Pacific) presenting vitiligoides spots in symetrical parts of the body, it seeming Pinta, named Safú. Munch, quoted by Montoya and Flores, has described between the arcos from Turkestan an dischromic affection, called vitiligo of Turkestan. In opinion of Montoya, it seems to be carate."

The conspicuous pintólogo and caratólogo, continue:

"Now, something about the words Pinta and Carate. The word Pinta appeared written for the first time in a letter that the north american McClellan sent at the American Medical Review and Journal and reproduced in Edimburgo Medical Science, N° 4, 1826, in Calcuta Medical Transaccions (6: 62: 1834); the english authors took the word of these megazines. It is curious that Mc Clellan living for a while in México where he saw the disease, wrote Pinta and not Pinto, because in México the first of these words is used in cases of *tabardillo* or exanthematic typhus, and the Mal del Pinto, as is current in State of Guerrero, where the sickness called his attention. We believe that Mc Clellan confounded the words or that wrote in his letter *pinto* and by an error typographical appeared *pinta*. This error of Mc Clellan or typographical error has been spreaded between the hispano-americans authors. The translator of the article of Muller, named pinto and the *mal de la pinta*. Hercelles, Peña Chavarría and Shipley and the north-American and English authors. In Cuba the word indicated in the treponemosis that we study, was introduced by Fox (1929)."

"The first european that wrote the word carate was Fernández de Oviedo y Valdéz in 1535, who heared it directly of mouth of the caribbeans. They used it for distinguish some indians affected by cutaneous spots, that probably is the same disease we know today."

León i Blanco continues:

"In Cuba the cases of carate are very scarce and come from the six provinces, places where never have been found focus or zones caratosas. Is good to know that some of our cases never have been gone out the capital of the Republic and always have lived in the center of the country. This opinion is very important, because always has been accepted that the carate is a rural disease; also is very interesting the rare transmission of the sickness; and so the patients suffering it does not remember contacts with

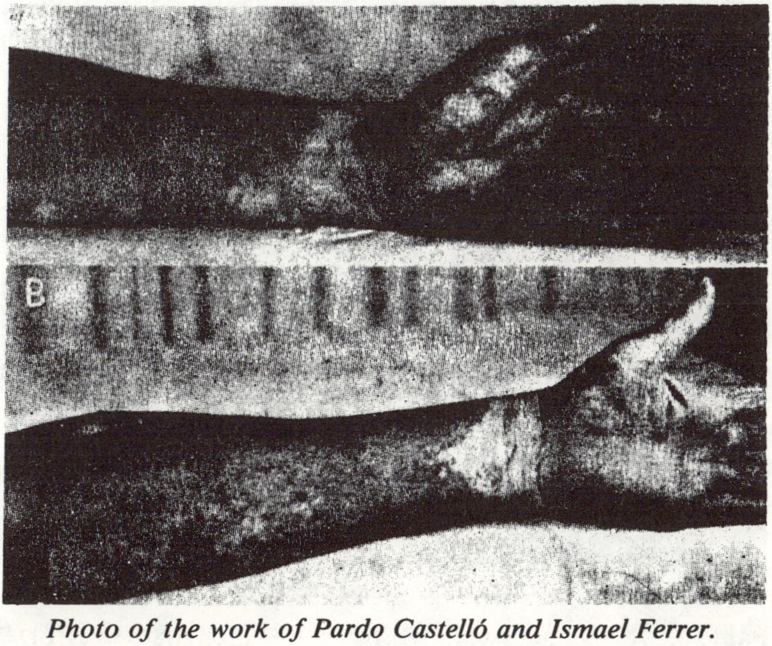

Photo of the work of Pardo Castelló and Ismael Ferrer.

persons infected and it is possible a reservoir extra human being of Treponema carateum or Treponema herrejoni and the infection from this deposit to the man by an unknown way."

"The total number of cases reported in Cuba are around two hundreds. It is difficult to say the exact, because one case has been reported twice; but attending to Grau Triana, Pardo Castelló and Pardo Castelló and Ferrer, in Cuba have been described 86 cases."

León i Blanco, follows: "In Mexico, according the first census about Mal del Pinto, realized by the Department of Public Health, exist, approximately, 270.685 *pintos*, number very conservator taking in account the epoch when was made where were unknown the initial lesion, the *pintides*, described years later, by León i Blanco."

"The cases are distributed in certain rural zones, called by González Herrejón *zones pintógenas*; the principal is located in the big hydrographical depression of river Balsas including the northeast of Oaxaca; north of Guerrero; a part of Veracruz; almost all the State of Morelos; the South of the States Mexico, Puebla and Michoacán. Besides, exist another small focus in the States Nayarit, Tabasco and Chiapas."

"Taking in account the population of the nation, are attacked approximately, the 1.5% of the total population."

"In Colombia the carate is endemic in all the valleys of the country, chiefly in the border of the large rivers. In account of Peña Chavarría and Shipley there are, nearly, 400.000, although never has been made a census. That number correspond to the 6% of the population."

"In Venezuela, there are around 50.000 caratosos (Iriarte), spreaded in the States Barinas, Apure, Mérida, Táchira, Trujillo, Lara, Zulia, Portuguesa, Falcón, Bolívar, Yaracuy, Carabobo and the Territories Amacuro and Amazonas."

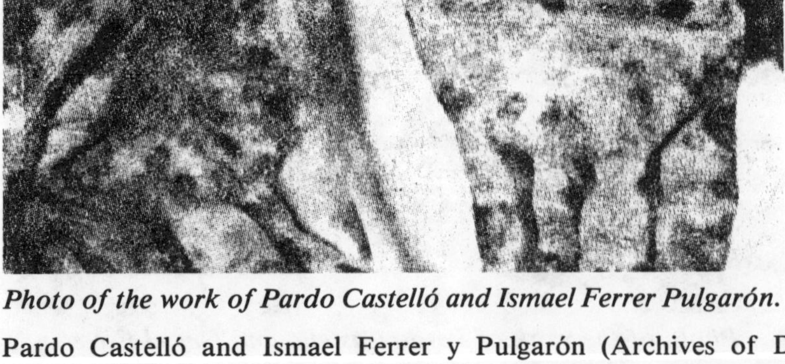

Photo of the work of Pardo Castelló and Ismael Ferrer Pulgarón.

Pardo Castelló and Ismael Ferrer y Pulgarón (Archives of Dermatology and Syphilology, may 1942, vol. 45, pages 843-864), in Pinta, Mal del Pinto, Carate, accompanied of photos, expose: "For several years we had observed in Cuba a number of Negro patients, suffering from a dyschromic dermatosis, which was considered a former of dermatophytosis in spite of the fact that pathogenic fungi could not be isolated. When the reports of Menk, González Herrejón and Fox became known to us, we thought that the condition observed in Cuba was similar to the one reported by these investigators, opinion that was strengthened when the serologic reactions (Wassermann and Kahn) in all our cases proved to be positive. However, having no experience with the clinical aspects of Mal del Pinto in México or of Carate in South America, we hesitated between considering the disease observing in Cuba as a type of dyschromic syphilis or a clinical form of Pinta. These doubts were finally dispelled when Fox attending the meeting of the American Dermatological Association in Havana, in 1932, studied some of the cases presented and thought that they were cases of Pinta. In spite of these general Cuban dermatologists still considered that pinta was a parasitic disease or a form of syphilis as late at 1937. One of us (V.P.C.) reported a number of cases in 1936 and affirmed the spirochetal nature of the disease in accord with González Herrejón and Fox. It might be of interest to mention that Fox recognized the first case of Pinta in Cuba when attending a meeting of the Cuban Dermatological Society in January 1928."

"Palmar and plantar hyperkeratosis of either diffuse or punctate type and with or without the formation of fissures are common in Cuba and rather unusual in México."

"We have seen lesions on the scrotum coincident with typical manifestations on the hands and feet; the lesions of the scrotum were indistinguishable from those of vitiligo, but the spirochete of pinta was recovered from the lymph the affected scrotal areas."

"Mal del Pinto in México and carate in South America are limited to certain regions, specially the river valleys. In Cuba the disease is endemic, but the patients come from the most diverse parts of the country and no *pinta zones* have been delimited. Furthermore, the manifestations of the disease in Cuba are practically limited to the dyschromic type of the late stage, and seldom have the early lesions been observed, the patients usually saying they have not previously had any disease of the skin. The majority of Cubans patients, are negroes, while in México, Venezuela, Colombia and Ecuador persons of the Indians race and mestizos are the most frequent sufferers. The white race is not inmune, but evidently the disease is rare in white persons. It occured in white in about 12 per cent of our Cuban cases. Children are often affected in México, but the disease is not transmitted to the offspring. In Cuba the youngest of our patients was 23, but we know of children about 10 years old in cases of some of our colleagues."

Alberto Oteiza Setien, Revista de Sifilografía, Leprología y Dermatología, Año 2, enero 1945, in "La lesión inicial experimental de la Pinta,

Mal del Pinto o Carare en Cuba'', says: ''Como León i Blanco ha reiterado sus dudas de que todo lo que se ha descrito en Cuba con el nombre de Pinta, sea en realidad la enfermedad producida por Treponema herrejoni; esto es, la afección que en la América Latina se conoce con los nombres de Pinta, Mal del Pinto o Carate.''

Are so many the doubts of León i Blanco that in his book ''El Mal del Pinto (México 1942), that as Cuban has owing to call La Pinta, in the Chapter I, doing the definition, finish that paragraph, so: ''It is produced by a treponema specific: Treponema herrejoni or Treponema carateum.''

The Pontiff of the carate, Salvador González Herrejón, in ''Mal del Pinto'', Leverkusen - Alemania, 1938, wrote: ''In the hand and also in the foot, never are affected the spaces between the fingers, neither the palms and plants.''

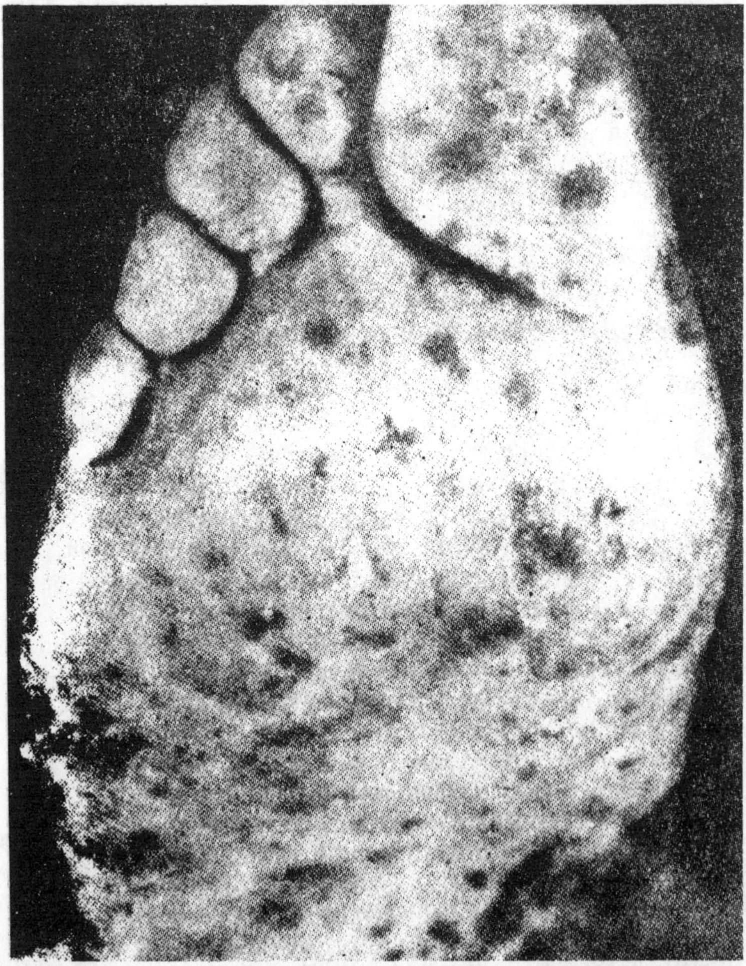

Photo of the communication of Pardo Castelló and Ismael Ferrer.

"In the cases of pinto reported by Pardo Castelló and Grau Triana, in Cuba the spots exist usually in the palms and plants, or at least preferably these areas, being a localization very unusual here in Mexico and also in Colombia."

Successively in his post-scriptum, add: "Who have read the former pages, will remember that in Cuba exist some hyperkeratosis stages of the palm of the hands and plants of the feet, with pigmentation grayish, of limited border, pinkish, etc. Now, then, that dermatosis was diagnosted as *tiña albígena* of Jenaselme. After, thought, chiefly Professor Sáenz, in late syphilitic lesions. In January, 1929, visited Cuba the north-american dermatologist Howard Fox, having the opportunity of seen one of these cases, saying that found the case very similar with the carate that he recently had seen in Colombia."

This opinion of Fox not impressed the Cuban dermatologist. At the end of the same year (1929), Braulio Sáenz loyal to his etiologycal concept published in the Bulletin of the Cuban Society of Dermatology and Syphilology (Vol. I, N° 3, pag. 198, october 1929), an article: "Sobre una forma rara de sífilis cutánea tardía, eritemo-atrofiante. Consideraciones diagnósticas" in which exposed his judgment.

"In 1932, the opinion of Professor Pardo Castelló was doubtful. Presented to the American Dermatological Association several clinical histories, with the name: "Leucodermia syphilitic?", and newly Fox, who attended this meeting, insisted were patients with Mal del Pinto."

Later, according Grau and Triana, yet wrote about a case: "En una mujer blanca, heredo-luética, con tres hermanos sifilíticos, uno de los cuales murió de sífilis maligna ósea."

Nothing more wrote Professor Sáenz, but his adjunt in the Service of Dermatology of the Hospital Our Lady of Las Mercedes in Havana, the doctor Grau y Triana, published in 1937, a communication: "Estudios de la Pinta o Carate en Cuba", and said "that the hyperkeratosis of the palms and plants were really *pinto*, and refused the theory spirochetal, believing in fungi.

"He thinks in the syphilitic origin and still that the visceral lesions, the positivy of the tests, and the success of the arsenic comes in approval. The search of spirochetes in lymph of the border of the lesions, the blood and tissues were always negative."

"In the works made in the Service of the Hospital Our Lady Las Mercedes, presented to the VII Congress of the Pan-American Association, held in Cuba that year, only two cases of Dr. Oteiza, lightly described, were exposed, with the name: ¿Pinta or Carate?"

"In this condition, arrived to Dr. Sáenz' service a new case, and taking the lymph of the border of the lesions in the hands, in dark field, Dr. Alfonso, Assistant of the Service, saw a treponema. That examination was accidental, but he was not in charge of that kind of investigations, and that afternoon or at the following day, was informed Professor Sáenz of the finding."

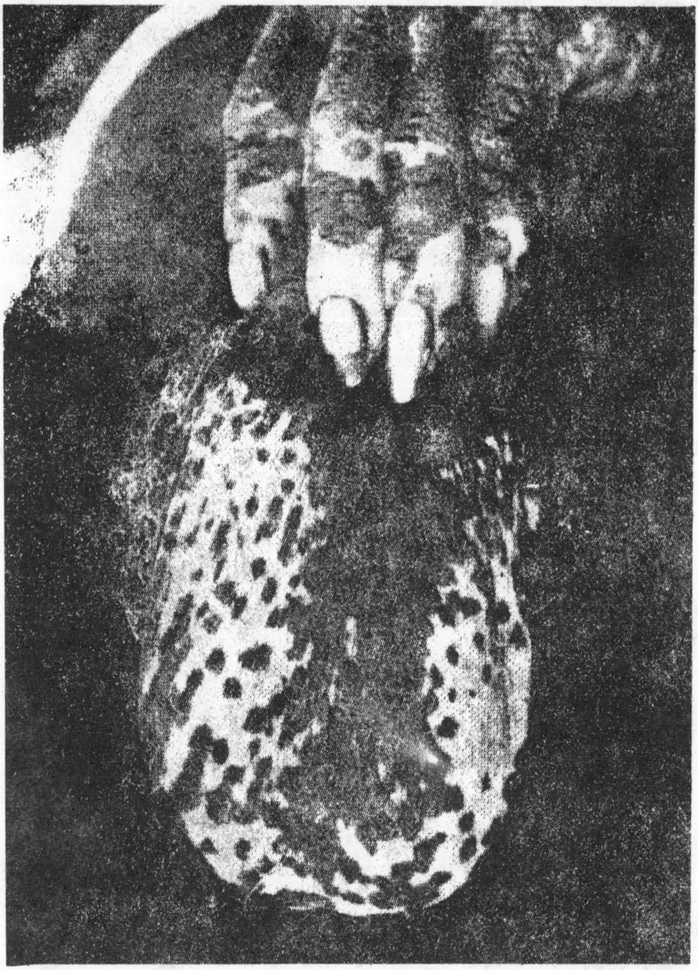

Photo of the work of Pardo Castelló and Ismael Ferrer.

"The case was presented to the Society of Dermatology and Syphilology of Cuba and we do not know the diagnosis, because to that moment Professor Sáenz believed in syphilitic origin; others thought the finding was the pathogenic cause of the Pinto."

"Let us finally a commentary about the finding and so we always say, intentionally, the word finding and not discovery."

In effect, we believe by the antecedents and documentation existing, the true of to find a treponema in a lesion of the hand, in a center where not were sure if the case belonging to Mal del Pinto, but thought in late manifestation of syphilis or in mycotic dermatosis and denied often the spirochetal theory, was simply a chance event, and not the result of organized labor seeking a purpose. Moreover, looking for always spirochetes in those lesions, was the T. pallida, trying to be in accord with Sáenz and Grau Triana. In the scientific investigation, looking for a thing

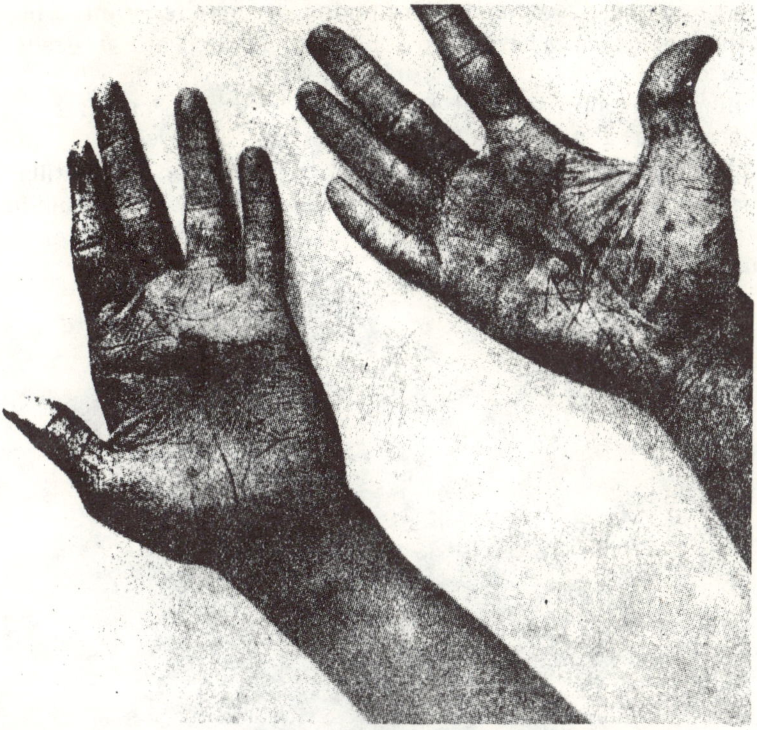

Exceptional case with spots in palms of the hands that are very rare. Photo of the work of González Herrejón.

and finding another one is very frequent, and for the Science the important is not the intention, is the thing found."

* * *

With all the former documentation exposed, we believe think and conclude that the *Pinta* of Cuba is not the Carate that everybody knows. The Cuban disease without doubt is a treponemosis, but totally different.

The *Pinta* is a sickness very scarce in Cuba, it is not a rural disease as the Carate, rather an urban disease with rebounded lesions hyperkeratosics in hands and feet and a pigmentation punctate type in those sites, details very rare in the *Carate*, as is seen in the photos of González Herrejón and Medina, making emphasis of it. Is an affection with a high percentage in the negroes, rare detail in the *Carate*. In our last visit to Havana, requested to our good friends Basnuevo and Sotolongo, that we should wish, before the departure to see a case of *Pinta*, and answered: "is an affection very scarce in Cuba; sometimes comes a case" and we told: "in Venezuela, when you like to see Carate is very common." The colleagues that spoke were Professors of the Institute of Tropical Diseases and Parasitology "Carlos Finlay" of the University of Havana.

The *Pinta*, according to our opinion, are manifestations syphilitics or perhaps yaws, as believed and considered Sáenz, Pardo Castelló, León i Blanco and others, till the visit of Fox to Cuba, telling them that was similar to the affection that he just had seen in a recent trip to Colombia; or either, the *Pinta* can be a treponematosis X, carried in the bouts slave traders, that has remained in Cuba. If in the Perla de las Antillas has existed *Carate*, as in Mexico, Colombia and Venezuela, we should have seen large focus in the groups working and living in the plantations of sugar cane.

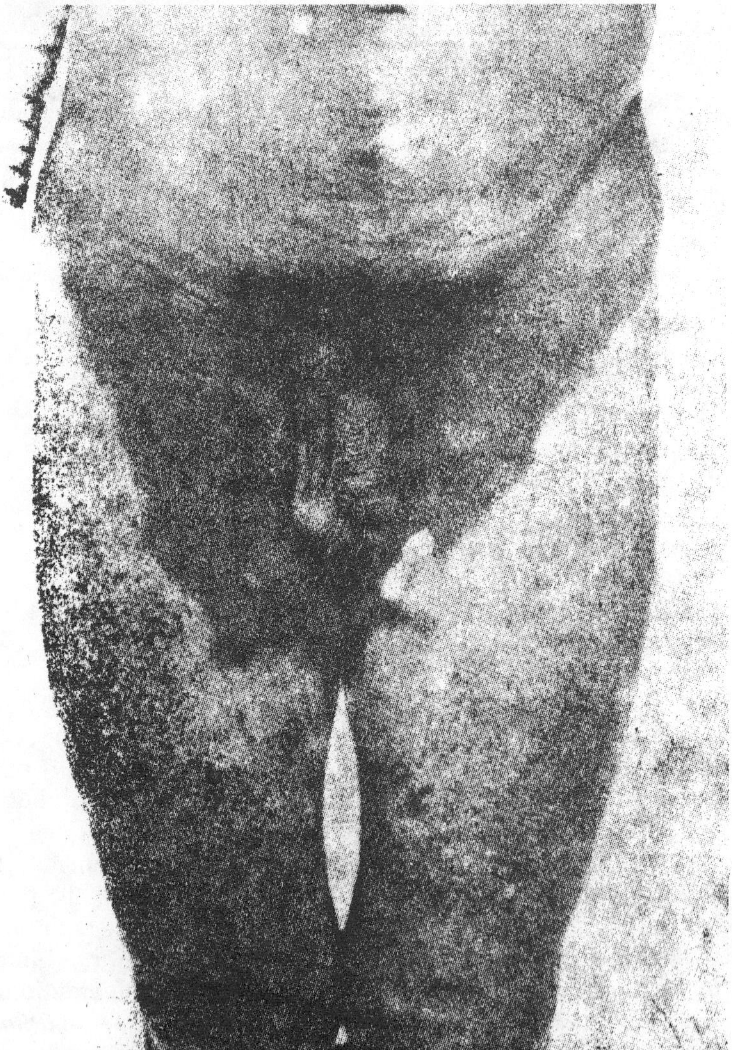

Internal surface of the thighs and genital region. Photo of the work of González Herrejón.

Between us were the Cuban investigators Francisco León i Blanco, notable pintologist and caratologist; Alberto Oteiza Setien, known dermatologist that was Minister of Health in the Government of Prío Socarrás, and the dermatologist and venereologist Ismael Ferrer y Pulgarón. Now then, an afternoon dialogizing with León i Blanco in one of the terraces of the Hotel Tamanaco, having by witness the mountain El Avila, during our conversation, I asked him: —"tell me a thing, do you believe that the *Pinta* is the *Carate*?", and he answered: —"Iriarte, the Pinta is not Carate, when I went to Mexico and now here in your country, I came to know the Carate."

Oteiza Setien arrived with the same doubts; interested to see Carate, Briceño Rossi and us prepared for him a meeting of the ancient Society of Microbiology, Parasitology and Tropical Medicine, saw the film that Briceño Rossi and us, together made when he was Director of Salubrity. After, he said to us: "The Pinta, it is not Carate." To the same conclusion arrived Ferrer y Pulgarón.

We propose that the treponema, perhaps, hastily had classified our remembered Master the wise Professor Brumpt as Treponema carateum Brumpt 1938, must be called Treponema pintae Iriarte 1966, referring to the finding in the Pinta, and that the Treponema found by León y Blanco in Mexico, in true Carate, be named Treponema herrejoni León y Blanco, 1938, because the Treponema carateum of Brumpt was found in a disease that not was Carate.

* * *

We regret these considerations in difficult moments for the Cuban science. Some years, we have kept these opinions waiting not wound susceptibilities and has requested to friend dermatologists expose our opinions.

We have good ties and deep estimation for the Cuban medicine; we know the numerous group of investigators, health officers and tropicalists, parasitologists, since the epoch of Finlay, Agramonte and Guiteras, till today; writers of prologues of one of our books are the Professor Kouri and Basnuevo; and in the meeting bi-anual of Cuban Laboratory Physicians, we had the honor, together with the Professor Rodríguez from México, being the only two invited of all America, having the official representation of Venezuela.

When the finding of the Treponema in Cuba, was a lenitive and stimulus for the Professor Sáenz, because his wife and three sons just disappeared in the shipwreck of the "Morro Castle", and after the death of León i Blanco y Ferrer i Pulgarón, who could have given yet a great deal to its native country and the Science. It seems to be the study of the Pinta has a fatidic sign.

If León i Blanco does not go to México, Briceño Rossi and us would have been the discoverers of the *Treponema*. The report of Professor Sáenz and his school was August 3 1938. León i Blanco went to México and published the finding of the Treponema in Mexican patients, October 13 1938, in Medicina, vol. 18, pages 617-618. Briceño Rossi and us found it here, in Venezuela, February 17 1939, four months and four days after León i Blanco.

Without any doubt the Cubans discovered, perhaps, a new *treponemosis*. Although the *Pinta* can be manifestation Syphilitics or yaws, and spoke about test with *Treponema carateum* positive in syphilis and yaws, were the Cubans who gave the alert and guide lines to seek and find the *Treponema*. Always the glory of the discovery is in hands of a *Cuban*, if our opinions are not mistaken.

November 1966

SUMMARY

Dr. David R. Iriarte, from Caracas (Venezuela) presents an important and exciting scientific work entitled "El Carate - La Pinta de Cuba no es el Carate".

Since thirty years ago Dr. Iriarte has studied and occupied about the disease. He has published many communications in connection with this subject, one of them is Paris, and in 1938 discovered, in association with Dr. Briceño Rossi, the Treponema of the Carate in Venezuela.

The author does an extensive exposition concerning the history, terminology, geographic distribution and etiology. In Venezuela this complain is nominated: "Carate, Carare and Cute", notwithstanding, Iriarte thinks the last nomination is applicated to different pigmentations of the skin.

There are infected cases in almost all the States of the country. A map is given showing the large and small focus where the illness exists. In Venezuela the Treponema was found, for the first time, in a patient of Guarenas, region of a little focus, situated one hour and a half from Caracas and was presented to the Academy of Medicine.

Iriarte believes that the Pinta of Cuba is completely different from the Carate of Mexico, Colombia, Venezuela and other countries. La Pinta is very rare. The author, in more than one occasion, in visit to La Habana has tried to see a case and has been impossible. With an enlarged documentation try to demonstrate that are two diseases.

Iriarte suggests that the Treponema, whose classification was made by Professor Brumpt, in Pinta of Cuba, as "carateum" Brumpt 1938, must be called Treponema "pintae" Iriarte 1966, and the Treponema found by León y Blanco, in Mexico, that it is the true germ and was discovered four months before us, must be nominated "herrejoni", León y Blanco 1938.

Several years ago, the author wished to expose these ideas, but his friendship and esteem for the Cuban colleagues and science had prevented him to do it.

SOMETHING MORE ABOUT CARATE*

By reason of the publication of our work "EL CARATE - LA PINTA de Cuba no es el Carate" read in this distinguished Academy on November 17, 1967 and presented to the VI Congress Ibero-Latino-Americano of Dermatology held in Barcelona, Spain, from the 24 to the 27 of June 1968, we have had the pleasure of receiving from several scientific men of different countries of America, some of them Mexicans, that we consider the most versed in this field, words of congratulations and encouragement and also observations about our appreciations.

An old friend Professor Gerardo Varela says that he should wish not to hear again as succeeded in the meeting about Treponemiasis in Washington 1964: "the pinto or carate has had many errors and contradictions in the hands of Latin-Americans".

The zealous investigator Luis Mazzotti, ancient chief of the Parasitology Laboratory of the Institute of Tropical Diseases of Mexico, in the Chapter "Carate" of the Section of Infection Diseases of the Encyclopedia Medico-Surgical (Paris) wrote the following historical details:

"The testimonies accumulate by León y Blanco try to prove that the carate existed in the intertropical America before the discovery.

Moziño, in 1798, showed the hyperchromatic spots cured with mercurio rubbings, not obtaining the same in the white stains.

On 1811, Beracoechea was doubtful about the contagion of the illness saying that the infants not adquired the disease and besides between the marriages, often one of them, only presents carate.

At the same time, Corona, make known that the carate start and show some lesions called *"empeines"*.

Tellez, in 1890, could perform cutaneous inoculations from infected persons to another undamaged got the transmission of the disease.

Ruiz Sandoval and Montoya Flores, in 1881, accused the fungi as the producer of the carate.

In the present century, Tussaint has worked about the pathology and in 1913, Grutz, discovered the specific action of the salvarsan".

* Published in Gaceta Médica de Caracas año LXXVII - Julio-Septiembre - Nº 7 a 9 - 1969.

REPLY TO THE CRITIQUE OF DR. J. ALFONSO ARMENTEROS FROM CUBA TO MY WORK "EL CARATE - LA PINTA DE CUBA NO ES EL CARATE" *

We have received, some time ago, something retrased, a critique appeared in the "Revista de Medicina Tropical", Vol. 21, N°'s 1, 2 and 3, December 1969. Moreover of the copy sent, Dr. Arturo Luis Berti, had the kindness of sending us another copy that he had received. One is in our poor library and another one in the donation that we made to this Institution.

It is a long, tedious and insubstantial censure that at times has details *anatolescos,* but always in a high climate, perhaps, by his status of physician and to the rigidity commanding in that country. As a good Cuban, we throw the glove and he must return it. We regret of that sympathetic land, where we have had agreeable moments and many good friends, thinking of the bad conditions of the present time.

In our visit to Havana we did not have the honor to meet the Professor Alfonso-Armenteros, but we believe, if we are not mistaken, that it was in that epoch a technician in the laboratoy in the Dermatological Service of Professor Braulio Sáenz, and he went who saw, accidentally, as refers the Professor González Herrejon and says the history, without seeking it, without thinking of it, appeared a spirochete in the lymph of a dyschromic lesion of the skin in a patient with hyperkeratosis palmplantar. This is not reprehensible, not loose merits the finding; many notable discoveries, very useful for the mankind have been obtained by the hazard.

We are very glad Dr. Oteiza Setien, our old friend, to whom include in the *sino* fatidic of the Cuban pintólogos, we knew through the academic Dr. Kerdel Vegas, that is living healthy in Puerto Rico.

The stage of isolation of his country is the cause of these errors. Lamentably, we were sure referring Sáenz, Grau-Triana, León y Blanco.

When we said: "always the glory of the discovery belong to a Cuban: Francisco León y Blanco". Armenteros, by chance, found a spirochete, moving, in the lymph of a lesion of the skin of a patient in Havana, in the Service of Professor Sáenz, was an accidental finding in a person that was not *caratosa;* this found thing, made enthusiastic to León y Blanco, going to Mexico, knowing zones of true *carate,* finding always a spriochete in the Mexican *caratosos,* and did a clinical description of the disease, inoculating it himself; spirochete found some days later by Briceño Rossi and us, here in Venezuela. Brumpt classified the germ as Treponema

* Read it in the meeting of the National Academy of Medicine (9-12-71)

carateum in mexican material sent by two ways: Mazzotti and González Herrejón. Professor Armenteros finding unexpected, unreasonable, by chance, by *carambola* is involucred in the discovery of the germ of *Carate.*

Alfonso-Armenteros, more than one time, said that we think and write very different than we said in former stage of epoch, but it is good that the distiguished investigator accept: that today we think of a mannner and tomorrow of other mode. Just, his finding, touched the old platform, brought new ideas, about this rare sickness called *carate.*

You, Professor Armenteros, distracting, entertaining, looking in dark field for a drop of lymph, saw a spirochete, believing by suspicions, that in that moment were not present the Professors Sáenz and Grau-Triana, has the merit that a found thing, did open the eyes and think that the *carate* was a treponemosis, as said Mazzotti, although either had suspicions by the works of Menck in 1926 and of González Herrejón 1927.

You say that we raise a cloud of dust supporting foreign proofs, without no contribution; without bringing personal tests; notwithstanding, you yourself, boast of *factotum* in the etiology of the carate, tells: "in nine years, in his dermatologyical statistic, has seen five cases, and one of them was a man of yellow race", and affirm, that in total, perhaps, the cases of Pinta presented arrive to 200. You come to Venezuela, go to Colombia, Ecuador, chiefly Mexico, with a bigger population, trip that we believe you did, and if you want to know the carate will see hundreds and thousands of cases, not five in nine years as you say.

It is not true, as you assert "that I have consulted a reduced bibliography of the communications published in some magazines, chiefly cubans". In our library there is a large bibliography about this theme and perhaps, will be very few the works that have not seen, read and consulted.

Professor Armenteros, you accept differences referring to etiology, clinical aspects and have a paragraph, as this: "at the end it is convenient to explain that about this affair have not been realized in Cuba works absolutely scientifics, either no investigator has gone to the regions from where the patients come from, and so can realize - in the adequate places -the investigation of cases, the study of the ambient, etc." or this: "the differences morphological that exist between the *Pinta* and the *Carate* are not a solid argument in order to consider it as different nosological entities. The cause of those differences are unknown, be possible regional conditions, direct or indirect, have important intervention in this affair."

Or this: "Without doubts, exist remarkable differences in relation with the number of cases and the existence of zones pintosas or caratosas in the different countries mentioned before as it happened in Cuba"; or this another: "In our country has not been reports till today none *zona pintosa*, because the patients coming from different places, almost always rurals. In consequence, we are in accord that referring to this aspect, there are differences between *Pinta* and *Carate, but we do not in accord when this one utilize this fact making the segregation to Pinta* of the *Carate*".

SODOKU IN VENEZUELA *

Sodoku is a disease, suspicious, long time ago, between us, but that had not been found in our country. As something published about this problem, exist only a communication of Dr. Tejera, of the year 1924, entitled: "The spirochete morsus muris, microbe of sodoku in the rats of Caracas". Dr. Tejera said: "exist in 10% of rats of Caracas the spirochete morsus muris, agent producing the sickness known with the name of sodoku, making to think that the disease must exist in Venezuela, probably confounded with another pyrexias".

Our patient says that when killing a rat in her home was bitten by the animal in one of the fingers of the right hand, feeling pain in the site of the bite. Fifteen days later, new pain and inflammation in the hand, high fever. The following day, feverish, appearance of a rash in the whole body, obliged her to go to the Hospital Vargas, on 29-8-39.

The diagnosis of entrance said cholecystopathy, but rapidly was done the clinical diagnosis of sodoku, doing herself an autodiagnosis.

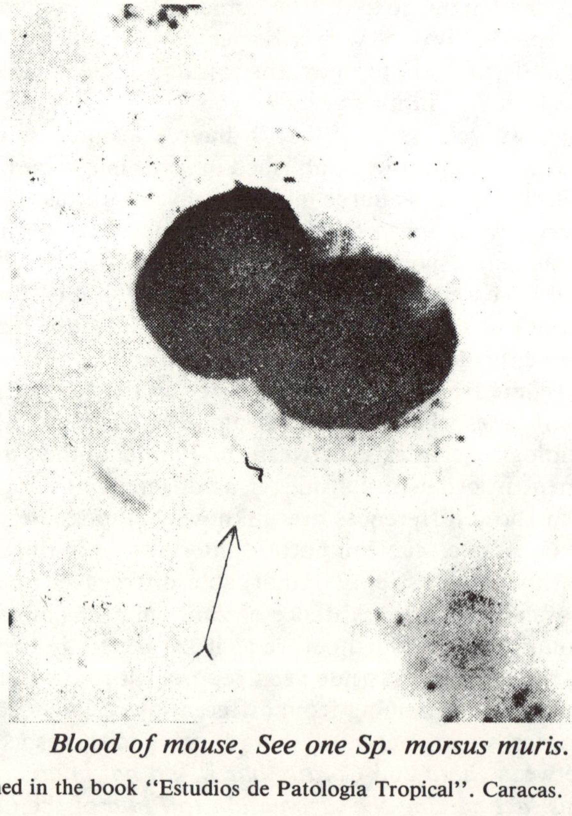

Blood of mouse. See one Sp. morsus muris.

* Published in the book "Estudios de Patología Tropical". Caracas. 1942.

Were made the following tests:

Radiography of the thorax: the right vertex is less clear than the left. Pulmonary fields clear. Calcified ganglions in the left lung.

Hemoculture in glucose broth	negative
Serum-diagnosis Widal	negative
R. Wassermann	negative
R. Kahn	negative
Glucose	0.76
Urea	0.23
Hematozoic Laveran	negative
White cells	14.300 m.m.
Differential count white cells	
Neutrophyles	90%
Eosinophyles	0%
Basophyles	0%
Lymphocytes	10%
Monocytes	0%

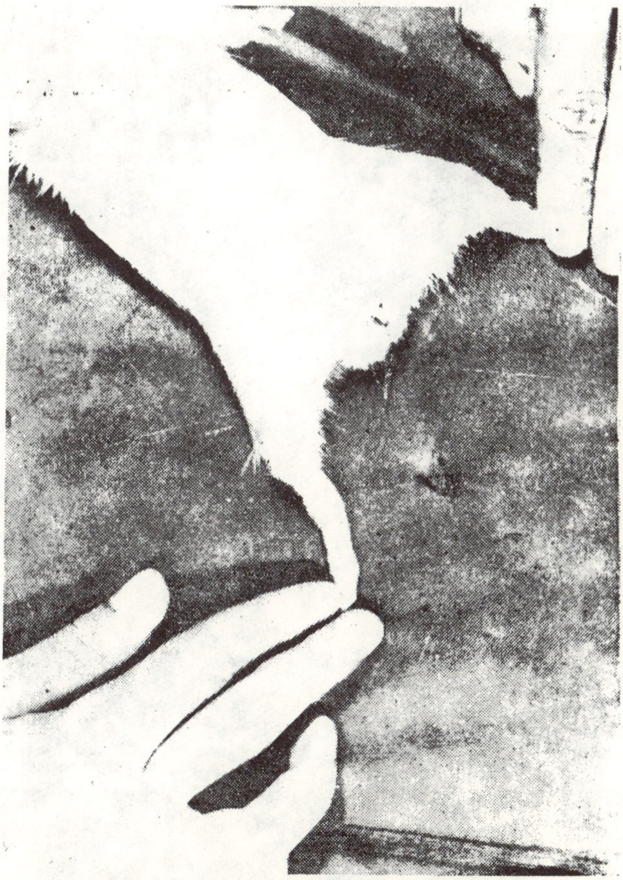

Mooser of one side symptomatic

Feces cysts of amoeba coli and dysenteric	
Urine albumin	slight positivity
P. bilious	positive
Uribilin	strong positive

Sediment white cells-corpuscles of pus, renal cells abundant (29-8-39).
Urine (30-8-39) albumin slightly positive, scarce red cells, white cells, vesical cells. No cylinders, no corpuscles pus.

On 1-9-39, we did the test of blood to the dark field and smears with the method Pappenheim, and the searches of spirochetes was negative. At the same we did the inoculation of blood, 2.5 cc to each animal, intraperitoneally, one guinea pig and one white mouse.

On 9-9-39, the examination of the blood in fresh to dark field, we saw germs of 3 or 4 microns, appreciating well the spires and with no rapid movement. On 11-9-39, the germs have increased in number and is possible to see flagellums in the ends. The average size is around the half of a red cell (3 or 4 microns), as has been verified in the smears, but in dark fields, we have rarely seen spirochetes with 6 or 7 microns.

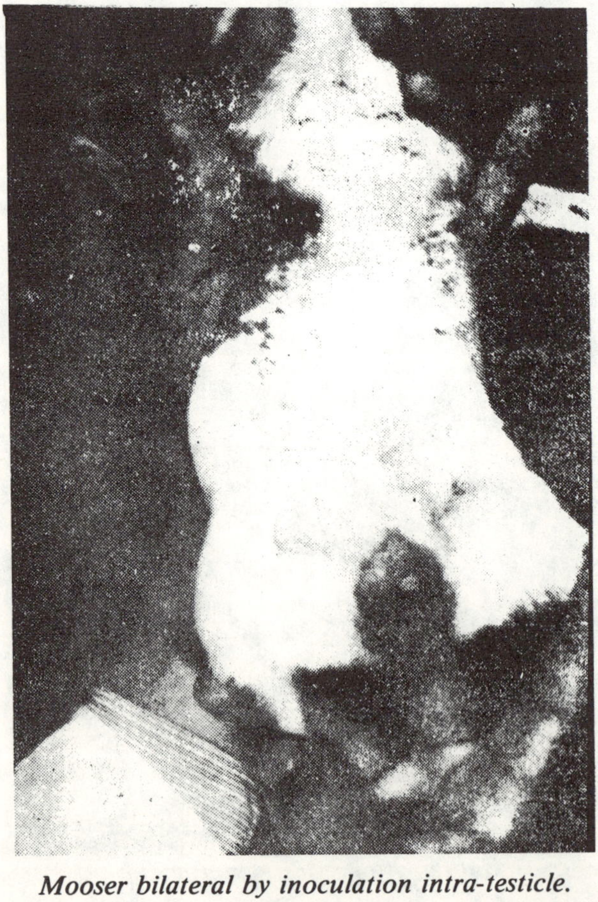

Mooser bilateral by inoculation intra-testicle.

In the same date with diluated blood in saline solution we inoculated another mouse intra-peritoneal.

On 13-9-39 in dark field the blood of the first mouse is positive with 2 or 3 spirochetes for field and with some drops of this blood diluted in saline solution, we have inoculated, with 2 c.c., each one, intraperitoneal, two guinea pigs trying to produce the phenomenon of Mooser.

On 16-9-39, we continue observing the two mice and two guinea pigs. The first mouse presents some spirochetes; the second, scarces (one, each 3 or 4 fields), we think, then, to search the spirochetes in the sublingual region as have demonstrated other researchers, and in effect, in a drop of lymph-blood taken under the tongue we found thousands of spirochetes when in the peripheric blood were rare, and for the first time we appreciate clearly the flagellums, but not for smears and Pappenheim. We appreciate also the pasive movement.

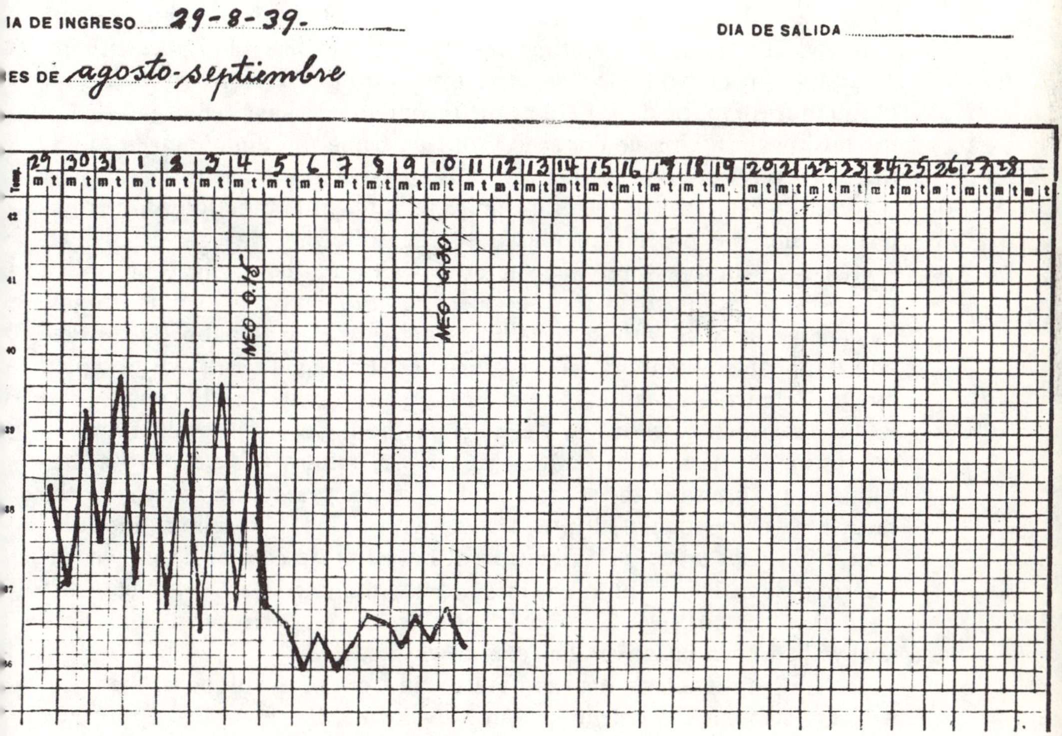

Curve thermic where it is possible to see the swift fall to the first injection of neosalvarsan.

On 18-9-39 testing in dark field the blood of the two guinea pigs, one of them, presented scarces (1 or 2 for each 4 or 5 fields). The searching in blood of the sublingual region of the first mouse by smears was positive. Testing the spittle and urine of this mouse, the first was positive and negative the second.

On 21-9-39, we did newly the examination of the animals, not presenting symptoms of peri-orchitis, the curve of temperature, morning and afternoon, was normal.

The following day we did assays of cultures, taking blood positive of the first mouse. The cultures were made in medium of Kast, modified for spirochetes.

The result of these trials was negative, only was development of bacteries and fungi. In this date, we inoculate with blood diluted of this same animal, intraperitoneal, a young rabbit that we had in observation till it died (3-10-39). The test of the blood of the heart by smears and Pappenheim, revealed scarce germs. The tests of this animal in fresh and dark field had been negative.

On 26-9-39, the first mouse was killed inoculated, in the Service of Anatomopathology of the Hospital Vargas, not finding nothing to the autopsy. The research of spirochetes in sections of several organs with impregnation of Levaditi gave negative results. In this date, test of a drop of blood in fresh to the dark field of the second mouse has been negative, but the positive in the tissue under the tongue, being this animal given to Dr. Mir for assays of sodoku-therapy in the Psychiatric Hospital.

On 27-9-39, one of the guinea pigs presents inflammation of the right testicle and the process increased to the following day, fever of 39°, grimaces to the pressure, there is no luxation of the organ; were taken photos and sacrificed in the Service of Pathology of Hospital Vargas. Smears made by us with material of scraping of the vaginal of the testicle and Pappenheim method, gave spirochetes. The same result was obtained by Dr. Potenza. The cuttings of several organs revealed nothing abnormal and the research of germs by Levaditi' method, gave null result. It is very interesting the peri-orchitis of this guinea pig, because it is a Mooser symptomatic. In this date, the second guinea pig not presenting nothing of the testicles. was reinoculated intra-testicle with blood diluted in saline solution; eight days later, inflammation of both testicles, process that was increasing. Sacrified the animal, the smears with material of scraping of the vaginal, were positive. The blood of this animal in fresh in dark field always had been negative. The sperm was negative.

Often in these tests the examination in fresh of the blood of the mice, we have seen large elements, rapid movements, that avoid to appreciate the morphology, displacement of the red cells, thinking, maybe, in Trypanosoma duttoni. However, the numerous smears has not been possible to verify these suspicions.

How all these searchs delay a long time, the patient feeling bad, high temperature, we did an injection of neosalvarsan (arsenic) of 0.15. Immediately, she was better, the fever disappeared and everything changed. For increases the therapeutic action we did another injection of 0.30 on

10-10-39. The treatment verified clearly the diagnosis of spirochetosis morsus muris.

CONCLUSIONS

1.- The first case of Sodoku in Venezuela comes under observation. The clinical diagnosis as quickly made on hearing the patient's story. The infection was caused by a rat-bite.
2.- The inoculations were positive in white mice, guinea pigs and rabbits, the clearest and highest percentage of infection being in the mice.
3.- Many times in the investigation of spirochetes in the peripheric blood by dark field examination the result has been negative, whereas they have been found very abundantly in the bloody lymph of the cellular tissue under the tongue.
4.- Of two guinea pigs inoculated intraperitoneally with a mouse blood dilution one showed symptomatic unilateral Mooser; the other reinoculated in the testicles gave a bilateral Mooser. In both cases the investigation of spirochetes by scrapings from tunica vaginalis has been positive.
5.- The experiments of cultures in modified Kast medium were null.
6.- The histopathological studies of sections from several organs, as well as the search for germs by the Levaditi method, were negative.
7.- The patient was treated with neosalvarsan. The first injection of 0.15 was enough to cause the temperature to disappear and the course of the disease to change from night to morning.

STUDIES ABOUT AVIAN EPIZOÖTY *
(SPIROCHETOSIS GALLINARUM)

In Ciudad Bolívar (State Bolívar), in a country seat of the place "Los Morichales", we knew it had an epizoöty among the hens, since two years ago, killing around 200 animals; epizoöty coming to be stronger in the former months to our arrival in December 1941.

The person in charge to take care of these animals had found in holes and crevices of the trunks of plum trees, where the hens accustomed to sleep, numerous exemplaries of ticks. Some of these plum trees had been burned trying to destroy the habitat of those acarus.

The examination of the blood of a hen that was sad the day of our visit, presenting a symptomatological similar picture, resulted negative. Observing this hen that died ten days later and testing newly the blood was equally negative, referring to spirochetes.

Inoculated four chickens with a crushing of more or less 50 ticks; one of them died with septicemia, probably, and others testing the blood in several occasions by smears or dark field, we could not find spirochetes.

The ticks sent to United States (Washington) have been classified as Argas persicus.

One of the chickens inoculated was also submitted to stings of the acarus.

Now, we have received ticks from a poultry yard situated in San José del Avila, that we have in observation. The bearer said we had produced the death of many hens.

According to Briceño Rossi, he found in december 1941, in a poultry yard of a house, placed in Santa Rosalía (Los Rosales) in a sick hen, in smears of blood, Giemsa' method, long spirochetes, around 30 microns of length, probably S. anserinum (Sakharoff 1891), S. gallinarum (Marchoux and Salimbeni 1903).

SUMMARY

1st - We have not found S. gallinarum.
2nd - We have found ticks in poulterers of Caracas and Ciudad Bolívar.
3rd - There are in both sites an history of epizoöty among those animals.

* Reprinted from "Boletín del Laboratorio de la Clínica Luis Razetti". Año III. N° 7. Abril 1942.

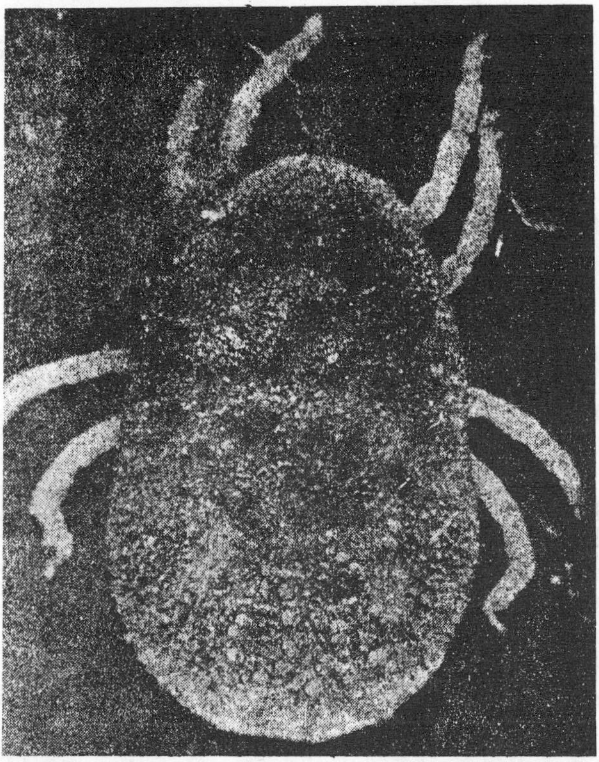

Argas miniatus (Koch 1844) caught by Briceño Rossi in Los Rosales, parish Santa Rosalía, as host transmissor of the avian epizoöty (S. gallinarum).

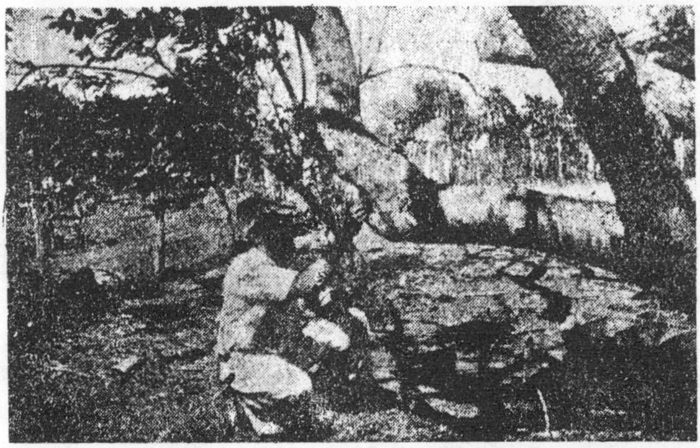

Seeking ticks in the fissures of the trunk of the plum trees (Spondias purpurea L.) in Ciudad Bolívar. (Photo Iriarte).

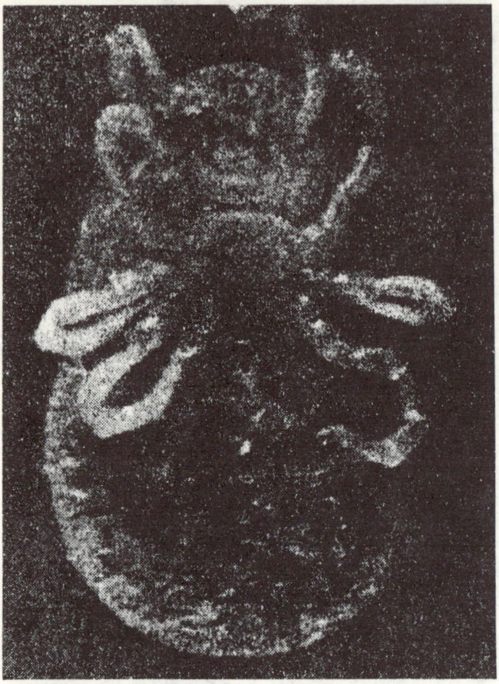

The same species (Argas miniatus).

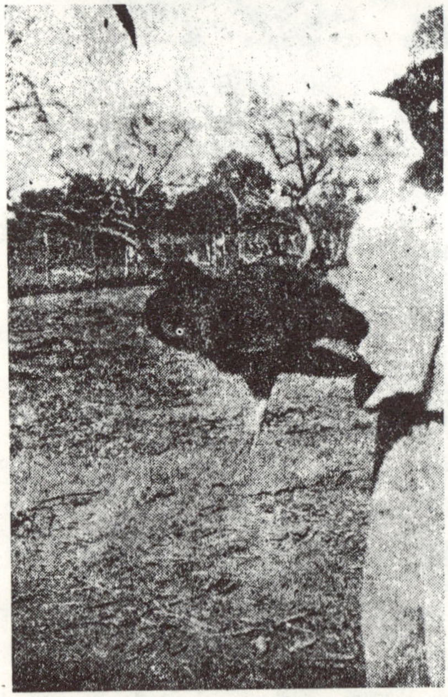

Hen in Ciudad Bolívar examined by Dr. Iriarte, suspicious of spirochetosis.

A NEW CASE OF SPOROTRICHOSIS *

The following observation has not a great importance; only is a new case seen in the country. It has two details: the characteristic of the affection, with its point of entrance and its lymphatic way. Besides, the cultures had not pigmentation, having been necessary to send cultures to Mackinnon in Uruguay, who had obtained, losing our enthusiasm believing to have in hands a new variety.

It is a patient that was sent to the Laboratory by Dr. Barrios Padrón, thinking in mycotic origin, coming from El Hatillo and with a long evolution.

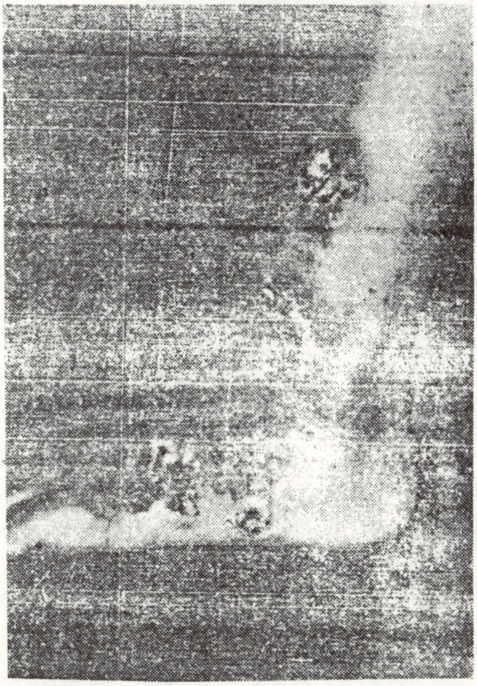

Case of sporotrichosis seeing the point of entrance.

The aspect of the young sick had done to think in sporotrichosis. The cultures in Sabouraud' medium gave to our distinguished mycologist Lorenzo de Montemayor of the Institute of Hygiene, to whom we give our acknowledgement, revealed the presence of Rhinocladium or Sporotrichum schencki-bermanni.

The treatment with local iodine was given and had a great improvement, but unknown the definitive result.

* Reprinted from "Boletín del Laboratorio de la Clínica Luis Razetti" - Año XIV - Vol. XVI - N° 39 - 40 - 1953.

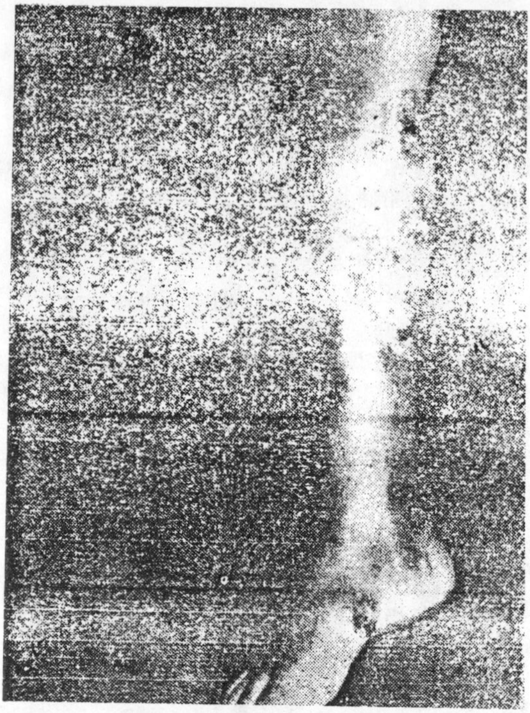

Other photo of the same patient, showing the lymphatic way.

PRESENCE OF FUNGI IN THE TONSILS *

(Its relation with the etiology of the actinomycosis)

(Work presented to the VI Venezuelan Congress of Medical Sciences and V Meeting bi-annual of the Asociación de Médicos Laboratoristas. Havana, Cuba.)

When the fact of Bostroem isolating an anaerobic strain, on thought that the soil and the plants, host of many saprophytic species, should be the source of infection of the actinomycosis.

Harz in 1877, discovered micro-aerophil species, in abdomen and maxillary bone, that should be the actinomyces bovis Harz (1877), species cultivated later, by Wolfand Israel (1891).

This work could be realized with the help and advices of the competent mycologist Lorenzo de Montemayor, of the National Institute of Hygiene, who did all the mycological part. Equally, also have helped for the Departments of Histo-pathology and Photography. For everything our acknowledgement.

To the old etiologic concept of the actinomycosis (plants and soil), some investigators starting by Lord, at the beginning of 1910, issued the hypothesis that seeing the difficult development of the actinomycosis hors human being, and not very contagious, presenting lesions in maxillary bone and neck, thought that possibly deposits of actinomyces were in teeth and tonsils, having obtained from dental caries and tonsillar crypts positive cultures of anaerobic species.

After, Lord and Trevett, doing cultures in 90 patients with material of caries and tartar on teeth, obtained suspicious colonies in 20%, but only four strains in pure culture. Naeslund in 1931, isolated strains indistinguished of israeli type, with bucal material, getting positive inoculations.

In the Mayo Clinic in Rochester, Figi and Cutts appointed 14 cases of actunomycosis in children with antecedents of tonsilitis and caries in teeth.

Davies did studies about the granules found in crypts of the tonsils, very similar to the "granules of sulphur" of the actinomycosis, not finding in them actinomyces, but an abundance of bacterial and spirilar flora, streptococcus and fusiform bacillus.

The well known mycologist Emmons, took the name granules from the tonsillar crypts or from the tonsils operated (100 cases) in the Services of the Presbiterian Hospital and Hospital Universitario in San Juan de Puerto Rico.

* Reprinted from the "Boletín of the Laboratorio de la Clínica Luis Razettti" - Año XV - N° 45 - 46 - 1955.

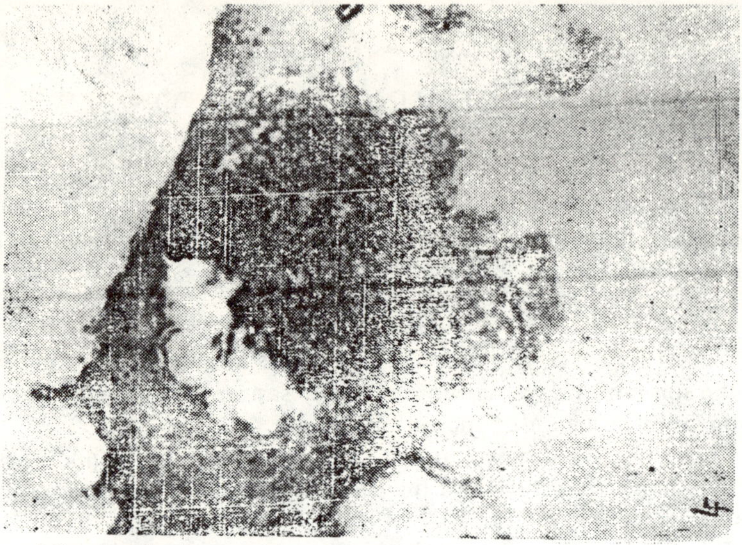

Micro-photo - Cutting of tonsil Hemalum-eosin coloration - Nodule simulating a botryomycoma.

The material was taken in boxes of Petri and the grains sectional: the half, studied in plates with Gram's method, and the other half in cultures. Few colonies of actinomyces gave the cultures, but in ten cases was isolate the Actinomyces bovis. Histologic cuttings of the tonsils presenting suspicious granules were negative. Emmons gave the following results:

Number of tonsils	100 couples
Actinomyces direct examination	47%
Actinomyces in cultures not pure	23%
Actinomyces in cultures pure	10%

Conclusion: "the organism found in these tonsillar granules is a strain of the pathogenic species Actinomyces bovis; that it is harbored in the tonsils where usually does not cause disease; and that the granules which are periodically discharged from the crypts of the tonsils are probably capable of lodging elsewhere in a tissue more susceptible to invasion by this organism and giving rise to true actinomycosis particulary of the abdominal type".

From the work of Lord and Trevett is the following paragraph: " Naeslund has succeeded in isolating from the normal mouth anaerobic organisms morphologically and culturally like the actinomyces of the Wolf-Israel type and capable of giving rise in the animals to characteristic actinomycotic lesions. The presence in the normal mouth of the actinomyces of the Wolf-Israel type has thus been established."

"So far as our observations are concerned, the aerobic-anaerobic organisms isolated by us from the normal mouth appear to be identical with the actinomyces of the Wolf-Israel type in morphology and staining reaction."

"The character of their initial growth in bouillon, the readiness in which growth occurs under aerobic conditions and failure to produce lesions characteristic of actinomycosis in animals make it impossible to classify them as belonging to the group of the actinomyces of the Wolf-Israel type."

"Organisms of the Wolf-Israel type have not been demonstrated outside the human or animal body and in view of their biologic character, it is unlikely that multiplication takes place in the outside world under any ordinary conditions. Implantation of the parasite within the tissue through injury by a foreign body may be a factor. There are many instances recorded in the literature of the presence in the lesions of foreign bodies most of vegetable nature, but in the majority of cases there is not history of a foreign body and none is found in the lesions. As the most common site of the disease is the region about the head and neck, with abdominal involvement next in frequency, and the buccal cavity is to be regarded as the portal of entry with secondary invasion of the neighborhood by direct extension and the abdomen and lungs through swallowed or inhaled organism."

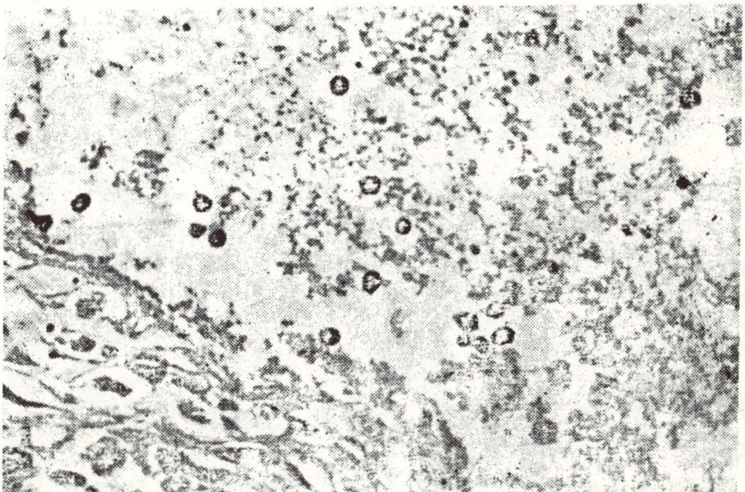

Microphoto - Cutting of tonsil - Hemalum-eosin staining -Showing numerous blastospores of yeasts, some in gemmation.

The work made by Pomales Lebron about the bacterial flora of the throat in Puerto Rico, found in a 97% of the cultures done with material of the tonsillar crypts, a positivity for streptococcus hemolytic. In a case of white membranes on the tongue and pharyngitis, isolated in abundance Monilia psilosis (Ashford), succeeding pure cultures.

In two patients with actinomycosis generalized studied by Carrion in Puerto Rico, in none of both was possible to find the portal of entry, to have food attention and care doing in some cases the diagnosis.

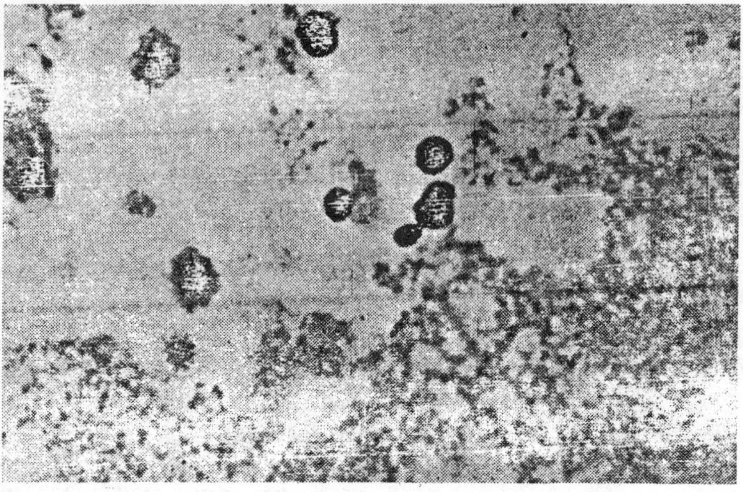

Micro-photo - Section of tonsil - Hemalum-eosin staining -Blastospores of yeast within the tissue (magnified).

* * *

The study was made about 200 couples of tonsils extirpated by us and other fellows oto-rhino-laryngologists in the "Clínica González Lugo."

After the surgical extirpation, the tonsils were placed inside of little bottles with glycerine pure, for the cultures; other part, was placed in formaldehyde to 10% for histological study; also was taken a small piece for aposition smears.

The research was divided in three ways:

a) Study for smears.

b) Histological study.

c) Study for cultures.

The smears for aposition were always stained for Gram and Giemsa's methods.

The material for histological study, already fixed, was dehydrated through alcohol and included in paraffin; the sections done were 5 to 7, and the orientation of them following the tonsillar crypts.

The staining methods were: hemalum-eosin, Gram's method applied to cuttings; sometimes specific stainings for fungi: Shiff, Gemori and derivatives, etc.

Referring to cultures, the material was crushed in small morter, rearing it directly or treating it before for the method of Almeida. As common medium was utilized the Sabouraud with light modification (2% of glucose and ph 7.2 to 7.6). Were used also, the Loeffler's medium, gelose Veillon, Norris and Raulin's methods, etc.

The microscopic result of the material studied for histological cuttings is the following:

Formationns with aspect of botriomycome	5 cases
Actinomyces	3 cases
Fungi blastospored	20 cases

In the cultures we have found numerous saprophytic fungi (moss). The study of these was impossible, needing time and extended bibliography. These fungi almost always were contaminated coming from the air and had not importance in the tonsils.

Our attention was mostly on those pathogenic fungi, as the yeasts of the group Candida: albicans and tropicalis, about those saprophytic fungi that could to enter in the organism.

The strains studied gave the following results:

Yeast anascoporeted	35 strains
Fungi hyphomycetes (filamentous)	32 strains
Total	67 strains

Were classified as follows:

Candida albicans	16 strains
Candida tropicalis	13 strains
Candida krusei	1 strain
Sacharomyces sp.	1 strain
Geotridum sp.	4 strains
Trichosporon sp.	3 strains
Actinomyces sp.	3 strains
Rhodotorula rubra	4 strains
Mucor sp.	6 strains
Rhizopus nigricans	6 strains
Demantiaceae	10 strains
Total	67 strains

DEDUCTIONS

In our medium, the mycologic flora of the tonsils seems to be relatively scarce. Among the yeasts, the most frequent is the Candida albicans, following in importance the Candida tropicalis. This last has been isolated at the Children Hospital by Potenza from esophagus and bronco-pulmonary lesions. The Candida krusei is seldom found in tonsils. Trichosporum and Geotrichum have been found.

It was possible to isolate only 3 strains of actinomyces, two of them aerobian of the group albus, and one anaerobian of biological and morphological qualities similar to Actinomyces bovis.

A point of interest is the matter of the nodules or formations in the shape of botriomicoma. In our cases it can not be determined whether they are the result of fungus or bacteria. It is evident that we have not found typical grains of actinomyces, with or without cudgels. There have been authors who have created formations similar to the botriomicomas as the results of experiments on rabbits, using Candida albicans for the inoculation.

Our results do not agree with those arrived at by foreign authors who have studied this same subject. In fact, they have found high percentages of Actinomyces in teeth, tonsils and buco-pharynx, but ours, which are poor, seems to sustain what has been observed in the actinomycosis clinic in our medium. The typical actinomycosis cervico-facial due to anaerobic stubs, type A. bovis, is extraordinarily rare among us; as it is well known, this type of affection is of endogenous origin. In countries where anaerobic strains of actinomyces are abundant in organs and sections mentioned, cases of actinomycosis cervico-facial-thoracic of exogenous origin are frequent.

Possibly the cases studied among us may be of exogenous origin due to actinomyces aerobian, group Actinomyces asteroides, as found in Dr. Velutini's patient by Montemayor.

BIBLIOGRAPHY

1.-*Lord F.T.*-A contribution to the etiology of actinomycosis. The experimental production of actinomycosis in guinea pigs inoculated with the contents of carious teeth. Boston Med. Surg. Journal - 163: 82-85 - 1910.

2.-*Lord F.T.*-The etiology of actinomycosis. The presence of actinomycosis in the contents of carious teeth and the tonsillar cripts of patients without actinomycosis. Jour. A.M.A. 55: 1261-3 - 1910.

3.-*Lord F.T. and Trevett L.D.*-The patogenesis of actinomycosis. Recovery of actinomyces-like granules from the normal mouth. Journ. of Infect. Dis. 58: 1 - 115-120 - 1936.

4.-*Naeslund, Carl.*-Experimentelle studien "Uber die Ätiologie und pathogenese der Aktinomycose. Acta Path. et Microbiolog. Scand. Suppl. VI. 8 = 1-156 - 1931.

5.-*Figi, F.A. and Cutts, R.A.*-Actinomycosis in childhood. Am. Journ. Dis. Chil. 42 : 279. 1951.

6.-*Davis, David J.*-The actinomyces-like granules in tonsils. Journ. Infect. Dis. 14 : 144-158. 1914.

7.-*Emmons, C.W.*-Actinomyces and Actinomycosis. Pto. Rico Journ. Pub. Health Trop. Med. 11 : 63-76. 1935.

8.-*Emmons, C.W.*-Razas de Actinomyces bovis aisladas en las amígdalas. Pto. Rico Journ. Pub. Health and Trop. Med. 11 : 728-735. 1936.

9.-*Carrion, A.L.*-Actinomicosis en Puerto Rico. The Puerto Rico Journal of Pub. Health and Tropical Medicine. 13 : 383-389 - 1938.

10.-*Pomales Lebron, Américo.*-Estudio verificado en Puerto Rico de la Flora microbiana de la gargante de sujetos normalees i enfermos i en amígdalas después de operadas. The Pto. Rico Journ. of Pub. Health and Trop. Med. 11 : 3 - 1936.

11.-*Mariat, F.*-Physiologie des actinomycètes aérobiès pathogènes. - I - Expèriences prèliminaires. Ann. de l'Institut Pasteur - T. 86. N°. 4 - 1954.

12.-*Jiménez, Juán B.*-Nota clínica acerca de tres casos de actinomicosis humana.- Memorias del IV Congreso Venezolano de Medicina. I - 123-127 p 1925.

13.-*De Bellard, E.P.*-Sobre un caso de actinomicosis humana. Gaceta Médica de Caracas. 8 : 116-117. 1924.

14.-*Rangel, Rafael.*-Observaciones sobre actinomicosis i epitelioma de la mandíbula inferior (con ocho preparaciones microscópicas). Gaceta Médica de Caracas. 6 : 61-62 - 1909.

15.-*Risquez, Jesús R.*-Nota sobre la actinomicosis en Venezuela. Gaceta Médica de Caracas. 10: 71-72. 1916.

16.-*Fonseca, Manuel A.*-Conferencia sobre Actinomicosis leída el 14 de agosto de 1908. Gaceta Médica de Caracas 10 : 72-77. 1916.

17.-*Velutini, Luis Alberto.*-Sobre un caso de actinomicosis abdominal primitiva de la piel. Memoria de las II Jornadas Venezolanas de Venereología, Dermatología i Lepra. 519-524. 1955.

18.-*Conant, Smith, Baer, Callaway, Martin.*-Manual of Clinical Mycology. 1954.

OTOMYCOSIS *

One of the superficial mycosis more frequent in the field of the oto-rhino-laryngology are the external otitis mycotic often ingrafted on eczemas of the auditory duct.

In accord Wolf (1) was Mayer who accused for the first time the presence of a "mycotic parasite in the pus of a draining ear" and the Professor Schwartz of Halle in 1867, according Hall (2), was who for the first time cited an Aspergillus. In recent works about this question, arrived to 53, the number of species appointed till now.

Exist different opinions among otologists, mycologists and bacteriologists about the action of these fungi, referring to a primary röle or are secondary elements.

Some investigators believe that an eczema or a chronic draining should help to the development of the fungi. It seems to be that the presence of a fungus in the external ear does not means to be exactly an otomycosis; it is necessary to take in account the clinical first, after the report of laboratory. A patient revealing in various time presence of fungi in the external duct, presenting lesions, accompanied for scales, secretion, itching, it is possible to do the diagnosis of otomycosis.

Da Silva Lacaz (3) found fungi in wrinkle, 3 cases; pavillion, 5 cases, duct, 6 cases.

The fungous and bacterial flora is very interesting referring to the treatment. The fungi have resistance to the sulfas, while the bacterium are very sensitive. According Conley (4), the fungus needs of the association with bacterium, and so has been found commonly the genus Pseudomonas, chiefly the species aeroginosa. Besides of the communications of Silverton (5) and Selvin (6) it is necessary to continue the research in this way.

Investigations of Haley (7), relating both floras found, excepting three cases, in the others always saw bacterium and fungi together. This author thinks that the fungi are capable alone of producing otomycosis, without to take in account the different bacterial species.

It seems difficult to do the clinical diagnosis, among an otomycosis, an eczema, a chronic seborrhea dermatitis, because these affections have itching, pain, inflammation, exfoliation and exudate white or yellowish.

In some patients, rarely there is an allergic reaction and in many cases with bacterial otitis, can give a cutaneous test positive (antigen). Sulzberger (8) believes that the test is convenient to make it near the ill region. Rudolph and Cohen (9) think in the nature of the tissue.

Singer and asst. said: (10) "The former research published about the etiology calling attention on the fungi. Among the military physicians in

* Reprinted from the "Boletín del Laboratorio de la Clínica Luis Razetti" - Año XV - N° 43-44 - Vol. XVI - 1955.

South Pacific, the main opinion was considering the external otitis of mycotic nature. The recent studies, among them ours, the opinion is different thinking has been given an excessive importance to the fungi, seeking in the Gram negative flora, appointing the röle of the Pseudomonas, as cause of this disease."

In the Venezuelan literature only appear our work in this field. In the year 1928 (11) we published the first case of otomycosis, fungus that was studied by us in the Laboratory of Hospital Vargas, classified as Aspergillus niger, classification approved by Maxon of the Department of Agriculture in Washington.

In February 1929 (12) we presented to the Medical Surgical Society of Zulia a new case, where the fungus was not classified, but we told it does not belonged to genus Aspergillus, and thought, may be, in the genus Lichteima Wuillemin; thus, we emit the idea of that another fungus, out of the genus Aspergillus, could produce otomycosis.

The following year, 1930 (13), in the same city of Maracaibo we found two new cases, whose fungi were sent to United States, and classified by Thom, of Washington, as Aspergillus flavus.

Later, 1943 (14), studied in the Service of ears, nose and throat of the Hospital Vargas a new patient, whose material from ears, cultures in Sabouraud's medium, gave a fungus that sent to Carrion of the School of Tropical Medicine, was classified as Aspegillus fumigatus.

We bring to this communication six new cases observed:

1 case for Penicillium (group notatum).

1 case for Aspergillus terreus (variedad flocconosa).

1 case for Aspergillus ochraceus.

2 cases for Aspergillus niger.

1 case for Aspergillus sp. *

We did not find inmersion baths in the history and only two of them had used swabs.

Among the symptoms are light deafness, giving the sensation of full of water, light noises, itching, light exudates. With the otoscopy is easy to see small concretions, little membranes, sometimes as dusty, scales mixed to granules of wax.

During the III Congress Latin-American of oto-rhino-laryngology was presented a work by Richarson (15) from Trinidad Island, showing 13 patients, finding in the majority of them Asp. flavus; in two, Candida parapsilosis and in one, Asp. chevalieri.

We have used silver salts, boric acid alcohol. With suspicions of bacterial infection acetic acid 2%. With the research of Turner (17), 1946, we have used widely the tincture of merthiolate of Lilly to 1 x 1000 with very good results and lastly the solution of bright green in water or alcohol (verdillon) with success. Marshall (18) and Almeida (19) studied the

* The classification of these strains was realized in the Section of Mycology of National Institute of Hygiene by the able mycologist Lorenzo de Montemayor, to whom express our acknowledgment.

fungicide power of all these substances (in vitro) on the Coccidioides inmitis and the Paracoccidioides brasiliensis.

SUMMARY

It is made a short exposition, up today, of the problem of the Otomycosis, history, etiology, symptomatology, parasitology and therapy, reporting six cases. For the first time are found, among us, the species ochraceus and terreus, var. flocconosa.

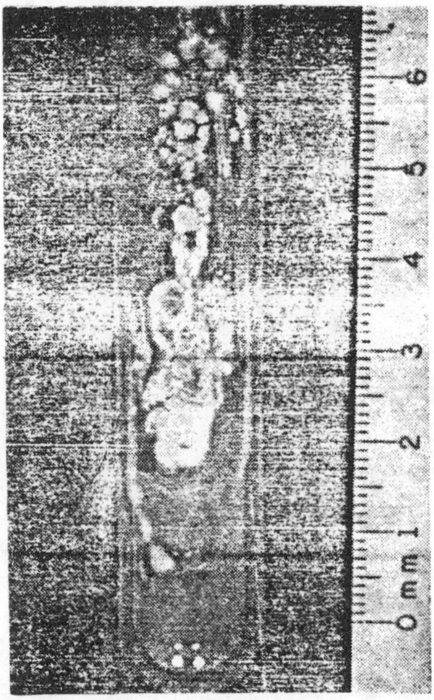

Penicilium sp. group notatum - Saboraud conservation - Temp. ambient.

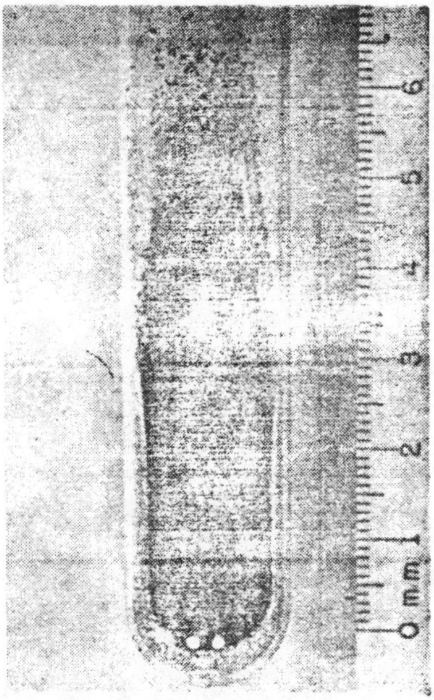

Aspergillus nigger Sabouraud conservation Temp. ambient.

BIBLIOGRAPHY

(1) *Wolf F.T.*-The relation of various fungi to Otomycosis.-Arch. Otoloaryngology - 43 361 -(Sept.) 1947.

(2) *Hall L.B.*-Aspergillus in the ear. Am. J. M. Sc. - 73 - 559 - 1877.

(3) *Da Silva Lacaz Carlos.*-Otomicoses por bolores e levaduras.

(4) *Conley J.J.*-Evaluation of fungous disease of the external auditory canal.-Arch. of Otolaryngology.- 47 - 721 - 1948.

(5) *Silverton J.T., Hess W.R. i Krafchuk J.K.*-Otitis externa: clinical observation and microbiological flora.-Arch. Otolaryngology 43 - 213 - marzo - 1946.

(6) *Salvin S.B. i Lewis M.L.*-External otitis, with additional studies on the genus Pseudomonas.-J.Bact. 51 - 495 - abril - 1946.

(7) *Haley Leanor D.*-Etiology of Otomycosis-Arch. of Otolaryngology - 52 - 208: 213 -1950.

(8) *Sulzberger M.B.*-Allergy in dermatology. Critical review of some recent contributions.-J.Allergy - 8 - 385 - mayo - 1937

(9) *Rudolph J.A. i Cohen M.B.*-Vasomotor rhinitis with negative skin tests: a local nasal allergy - 5: 476 - julio - 1933.
(10) *Singer David E., Freeman Elizabeth y otros.*-Otitis externa. Bacteriological and Mycological studies. Ann. of Otology, Rhinology and Laryngology- 61 - 317-30 - junio - 1952.
(11) *Iriarte David R.*-Nota preliminar sobre las otomicosis en Venezuela y sobre un hongo de la Euphorbia hypericifolia.-Gaceta Médica de Caracas - XXV (17): 258 - sept. - 1928.
(12) *Iriarte David R.*-Sobre un caso de otomicosis-Rev. de la Soc. Méd. Quir. del Zulia.- III (2): 15-17 - 1929.
(13) *Iriarte David R.*-Rev. de la Soc. Méd. Quir. del Zulia - IV (2): 143-144 - febrero - 1930.
(14) *Iriarte David R.*-Aspergillosis auricular por Aspergillus fumigatus Fresenius 1863 -Arch. Ven. Soc. O. R. L., Oftalm. Neur. IV (1): 33-36 y Boletín del Lab. de la Clí. Razetti. VI (10): 173-173 - mayo - 1943.
(15) *Richardson E.C.*-Report on the treatment of 13 cases of Otomycosis with comirin. III Cong. Lat. Amer. O. R. L.- 1953 - (16) loc. cit.
(17) *Turner J.S. y asociados.* Tropic-proofing of optical instruments by a fungicide - Nature -158 - 43 - 1946.
(18) *Marshall M.S.*-Merthiolate new antiseptic.-California & West med. 35 - 43 - 1931.
(19) *Almeida F. y asociados.*-Accao do "Yatren" e do "Merthiolate"in vitro sobre o Paracoccidioides brasiliensis-Arch. Brasil med. 36 - 41 - 1946.

ASPERGILLOMYCOSIS OF THE EARS FOR ASPERGILLUS FUMIGATUS FRESENIUS (1863)

In September 1928 we published in the Gaceta Médica de Caracas, the first case of Otomycosis in Venezuela, entitled "Nota Preliminar sobre las Otomicosis en Venezuela." Fungi studied by us in the Laboratory of Hospital Vargas, arriving to the classification as Aspergillus nigger, determination verified for the mycologist Dr. Maxon, of the Department of Agriculture of Washington.

Later, in February 1929, we presented to the Medical Surgery Society of Zulia, a new case, in which the fungus was not classified, but we told that the fungus was not Aspergillus, genus found in the 80% of the patients with otomycosis. We thought in the genus Licht heimia Vuillemin, perhaps, as producer.

The following year, 1930, in the same city of Maracaibo, we found two new cases, whose fungi sent to United States and classified by Thom, coming to be Aspergillus flavus.

Lastly, in the Service of ears, nose and throat of the Hospital Vargas, we had the opportunity to do a new observation of auricular mycosis in a patient of 40 years old, with troubles in the left ear (deafness, light pains, itching, hummings). We made cultures of the material in Sabouraud gave colonies of a fungus of aspergillar type that sent to Dr. Carrion of the School of Tropical Medicine of Puerto Rico, resulting to be Aspergillus fumigatus.

COMMENTARIES

The auricular mycosis does not seems to be very frequent among us, taking in account the errors of diagnosis; however, Galloway in 1929, according to Brumpt, believed that the 70% of the auricular affections between european people in the islands of Malaysia (Malay Archipelago) are of mycotic origin. Our patients are not of low age, not rural people and no history of baths in river.

The Aspergillus nigger Van Tieghem 1867 (Sterigmatocystis nigra Van Tieghem 1877), producer of our first observation has been accused in the world as causing affections of this type. Bergeen, 1929, in the School of Veterinary of Hanoi (Indochina) cited two cases of auricular mycosis in animals, ox and deer, produced by this fungus.

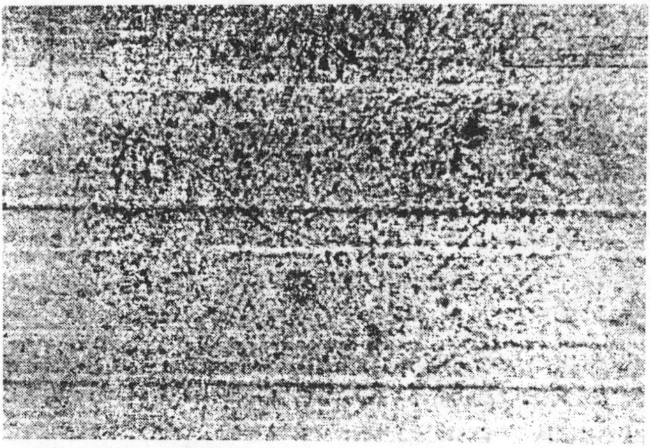

Micro-photo-Aspergillus fumigatus

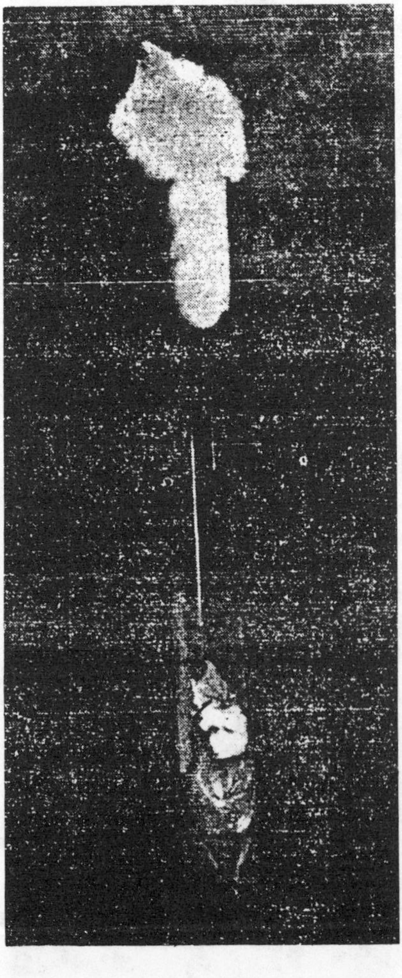

Photo-Culture of Candida (Monilia) albicans in Sabouraud medium.

The Aspergillus (Eurotium) flavus Link 1807, referring Siebermann is the same appointed by Wreden in 1874 with the name of Aspergillus flavescens in otomycosis. The A. flavus has been the cause of the two cases found by us in 1930 in Maracaibo. This fungus has been found in corneal ulcers in United States by Zentmayer in 1812.

The fungus important today in this field is the Aspergillus fumigatus Fresenius 1863, one of the species more spreaded, more pathogenic and more studied. The spores of this Aspergillus are very spreaded in the ambient, on seeds, soil, atmospheric dusty.

It has been found also on doves, hens, turkeys, canaries, parrots and other animals in zoological gardens, producing the death in ravens, pheasants, white stork, penguins. According Siebermann of 36 patients studied for him, 16 of them were produced for the species fumigatus.

In all our patients as treatment we have employed auricular douches for extracting the mycelar plugs and instillations of silver nitrate to 1% with success.

CONCLUSIONS

1.- A new case is presented of Otomycosis produced by Aspergillus fumigatus Fresenius 1863.

2.- Formerly, we had presented another 4 observations, one of them the first in Venezuela, whose fungi were: Aspergillus nigger; Sterigmatocystis (Diplo stephanus nigra Van Tieghem 1867); Aspergillus (Eurotium) flaves Link 1807. One of these fungi could not be classsified, but this fact demonstrated that in Venezuela there are cases of otomycosis not produced by the genus Aspergillus.

3.- The age of the patients was always higher than 20 years old, are not rural people, no history of immersion baths.

4.- The treatment used in all the cases has been the solution of silver nitrate 1% with success.

THE PHARYNGEAL MYCOSIS * **

At the end of the last century, in 1872, the German Fraenkel created the term of *pharyngeal mycosis* for the tonsillar infection for Leptotrix bucalis, filling chapters in the books of oto-rhino-laryngology with the name of *pharyngeal mycosis.*

When we were students and later physicians working always in these problems of O.R.L., we saw patients, men or women, suffering of the throat and to the examination we observed on the tonsillar surface of both sides, on the lymphatic follicles of the rear wall and sometimes on uvula and pillars, some hard whitish excrescences attached to the sites of implantation; formations that, in accord to some authors, extended to larynx, but that we have not seen.

This symptomatology was that we knew when we were students, and thus, in 1943, studied and published in the Boletín del Laboratorio de la Clínica Luis Razetti, Año IV, N° 10, a case entitled: "Faringomicosis a Candida (Monilia) albicans"; observation that was later reprinted for a Cuban review, saying the following: (***)

"To our consultation of the Service of ears, nose and throat of the Hospital Vargas, went, various months ago, an ill of 30 years old, suffering of troubles in the throat".

"To the examination of the pharynx we saw numerous white, small concretions, like the granules of rice, hard, excelling on the surface of the tonsils".

"Immediately we did the diagnosis of pharyngeal mycosis, verified after for the direct examination of the granules and cultures in Sabouraud, where 48 hours later appeared a fungus colony".

"Cultures of this material sent to our friend and competent mycologist Dr. Carrion of the School of Tropical Medicine of Puerto Rico, who gently answered the following: the characteristics of this organism are very similar with the species Candida (Monilia) albicans. Did the diagnosis for the aspect of the colonies in agar glucose to 4%, in the microscopic morphology, in the fermetation of the sugars and in the reactions of agglutination".

"Our patient was submitted to surgery and one of the tonsils was sent to the Service of Histo-pathology, receiving the following result: nothing abnormal."

* Conde Jahn and Briceño Iragorry presented to the Second South-American Congress of Oto-rhino-larynogology, a communication about this same question, entitled: "Hiperqueratosis folicular amigdalina", published in the Memories of that Congress.

** Reprinted from the "Boletín del Laboratorio de la Clínica Luis Razetti"-Año VII-N°'s 21-22 1946.

(***) Revista de Medicina Tropical, Parasitología, Clínica i Laboratorio. Habana - Cuba -Vol. X - N° 1 - 1944.

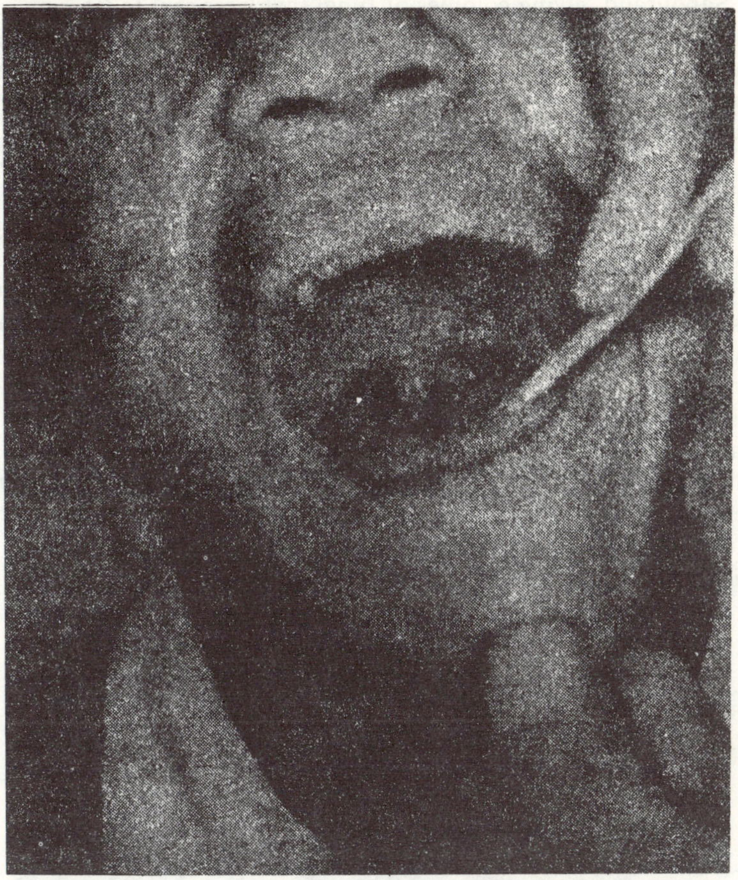

Patient whose cultures gave Candida albicans.

To the old concept that we have come exposing since a long time ago, are the opinions of notables in this field, as the Australian Wesseley, the French Baldenweek and the North-American Imperatori, telling that the fungi grafting secondary and they have no importance.

At present time with these new concepts, we resolved to study cases from the consultations of Hospital Vargas, Center Antituberculosis and Center of the Social Insurance.

We took four patients of these Services in order to submit them to mycologic histo-pathologic studies, gently helped by the Hospital Vargas and Carrion and Koppisch of the School of Tropical Medicine of Puerto Rico, to whom we gave our acknowledgment.

These choosen cases were submitted to surgery, taking the small excrescences for the mycologic study and the tonsillar tissue for the histopathology.

Material of the granules was examined in fresh, in plates, finding myceliums of fungi, superficial cells and cellular detritus; we did cultures in Sabouraud, giving colonies of fungi that were sent to Carrion, classifying fungi of the genus Penicillium and Candida, arriving to the Candida (Monilia) krusei; besides, a fungus like interesting, that Carrion continues studying. In some cultures it is possible to find two different strains, as in case 3: Penicillium and Candida krusei.

The following histo-pathological reports were done by Koppisch, from Pto. Rico:

Case 1 - Microscopic: the germinative center of the tonsils are very large. Among the lymphocytes there is numerous plasmatic cells. Within the crypts there are some polimorpho nuclears, infiltrating the epitellium and also bacterial colonies, but not fungi, nor myceliums. The connective tissue around the gland is edematous. In some fields is infiltrated for plasmanophiles.

Diagnosis: Tonsilitis chronic.

Case 2 - Microscopic: There are wide fields of fibrosis invading the tonsillar tissue. The crypts are enlarged and filled of epithelium with keratosis. There is in the cutting small part of pharyngeal muscle. The fungi were not found.

Diagnosis: Chronic tonsilitis with fibrosis.

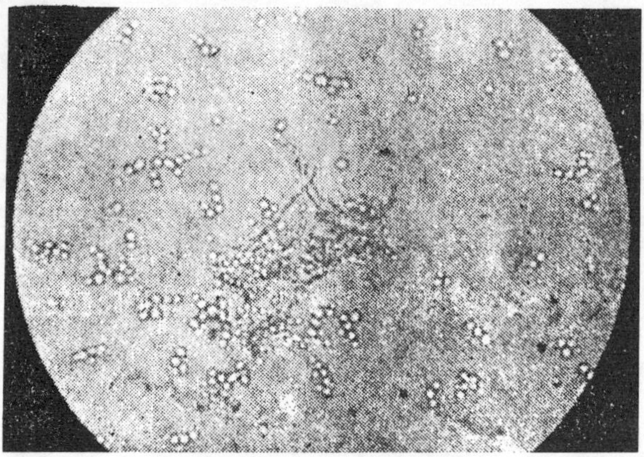

Micro-photo - Showing Candida albicans of the patient 1 - Cultures in Sabouraud.

Case 3 - Microscopic. The surface is covert epithelium scaly with signs of parakeratosis. The epithelium is hypertrophic and toward the end. There are cords anastomosed and formations isolated invading the deep of the connective tissue. The mitosis are scarce and the nucleus are normal in form, size and staining. The connective tissues are infiltrated of histiocytes, lymphocytes and plasmatic cells. In one or two places there are giant cells, but not fungi. Toward the end of more hyperplasia there is an ulcer. Ziehl-Neelsen method: no presence of bacillus acid-resistents.

Diagnosis: inflammation acute and chronic, with ulceration.

Case 4 - Microscopic: Some of the crypts are very enlarged, because inside

of them there are numerous cells for exfoliation and keratosis. The tonsillar tissue has plasmatic cells, very abundant. The epithelium of the surface is normal.
Diagnosis: chronic tonsilitis.

For former exposition it is easy to see that in all the cases there are chronic tonsilitis and never the presence of fungi within the tonsillar tissue; thus, for these reasons, we are in accord with the modern concepts referring to do not acceptance of the pharyngeal mycosis, but, simply an hyperkeratosis tonsillar follicular, having the fungi found a secondary importance.

CONCLUSIONS

1.- We expose a little of history about the denomination in O. R. L. of pharyngeal mycosis.
2.- We explained the two concepts in opposition. It is reprinted the history of a case either published and are studied various patients observed lastly.
3.- We practiced examination in fresh, giving account of the presence of fungi, and cultures in Sabouraud, cultures sent to Carrion of Puerto Rico succeeding the classification of fungi of the genus Penicillium and Candida, arriving to the species C. krusei. There was a fungus not classified yet and Dr. Carrion continues researching about it.
4.- The studies histo-pathological revealed in the four cases a chronic tonsilitis. In none of the sections was it possible to find fungi.

PARACOCCIDIOIDOMYCOSIS OR BLASTOMYCOSIS BRASILIENSIS

(Work presented to the I South-American Congress of Oto-rhino-laringology and published in the Proceedings of the same meeting)

The initial lesions representing the primary localization of the paracoccidioidomycosis often are situated on the tonsil and the buccal pharyngeal mucous. The literature about this subject and the clinical observations of the oto-rhino-laryngologist verify this opinion.

The initial lesion can be an ulceration of the gun, tongue, lips, cheeks, palate or floor of the mouth, attacking any site of this mucous, invading rarely to the pharinx and larynx. These lesions are painless and produce abundant salivation.

Exist an aspect of manifestation very frequently described by Pupo and Cunha Motta, called "estomatitis ulcerosa muriforme", characterized for ulcerations of various forms and sizes, not very deep, showing in

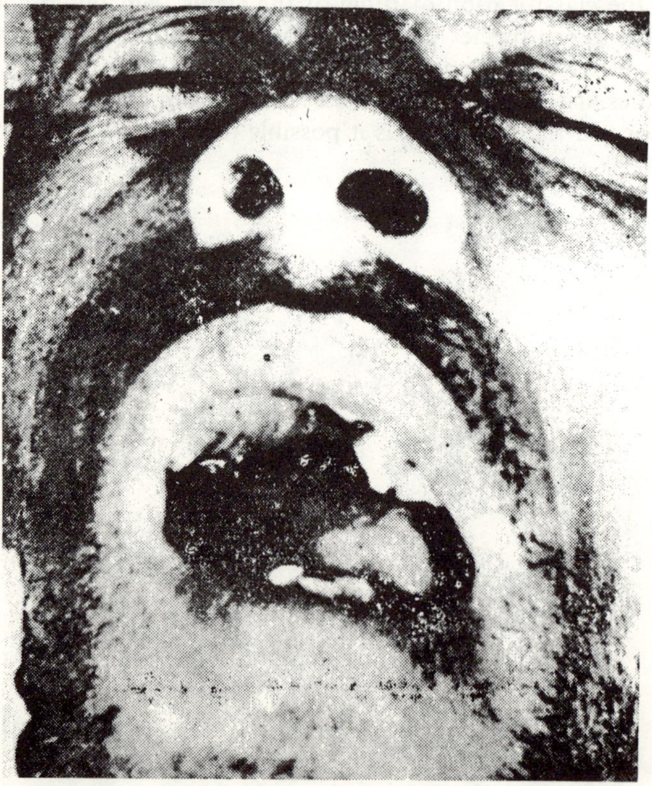

Photo of the patient showing the lesions.

the surface numerous and little granulations covert of an exudate pustulous. The papule form is scarce and the induration is yet more rare.

Pupo, cited by da Cunha Motta, called to attention the hidden infections in tonsils, that could appear by ganglionic primitive forms, characterized for cervical adenopathies supraclavicle and till axillars.

In the tonsillar tissue the fungi should find a place appropriate for their development and multiplication, invading pillars, uvula, epiglotis, larynx, and for lymphatic way, should arrive to all the organs; later the death.

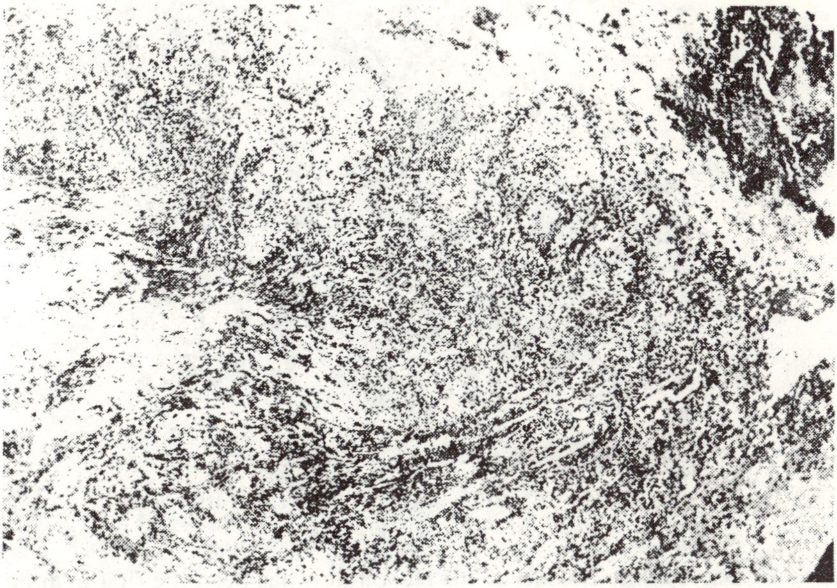

Cutting of tonsil. General aspect. Upper, epithelium spino-celullar. Low, glandular buccal debris. Under the epithelium giant cells of various sizes. Magnify 12 D.

Our patient is a man 38 years old, born in Los Teques (State Miranda), agriculturist and native, going to the Service of Oto-rhino-laryngology of Hospital Vargas, suffering since five months before, little touble in the throat, chiefly when he swallowed, sometimes accompanied by fever.

To the oto-rhino-laryngologist test we found on the right tonsil, a little ulceration, of irregular borders, prominent surface, invading anterior pillar and part of the neighbor membrane; painless lesions; abundant secretion of salive. To the inspection and palpation of the neck, we saw a right packet of infarted ganglions, some isolated.

The patient went three times to our consultation, in one of them we did the extirpation of a ganglion of the neck, but in opinion of Dr. Jaffe, not found fungi in sections, only an inflammatory stage. As in all these chronic cases he has been lost; almost sure will come again in fatal condition.

As till today the treatment of the paracoccidioidomycosis is null, we simply, prescribed iodine and injections of Gadusan. The result was unknown to us.

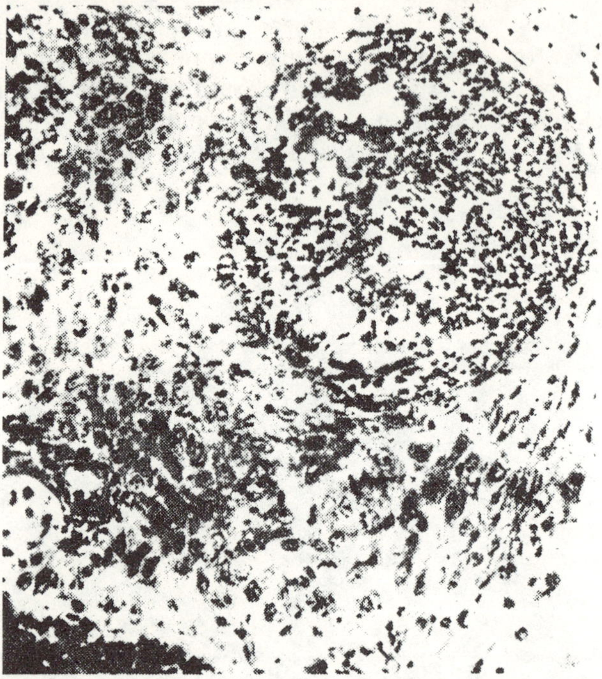

Micro-photo-Giant cell with inclusions of paracoccidioides - Magnify 280 D.

O'Daly, in the Boletín de los Hospitales, has been the first in appointing this affection in our country, describing three cases in authopsies. Our case is the first found *in vivo* and the fourth published.

CONCLUSIONS

1.- A case of paracoccidioidosis is presented in a man 38 years old, a mulatto agriculturist from Los Teques in the State of Miranda. The initial lesion was situated on the right tonsil invading the anterior pillar and the mucous membrane of the cheek.

2.- O'Daly has been the first person to call attention to this affection in this country by citing three cases in authopsies. This is therefore the 4th case published among us and the first found in living person.

3.- The fungus was found by smears with material taken from the surface of the lesion and by histopathological sections. The experiment of cultures were negative.

4.- As the patient showed right cervical ganglionic infarct, one of these ganglions was extirpated. In sections made in the Serv. of Path. Anat. of Hospital Vargas they found no paracoccidioides. but only an inflammatory process.

REGARDS ABOUT PARACOCCIDIOIDOMYCOSIS *

(Service of Hospital Vargas-Chief Professor Conde Jahn)

Dr. Iriarte spoke about a series of considerations about the paracoccidiosis brasiliensis in Venezuela. He mentioned that the first cases were observed by O'Daly 1937, in authopsies; later, the expounder in collaboration with César Rodríguez 1939, found the first case *in vivo;* after, appeared the observations of Guerra 1940 presented to the Jornadas de Tuberculosis held in San Cristóbal, and finishing the communication of Celis Pérez 1941 about cases in Valencia, entitled "The lacalizations buccal-pharynx, laryngeal of the granuloma paracoccidioidal".

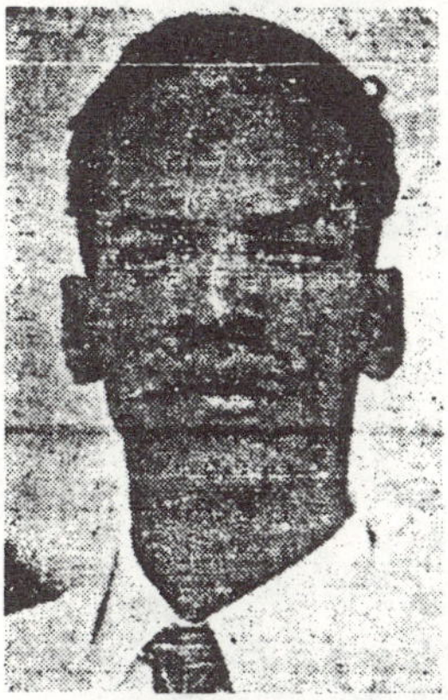

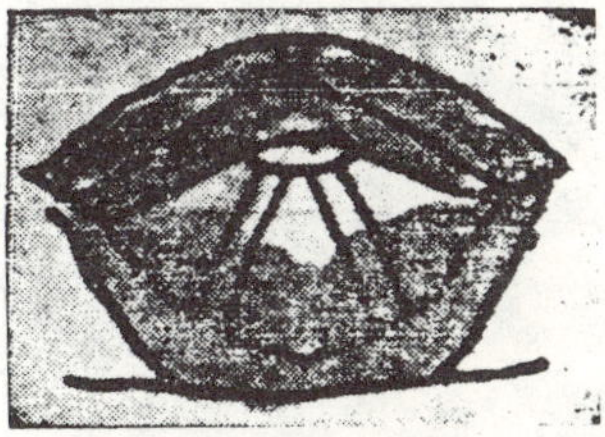

J.G. Schema of the laryngeal lesions.

J.G. observed a case showing the infiltration of the lips.

Dr. Iriarte said about the frequency of this affection between us, considering the number of cases seen in the Service of ears, nose and throat of the Hospital Vargas and for the news from various patients observed in the Service of Dermatology of the same Hospital, Professor Guerra and his school.

The sites of localization are lips, mouth in general, including tongue and palate, pharynx and larynx. Told about the aspect of the commmissures and about the infiltration and hardness of the lips, as is possible to see in the patient Sangrone (photo).

He said to have seen pulmonary lesions in both cases presented, and there was nothing special in the radiologic aspect; however, exposed that the radiologic images, in accord to the opinion of Dr. Criollo Rivas, are of

* Reprinted from "Boletín del Laboratorio de la Clínica Luis Razetti" - Año VI - N° 16 -1945.

nodular big type, being interesting the nodular small that revealed the second case.

Also, called the attention that the bases, according to Dr. Soulés Baldó are undamaged and it seems to be that the tisiologists should wish to establish in this image a radiologic sign of the paracoccidioidomycosis, because in the hematogenic tuberculous rearings all the lungs, including the bases are invaded; notwithstanding, according to Missici and Nazzi the pulmonary mycosis are situated in hilum and bases, while the tubercules in apexs. He said that according to Pupo in 33 cases studied, in none found pulmonary lesions.

He spoke that yet it is not possible to know if this affection has a pulmonary beginning infecting later superior sites (larynx, pharynx, mouth, etc), as happen in tuberculosis; or could be, on the contrary,

Radio Nº 1.

descending. To this last hypothesis is partisan the expounder according to his experience.

The examination of the spittle investigating B. de Koch, has been made in series in both cases with negative result and in the two patients the larynx has been taken. He did emphasis to the inefficiency of the treatment, however, praised the improvement observed with the sulfas. He did mention the old treatment with iodine.

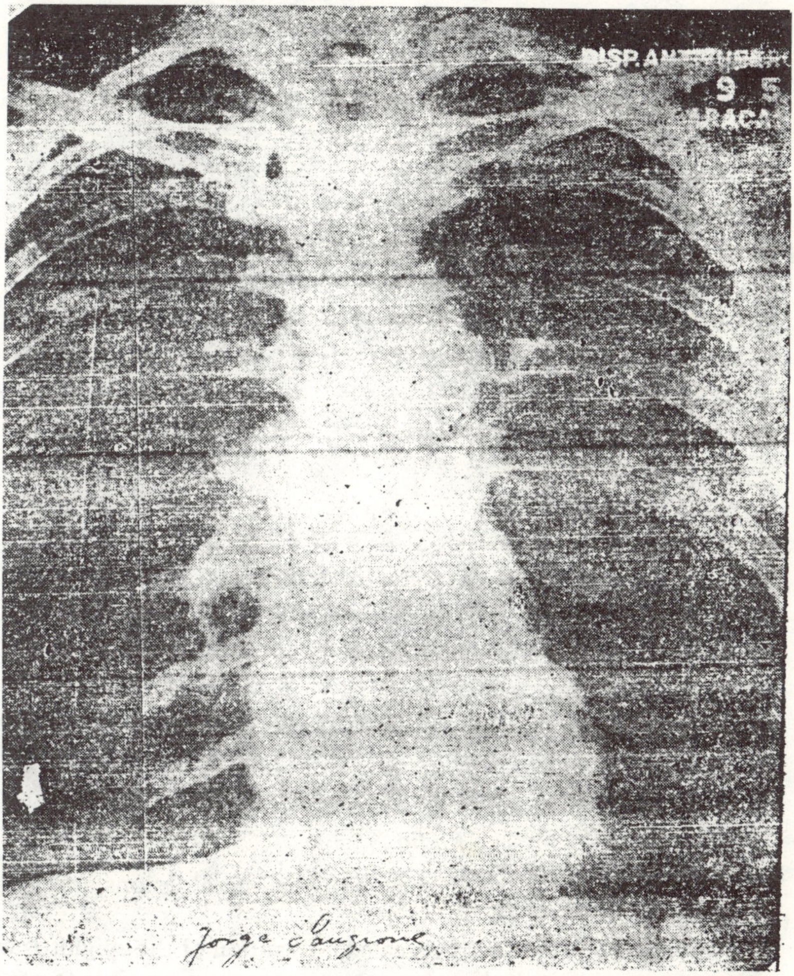

Radio Nº 2.

The short histories of the cases are: J.G., 32 years old, color people, single, born in Puerto Cabello.

Ten months before, ulceration in lower lip, near the left commissure; after upper lip; later, lesions in the gums and next mucous membranes. Six months with hoarseness, and strong pain when swallowed.

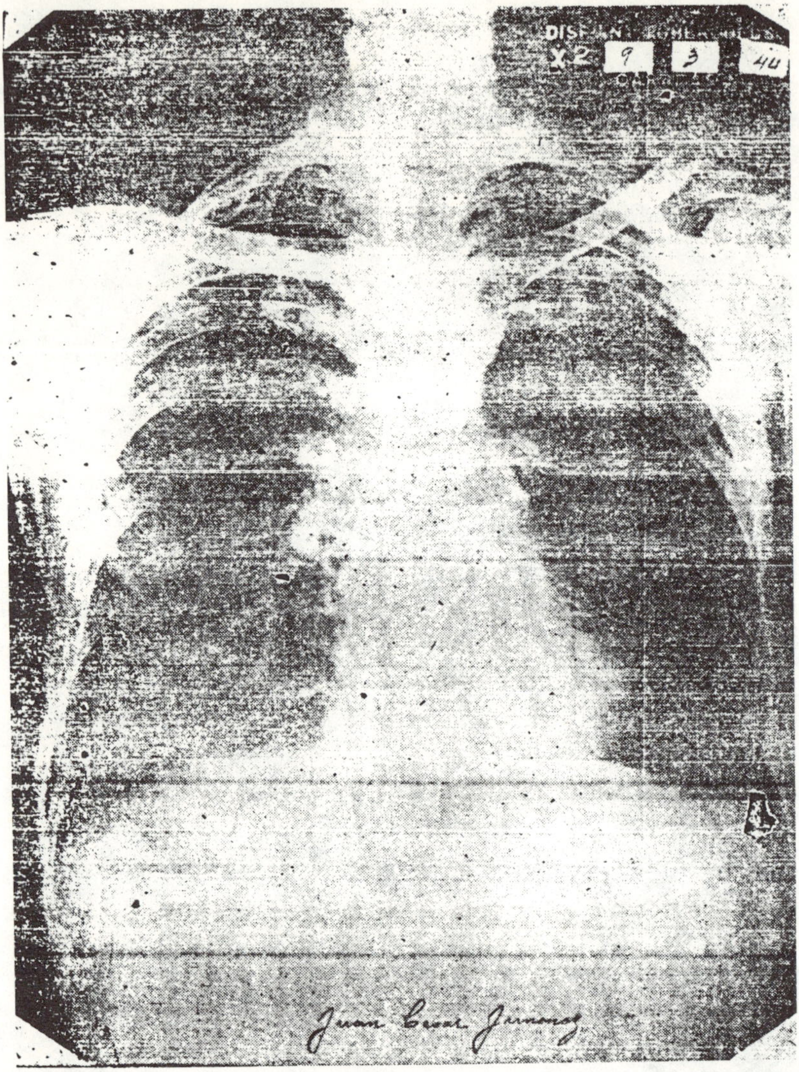

Radio N° 3.

Paracoccidioides positive in smears of the buccal lesions and biopsy of the epiglottis.

The laryngoscopy indirectly revealed infiltration of the epiglottis with ulceration; arytenoids with the same aspect; it was not possible to see the endolarynx.

Treatment: sulparidine (Dagenan). With 38 tablets the patient had a notable improvement, cicatrization of the lesions, the infiltration of the lips decreased, when swallowing very light pain, the hoarseness diminished, living in the hospital.

The second case - C.J., 61 years old, white, single, born in Montalbán (State Carabobo).

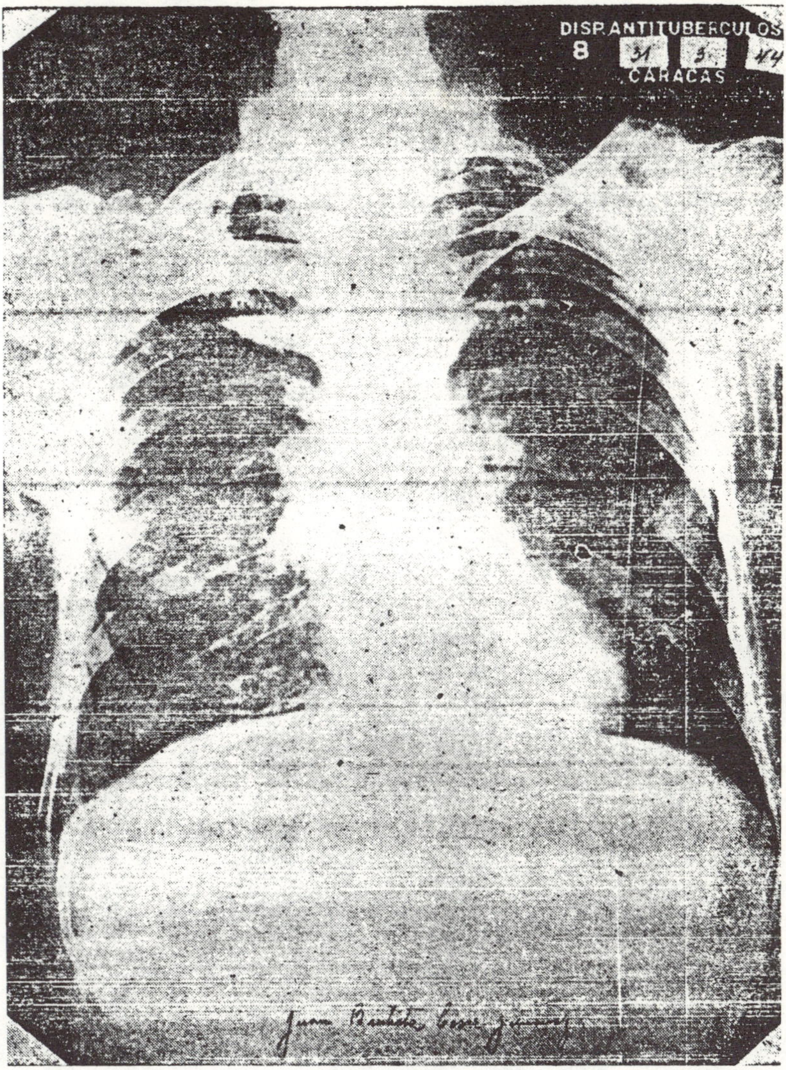

Radio Nº 4.

The affection started one year before for an ulceration of the upper lip, after, lesion in the mocous membrane of the mouth, hard and soft palate. Three months ago hoarseness and later pain to swallow. The examination to the entry at the hospital gave: ulceration right nostril, buccal mucous, palate (hard and soft), infiltration and ulceration of the arytenoids; it was not possible to see inside the larynx.

Kahn	negative
Spittle	negative
Smear	paracoccidioides positive
Biopsy	granuloma to paracoccidioides

Globular sedimentation: lst hour 30 - 2nd 32 17. 5 unidades Westergreen.

Blood count: lymphocytes 30, polynuclears 64, eosinophiles 6.
Treatment: Sulfathiazole 120 tablets, corresponding 60 grams. Hematic control done during the treatment gave: 3.840.000 red cells. The improvement was notable. The extense buccal ulceration almost had disappeared. The laryngoscopy revealed improvement of the lesions. The voice was more clear and eating was not inconvenient.

The expounder showed two radiographs: one, made to the entry and the other one after the treatment of 60 grams of sulfathiazole.

RHINO - SCLEROMA IN VENEZUELA *

Some time ago we presented in the corresponding meeting of the Service O. R. L. of the Hospital Vargas the first case of rhinoscleroma observed in the country, with the collaboration of Gedeón. A woman, 23 years old, native, born in Carache (State Táchira). In the cuttings of the lesion were found the characteristic cells of Mikuliks. In the cultures it was not possible to verify the Frisch' bacillus, but in the smears we found germs in form of diplo-bacillus with capsule. Today we expose a second case of the same affection. Clinically not a very typical case, but suspicious, verified for the histo-pathological study.

The present patient was born in Boconó (State Trujillo), 20 years old and agriculturist. He says that several years before began to feel obstruction in both sides of the nose, abundant secretion, consulting a colleague in the interior and being operated with diagnosis of polyps. Remember that patient that had a light improvement, resolving after, to come to Caracas to get entrance to the Service O. R. L. of the Hospital Vargas.

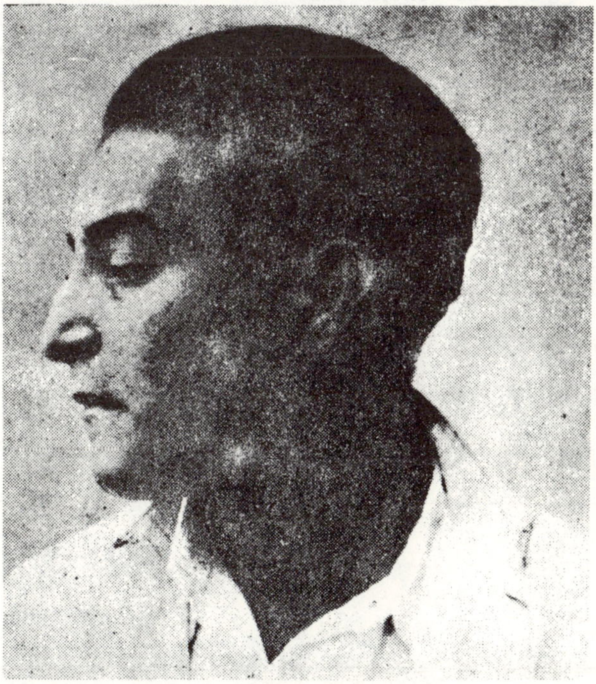

Profile of the patient. It is possible to appreciate a light deformation of the nasal pyramid.

* Reprinted from "Estudios de Patología Tropical" book. 1942.

The oto-rhino-laryngeal examination permitted to see the nasal obstruction owned to formations of pink color, process extended to the pharynx and tonsils, neo-formations of the same aspect and color. The posterior laryngoscopy permitted us to see the cavum filled by the tissue mentioned.

When a biopsy was taken of the nose (12-2-39), the diagnosis oscillated among lymphosarcoma, lymphoangioadenoma and other affection. Wassermann and Kahn' tests were positive (+ + +). Taking in account this positivity was treated with arsenic and bismuth without no improvement.

A secondary biopsy (10-4-39) brought the report of rhino-scleroma. Seeing it difficult to treat this patient, he was sent to the Anticancerous institute "Luis Razetti", under the attention of Drs. Landaeta Sojo y Pallares, sending us later the following report:

TREATMENT

PLAN DE TRATAMIENTO

Fecha	diaria	r	kv voltaje	Ma	Filtro	Df	Campo	Dosis
13-6-39		300	200 r	5	0,75 Cu - 1 al	50	10x 10	3.600

TRATAMIENTO

Fecha	Rayos X	Radium
13-6-39	300 r	30-5-39 20 mg. ra. en tubos de aluminio 9 a. m. Se leva las 5.30 p. m. del mismo día.
14-6-39	300 r	6-7-39 20 mg. ra. en dos tubos de platino intranasal.
15-6-39	300 r	8-7-39 Levantamiento a las 9 a. m.
16-6-39	300 r	
17-6-39	300 r	
19-6-39	300 r	
20-6-39	300 r	
22-6-39	300 r	
23-6-39	300 r	
24-6-39	300 r	

Finished the treatment, the nasal permeability had improved notably and the neoformations in the pharyx were stopped. Later, news coming from him saying he was feeling well.

CONCLUSIONS

1.- A new case of rhinoscleroma is presented, the patient being a man 20 years old, a white agriculturist from Boconó in the State of Trujillo. Iriarte a short time ago called attention to the first case published in Venezuela.

2.- The clinical diagnosis was suspected, being subsequently corroborated by the histopathological report of the Serv. of Path. Anat of Hospital Vargas and that of Koppisch of the School of Tropical Medicine of Pto. Rico.

3.- As the patient had a positive serology and one of the histopathological diagnosis of the first biopsy was granuloma venereum, a bismuth-arsenic treatment was tried and subsequently an intravenous series of tartar emetic, but no modification of the process was observed.

4.- The patient having been transferred to the anticancerous institute "Luis Razetti" and treated with X rays and radium by Drs. Landaeta (Sojo and Pallares) his improvement was remarkable.

BILHARZIOSIS - SNAILS

SUSPICIONS OF FOCUS OF BILHARZIOSIS IN THE EAST OF THE COUNTRY *

In some days of vacation staying lastly in the city of Cumaná, the colleagues (Rodríguez, Vargas Camero, Noguera), spoke of patients with a dysenteric syndrome, rebellious to any treatment used in that epoch: emetine, yatren 105, treparsol, estovarsol, ipecacuanha, enterovioformo, opran, etc.. Desperate, hopeless in front of these ills, they injected emetic and the patients showed notable improvement.

When we arrived there, Dr. Julio Rodríquez had in observation one of these cases. The examination of feces that we did was positive for eggs of bilharzia.

The present patient is a woman 42 years old, having lived all her life in the State Sucre, never going out, suffering since around one year of a crisis of diarrhea, pain in the right hypochondrium, dizziness, tenesmus.

Asking about the places were she could have been infected, she tells us that she bathed in the river Bordones and in the stream of Tataracual, village between Cumaná and Cumanacoa. The first of these sites was visited by us, not finding snails of the family Planorbidae, only Ampularidae that they call commonly *cuibas.* We had no time to visit the second place.

Speaking with Dr. Bougrat in Margarita (Juan Griego), told us he had observed several cases of bilharziosis, from the zone Golfo de Cariaco, place where exists a lagoon and probably site of the infection. Seeking mollusks was not possible, perhaps the strong droughts will not be favorable to the development of malacological fauna.

SUMMARY

1.- Verified the suspicions of colleagues of the presence of bilharziosis in the State Sucre. Besides Sucre, perhaps another State. According to Potenza, belonging to the Anatomo-pathological Service of Hospital Vargas, in biopsies of liver coming from State Bolívar seeking yellow fever, have found typical lesions of bilharziosis.

2.- The verification has been done for the examination of feces in a lady with intestinal troubles, of 42 years old, never going out of State Sucre.

3.- We could not find mollusks of the family Planorbidae, only Ampullaridae that the people call cuibas. For the data obtained the focus of infection should be perhaps, in Tataracual and the lagoon of Cariaco.

4.- The physicians of those regions will seek te mollusks, the places where are found, the percentage of infestation, examinaton of the feces, etc., in the suspitious cases.

***Reprinted from the Boletín del Laboratorio de la Clínica Luis Razetti - Año I - N° I - 1940.**

MALACOLOGICAL COMMENTARIES *

Since an old friend, colleague and fellow of the Academy, Dr. Antonio Leocadio Briceño Rossi, read in one of the weekly session of this Institution, a work entitled "Nueva Nomenclatura para el huésped intermedio del Schsitosoma mansoni in Venezuela", appeared in one of the last numbers of the Gaceta Médica de Caracas (april-june 1961), we have been interested, chiefly, we have worked formerly in the compilation of mollusks and also in our antique affections in affairs of parasitology and tropical medicine.

Around the year 1923, when we began making practices of laboratory in the Section of Bacteriology and Parasitology of the disappeared Dirección de Sanidad Nacional, headed by Tejera, we observed and helped in the rearings of these mollusks.

The malacological fauna it seems not to be much rich. We had heard this opinion, coming from our remembered friend Professor Pittier, who doing frequent trips through the country, sought always snails for request of American malacologists. We could verify later, in our travels for eighteen of the twenty States of the nation. Lastly, members of the Natural History Society of the School LaSalle have made interesting findings in this field.

Briceño Rossi did reference to the work: "Studies on Venezuelan Planorbidae" of Bengt Hubendick, from Gotenburgo, dedicated to our failed and able fellow of Course Carlos Ottolina, saying: "In so interesting work, Hubendick assures, irrefutable, that the genus Australorbis, Biomphalaria, Platytaphius, Taphius and Tropicorbis are an alone genus, that for priority corresponding to genus Taphius Adams and Adams, 1855; assures also that must not take in account the priority of the subgenus Planorbina of Haldeman, 1842, owned to the several proofs. In this way, Pilsbry, 1934, and Vianna Martins, 1938, had separated the Sub-American species of the genus Planorbis, incorporating it for priority to the genus Australorbis."

"In this stage, the specie glabratus Say, 1818, now is denominated Australorbis glabratus Say; but now, with the work of Hubendick, with the catalogue, on will call Taphius glabratus Say, according to rigid laws of the zoological nomenclature, affair discused for Barbosa, Hubendick, Malek and Wright in the International Commission of the Zoological Nomenclature, 1958."

* * *

It is necessary a correct systematization of invertebrate hosts of the

* Reprinted from Gaceta Médica de Caracas.- Año IXX 1 - 2 - 1962.

billarziosis, disease not only of the center of the country, but also, possibly, extended to another zones, already that we in Boletín del Laboratorio de la Clínica Luis Razetti, Año I, N° 1, gave the alert that probably existed in the State Sucre; Briceño Iragorry, in the same review, studied a case probably autochthonous from State Monagas; Potenza, in hepatic biopsies coming from different regions found lesions, characteristic of the bilharziosis, and Luttermosser, in shells brought from the East States, found shells of Planorbidae. This necessity was evident in the first meeting of the mixed group O I H P and O M S, gathered in Egypt in 1950, as follows: "determination of the geographical distribution of the vector snails, adopting an uniform classification and nomenclature, based in the internal morphology and ecological characteristics of the mollusks, in change, of the external characteristics of the shells."

The snails hosts of the Bilharziosis mansoni are of the class Gasteropod, order of the Pulmonate, sub-order Basomatoforos, comprising five families: Lymacidae, Planorbidae, Physidae, Ancylidae and Bulinidae. The Planorbidae comprise four sub-families: Segmentininae, Planorbinae, Helisomatinae and Planorbulinae. The planorbinae comprise ten genus, including two of them, species in relation with human pathology, as follows: Australorbis Pilsbry, 1934 and Tropicorbis Pilsbry and Brown, 1914.

Lucena and Pessoa give clefs for the differentiation of both genus. The Australorbis host specially in the Antilles and South America, comprise: Australorbis glabratus Say, Australorbis olivaceus Spix, Australorbis camerunensis Boettger, Australorbis inmunis Lutz, Australorbis tenegophilus d'Orbigny, Australorbis bahiensis Dunker. The Tropicorbis, also American, comprise: Tropicorbis stramineus Dunker, Tropicorbis janeirensis Clessin and Tropicorbis nordestensis Lucena. Juan Iturbe, 1955, wrote the following: "Of these molluks are very interesting for us the genus Planorbis and specially the sub-genus Planorbina Haldeman, 1842, natives from the Antilles and South America, and in that group are the hosts invertebrates of the Schistosoma mansoni in our country. It is well advise that the modern malacologists Pilsbry (1934) and Vianna Martins (1938) have separated from the genus Planorbis the South-American species and among them has priority the name Planorbis glabratus Say (1818), corresponding it now: Australorbis glabratus Say 1818. Planorbis glabratus Say 1818, Planorbis guadalupensis Sowerby 1822, Planorbis striatulus 1827, Planorbis xerampelinus Drouet 1859, etc. The main intermediate host of the Schistosoma mansoni in Venezuela, as experimentally we demonstrate (1916), it has six spirals and can arrive in the adult stage 24 m.m. of width and 7 m.m. of height. It is not salient in its distal end; the spirals sink in a conic depression; its inferior face is less depressed; its teeth are placed regularly and has filiform tentacles. The specimens more developed look likes to Planorbis olivaceus, but are distinguished by the size and for the flattening of the last spiral. The color of the adult specimens caught by us in the streams of the surroundings of Caracas is brown yellowish; this color something more pale in the specimens from Puerto Rico, according Martens (1873). In the material of mollusks from this island sent to us by Gutiérrez Ingaravidez (1917), we could easily identify many specimens of Planorbis guadalupensis, much of them infected with Schistosoma mansoni. Our research, in accord González Martínez, 1928, were accepted favorable for all the scientists of the School of Tropical Medicine, and two years later verified for Brumpt 1920, and his assistant Langeron, who had the opportunity of examine widely specimens taken to Paris for González Martínez, who in his interesting work, said the following: "before Hoffman, Iturbe in 1917 and Brumpt, 1920, have found the Planorbis guadalupensis as the intermediate host of trematode of the island, fact verified by us in 1931."

Iturbe said that the first work about the molluks of our country was done for the German Karsten 1860, with the study and revision of collections from Zoological Museum of Berlín; years later, Von Martens did a wide communication utilizing material caught and sent for Appun and Ernst and that Vicente Marcano in 1889, doing etnographic explorations in the State Aragua, in the place Los Cerritos, near Valencia's lake, in pre-Colombian tombs, found shells of snails classified with the help of Fischer, resulting some of it as Planorbis olivaceus Spix 1827, specie that was considered as native of Brazil.

Referring the genus Tropicorbis, the specie Tropicorbis havanensis Pfeiffer, was accused by Gram and Files (1946), having obtained the infection for Schistosoma mansoni in a percentage of 9% in specimens collected in Baton Rouge, in the State of Louisiana. Luis Manuel Peñalver, our Assistant Professor of our chair of Tropical Pathology, during his stay in Havana, observed (1949) cases not autochthonous of bilharziosis, and did an interesting experimental work utilizing Cuban mollusks of sweet water, belonging the genus and species following: Helisoma, Lymnaea cubensis, Marisa cornuspira and Pomacea paludosa. With none of these species got experimental infection. It was attraction and penetration miracodium in Tropicorbis havanensis, Lymnaea cubensis, Physa cubensis and Helisoma caribaeus, but not evolution in the mollusk.

F. S. Barbosa, authority in this field, from the National Institute of Rural Diseases of Recife (Brazil), suggested that the species of genus Taphius of the Titicaca's lake in Bolivia 1955, studied by Hubendick, did not presented generic delimitation among Australorbis, Tropicorbis; the same, among African genus Biomphalaria and American genus Tropicorbis and Australorbis; that the opinion of Hubendick placing in Biomphalaria the hosts of African and American schistosomiasis required consideration and fitting of the nomenclature, and told that the hosts temporaly could be classified in the genus Biomphalaria, Tropicorbis and Australorbis.

Referring the problem of the discriminate species of the Planorbidae, Barbosa believes that up today could be individualized: Australorbis glabratus Say, Australorbis nigricans Spix, Australorbis incertus Lutz,

Tropicorbis centrimetralis Lutz and Tropicorbis janeirensis Clessin.

In our American continent till up today there are three species very spreaded and host of the Bilharzia mansoni: Australorbis glabratus Say, called Australorbis olivaceus or Australobis guadeloupensis; the Tropicorbis centrimetralis, called equally stramineus, argentinensis or patagonicus and the Australorbis nigricans, nominated also inmunis, and two potential species: Tropicorbis havanensis, accused by Gram and others 1945, and Tropicorbis chilensis, accused by Barbosa and Barbosa 1957, as receptive to a group of Brazilian trematodes.

Research of Files have revealed that exist physiological differences between snails and trematodes of different Continents. The Tropicorbis centrimetralis is not an efficient host of the Schistosoma mansoni but it is considered the spreader in the North-east of Brazil and Australorbis nigricans is receptive to some group, while is refractory to others. Australorbis glabratus, remains then as the true host of the Bilharzia mansoni in América.

* * *

For all these considerations, we continue having to Taphius as a genus of the sub-family Planorbinae and will call always to our intermediate host of the bilharziosis: Australorbis glabratus Say 1818, Pilsbry 1934.

THE BREADFRUIT TREE
(ARTOCARPUS COMMUNIS FORST)
ANALYSIS OF ITS FRUIT SINCE THE NOURISHING VANISHING POINT *

I

CLASSIFICATION

The following is the classification made by H. Pittier, took it from his book "Manual de las Plantas Usuales de Venezuela." 1926: "Arbol de Pan. Moráceas. Artocarpus communis Forst. Chart. Gen. 102. 1776. Sin: árbol de pan (general); fruta de pan; pan de pobre (Barinas, Falcón, Trujillo); pan de todo el año (Barinas); topan (Yaracuy)."

"Arbol muy ornamental, lactífero, de mediano tamaño, con hojas anchas, lobuladas o pinatifidas. Es especie monaica, apétala, las flores masculinas con cáliz de dos sépalos e insertas en un receptáculo alargado y claviforme; las femeninas de cáliz tubuloso, formando en su conjunto una cabezuela esférica. Los frutos redondos u ovalados adquieren las dimensiones de una cabeza de niño y se presentan en dos variedades, la una con, la otra sin semillas".

"En otros países ambas variedades desempeñan un papel no despreciable en la alimentación de la gente de los campos, pero en Venezuela no son muy populares. Las semillas se comen hervidas en agua con sal, como las castañas europeas; la fruta estéril se come antes de su completa madurez, hervida en agua o tostada en tajadas, sea en un horno, o del mismo modo que las arepas. Los habitantes de la Polinesia, en donde el árbol parece ser indígena, también lo aderezan de varios modos, pero siempre constituye un alimento sano y de provecho. Usaban en un tiempo la corteza para hacer uno de los tejidos con que se vestían; la leche da una cola fuerte y la emplean además en el calafateo de sus botes, así también, como elemento de sus varios afeites y pinturas. La madera es amarillenta y de una dureza mediana; se dice que no la ataca el comején."

"La variedad de semillas se reproduce por medio de éstas y se propaga espontáneamente en la tierra caliente de los trópicos. La variedad estéril, que sólo se encuentra en estado de cultivo, se multiplica artificialmente por medio de los retoños arraigados que crecen en la base del tronco o en las raíces, cuando éstas son muy superficiales."

CHEMICAL ANALYSIS

The chemist analysis has been divided in two parts, englobing in the

* Reprinted from the book "Trabajos Científicos." 1937 Thesis of baccalaureate.

first, the processes done about the row fruit, as is taken from the trees; and in the second, the made about the boiled fruit, as often eaten.

FIRST PART

In this are included humidity and starch.

At the begining we made a trituration using a machine to grind, but the crushing resulted very thick, but then we used a grater, obtaining something alike to the coconut, giving a similar to the potato or benne.

HUMIDITY

In order to know the humidity we took a known amount of the grating and placed it inside the stove during 24 hours and later in the dryer of S 04 H2 during 12 hours, obtaining the figures:

Amount of water 60.365%

Amount of solid 39.635%

for the potato the amount of water according Balland, should be of 80.60%.

STARCH

We took 110 grams of the grating, added a certain quantity of CO3HNa, waiting for several hours, later, added H2O and sifted, receiving in conic vase in order to decant, and a liquid volume of 500 c.c. gave a feculent deposit of around 80 c.c.

Later, treated with HC1, producing great effervescence for the presence of CO3HNa and we decanted newly; right after that, added H2O and we did the former; inmediately solution of sodium sulfite in order to whitten the starch and lastly added C2H50H, to extract a resinous substance, perhaps coming from the seeds.

Seeing the fecula to the microscope has semi-spheric forms very abundant and also, in polygonal forms; almost always hexagonal, liking the manihot (yuca) starch. Looking to the figures is easy to see the similarity, but in size the yuca is bigger.

The slides have been made in a mixed of water and glycerine, substance that has the properties of avoid the dessication and enlarge, showing it in true form. In slides in the book of Willey (Foods and their adulteration. 3a. edition), the similarity is large.

The polarization cross is less thick in relation with the cross of the yucca (manihot).

These drawings have been made with the camera lucida of the eyepiece of drawing of Leitz (model 2° for inclined microscope in accord Langeron).

FUNGUS

Some fruits that remained three days within the ice box procuring the conservation, was on the development of fungi and thinking should be important in the future exporting this fruit, because in many places is essential in the base of the feeding, replacing the potato as in Korea, having sent some cultures to United States waiting answer, but examined for Nogueira Gómez is an Aspergillus, type orizae.

SECOND PART

In this second part are the rest of the analysis practiced with the flour of the fruit, obtained: boiling, grating, 24 hours in the stove, pulverized and sifted.

PROTEINS

The dosage of the proteins was made proportioning the total nitrogen for the Kjeldahl' method, and for transforming in proteins multiply for the coefficient 6.25. The result was of 11.025%. This figure it seems good to us, if we compared with the potato, that Balland said has a maximum of 2.81% and a minimum of 1.43%.

Comparing with cereals, please to see the following amount, taken from Leach (Foods inspection and analysis): barley, 11.52%; corn (medium figure) 9.88%; rice (polished), 7.18%; rice (without polished), 8.02%; oat (medium figure), 12.15%; almond, 20%; peanut, 11.00%.

STARCH AND SUGAR

With the chemical procedures, using the Fehling's liquor, on obtained the following figures: glucosa, 64.19%, multiplied for the coefficient 0.9

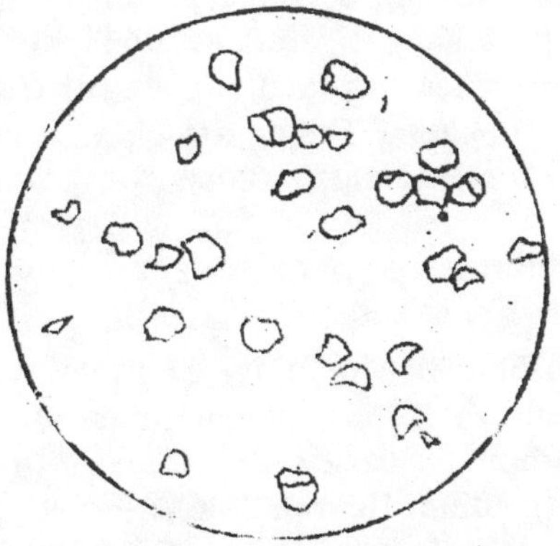

Fécula. Arbol del pan.
Obj. 6. Leitz.

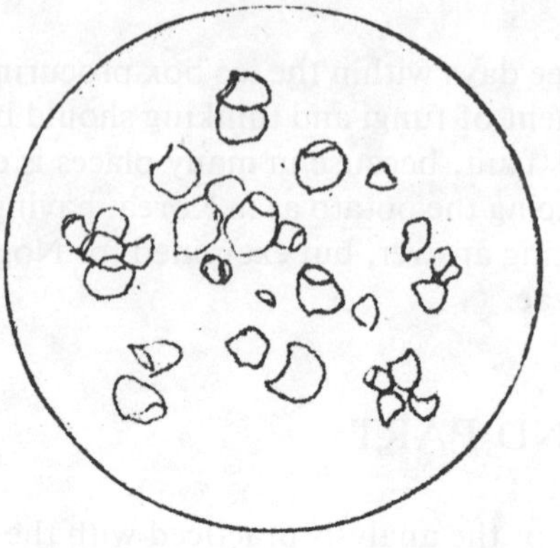

Fécula. Jatropha manihot.
Obj. 6. Leitz.

gave a total of 57.771% in starch, including in this figure the sugar of the seed, is called starch and sugar. In relation with the potato, this one contains, according Balland an amount of sugar and fecula: minimum, 15.58/ and maximum, 29.85%. Quantities of carbohydrates, according Atwater and Boyant: banana, 22.00%; orange, 11.60%; pineapple, 9.75%; grapes, 19.20%.

GREASES

The dosage was made for the Soxhlet's method and we worked with 10 grams. The result was the following: amount of greases, 5.57%.

The potato contains a quantity of grease very reduced, with a minimum of 0.04% and a maximum of 0.14%. Now, compared with almond 54.9%; peanut, 71.2%, the greases will be poor for the fruit of our study.

CELLULOSE

We did the Balland's method: 25 grams of flour is mixed in 150 c.c. of acidulated water with HC1, boiling during 20 minutes, sift it and the residue treat it with a solution potassium hydrate to 10% during 20 minutes, to filter, to wash with hot water and finally, treat for C2H50H and (C2H5) 20. The result was of 10.420%. The potato gives, according Balland a minimum of 0.37% and a maximum of 0.68%.

ASHES

The Artocarpus communis produces a quantity of ashes equal to 3.30%. The potato gives a maximum of 1.18% and a minimum of 0.44%. The following cereals give these amounts: barley, 28.7%; corn (medium figure), 1.36%; rice, 0.46%; oat, (medium figure), 3.46%.

In the ashes was made the dosage of silex in Si 02, the potassium in

K_2O, the sodium in Na_2O, the calcium CaO, the magnesium in Mg O, the iron in Fe_2O_3, and the phosphoric and sulfuric acids under the form of anhydrides P_2O_5 and SO_3, the chlorine in Cl.

SiO_2

The quantity of silex obtained was of 1.30%. Working on 1 gram of ashes, the potato contains 2.13%.

K_2O and Na_2O

Obtained the chloride of potassium and sodium were treated for the chlorine of platinum to transform the KCl in Pt $(KCl)_2$ and to separate the NaCl. For computation were changed in its oxides and so the K appreciated in K_2O was of 32.60% and the Na in Na_2O was of 40.08%. The potato contains K_2O, a 60.37% and Na_2O, 2.62%.

CaO and MgO

The amount of CaO obtained was of 9.80% and of MgO, 1.10%. The potato gives: CaO, 2.57% and MgO, 4.68%.

Fe_2O_3

The weight of Fe_2O_3 was of 1.30%. For the potato the figure is of 1.18%.

P_2O_5 and SO_3

It was obtained a regular quantity in the dosage of the P_2O_5 and was of 16.50%. The potato advanced slightly and in accord the analysis made in this last one has given a quantity of 17.33%.

For the SO_3 we added chloride of barium to transform all the SO_4Ba to calcine and to appreciate SO_3, we multiplied for the coefficient 0.3433. The result was of 1.85%. According to the analysis the potato contains 6.49%.

Cl

The dosage was done on 50 centigrams of flour and using NO_3Ag, obtaining the figure of 4.26%. The potato gave the figure 3.11%.

Please see the results in the two following columns:

Ashes of the breadfruit

SiO_2	1.30%
K_2O	32.60%
Na_2O	40.08%

CaO	9.80%
MgO	1.10%
Fe_2O_3	1.30%
P_2O_5	16.50%
SO_3	1.85%
Cl	4.26

Ashes of the potato, according Wiley

SiO_2	2.13%
K_2O	60.37%
Na_2O	2.62%
CaO	2.57%
MgO	4.69
Fe_2O_3	1.18%
P_2O_5	17.33%
SO_3	6.49%
Cl	3.11%

We see that the essential elements: P_2O_5, K_2O, Fe_2O_3 and CaO, the amounts found are not very straggler. In the place almost are equals; in the second place our fruit is a little behind, but in change in the last two places the figures are advanced in relation with the potato.

For then, the breadfruit is not poor for feeding, according with all the proofs, as we have read in "Geografía Médica. del Zulia", telling that the breadfruit produces something, like the chestnut, that roasted, are not very nourishing, but pleasing to the taste, and Lanessan (Les Plantes utiles des Colonies Francaises), saying, referring to the "igname" variety, as agreeable food, but low in nutrition.

Perhaps, this one will be the first analysis made about the "châtaigne" variety of the breadfruit (very possible that in the United States the analysis of this fruit has been made), because we have looked in many books and reviews.

Now, about the *igname* variety, Pellerin (L'Expert chimiste), brings the following:

Water	Sub-nitrogenous	Grease	Sugar	Starchy or extr.	Cellulose	Salts
14.20%	2.84%	0.90%	14.76%	60.50%	4.41%	2.40%

CALCULATION OF THE CALORIES

Accepting the coefficients of Hugounenq (Chimie physiologique et pathologique): carbohydrates, 4.1%; proteins, 4.1%; greases, 9.4%; and knowing already the quantities of 57.771, 11.025 and 5.57, obtained in these analysis for each one of those foods, respectively, we will have the following calculations:

57.771 X 4.1 — 11.025 X 4.1 — 5.57 X 9.4

for each 100 grams of fruit will obtain the following figures i calories:

Carbo-hydrates 326.86: proteins 45.20; greases 52.358.

Our acknowledgement to *DR.NOGUERA GOMEZ* under whose wise patronage has been possible to do this work.

ENTOMOLOGIA

ANNOTATION ABOUT A NEW SPECIE OF SIMULIIDAE IN THE COUNTRY (Simulium limbatum Knab 1915-16) *

Here the following paragraphs of the Chapter "Introduction" of the work of Pinto "Simuliidae da America Central e do Sul (Diptera)", make to see the importance of these arthropoda:

"The principal pathogenic interesting of these insects, mainly in he transmission of sickness, started with the research of Professor D.B. Blacklock, demonstrating that the sting of Simulium damnosum Theobald, transmitted the Onchocerca volvulus, in Africa".

"The scientists from Mexico, C.C. Hoffmann and others, began research about the spread of the Onchocerca caecutiens and verified that the filaria will develop in the muscles of the thorax of Eusimulium mooseri Dampf, and for as much could be the transmissor of the disease in Mexico".

"During some time the simuliidae, according to the theory of Marchoux and others, raising suspicions of transmitting the leprosy. Doubts that never were verified, with the argumentation that among the inhabitants of Hawaii, where the leprosy is frequent; however, there are no simuliidae".

"Sambon thought they were the spreaders of the pellagra; Jennings and other researchers never could verify".

"Probably so diptera, as hematophagous insects, spread parasites, either in man of among the animals".

"In Brazil, the people believe that pemphigus and other illness' are transmitted by simuliidae".

In Sud America are unknown species capable of killing animals as has been seen in Europe; however, in certain regions are very numerous, annoyings, big prickers, and some of them can pursuit the man still six kilometers from the border of the river".

"In some places, as has been observed by Lutz in Isla Grande and by Neiva in villages of Sao Paulo, causing despair among the rural people".

Pinto forgot among the ravages of simuliidae as probable spreaders of *carate* or *carare.* We have published that Montoya y Flores, at the end of the last century accused these insects as transmissors, and here, between us, the people think in the indirect contagion through insects, called *mosquitos* or *plaga,* because the name of *jejen,* cited for Philippi in Chile is used for the ceratopogonidae, as said Knab for the same country and as we have it verified, between us.

In our book "Estudios de Patología Tropical" we appointed another

* Reprinted from "Boletín del Laboratorio de la Clínica Luis Razetti" - Año III - N° 8 -1942

specie of simuliidae for the region of Guarenas (Simulium exiguum) of State Miranda, species mentioned in 1906 as captured in Alto Sarare. With this specie we did some trails about the transmission of *carate,* but these insects in captivity frequently died and the sting is difficult. In Mexico, after the puncture sucking blood in patients *caratosos,* in the test of blood in dark field, have been seen spirochetes.

On Christmas vacation (1941) in the State Bolívar, to the border of a waterfall, to 50 km, from Ciudad Bolívar, called La Candelaria, we caught some specimens of simuliidae, stinging on the back of two young fishermen, and they were sent to the Department of Agriculture in Washington and were classified by Stone as Simulium limbatum Knab. This specie was found by this last researcher to the border of the river Riponumi in British Guayane, and it seems to be very similar to the species amazonicum of Goeldi (1905). Up till today there has been found in the country, including the present, thirteen species, as following:

S. amazonicum Goeldi, 1905 (lutzi, minusculum, nitidum)
S. lugubre Lutz and Nuñez Tovar, 1928
S. incrustatum Lutz 1910
S. lutzianus Pinto 1931 (rubrithorax Lutz, 1909)
S. rubrithorax Lutz, 1909
S. subnigrum Lutz, 1910
S. versicolor Lutz and Núñez Tovar, 1928
S. exiguum Roubaud, 1906
E. ochraceum Walker, 1860
E. paraguayense Schrojtky, 1909
S. metallicum Bellardi, 1859
S. pulverulentum Knab, 1914
S. limbatum Knab, 1015-16

In April, during the days of holyweek, we went to the region of Choroni (State Aragua) making an abundant capture, places visited by Lutz and Núñez Tovar.

The material sent to Washington to our friend Dr. Allan Stone, has been classified.

Small river Curucurumbo, 16 km. from Maracay (State Aragua) and 550 m. of height. Capture: S. metallicum Bell. and S. exiguum Roubaud.

Small river La Quebrada, in the surroundings of the village Choroní. Capture: S. metallicum Bell. and S. incrustatum Lutz.

River Choroní, place Los Cerritos (State Aragua). Capture: S. metallicum Bell. and S. incrustatum Lutz.

River Choroní, place El Parnaso (State Aragua). Capture: S. incrustatum Lutz and S. rubrithorax Lutz.

SUMMARY

It is presented a new species of the family Simuliidae for Venezuela (Simulium limbatum Knab 1915-16). The specimens were caught on the border of a waterfall, situated 50 km. from Ciudad Bolívar, called La Candelaria. With this species is increased to thirteen the number of Simuliidae appointed in the country up till today. Have been found in the region of Choroní (State Aragua); S. exiguum Roubaud, S. metallicum Bell., S. incrustatum Lutz and S. rubrithorax Lutz.

BIBLIOGRAPHY CONSULTED

1.-*Lutz.*-Contribuicao para o conhecimento das especies brazileiras do genero "Simulium" Mem. do Inst. O. Cruz. - Tomo I. - Fac. II. 1909.

2.-*Lutz.*-Segunda contribuicao para o conhecimento das especies brazileiras do genero "Simulium". Mem. do Inst. O. Cruz. - Tomo II. - Fac. II. 1910.

3.-*Lutz.*-Terceira contribuicao para o conhecimento das especies brazilieras do genero "Simulium". Mem. do Inst. O. Cruz. - Tomo IX. - Fac. I. 1917.

4.-*Lutz, Souza Araugo e O. da Fonseca filho.*-Viagem scientifica no Rio Paraná e a Assuncion com volta por Buenos Aires, Motevideo e Río Grande. - Mem. do Inst. O. Cruz. - Tomo X. - Fac. II. 1918.

5.-*Lutz y Núñez Tovar.*-Estudios de Zoología y Parasitología Venezolanas. -Obra, 1928.

6.-*Pinto.*-Simuliidae da America Central e do Sul (Diptera) VII reunión de la Sociedad Argentina de Patología Regional del Norte, 1931.

7.-*Pinto.*-Zoo-parasitos de Interesse Medico e Veterinario. - Obra, 1938.

8.-*Strong, Sandground, Bequaert. Ochoa.*-Onchocerciasis. - Harvard University Press., 1934.

9.-*Strong, Bequaert, Shattuck, Wheeler.*-Medical Report of the Hamilton Rice Seventh Expedition to the Amazon 1924-1925, (1926).

10.-*Carbonell.*-La Parasitología en Venezuela y los Trabajos del Dr. Núñez Tovar. - Obra, 1938.

11.-*Briceño Iragorry.*-Nota sobre Simuliidae (Diptera) con citación de una nueva expecie para el país y lista de las conocidas en Venezuela.-Boletín del Laboratorio de la Clínica Luis Razetti. - Año II. - N° 6. - 1941.

12.-*Briceño Iragorry.*-Nota sobre Simulium pulverulentum Knab, 1914.-Boletín del Laboratorio de la Clínica Luis Razetti. - Año III - Vol. II. - N° 7.

13.-*Orfila.*-Simuliidae (Diptera) de la República Argentina, IX reunión de la Sociedad Argentina de Patología Regional. Tomo III, 1939.

14.-*Surcouf y González Rincones.*-Les diptères vulnérants du Venezuela. Primera parte, 1910.

15.-*Iriarte.*-Estudios de Patologia Tropical. - Obra, 1942.

CONTRIBUTION TO THE VENEZUELAN FAUNA *

We give here the classified material that we have found since a long time ago till today, material collected in trips from almost the whole country, in different months of the year. These classifications have had the help of the staff of the Department of Argriculture of Washington, mainly to Dr. Allan Stone, and the Professor Joseph C. Bequaert of the School of Harvard in Boston, to whom we give our acknowledgment.

ARTROPODOS
INSECTA (clase)
(hexápoda)

Corrodentia (orden)
Psoquillidae (familia)

Phoquilla sp.	det. Gurney

Anoplura (orden)
Haematopinidae

Haematopinus suis L.	det. Bequaert sitio de captura: Cumaná (Edo Sucre).

Homoptera (orden)
Fulgoridae

Oliarus sp.	det. Sainer s. de c. Estado Barinas.

Hemiptera (orden)
Reduviidae

Brontostoma notata Stal	det. Barber s. de c. Caracas.
Eutriatoma maculata Erich.	det. Barber s. de c. Estados Bolívar, Barinas, Falcón, Anzoátegui, Guárico y Zulia.
Panstrongylus geniculatus Latr.	det. Barber s. de c. El Valle (Dto. Federal) y Caracas: El Calvario, Catia, Los Chorros, Guarenas (Edo. Miranda).
Psammolestes arthuri Pinto	det. Barber s. de c. Estados Aragua, Cojedes y Guárico.
Rhodnius prolixus Stal.	det. Barber s. de c. Estados Anzoátegui, Portuguesa, Guárico, Trujillo, Mona-

* Reprinted from the "Boletín del Laboratorio de la Clínica Luis Razetti" - Año IV - N° 11 -1943.

	gas, Miranda y Sucre.
Spiniger rubropictus H.S.	det. Barber s. de c. alrededores de Maracaibo (Edo. Zulia).
Coreidae	
Corizus sidae Fab.	det. Dpto. Agric. de Washington s. de c. alrededores de Caracas: Hospital Vargas, Los Chorros, El Paraíso.
Leptoglossus gonagra F.	det. Barber s. de c. alrededores de Villa de Cura (Edo. Aragua).
Pyrrhocoridae	
Dysdercus maurus Dist.	det. Dpto. Agric. de Washinton s. de c. Acarigua (Edo. Portuguesa).
Dysdercus fernaldi Ballou	det. Sailer s. de c. Estado Barinas.
Lygacidae	
Orthaca bilobata Say.	det. Malloch s. de c. Caracas y Maracaibo (Edo. Zulia).
Pentatomidae	
Nezara stictica Dallas	det. Zetek s. de c. Caracas.
Miridae	
Dicyphus notatus Dist.	det. Barber
Trichoptera (orden)	
Hydropsichidae	
Género? especie?	det. Townes s. de c. Guarenas (Edo. Miranda).
Leptocoridae	
Género? especie?	det. Townes s. de c. Guarenas (Edo. Miranda).
Lepidoptera (orden)	
Phalaeniaae	
Laphygma frugiperda S. & A.	det. Clarke s. de c. Caracas.
Amalidae	
Cosmosoma sp.	det. Field s. de c. Estado Barinas.

Diptera (orden)

Simuliidae

Eusimulium ochraceum W.	det. Stone
E. bicoloratum Mall.	det. Stone
E. lutzianus Pinto	det. Stone
E. lugubre Lutz y Núñez Tovar	det. Stone
Simulium haematopotum Mall.	det. Stone
S. exiguum Roub.	det. Stone y Bequaert
S. sanguineum Knab	det. Fairchild
S. metallicum Bell.	det. Stone
S. limbatum Knab.	det. Stone
S. rubrithorax Lutz.	det. Stone
S. incrustatum Lutz.	det. Stone
S. sp.?	det. Greene
S. sp.?	det. Greene
	s. de c. las capturas de toda esta familia Simuliidae se han hecho en 10 Estados y el Distrito Federal.

Chironomidae

Chironomus sp.	det. Stone
Coelotanipus sp.	det. Stone
Pentaneura sp.	det. Stone
Tendipes sp.	det. Stone
	s. de c. capturas de estos cuatro géneros han sido efectuadas en varias regiones del país.

Ceratopogonidae

Culicoides paraensis G.	det. Stone
	s. de c. El Hatillo y Guarenas (Miranda), Macuto (D. F.) y Edo. Barinas.
Culicoides variipennis Coq.	det. Stone
	s. de c. Caracas.
Culicoides stellifer Coq.	det. Stone
	s. de c. Macuto (Dpto. Vargas, Dto. Federal).
Culicoides sp.	det. Stone
Culicoides sp.	det. Stone
Atrichopogon sp.	det. Stone
Atrichopogon sp.	det. Stone
Lasiohelea sp.	det. Stone
Lasiohelea sp.	det. Stone
Lasiohelea sp.	det. Stone
Lasiohelea sp.	det. Stone
	s. de c. los géneros Atrichopogon y Lasiohelea han sido recogidos en varios sitios del país.

Psychodidae

Phlebotomus migonei F.	det. Stone s. de c. Caracas.
Phlebotomus evansi N. T.	det. Stone s. de c. Macuto (Dto. Federal) San Mateo (Edo. Aragua).
Phlebotomus sp.	det. Stone
Phlebotomus sp.	det. Stone

Culicidae

Anopheles pessoai G. & L.	det. Stone s. de c. Río Curbati (Estado Barinas).
Anopheles sp. (grupo oswaldoi)	det. Stone s. de c. Río Curbati (Estado Barinas).
Anopheles (Nyssorhynchus) sp.	det. Stone s. de c. Río Curbati (Estado Barinas).
Aedes aegypti L.	det. Stone s. de c. Caracas.
Aedes sp.	det. Stone s. de c. Río Curbati (Estado Barinas).
Culex sp.	det. Stone s. de c. Río Curbati (Estado Barinas).
Psorophora confinnis L. A.	det. Stone s. de c. Río Curbati (Estado Barinas).

Cecidomyiidae

Mycodiplosis sp.	det. Greene

Mycetophilidae (Sciaridae)

Lycoria sp.	det. Dpto. Agric. de Washington.

Tabanidae

Chrysops laeta F.	det. Stone s. de c. Estado Barinas.
Chrysops variegata Deg.	det. Stone s. de c. Estado Barinas.
Dichelacera sp.	det. Stone
Stenotabanus sp.	det. Stone s. de c. Estado Barinas.
Tabanus sp. cercano a subruber Bell.	det. Stone

Tabanus lineola F.	det. Stone s. de c. Estado Barinas.
Tabanus cajennensis F.	det. Stone s. de c. Estado Barinas.
Phoridae	
Megaselia sp.	det. Greene
Dolichopodidae	
Psilopus sp.	det. James s. de c. Estado Barinas.
Syrphidae	
Volucella (Ornidia) obesa F.	det. Greene
Volucella tricincta Big.	det. Greene
Baccha sp.	det. Greene s. de c. Estado Barinas.
Chloropidae	
Hippelates sp.	det. Hall
Hippelates sp.	det. Bequaert s. de c. los Hippelates sp. han sido capturados en Guarenas (Estado Miranda) y Macuto (Dto. Federal).
Hippelates nobilis Lw.	det. M. T. James s. de c. Estado Barinas.
Oscinella sp.	det. Greene
Oscinella sp.	det. Greene
Oscinella sp.	det. Greene
Ephydridae	
Género? especie?	det. Greene
Agromyzidae	
Agromyza sp.	det. Greene s. de c. Estado Barinas.
Anthomyiidae	
Anthomyiinae (subfamilia)	det. Hall.
Muscidae	
Stomoxys calcitrans L.	det. James s. de c. Caracas.
Charadrella macrosoma V. W.	det. Greene
Neomuscina pictipennis Big.	det. Greene
Callyphoridae	
Cochliomyia americana	

Cush. y Patt.	det. Hall.
Cochliomyia sp.	det. Hall.
Cochliomyia macellaria F.	det. Greene
Lucilia purpurascens Fab.	det. Greene
Lucilia eximia Wd.	det. James.
Sarcophagidae	
Sarcophaga sp.	det. James
Sarcophaga plinthopyga Wd.	det. James s. de c. Estado Barinas.
Sarcophaga sp.	det. Greene
Sarcophaga sp.	det. Hall
Sarcophaga sp.	det. Hall
Sarcopromusca arcuata Tns.	det. Greene
Harpagopyga n. sp. cercana a divergens Curr.	det. Hall s. de c. de un caso de nasomiasis del Hosp. Vargas.
Hyppoboscidae	
Pseudolynchia canariensis Macq.	det. Bequaert s. de c. encontrada en aves del Estado Guárico.
Coleoptera (orden)	
Anobiidae	
Calymaderus sp.	det. Fisher
Scarabacidae	
Phaneus sp.	det. Chapin s. de c. Estado Barinas.
Scolytidae	
Xyloborus sp.	det. Blackman s. de c. atacando cocoteros en Cumaná (Edo. Sucre).
Hymenoptera (orden)	
Ichneumonidae	
Ephialtes semisanguineus Cress.	det. Cushman s. de c. Estado Barinas
Vespidae	
Chartergus sp.	det. Townes s. de c. Estado Barinas

Gymnopolybia pallidipes Oliv.	det. Townes s. de c. Estado Barinas

Sphecidae

Stictia pantherina Handl.	det. Townes s. de c. Estado Barinas

Formicidae

Atta sp.	det. Smith
Brachymyrmex sp.	det. Bequaert
Cephalotes sp.	det. Smith
Crematogaster brevispinosa Mayr.	det. Bequaert
Crematogaster (Orthocrema) sp.	det. Smith
Dorymyrmex pyramicus Roger	det. Smith
Monomorium pharaonis L.	det. Bequaert
Pachycondyla crassinoda Latr.	det. Smith
Pheidole sp.	det. Bequaert
Pheidole sp.	det. Smith
Paratrechina longicornis Latr.	det. Bequaert
Solenopsis sp.	det. Bequaert
Tetramorium guineense F.	det. Smith
Tapinoma melano cephalum F.	det. Bequaert s. de c. a excepción de Atta sp. Cephalopes sp. i Pachycondyla erassinoda L., que fueron capturadas en el Edo. Barinas, las restantes son colectadas en Caracas.

Apidae

Trigona sp.	det. Crawford s. de c. Estado Barinas

ARACHNIDA (clase)
(octópoda)

Chelonethidae (orden)

Cheliferidae

Chelifer sp.	det. Bequaert s. de c. nidos de pájaros en los Estados Aragua y Guárico.

Acarina (orden)

Argasidae

Ornithodorus sp. cercana a talaje Guer-Men.	det. Ewing

	s. de c. San Cristóbal (Edo Táchira)
Argas persicus Oken	det. Ewing
	s. de c. Ciudad Bolívar (Edo. Bolívar).
Ixodidae	
Amblyomma sp.	det. Ewing
	s. de c. sobre una serpiente en Ciudad Bolívar (Edo. Bolívar).
Amblyomma curruca Schulze	det. Bequaert
	s. de c. sobre un venado
Boophilus annulatus Say	det. Ewing
	s. de c. sobre un venado en Ciudad Bolívar (Edo. Bolívar).

MOLUSCOS

Ampullariidae	
Ampullaria (Ceratodes) cornuarietis L.	det. Ravenel
	s. de c. Distrito Federal
Pomacea glauca L.	det. Bequaert
	s. de c. Estados Miranda, Sucre, Nueva Esparta y Distrito Federal.
Pomaca (Effusa) dubia Guilding	det. Bequaert
	s. de c. Guarenas (Edo. Miranda).
Lymnaecidae	
Lymnacea cubensis Pf.	det. Bequaert
	s. de c. El Valle (Dto. Federal).
Melaniidae	
Pachycheilus laevissimus Sow.	det. Bequart
	s. de c. Estado Cojedes.
Planorbidae	
Australorbis olivaceus S.	det. Bequaert
	s. de c. El Paraíso (Caracas).
Physidae	
Aplexa marmorata G.	det. Bequaert
	s. de c. Distrito Federal.
Subulina octona Brug	det. Bequaert
	s. de c. Caracas.
Poteria popayana Lea	det. Bequaert.

AVES

Furnaridae
Phallecodomus rufifrons
inornatus Ridgway — det. Greenway
s. de c. San Mateo (Edo. Aragua).

Icteridae
Icterus nigrogularis heliolides C. — det. Escuela de Harvard (Boston)
s. de c. San Mateo (Edo. Aragua).

Troglodytidae
Troglodytes musculus clarus
Berlepsch y Hartert — det. Greenway
s. de c. San Mateo (Edo. Aragua).

MAMIFEROS

Quiropteros
Desmodontidae
Desmodus rotundus Geo. — det. Allen
s. de c. San Mateo (Edo. Aragua).

Filostomidae
Glossophaga soricina Pallas — det. Allen
s. de c. San Mateo (Edo Aragua).

COMMENTARIES

We present a list of 140 specimens. In 82 of them we give genus and specie, in 55, the genus, in 1, the subfamily and in 2, the family.

Between the arthropoda, the class Insecta with nine orders: Corrodentia, Anoplura, Homoptera, Hemiptera, Trichoptera, Lepidoptera, Diptera, Coleoptera e Himenoptera. In the order Corrodentia: one family, one genus and one species, indeterminated; in Anoplura: one genus and one species; in Hemiptera; one genus and one indeterminated species; in Hemóptera; one genus and one indeterminated species; in Hemiptera; one family, six genus and seven species; in Trichóptera; two families, with indeterminated genus and species; in Lepidóptera; two families, two genus, one specie and another one indeterminated; in Díptera: eighteen families, thirty seven genus and forty one species; besides, thirty two species and one genus, indeterminated.

In the class Arachnida, two orders: chelonethida and acarina. In the Chelonethida; one family, one genus, one indeterminated species, and in the order Acarina; two families, four genus and four species.

Hematopinus suis L. has been caught by us on pigs from Cumaná (State Sucre). It can live on man.

The reduviidae have very much importance in America, because they are the transmissors of the Chagas disease, one of the principal rural endemic sickness between us. P. geniculatus has been found in El Valle (Dto. Federal), surroundings of Caracas (Catia, El Calvario, Los Chorros) and Guarenas (State Miranda); E. maculata in several States: Bolívar, Barinas, Anzoátegui, Falcón, Guárico and Zulia; P. arthuri in Aragua, Guárico and Cojedes; S. rubropictus in Maracaibo (State Zulia); B. notata in Caracas.

Corizus sidae has been found in Caracas and we have demonstrated it to be the transmissor of the flagellosis of the plants (Euphorbiaceaes) in Venezuela.

Leptoglossus gonagra collected in roofs of huts of the surroundings of Villa de Cura (State Aragua) living together R. prolixus. It is a phytophagous insect. They are accused of attacking the tomato and the sunflower.

Dysdercus maurus and Dysdercus fernaldi are of the genus that are aggressors of the cotton. Orthaea bilobata found in Caracas and Maracaibo have been accused as the transmissors of flagellates of plants in Martinica. Between us, it is common to find Dysdercus fernaldi (Ballou), living in malváceas.

Nezara stictica found in Caracas has been utilized by us, in research about the spread of protozoa in plants. The species viridicula L. existing also in the country, attack the soybean, beans, spurge, benne and cotton.

Dicyphus notatus belong to the family of the mosquito of the tabacco, Cyrtopeltis notatus Dist. They suck the sap of the leaves, producing lesions, perhaps, for causing action of the spittle.

The larves of hydropsychideos are good for the feeding of the fishes.

Laphygma frugiperda is one of the whip of the Venezuelan agriculture, their larves are destroyers, every year, of plantations. It has been caught by us in Caracas, in larval stage living on P. maximum. When it attacks the corn it is called "cogollero"; other people say "mariposita de San Juan". The adult is gray, nocturnal and attracted to the light.

Simuliidae have a principal importance in relation with men and animals, transmitting the O. volvulus and caecutiens and the L. anatis and smithi, and possibly, one of our rural endemic diseases: the *carate.*

The larves of chironomidae are aquatic, and Pinto has found a species as parasite of nymphs of simuliidae.

Ceratoponidae, including the three genus that we present, inclose the group pricker called by our people "jején". They are accused as being the transmissors of human and animal parasites.

Phlebotomidae are very interesting being the transmissors of the leishmaniasis, one of our rural sickness. We present two species: evansi, collected in Macuto and San Mateo (State Aragua), and migonei, caught in our laboratory of the Clínica Luis Razetti. This group is called by our people "angoletas", "palomillas" or "balandras".

Culicidae in our list is represented by the old transmissor of the yellow fever, the common aegypti, and some anopheles. It is very known the importance of this family.

The genus Mycodiplosis attacks some plants producing gallnuts.

Tabanidae are interesting as prickers. We present a new species for Venezuela, according to the Pechunom' list. They have importance refering as transmissors of tularemia, the filaria Loa-loa and trypanomomas between echinus and bovines. All the specimens have been caught in trips to the interior of the country.

Phoridae lives in larval stages as commensals of ants and bees. One species parasite eggs of frogs.

The larves of Syrphidae are useful to the agriculture and horticulture destroying the green flies.

Chloropidae lastly have much importance since the medical studies of Kumm in Jamaica, referring to the transmission of yaws. In our monograph about this disease we reported findings of these insects in Macuto and Guarenas (State Miranda).

Anthomyiidae attacks the wheat, the corn, onion, spinach, the roots of the cruciferae (cabbage, radish, turnip, watercress, etc.).

Stomoxys are voraceous prickers, suspicious of transmitting human and animal diseases. They have been caught in the garden of my home, in the Park Los Caobos.

The genus Cochliomyia and Lucilia attacks the men, developmenting their larves, producing myasis cutaneous or of cavities; either the same in animals. Our specimens have been obtained of larves taken of nasal myasis, in rural workers going to consultation in the Hospital Vargas.

Sarcophagidae producing also several myasis in men and animals, harming the leathers of the last. We have found a new species for the world in the genus Harpapopyga whose larves were taken of a case of nasal myasis. It seems to be that these dipterous had not been accused before as producing myasis.

Hyppoboscidae are the transmissors of Haemoproteus columbae. Our specimens are from birds caught in trips to the interior of the country.

Between the Coleoptera we have found in Cumaná one species of the genus Xyloborus attacking the coconut plantations. The Department of Agriculture in Washington was very interested for this finding. The genus Calymaderus is destroyer of woods, books, etc.

The ants, some of them have medical importance, because as we have demonstrated should be very useful in the biological fight against the reduviidae, transmissors of Chagas' disease.

In Arachnida, in the family Cheliferidae, we have found a chelifer that according to the opinion of Anduze, possibly should be the species cancroides, living in the nests of Phallecodomus rufifrons inornatus Ridgway, as hyperparasite of P. arthuri.

In Acarina, family Argasidae, we have tound O. talaje, transmissor of the spirochetosis of the hens, that accompanied by Briceño Rossi we have found, for the first time, in the country.

In Ixodidae caught Amblyomma curruca Schulze, appointed for the second time in the world, and B. annulatus, transmissor of the pyroplasmosis of the bovines, whose larves live, many times , on man.

* * *

In the list of Molluscan, in relation with medical aspects, the two more important are L. cubensis that possibly should be the intermediary host of F. hepatica between us, and A. olivaceus, intermediary host of B. mansoni in Caracas valley.

In chiropterous, the Desmodus is sucker. Today the bats have human and animal importance, because they lodge schyzotrypanum, may be, perhaps, cruzi, and possibly are transmissors of paralytic rabies.

CONCLUSIONS

We show here a list of 140 specimens between arthropoda, molluscan, birds and mammals, collected during some time and in different places of the country and different epochs of the year. Most of them have a medical and veterinary importance, either as prickers, transmissors, intermediary hosts, reservation of virus, useful for the biological fight, etc. Some of them have a narrow relation with agriculture, either, as destroyers of plagues, as aggressors of plants or as transmissors of diseases.

In Simuliidae we give three new species for Venezuela: S. haematopotum Mall., S. bicoloratum Mall., and S. sanguineum Knab. In Ceratopogonidae, a new species for Venezuela, Culicoides stellifer Coq. In Tabanidae, other new species for us, Tabanus subruber Bell. In the genus Harpagopyga of the Sarcophagidae a new mundial species, like Harpagopyga divergens Curr.

We regret the lack of libraries between us, but we have almost the security that some of these specimens, probably, for the first time are appointed in Venezuela.

Our acknowledgement to Charles H. Ballou and Pablo J. Anduze for their entomological advices in the fancy work of these notes.

ABOUT A NEW SPECIES OF FLEBOTOMUS IN THE COUNTRY: PHLEBOTOMUS (BRUMPTOMYIA) SUIS. ROZEBOOM 1940. *

(Dedication to Dr. Luis Vargas, distinguished Mexican entomologist)

The family Psychodidae is very important in the medical entomology, because one of their genus: Flebotomus, has been accused of transmitting the fever of three days, the peruvian wart and mainly, the American leishmaniasis, a very common rural endemic between us.

Having worked in this field lastly we have had the opportunity of handling this group of insects, either that the researchers of the Sergent brothers, Adler and Theodor about the oriental buttom and those of Beaurepaire Aragao, in Brazil, with the Ph. intermedius for the American leishmaniasis, demonstrating the importance in the spreading of this endemic.

Just, here Pifano, making researches in the State Yaracuy, found the species longipalpis (Lutz and Neiva 1912) with natural infection for leptomonads.

The story of these dipteres in Venezuela, has relation with contributions of Tejera and Núñez Tovar, Brumpt, Nitzulescu and Costa Lima, Root and Hill, Lutz and Dyar, Anduze and Pifano, Briceño Iragorry, de la Plaza and Ortiz.

Still now our catchs in this field are reduced to District Federal and State Aragua, appointing four species: evansi, migonei, panamansis and a fourth *suis,* that is the main object of this communication.

The popular names of this kind of insects in Venezuela are the following: "angoleta", "palomilla", and "balandra"; however, we have seen the most used is "palomilla", but this nomination, and the other "angoleta", are applied to tabanidae of genus Chrysops. The name of "balandra" is unknown for us. According to Núñez Tovar the word "angoleta" is indian, but till today we had thought the nominations of "angoleta" and "balandra" was in relation with the wings of the animals, like the erectile sails of a vessel.

The species *evansi* seems to be very frequent in the center of the country, collecting it in Aragua and in Macuto (Dto. Federal); in this last site in July, raining, near an electric light and stinging in arms and legs we have captured around 50 specimens in a short time. This species was appointed for the first time by Núñez Tovar in 1923 and dedicated to Miss Evans of the Tropical Medicine School of Liverpool.

The species *migonei* Franca 1920 was caught by us in the interior of our Laboratory in Caracas, pricking one of hands at six in the afternoon.

* Reprinted from "Boletín del Laboratorio de la Clínica Luis Razetti" - Año V - N° 15 - Vol. IV - 1944.

The species *panamensis* Shannon 1926, has been caught in the farmer Aguacatal and surroundings (State Aragua). In accord with a letter from Rozeboom, he thinks that with the material that he has, and the different places of capture, his opinion is that *panamensis* may be the main species transmitting, first, the leishmaniasis.

The species *suis* has been caught also in farmer Aguacatal and surroundings (State Aragua) and classified by Rozeboom. This species has been found also by Anduze in State Barinas. We think that his catch was former to us. This material was classified by the same entomologist.

It seems to be that *suis,* found the first time in Panamá, in accord with the opinion of Rozeboom, may be synonymy of *gomezi* Nitzulescu 1931, appointed for State Táchira and collected by Tejera.

With this new species increase to thirteen the number of species found till today in the country, as follow:

1- Ph. atroclavatus Knab 1913
sin Ph. tejerae Larrouse 1921
2- Ph. maracayensis Núñez Tovar 1923
3- Ph. evansi Núñez Tovar 1924
4- Ph. longipalpis Lutz y Neiva 1912
sin. Ph. otamae Núñez Tovar y Tejera 1924
5- Ph. migonei Franca 1920
sin Ph. rangeli Núñez Tovar y Tejera 1924
6- Ph. panamensis Shannon 1926
7- Ph. gomezi Nitzulescu 1931
8- Ph. squamiventris (?) Lutz y Neiva 1912
sin. (?) Ph. evansi Núñez Tovar 1924
9- Ph. almazani Galliard 1934
10- Ph. intermedius Lutz y Neiva 1912
11- Ph. cruciatus Coquillet 1907
12- Ph. anduzei Rozeboom 1940

Here the original description of the species *suis:*

Flebotomus suis, a new *Flebotomus* from Panama (Diptera, Psychodidae). Amer. J. Hygiene 32 (1) 8-11. July, 1940.

Flebotomus (Brumptomyia) suis, n. sp.

Male. Color yellowish brown; eyes black; mesonotum infuscated. Palpal formula 1, 4, 3, 2, 5. Measurements, percentage lenght of palpal segments, and wing ratios are given in table 1.

Hypopygium (figure 1). Basal segment of upper clasper slightly more than three times as long as wide; with an inner basal tuft of about fifteen long setae arising from a group of prominent tubercles. Terminal segment of upper clasper three-fifths as long as the basal segment; with four strong, curving spines, one apical, one subapical, and two median. Lower clasper slender, as long as the basal joint of the upper clasper. Middle clasper somewhat shorter than lower clasper, with long, fine setae apically. Sub-median lamella broad, about as long as the middle clasper; with long fine setae apically and along the lower, outer border. Genital filaments long, extending beyond tip of lower clasper.

Female. Measurements, percentage lenghts of palpal segments, and wing ratios (figure 2) are given in table 1. Palpal formula 1, 4, 2, 3, 5 (figure 3).

Buccal armature (figure 4) with four strong horizontal teeth, and a row of small ventral teeth. No pigmented area.

Spermatheca (figure 5) carrot-shaped, with large head and about eight rings.

Flebotomus suis is very closely related to *Flebotomus diabolicus* Hall, but there are certain differences in the male hypopygium that separate the two species. Hall's (1936) figure of *F. diabolicus* terminalia shows three strong spines apically on the basal joint of the upper claspers; these are absent in F. suis. The four spines on the apical joint of the upper clasper of *F. diabolicus* are rather evenly spaced, while in *F. suis* they have the appearance of being paired. *F. suis* is larger than *F. diabolicus.*

F. suis is the third member of the subgenus *Brumptomyia* that has been collected in North and Central America; the other two are *F. vexator* Coquillett, and *F. diabolicus* Hall. It is easily separated from *F. vexator* by the spines of the apical joint of the upper clasper; *F. vexator* has five of these spines.

F. suis may be *F. gomezi* Nitzulescu (1931), which was collected in Venezuela. *F. gomezi* has a similar palpal formula, and there are small differences in the wing ratios. The buccal armature of the two forms is also very similar, but there are some differences in the structure of the spermathecae, which may be of specific value, but which may also be the result of distortion. Nitzulescu states that the spermathecae in *F. gomezi* "est crénelé et comme plissé en accordien, car les crénelures sont étroitement serrées et profundes. A l'extrémité distale il y a une large collerette, qui rend plus just encore l'image de la clochette que nous avons évoquée. Le bord de la collerette est herissée de petits poils renflés en tetes d'épingles a l'extrémité. Du fond de la collerette sort le cou tres court portant une tete a peine arrondie, surmontée de longs poils terminés égalment par des renflements en tetes d'épingles".

The structure of the spermatheca of the writer's allotype female can be seen clearly with a 3 millimeter oil immersion lens and a 10X ocular. The edges of rings appear rounded rather than pointed, so that the edge of the organ is not "notched"; furthermore, the head is not "covered with small hairs swollen into pin heads at the tip".

If subsequient work proves that the forms belong to the same species, *F. suis* will become a synonym of *F. gomezi*; in that case this paper, at any rate, presents a description of the male of *F. gomezi.*

The writer is reluctant to call this paper a description of the male of *F. gomezi,* as he is not certain that his specimens are *F. gomezi.* Certain groups of closely related insect species can be separated only by male characters, while the females are identical, and until the male of the Venezuelan *F. gomezi* is found, it seems best to give the Panamanian form

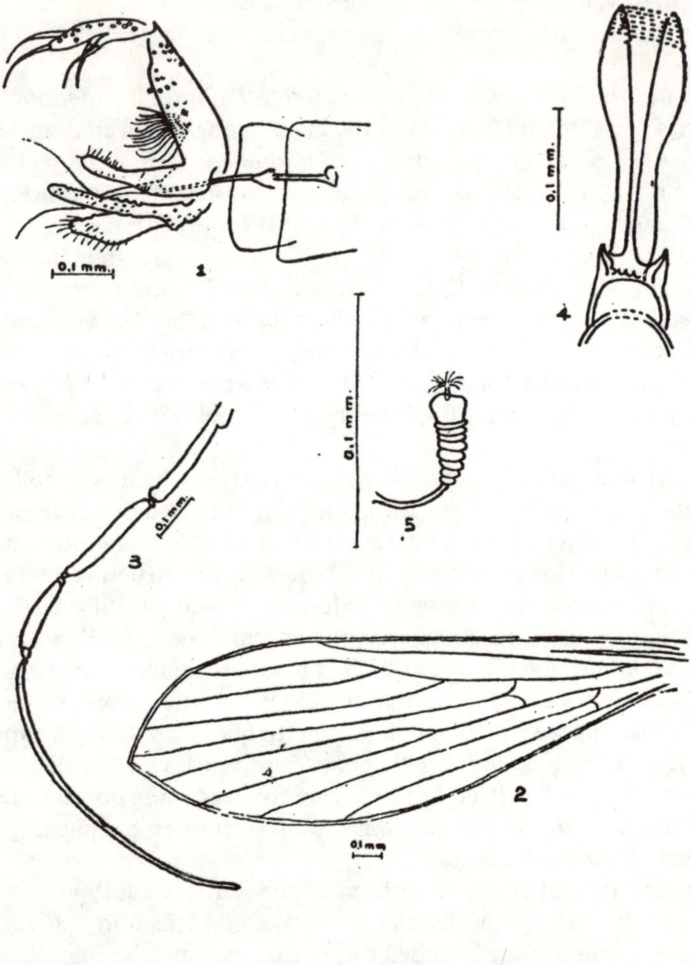

F. SUIS-EXPLANATION OF PLATE

Figure 1.- Hypopygium of type male.
Figure 2.- Wing of allotype female.
Figure 3.- Palp of paratype female.
Figure 4.- Buccopharynx of allotype female.
Figure 5.- Spermatheca of allotype female.
All drawings were made with a calibrated camera lucida.

a specific name.

The type slides have been deposited in the U.S. National Museum.

REFERENCES

Hall, D.G.-1936.-*Phlebotomus (Brumptomyia) diabolicus* a new species of biting gnat from Texas (Diptera: Psychodidae). Proc. Ent. Soc. Wash. 38: 27-29.

Nitzulescu, V.-1931.-Sur un Phlebotomus nouveau du Venezuela *Ph. gomezi* n. sp.-Ann. Parasit. Hum. Comp. 9: 247-255.

BIBIOGRAPHY (CONSULTED)

1924-*Núñez Tovar, Manuel.*-Mosquitos y flebotomos de Venezuela (trabajo al 4° Congreso Venezolano de Medicina).

1926-*Adler S. y Theodor O.*-Further observations on the transmission of cutaneous leishmaniasis to man from Ph. papatasii Ann. ot Trop. Med. and Paras. Vol. XX. No. 2.

1932-*Da Costa Lima, A.*-Sobre of phlebotomos americanos (Diptera: Psychodidae) Mem. do Inst. Osw. Cruz. Tomo XXVI. Fasc. I.

1934-*Brinceño Iragorry, L. y de La Plaza, G.*-Una nueva especie de flebotomo en Venezuela. Medical N° 8.

1942-*Rozeboom, L.E.*-Ph. Anduzei, a new phlebotomus from Venezuela. Bol. de Entomología Venezolana. Vol. I. N° 4.

1940-*Pifano, Félix.*-Sobre el desarrollo de leishmania trópica brasiliensis en flebotomos de Venezuela. Gaceta Médica de Caracas. N° 10.

1920-*Franca, C. y Parrot, L.*-Introduction a l'etude systematique des Dipteres du genre Phlebotomus. Bull. Soc. Path. Exot.

1927-*Beaurepaire Aragao, Henrique de.*-Leishmaniose tegumentar e sua transmissao pelo phlebotomos. Mem. do Inst. Osw. Cruz. Tomo XX. Fasc. II.

1938-*Soutwell, T. y Kirshner, A.*-On the Transmission of leishmaniasis. Ann. of Trop. Med. and Paras. Vol. 32. N° 1.

1939-*Adler, S. y Theodor, O.*-The behaviour of Leishmania chagasi in Phlebotomus papatasii. Ann. of. Trop. Med. and Paras. Vol. 33. No. 1.

1942-*Ortiz C., Ignacio.*-Revisión histórica de nuestros Phlebotomus con citación de una especie (Phlebotomus cruciatus Coq.) nueva para Venezuela. Bol. de la clín. Razetti. Vol. II. N° 9.

1940-*Ayrosa Galvao, A.L. y Coutinho, J.O.*-Contribuicao ao estudo dos flebótomos do Est. de S. Paulo. Arquivos de Hig. e Sau. Pública. Año V. N° 9.

1940-*Coutinho, J.O.*-Observacoes sobre algumas espécies de flebótomos com a descricao do macho de Phlebotomus Lloydi-Antunes. 1937. Arq. de Hig. e Sau. Pública. Año V. N° 9.

1940-*Pessao, S.B. y Pestana Bruno Rangel.*-Infeccao natural do Phlebotomus migonei por formas de leptomonas provavelmente da Leishmania brasiliensis. Arq. de Hig. e Sau. Pública. Año V. N° 9.

1940-*Carbonell, Diego.*-La Parasitología en Venezuela y la obra del Dr. Manuel Núñez Tovar. Obra. Caracas.

1940-*Rozeboom, L.E.*-Flebotomus suis, a new Flebotomus from Panama (Diptera-Psyschodidae). Am. Jour. Hygiene 32. 8-11. July.

NEW SPECIES OF SIMULIIDAE FOR VENEZUELA (Simulium samboni)

(This finding increase to 24 the number of species found till today) *

We have appointed this new species among us in material of nymphs and adults with the wise collaboration of Vargas, from Mexico, who has made the classificaiton.

The site of capture is named El Samán at the side of the road from Petare to Guarenas (State Miranda) at the borders of the river Guarenas. In this place, we have caught seven species, including this one.

The species that Dampf (1943) described as Simulium samboni inRev. Soc. Mex. Hist. Nat. and Hoffmann (1931) called formerly E. *ochraceum,* belongs to the species that Vargas named today in his monograph "Simulidos de México", Simulium (Lanea) *downsi* n. sp.

According to Vargas the true *samboni* and the *downsi* must be admitted to join to a subgenus, separated of that one including *ochraceum,* belonging to the genus *Cnephia* and must be called *Cnephia ochraceum.*

Here the original description of Jennings kindly sent it for Vargas:

"TWO NEW SPECIES OF SIMULIUM FROM TROPICAL AMERICA" **

A.H. Jennings.

SIMULIUM SAMBONI new species

Female. Occiput, frons and face black, brownish yellow, very gray pollinose. Antennae rather stout, brownish yellow, darker distally, the first two joints honey yellow and smooth, the others clothed with short whitish, pile. Palpi blackish. Mesonotum bright orange—ferruginous with four narrow, pollinose, grayish—silvery stripes, the outer ones at the lateral margins, the inner pair sinuate, extending nearly to the scutellum and dividing the disk into three nearly equal parts; vestiture of fine, evenly distributed golden hair—scales not forming regular series. Scutellum paler than mesonotum, honey yellow; transverse hair—scales on the disk golden, the marginal bristles—black. Postnotum ferruginous. Pleurae ocher—yellow, strongly infuscated on the mesosternum. Abdomen subcylindrical, black and gray; segments 2 to 5 black and with the margins and two longitudinal stripes gray, thus delimiting three series of large black spots; sixth segment shining, mostly gray. Anterior coxae yellow, the others infuscated. Legs bright ocher—yellow, the hind pair with the apices of the femora infuscated and the distal halves of the tibiae blackish,

* Reprinted from "Boletín del Laboratorio de la Clínica Luis Razetti" - Año VIII - Vol. XV -N° 23-24 - 1947

** 1915.-Proceedings of the Entomological Society of Washington, Vol. XVII; pág. 199-200.

their basal halves with whitish luster; front tarsi with the first joint pale, its distal fourth blackish, the second joint pale on basal half, the last three points wholly blackish: hind tarsi with the first joint pale, infuscated along its lower margin and on apical third, the second joint pale on basal half, the last three joints wholly blackish; appreseed hairscales partly pale and partly black, in correspondence with the ground-color. Claws simple, thickened at base. Wings hyaline, the venation normal; thick veins pale yellow; anal field without iridescent spot. Halteres pale yellow. Lenght: Body about 1.5 mm., wing 2mm.

Male. Holoptic. Antennae much more slender than in the female, Mesonotum strongly convex, the silvery pollinose ornamentation reduced to two short wedge-shaped spots at anterior margin and visible only in certain lights.

Empire, Canal Zone, Panama, reared from pupae taken from a small tributary of the Comacho River, October 4, 1913.

It gives me pleasure to dedicate this handsome species to Dr. Louis W. Sambon.

This fact is very interesting, because the first catch made (1929) for us in the border of the river Apón, District Perijá of State Zulia, the material was classified in Washington, giving the genus, but not the species. Now, with the help of Vargas, it is possible to see the large spreading of the S. metallicum, and we believed it was the first time found in the State Zulia.

CULICOIDES IRIARTEI
(NEW SPECIES) *

SIMULIUM IRIARTEI
(n. sp.) **

News arrived lastly gave account of a new Venezuelan specie of the genus Culicoides, it has been named, in honor of Dr. Iriarte, Culicoides iriartei.

Doing memory, in the century XVIII, another Iriarte, the Spanish diplomatic, born in Canarias Islands, was created in honor of him a genus of plants Iriartea, and is now, than in honor of another one, neither Spanish, but Venezuelan, in another branch of the Natural Sciences, has been given to two arthropoda, the names of Simulium iriartei and Culicoides iriartei.

The classification of these two new species of Simuliidae and Ceratopogonidae has been done for two remarkable and specialized entomologists.

CULICOIDES IRIARTEI NEW SPECIES
Fig. 6

Female.-About 1.3 mm. long. Eyes narrowly separated. Labrum very short, 0.123 mm. in length, ratio of labrum to clypeus plus frons 44:70. Antenna with segments 3-9 not beadlike but of about the same size and shape thereafter an abrupt change in size and the segments longer. Palpus slightly longer than the labrum, 0.134 mm. in length, third segment much longer than the first and second, expanded with a large deep sensory pit, fourth segment wider and shorter than the fifth (fig. 6, A). Mesonotal pattern unknown. Legs brown, first and second femora with distinct distal light rings, first and second tibiae with basal ones, and third tibiae with bith basal and distal ones; hind tibial comb with four robust bristles of which the first is the longest (fig. 6, B). Wing 0.98 by 0.41 mm. with abundant macrotrichia; second radial cell in a dark spot. Following the wide dark spot over the costal cell there are four-glass spots anterior to vein M_1, three of which are transverse and one is horizontal; the light spot adjoining the second radial cell is more or less hour-glass shaped, the one in the distal part of cell R_5 is "open" and expanded anteriorly, the horizontal

* Reprinted from "Annual of the Entomological Society of America" - Vol. 45. N° 3. 1952 (Six new neitropical species of Culicoides - Diptera - Ceratopogonidae by Irving FOX)

** Reprinted from "Revista del Instituto de Salubridad y Enfermedades Tropicales". - Vol. VII. 1943. N° 3 y Vol. XVII. 1957. N° 4. México D.F. (Luis Vargas, Martínez y A. Díaz Nájera) one begins near the white spot over the cross-vein and reaches to the edge of the wing; vein M_2 is straddled by a dark spot which separates two broad light spots; cells M_1 and M_2 each with a distal light spot, veins Cu_1 and Cu_2 bordered with lights areas and the light spot in cell Cu_1 is "open"; anal cell with two light spots of which the basal is double (fig. 6, C). Spermathacae double; large, oval, the ducts chitinized for a long distance (fig. 6, D).

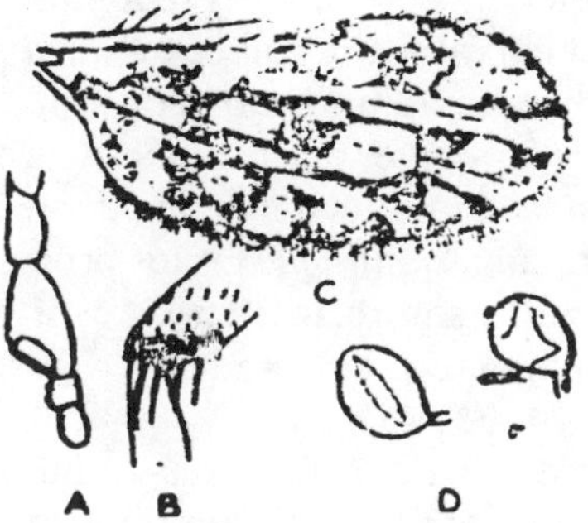

Fig. 6
Culicoides iriartei new species, female; A, palpus; B, hind tibial comb; C, wing; D, spermathecae.

Remarks.-In the pattern of the wing this species seems to be similar to *C. propinquus* Macfie from which it differs in that the light spot bordering vein M_1 originates more basally and also in the character of the light spots in cell Cu_1 and the anal cell. The species is named in honor of Dr. David R. Iriarte of Caracas, Venezuela.

Type Material.-Female holotype from La Salina (Edo. Zulia), Venezuela, collected by Ignacio Ortiz C. in March, 1949.

S. (Simulium) iriartei n. sp.

S. (Prosimulium) hirtipes Vargas, 1943 (nec Fries, 1824) Rev. Soc. Mex. Hist. Nat., 4: 143, 146: lám. VI, fig. I (pupa)

MACHO.-Holóptico, color negro. Cabeza.-Clípeo pequeño, negro, con luz de frente se ve blanco brillante, los pelos son negros; palpos negros; antenas negras, con once segmentos, con fina pubescencia amarillo pálido.

Tórax.-Longitud 1.2 mm. Escudo negro con pilosidad verdosa, todos sus bordes están ocupados por una banda polinosa de color verde metálico, dicha banda es más ancha en el borde anterior, en la zona posterior hay grupos de pelos erectos morenos que se confunden con los del escudete; éste es triangular de color más claro que el escudo, con pelos erectos morenos y pilosidad tendida plateada. Postnoto prominente, intensamente negro. Pleuras blanco-polinosas con mechón de pelos morenos. Balancines con el ápice blanco, el tallo y la base morenos. Alas sin célula discal, *Se* desnuda en toda su longitud, R_1 desnuda en su mitad basal, R_{2+3} simple, Cu_2 arqueada; longitud 2.8 mm., ancho 1.3 mm. Patas obscuras, excepto la primera coxa que es amarillo o morena y la cara anterior de la tibia del mismo par tiene abundante pilosidad blanca, el basitarso posterior tiene moderada forma de huso, con la mitad basal más clara, se observan escasas escamas en el fémur y la tibia; longitudes, par I: 3 mm., par II: 2.8 mm., par III: 3.2 mm.

Abdomen.-1 a cara dorsal es negra y la ventral amarillenta de la tercera a la séptima esternita hay manchas centrales morenas con acumulación de pelos, en la tercera y la cuarta tergita, lateralmente a la línea media, hay mechones de pelos negros erectos. Genitalia: pieza basal redondeada, tan ancha como larga; pinceta delgada, encorvada con fuerte espina distal, el proceso basal interno tiene su ápice cerrado; adminículo pequeño, aplanado lateralmente, en forma de V invertida, con el borde anterior proyectado, agudo, arqueado ventralmente, en la cara dorsal hay una depresión en forma de canal y en la ventral se forma una quilla pilosa; los procesos basales están muy separados, vistos de perfil son rectos, angostos. Los brazos del adminículo son de bases débilmente pigmentadas y rugosas con cinco dientes largos en la punta (figs. 74, 75, 76 y 77).

HEMBRA.-Dicóptica, del color del macho. Cabeza.-Frente ancha, negra. brillante; clípeo cuadrangular moreno obscuro, con finos pelos morenos; palpos negros; antenas infuscadas con fina pubescencia gris, de once segmentos, los dos basales son morenos.

Tórax.-Longitud 1.3 mm. Escudo negro con pilosidad verdosa y con tres líneas blanquecinas muy delgadas, las dos laterales tienen dilataciones anteriores triangulares, en el extremo posterior se tocan, aunque ya muy difusas, con la banda del mismo color que baja de los bordes laterales. Escudete triangular, amarillento, con cerdas erectas en su borde distal y pilosidad tendida amarilla brillante, en el centro. Postnoto negro con polinosidad gris. Balancines, pleuras y alas como en el macho, dimensiones de las alas, longitud: 3 mm., ancho 1.5 mm. Patas también como las del macho, pero la primera coxa más amarilla y la mitad basal del primer tarso medio, blanca; uñas normalmente encorvadas con un diente triangular en el último tercio, el espolón basal es moderado; calcipala y pedísulco presentes; longitudes, par I: 3 mm., par II: 2.7 mm., par III: 3.1 m.

Abdomen.-Obscuro, la segunda tergita tiene dos manchas morenas laterales en relación a la línea media, la tercera a la séptima tergita sólo tienen una mancha central que no resalta mucho de la coloración general, los últimos segmentos son brillantes. Genitalia: oviscaptos apenas marcados; lóbulos anales anchos con los bordes redondeados, terminados en punta moderada, en dirección apical; el mango de la horquilla es aplanado lateralmente, tiene una ligera dilatación en el extremo; los brazos de la horquilla son planos con el extremo terminal torcido, tienen una saliente triangular externa, los bordes internos forman ángulo agudo con incisión en el vértice (fig. 78).

La especie se dedica al *Sr. Dr. David R. Iriarte* de Caracas, Venezuela.

S. (Simulium) iriartei n. sp.
Larves

Longitud: 6.5 a 7 mm. Color amarillo grisáceo, el quinto segmento minal de algunas larvas presenta un aspecto rojizo. Lámina frontal con un dibujo en forma de tridente: antenas ligeramente más que el tallo del abanico, el segundo segmento se ve estriado: abanico cefálico con 37-45 ramas; submentón con nueve dientes en el margen anterior, la lámina ventral lleva seis a nueve pelos, generalmente siete, en cada lado. Octavo segmento abdominal sin tubérculos; no tiene escamas rectales; branquias anales como con diez lobulaciones en un tronco grueso; ventosa anal con 73-75 filas de ganchos. Difiere de *tricornis* porque la escotadura epicraneana tiene forma de triángulo equilátero (fig. 148), y de *parrai* porque carece de áreas claras en las láminas epicraneanas.

Localidad: Contreras, D.R., colectó A. Diaz Nájera, IV. 1944.

Lámina N° 3835, ejemplar montado en líquido de Berlese y veinte larvas de sexta muda conservadas en alcohol, se encuentran en la colección del Instituto de Salubridad y Enfermedades Tropicales.

LISTA DE LOS SIMULIDOS DE MEXICO *

Géneros:
CNEPHIA Enderlein, 1921.
GIGANTODAX Enderlein, 1925.
SIMULIUM Latreille, 1802.

Subgéneros de *Simulium*
BYSSODON Enderlein, 1925.
EUSIMULIUM Roubaud, 1906.
HEARLEA Rubzov, 1940.
HEMICNETHA Enderlein, 1934.
NEOSIMULIUM Rubzov, 1940.
NOTOLEPRIA Enderlein, 1930.
PSILOPELMIA Enderlein, 1933.
SIMULIUM s. str. Latreille, 1802.

Especies:
Cnephia aguirrei Dalmat, 1949.
Cnephia aguirrei Vargas y Díaz Nájera, 1948.
Gigantodax wrighti Vargas, Martínez y Díaz N., 1944.
Simulium (Byssodon) ganalesense Vargas, Martínez y Díaz N., 1946.
Simulium (Byssodon) quadrivittatum Loew, 1862.
Simulium (Eusimulium) aureum Fries, 1824.
Simulium (Eusimulium) pugetense Dyar & Shannon, 1927.
Simulium (Hearlea) ayrozai Vargas, 1945.
Simulium (Hearlea) canadense Hearle, 1935.
Simulium (Hearlea) capricornis De Léon, 1945.
Simulium (Hearlea) carolinae De Léon, 1945.
Simulium (Hearlea) dalmati Vargas y Díaz Nájera, 1948.
Simulium (Hearlea) delatorrei, Dalmat, 1950.
Simulium (Hearlea) deleoni Vargas, 1945.
Simulium (Hearlea) estevezi Vargas, 1945.
Simulium (Hearlea) ethelae Dalmat, 1950.

* Luis Vargas, Díaz Nájera and Martínez Palacios.

Simulium (Hearlea) gorirossii n. sp.
Simulium (Hearlea) johnsoni n. sp.
Simulium (Hearlea) juarezi n. sp.
Simulium (Hearlea) menchacai n. sp.
Simulium (Hemicnetha) briceñoi Vargas, Martínez y Díaz N., 1946.
Simulium (Hemicnetha) earlei Vargas, Martínez y Díaz N., 1946.
Simulium (Hemicnetha) freemani Vargas y Díaz N., 1949.
Simulium (Hemicnetha) guerrerense Vargas y Díaz N., 1956.
Simulium (Hemicnetha) hinmani Vargas, Martínez y Díaz N., 1946.
Simulium (Hemicnetha) mexicanum Bellardi, 1862.
Simulium (Hemicnetha) paynei Vargas, 1942.
Simulium (Hemicnetha) pulverulentum Knab, 1914.
Simulium (Hemicnetha) smarti Vargas, 1946.
Simulium (Hemicnetha) solarii Stone, 1948.
Simulium (Hemicnetha) virgatum Coquillett, 1903.
Simulium (Hemicnetha) yepocapense Dalmat, 1949.
Simulium (Neosimulium) argus Williston, 1893.
Simulium (Neosimulium) encisoi Vargas y Díaz N., 1949.
Simulium (Notolepria) gonzalezi Vargas y Díaz N., 1953.
Simulium (Psilopelmia) callidum Dyar & Shannon, 1927.
Simulium (Psilopelmia) d'andrettai Vargas, Martínez y Díaz N., 1946.
Simulium (Psilopelmia) downsi Vargas, Martínez y Díaz N., 1946.
Simulium (Psilopelmia) dugesi Vargas, Martínez y Díaz N., 1946.
Simulium (Psilopelmia) haematopotum Malloch, 1914.
Simulium (Psilopelmia) mangabeirai Vargas, 1945.
Simulium (Psilopelmia) mediovittatum Knab, 1915.
Simulium (Psilopelmia) ochoai Vargas, Martínez y Díaz N., 1946.
Simulium (Psilopelmia) samboní Jennings, 1915.
Simulium (Psilopelmia) trivittatum Malloch, 1914.
Simulium (Psilopelmia) veracruzanum Vargas, Martínez y Díaz N., 1946.
Simulium (Psilopelmia) zempoalense Vargas, Martínez y Díaz N., 1946.
Simulium (Simulium) anduzei Vargas y Díaz N., 1948.
Simulium (Simulium) bustosi Vargas, Martínez y Díaz N., 1946.
Simulium (Simulium) costa-limai Vargas, Martínez y Díaz N., 1946.
Simulium (Simulium) hechti Vargas, Martínez y Díaz N., 1946.
Simulium (Simulium) iriartei Vargas, Martínez y Díaz N., 1946.
Simulium (Simulium) jacumbae Dyar & Shannon, 1927.
Simulium (Simulium) jobbinsi Vargas, Martínez y Díaz N., 1946.
Simulium (Simulium) lassmanni Vargas, Martínez y Díaz N., 1946.
Simulium (Simulium) marquezi Vargas y Díaz N., 1957.
Simulium (Simulium) metallicum Bellardi, 1859.
Simulium (Simulium) ochraceum Walker, 1861.
Simulium (Simulium) parrai Vargas, Martínez y Díaz N., 1946.
Simulium (Simulium) puigi Vargas, Martínez y Díaz N., 1946.
Simulium (Simulium) raizi Vargas y Díaz N., 1948.

Simulium (Simulium) sayi Dyar & Shannon, 1927.
Simulium (Simulium) tuberosum Lundström, 1911.
Simulium (Simulium) tricornis Dr. Léon, 1945.

Las especies que se citan a continuación no están agrupados subgenéricamente ni se tienen datos amplios que permitan hacerlo; por lo tanto no se incluyen en las claves:

Simulium alticolum Dyar & Shannon, 1927.
Simulium coffeae Vargas, 1945.
Simulium diaz-najerai Vargas, 1943.
Simulium occidentale Townsend, 1891.

Huajuapam, 10-II-49. Col. F. Reyes.
Sta. Catarina, Acatepec, IV-53. Col. I. Reyes.
Agua Ancha, Teot., IV-53. Col. I. Reyes.
Eloxochitlán, Teot., IV-53. Col. I. Reyes.
San Antonio Eloxochitlán, Teot., IV-53. Col. I. Reyes.
Buenavista, Teot., IV-53. Col. I. Reyes.
Clemencia, Teot., s/f. Col. U. Velasco.
Montoya, 23-X-48. Col. F. Reyes.
Vista Hermosa, 20-X-48. Col. F. Reyes.
Rancho Manuel Torres, 5-XII-48. Col. F. Reyes.

Simulium (Psilopelmia) zempoalense
Temextitlán, 1949. Col. C. Martínez,

Simulium (Simulium) anduzei
Cerro de San Felipe del Agua, 23-II-48. Col. I. Córdova.
Tectitlán, 24-I-50. Col. I. Reyes.
Rancho Tarabundí, XI-49. Col. C. Martínez.
La Luz, Ixtlán, 22-XI-52. Col. P. Ramírez.
Totontepec Mixe, VIII-52. Col. C. Martínez.

Simulium (Simulium) bustosi
Tectitlán, 24-I-50. Col. I. Reyes.

Simulium (Simulium) costa-limai
Cerro San Felipe del Agua, 23-II-48. Col. I. Córdova.

Simulium (Simulium) iriartei
San Felipe del Agua, 11-XII-43. Col. A. Martínez.
Guelatao, 12-VIII-48. Col. A. Tort.
Comaltepec, 30-XI-48. Col. I. Córdova.
Rancho Manuel Torres, 5-XIII-48. Col. F. Reyes.
San Pedro Nolasco, 8-XII-48. Col. F. Reyes.
San Pablo, Etla, 21-I-49. Col. F. Reyes e I. Córdova.
Jaltianguis, Ixtlán, 16-V-50. Col. Dr. L. Vargas y A. Martínez.
Río de Ixtlán, 16-IV-50. Col. Dr. L. Vargas y A. Martínez.

Simulium (Simulium) jacumbae
San Sebastián, Etla, 12-XI-49. Col. I. Córdova y F. Reyes.

Simulium (Simulium) jobbinsi
Lalopa, 20-III-50. Col. C. Martínez.
Yagila, IV-50. Col. J. Hernández.
Fuente de Chapulapa, Cuic., 10-II-52. Col. C. Martínez.

Tarabundí, Ixtlán, VII-52. Col. M.L. Espinosa.

San Pedro Yaneria, Ixtlán, 4-X-52. Col. H. Pineda.

Rancho San Isidro, Istlán, V-52. Col. C. Martínez.

Totontepec, Mixe, VIII-52. Col. C. Martínez.

La Soledad, Ayutla, Teot., II-53. Col. Personal Oncocercosis.

Chiquihuitlán, Cuicatlán, II-53. Col. I. Reyes.

El Faro, Teotitlán, III-53. Col. I. Reyes.

Finca La Carlota, Ayutla. Teotitlán, III-53. Col. I. Reyes.

Simulium (Simulium) metallicum
Guelatao, Ixtlán, IX-42. Col. M. Macías.

Yagavila, IX-42. Col. M. Macías.

Simulium (Psilopelmia) haematopotum
Colima, Chiapas, Guerrero, Jalisco, Michoacán, Morelos, Nayarit, Oaxaca, Puebla, Sinaloa y Veracruz.

Simulium (Psilopelmia) mangabeirai
Distrito Federal, México, Michoacán Veracruz.

Simulium (Psilopelmia) mediovittatum
Chihuahan, San Luis Potosí, Tamaulipas y Veracruz.

Simulium (Psilopelmia) ochoai
Veracruz.

Simulium (Psilopelmia) samboni
Chiapas, Oaxaca, Tabasco y Veracruz.

Simulium (Psilopelmia) trivittatum
Coahuila, Colima, Chihuahua, Guanajuato, Guerrero, Jalisco, Michoacán, Morelos, Nuevo Léon, Oaxaca, Puebla, San Luis Potosí, Tamaulipas y Veracruz.

Simulium (Psilopelmia) veracruzanum
Colina, Chiapas, Durango, Jalisco, México, Michoacán, Morelos, Nayarit, Oaxaca y Veracruz.

Simulium (Psilopelmia) zempoalense
Morelos, Oaxaca y Veracruz.

Simulium (Simulium) anduzei
Distrito Federal, Morelos, Oaxaca y Veracruz.

Simulium (Simulium) bustosi
Oaxaca y Veracruz.

Simulium (Simulium) costa-limai
Morelos y Oaxaca.

Simulium (Simulium) hechti
Distrito Federal y Morelos.

Simulium (Simulium) iriartei
Districto Federal, Durango, Guerrero, Oaxaca y Veracruz.

Simulium (Simulium) jacumbae
Chiapas, Hidalgo, Jalisco, Michoacán, Oaxaca y Veracruz.

Simulium (Simulium) jobbinsi
Chiapas, Oaxaca y Veracruz.

Simulium (Simulium) lassmanni
Districto Federal, Guanajuato, México y Veracruz.

Simulium (Simulium) marquezi
Chihuahua, Districto Federal y México.

Simulium (Simulium) metallicum
Celima, Chiapas, Chihuahua, Durango, Guerrero, Hidalgo, Jalisco, México, Michoacán, Morelos, Nayarit, Nuevo Léon, Oaxaca, Puebla, San Luis Potosí, Sinaloa, Sonora, Tabasco y Veracruz.

Simulium (Simulium) ochraceum
Chiapas y Oaxaca.

Simulium (Simulium) parrai
Oaxaca y Veracruz.

Simulium (Simulium) puigi
Chiapas, Oaxaca y Veracruz.

LAMINA LIII

Simulium (Simulium) iriartei

417. Adminículo del macho, vista dorsal.
418. Branquias de la pupa.
419. Pieza basal y pinceta del macho.
420. Horquilla de la hembra.
421. Cerco y lóbulo anal de la hembra.
422. Bucofaringe de la hembra.
423. Capullo, visto dorsalmente.
424. Capullo, visto lateralmente.

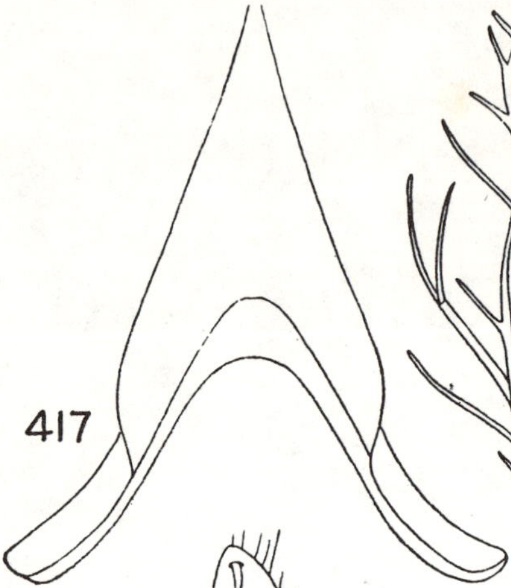
417

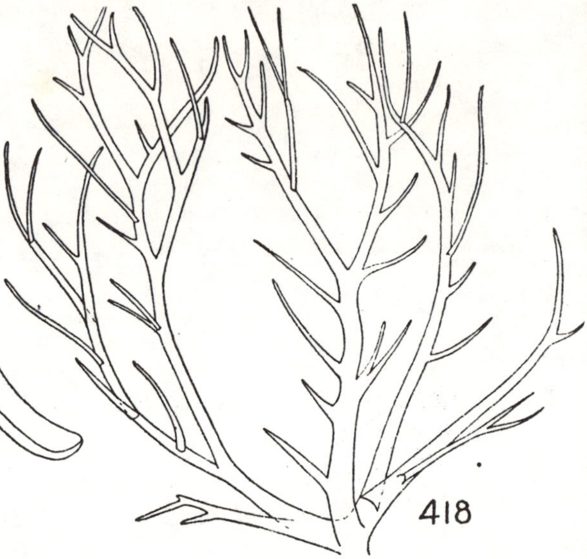
418

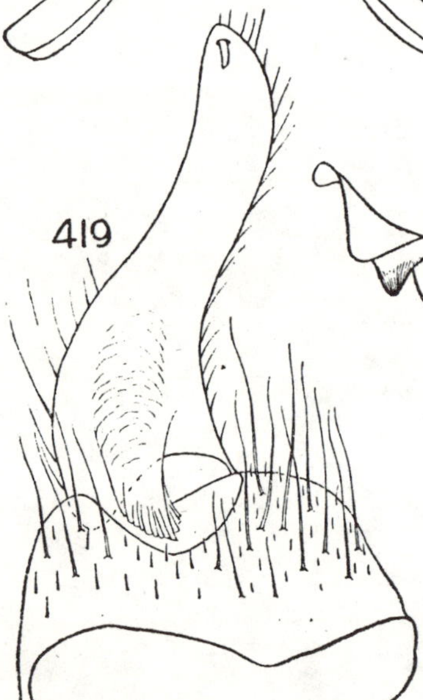
419

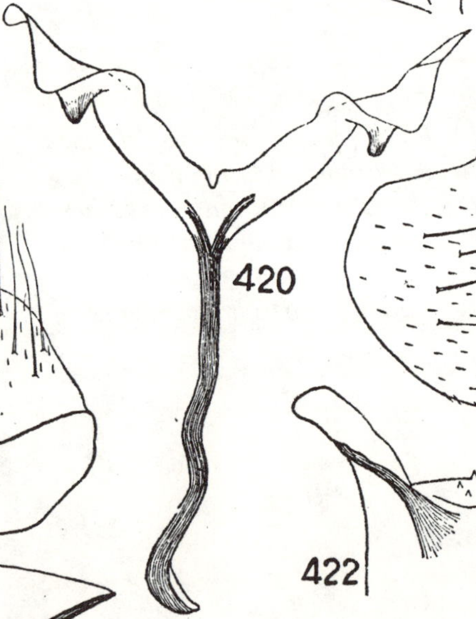
420

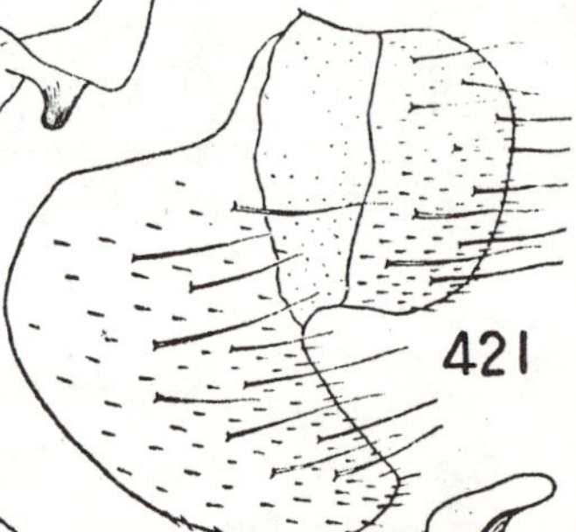
421

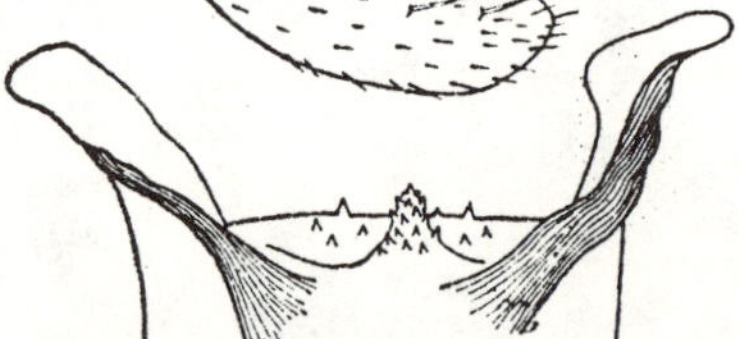
422

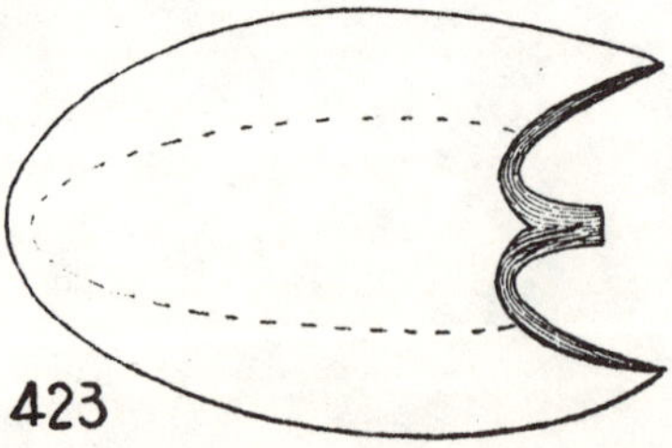
423

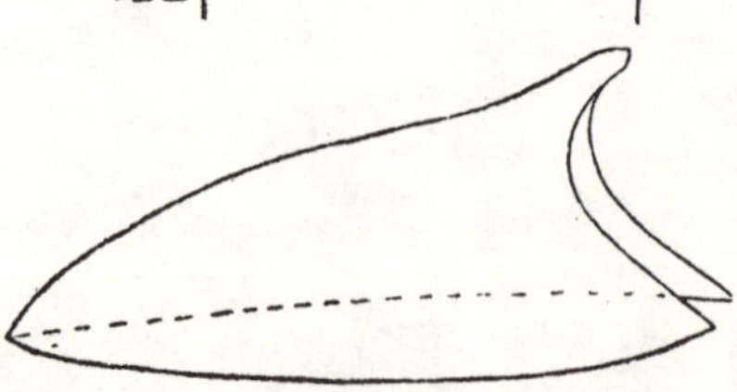
424

LIST OF THE PHLEBOTOMUS FOUND IN VENEZUELA *

1.- *Ph. almazani Galliard 1934.*
El Tinaco (Estado Cojedes) capturado por Briceño Iragorry i G. de La Plaza.
2.- *Ph. anduzei* Rozeboom 1943.
La Gran Sabana (Estado Bolivar) capturado por Anduze.
3.- *Ph. atroclavatus Knab 1913.*
Sin:
Ph. tejerae Larrouse 1921.
Ph. guadeloupensis Floch i Abonnenc 1945.
Mene Grande (Estado Zulia) capturado por Tejera.
Mene de Mauroa (Estado Falcón) capturado por Ortiz.
Sin indicar sitio, capturado por Anduze.
4.- *Ph. cayennensis* Floch i Abonnenc 1941.
Bachaquero i Rio Negro (Estado Zulia) capturado por Anduze.
Alrededores de San Felipe (Estado Yaracuy) capturado por Ortiz (comunicación verbal).
5.- *Ph. evansi* Núñez Tovar 1924.
Mariara (Estado Carabobo) capturado por Núñez Tovar.
Macuto (Distrito Federal) capturado por Iriarte.
Mene de Mauroa (Estado Falcón) capturado por Ortiz.
Altagracia de Orituco (Estado Guárico) capturado por Anduze.
Bachaquero, Selva de Tamanaco i Río Negro (Estado Zulia) capturado por Anduze.
Ocumare del Tuy (Estado Miranda) capturado por Ortiz (comunicación verbal).
San Mateo (Estado Aragua) capturado por Iriarte.
6.- *Ph. gomezi* Nitzulescu 1931.
Sin:
Ph. suis Rozeboom 1940.
Ph. japigny Floch i Abonnenc 1944.
San Cristóbal (Estado Táchira) capturado por Tejera.
Hacienda Aguacatal, alrededores de San Mateo (Estado Aragua) capturado por Iriarte.
San Felipe (Estado Yaracuy) capturado por Ortiz (comunicación verbal).
Churuguara (Estado Falcón) capturado por Ortiz (comunicación verbal).
Ocumare del Tuy (Estado Miranda) capturado por Ortiz (comunicación verbal).

* Reprinted from the "Boletín del Laboratorio de la Clínica Luis Razetti". Año XII. Vol. XVI. N° 35-36. 1952.

Caracas (Distrito Federal) capturado por Ortiz (comunicación verbal).
(Estado Barinas) capturado por Anduze (comunicación verbal).

7.- *Ph. intermedius* Lutz i Neiva 1922.
Sin:
Ph. lutzi Manson Bahr. 1925.
Ph. mazai Paterson 1926.
Ph. neivai Pinto 1926.
Valles del Yaracuy (Chino i Farriar) (Estado Yaracuy) capturado por Pifano.

8.- *Ph. lichyi* Floch i Abonnenc 1950.
Río Borburata (Estado Carabobo) capturado por Lichy.

9.- *Ph. longipalpis* Lutz i Neiva 1912.
Sin:
Ph. otomae Núñez Tovar i Tejera 1924.
Isla de Otama en el Lago de Valencia (Estado Carabobo) capturado por Tejera.
El Tinaco (Estado Cojedes) capturado por Briceño Iragorry i de La Plaza.
Mene de Mauroa (Estado Falcón) capturado por Ortiz.
Valles del Yaracuy (Farriar i El Chino) (Estado Yaracuy) capturado por Pifano.

10.- *Ph. migonei* Franca 1920.
Sin:
Ph. rangeli Núñez Tovar 1924.
Ph. araozi Paterson i Shannon 1926.
Choroni (Estado Aragua) capturado por Tejera.
Caracas (Districo Federal) capturado por Iriarte.
Valles del río Yaracuy (Estado Yaracuy) capturado por Pifano.

11.- *Ph. maracayensis* Núñez Tovar 1923.
Tucupido (Estado Aragua) capturado por Núñez Tovar.
Valles del río Yaracuy (Estado Yaracuy) capturado por Pifano.

12.- *Ph. punctigeniculatus* Floch i Abonnenc 1944.
Río Negro (Estado Zulia) capturado por Anduze.

13.- *Ph. panamensis* Shannon 1926.
Sin:
Ph. davisi Root 1934.
Barquisimeto (Estado Lara) capturado por Hill.
Ocumare de la Costa (Estado Aragua) capturado por Root.
Hacienda Aguacatal, alrededores de San Mateo (Estado Aragua) capturado por Iriarte.
Mene Mauron (Estado Falcón) capturado por Ortiz.
Ocumare del Tuy (Estado Miranda) capturado por Ortiz (comunicación verbal).
San Felipe (Estado Yaracuy) capturado por Ortiz (comunicación verbal).

Valles del río Yaracuy (Estado Yaracuy) capturado por Pifano.
Gran Sabana (Estado Bolívar) capturado por Anduze.
(Estado Barinas) capturado por Anduze.

14.- *Ph. squamiventris* Lutz i Neiva 1912.
No se sabe bien el sitio de captura, posiblemente (Estado Aragua).

15.- *Ph. trinidadensis* Newstead 1922.
Sin:
Ph. cruciatus Coquillet 1907 (descripción incompleta).
Ph. yucatenensis Galliard 1934.
Ph. baduelensis Floch i Abonnenc 1941.
Ph. villelai Mangabeira 1942.
Mene de Mauroa (Estado Falcón) capturado por Ortiz.
Bachaquero, Río Negro i Selva de Tamanaco (Estado Zulia) capturado por Anduze.

16.- *Ph. verrucarum* Townsend 1913.
Río Borburata (Estado Carabobo) capturado por Lichy.

17.- *Ph. venezuelensis* Floch i Abonnenc 1948.
Altagracia de Orituco (Estado Guárico) capturado por Anduze.
Río Negro i Selva de Tamanaco (Estado Zulia) capturado por Anduze.

18.- *Ph. zuliaensis* Floch i Abonnenc 1948.
Altagracia de Orituco (Estado Guárico) capturado por Anduze.
Bachaquero i Río Negro (Estado Zulia) capturado por Anduze.

SHORT NOTES ABOUT SIMULIUM LUTZIANUM PINTO (1931) *

As we know, this simuliidae was separated, for Pinto, from the Venezuelan material carried and studied by Lutz, of the group rubrithorax, as a new species.

Briceño Iragorry caught nymphs in Los Chorros, and obtained adults, that were studied by Briceño helped by Fairchild, description appeared in the N° 10, year 43, of our Bulletin.

In our work "La familia Simuliidae en Venezuela", we appointed have found this species in Tabay (State Mérida) and in the small river going at the side of the road between Petare to Guarenas, in the place El Samán.

Some time ago, Fernández Vautrai, expert in this kind of insects, because he helped in the Oswaldo Cruz in researches about this family, who carried with him from Colonia Tovar some pupae of respiratory tubes short and thick, collected in a conduit of sewage.

As not was possible to obtain adults coming from these pupae, exist the doubt among the persons that have studied simuliidae (Anduze, Briceño Iragorry and Iriarte) referring to what species should have come out from these pupae, either a new species or one of the described in other countries with pupae of this type.

Just, Anduze described the suspicous species in the Boletín de la Academia de Ciencias Físicas i Naturales, and taking in account the form of war clubs of the branchial tubes, has been nominated *mattea-branchia.*

Brinceño Iragorry and us, separated, visited Colonia Tovar, more or less 1.700 m. of altitude. Briceño Iragorry, the site called La Mariposa; Carrizales, near Los Teques and the hills of El Avila, a height of around 1.500 meters. Iriarte, profiting invitation Dr. Villoria, chief of coordination of I N O S, we were in the region of the dam Agua Fría, near Colonia Tovar, and arrived 1.700 m. of height.

The finding of Simuliidae in the small river of Agua Fría was difficult. Six persons staying for a while on the borders of the river, none being attacked by the insects and also it was not possible to find pupae; but, looking for a horse, pasturing on the grass, we saw that besides of stomoxys that pricking the animal, had scarce simuliidae stinging on the ears and caught several specimens that sent to Luis Vargas of Mexico, have been classified as S. lutzianum. According to Briceño Iragorry the captures of him in the places that we have appointed have given also S. lutzianum.

* Reprinted from "Boletín del Laboratorio de la Clínica Luis Razetti". Año IX - Vol. XV - N° 27-28 - 1948.

CONCLUSION:

1.- The adults that should have come out of the pupae of short and thick tubes, brought from Colonia Tovar, by Fernández Vautrai, continue being indeterminated. It is called *mattea-branchia* by the description of Anduze, and will be considered a new species, till to fall in synonymy with species described, having the same type of pupae.
2.- S. lutzianum seems to be an insect of high regions, was found in Los Chorros and Carrizales (Briceño Iragorry); in small river running at the side of way Petare-Guarenas, in the place El Samán (Iriarte); in the hills of El Avila (Briceño Iragorry); in Tabay (Iriarte) and the small river of Agua Fría (Iriarte).
3.- It has been found as much up today, in District Federal, State Miranda and State Mérida. The pupae separated for Pinto in material of Lutz, arise from Rio Castaño (State Aragua) and Smart speaks of pupae of this species in Guayana, about report given by Briceño Iragorry.
4.- It is a simuliidae of zoophyle customs in accord to the observations that we have made; however, according to Briceño has found female adults stinging people in the region Los Chorros.

CONTRIBUTION TO THE STUDY OF THE CERATOPOGONIDAE HEMATOPHAGOUS FOUND IN VENEZUELA *

FIRST PART

The Ceratopogonidos or Ceratopogoninas of Kieffer, equivalent to Ceratopogon of Meigen, sub-family of the Chironomidae, family of the sub-order Nematocera, order of the Diptera, are insects very frequent in some zones of the country and that the people call "jejenes".

All these insects were included in the genus Ceratopogon as was said by Meigen (1) in 1803, who does not accept the genus Culicoides of Latraille (2). Winnertz, 1852 (3), Schiner, 1862 (4) and others continued the instance of Meigen, till that Kieffer J.J., 1906 (5), restored the word Culicoides.

This author told that these insects were recognized easily by the macrotrichiasis, at least in a part of the wing, and in the empodia very reduced of the tarsal hooks; however, it was necessary that Malloch have given as typical the presence of sensory pits on the disk of mesonotum.

Genus related as Neoceratopogon and Leptoconops have the same auxiliaries, but not so developed. Cartes H.E., Ingram A. and Macfie J.W.S. give a complete description of Culicoides in work about species of the WEST Africa (6).

At first, these mosquitos, belonging to the genus Acanthoconops, Culicoides, Lasiohelea, Ceratopogon, Leptoconops and Heloconops, have called the attention for the voracity, with exceptions, as Lasiohelea grisea; however, it has been cited by Malloch as pricker. Referring to the effect on men and animals, they have been accused worse than the long shanked.

N.A. Dyce Sharp (7) (8) has verified the development of the Filaria perstans, or better, the old Filaria sanguinis hominis minor, found by Manson in 1890, in Culicoides austeni (Carter, Ingram and Macfie, 1920), in 95% to 100% of the specimens caught in the zone of Manfe, Camerún (Africa), and in C. grahami, a variety of Acanthocheiloneum perstans in six days. A 33% of the sauvage specimens were infected.

Buckley J.J.C. (9) demonstrated the development of Filaria ozardi, Manson 1897, different to pertans of the rear end sharper, in Culicoides furens Poey, doing cycle since the sting till the infected stage in proboscis in eight days; researches made in the Island of St. Vincent (West Indies).

Not only filarial found in the man, but also in animals, are capables the ceratopogonidae of the host, and so, Steward J.S. (10) (11), verified

* Reprinted from "Boletín del Laboratorio de la Clínica Luis Razetti". Año X - Vol. XV -N° 31-32 - 1950.

the infection and development in England, in Culicoides nubeculosis Mg. and C. obonsoletus Mg. of the Onchocerca cervicalis (Railliet and Henry 1910) of the horse; Buckley (12), cited formerly, appointed the development of O. gibsoni (Cleland and Johnston 1910) of the cattle in Malay Archipelago in Culicoides punges, succeeding to infect other species, experimentally.

Hoffmann (13) cited form of sausage in the thoracic muscles of Culicoides filariferus, that Vargas Luis (14), said to be the same C. diabolicus (Hoffmann 1925), very similar to C. guttatus (Coquillet 1904), different, chiefly, for the size of the wing; and Dampf A. spoke about 107 specimens for him.

Sambon L.W. (16) said that Simuliidae and Leptoconops could be the transmissors of the pellagra, and Willcocks F.C. (17) accused to L. kerteszi Kieffer and Culicoides sp.

Townsend C.H. (18) thought that the peruvian leishmaniasis called "Uta", could be transmitted for Forcipomyia utae.

Chatton E. and Blanc G. (19), referring the transmission of Toxoplasma gundii (Nicolle and Marceaux 1909); of the Ctenodactylus gundi by Leptoconops kerteszi; Sergent, Parrot and Donotien (20) found microfilarias in a ceratopogonidae from Algeria the Holoconops mediterraneus, and, at the last, Wanson M. (21) has suspicions that the red fever of the Congo, similar to dengue, could be transmitted by these insects.

* * *

The ceratopogoninae have various names, and so Lutz A. (22), for species to the border of the sea, in Brazil, named *marium* or *muruim,* being an indigenous word that the french have modified in maringouim; Goeldi brings *meruim,* but according to Lutz is a printing error. Also in portuguese are named *mosquitinhos do mangue,* that should be equivalent to mangrove fly, for living always near the plantations of those trees. For the brazilian species from the Interior, they say *mosquitos polvora,* for the resemblance with the granules of the explosive.

In english is used sandfly, that it seems to be originally referring to ceratopogonidae, but also is employed for to appoint the phlebotomes. The Germans say sandflige. In the english language they also say *midges* or *gnats,* for denomitate these insects, telling the German *gnitzen* in relation with the second. *Punkies* is used currently among the Anglo-saxons.

In Mexico, in accord with Vargas L. (23) says *chaquistes* or *jejenes;* in Cuba, it seems to be, calling them also jejenes; many persons englobe as jejen all little hematophagous, but the majority knows that they are the very little mosquitos, voraceous, whose pricking is painful, abundant in certain zones and certain months of the year.

* * *

Lutz A. (24) (25) in whose valuable works of the years 13 and 14, reported the description of several species and a series of details about these animals.

Hoffmann W.A. (26) published in the year 25 an interesting work bringing the description of 19 species, some of them new to the science.

Joahnnsen O.W.A. (27) is in accord with Edwards that C. ferrugineovitatus Zett., is a pallid variety of C. plumosus L.; C. hilaris Walker and C. Nephoterus Mitch., are the same; C. glacurus Wied. = = C. stigmaterus Say. Edwards F.W. (28) cited C. gymnopterus page 247. Mandoul A.H. (29) observed the C. perpungens Kieffer, stinging the man in the region of Burdeos, doing the classification Kieffer himself.

Winner Ant. (30), in work written in Czech, with summary in german, presented various species from Palestine, but said that the material was scarce.

Macfie J.W.S. (31) (32) in the islands of Society, caught 202 specimens of 9 species, representing 6 genus, including, so: Lasiohelea pacifica, Atrichopogon obscuripes, Culicoides insulanus and Dasyhelea pacifica, Dasyhelea var, pallida, Dasyhelea fulvicauda, Stilobezzia tenebrosa, S. maculipes.

The same Macfie (33) in the same year, in the Amazon region, in specimens caught in the Coast of the State of Piauhi, found: Lasiohelea louriei ♀, Atrichopogon glaber ♀, Atrichopogon insignieventris ♀. Atrichopogon flamineus ♀, Culicoides amazonicus, Dasyhelea hippolytae ♀, Dasyhelea penthesileae ♀, and Dasyhelea thalestris ♀.

Causey O.R. (34), during a stay in Siam, from August 1931 to July 1935, caught specimens of Culicoides, did a revision, describing new species from that zone.

Adamson A.M. (35), in the island of Trinidad, caught near the Coast, 7 specimens of Culicoides and 1 of Holoconops, pricking.

Roman E. (36), near to Lyon (France) said not to be stinging for the species Culicoides pulicaris var. ocellaris and var. edwardsianus, Culicoides minutissimus = = pumilus and Culicoides obsoletus, but Galli-Valerio accused it,, in that region, as pricker. Roman supposed then that the transmission of filarias as Ackanthocheilonema pertans through these insects should have a series of conditions.

Johansen O. (37) published in 1943 an important communication about this type of insects.

Vargas Luis (38), cited for Mexico 14 species: albomaculata, baueri, cockerelli, tristiatulus, copiosus, crepuscularis, dampfi, diabolicus, furens, haematopotus, luteovenus, piliferus, seopus, variipennis and yukonensis.

* * *

It seems to be, in accord with Edwards F.M., Oldroyd H. and Smart

J. (39), that the first description of a biologic cycle of a specie of Culicoides, probably was published in 1713 by W. Derhan, of Upminster in Essex, in work entitled: "Físco-teología or a demonstration of the human being and attributes of God, for his work of the Creation"; later, two centuries after.

Patton, in 1917, published with illustrations of the life of a specie from Hindustan, and Lutz, at the same time, gave to know his interesting works. The publications of Heeger in 1856, about the larves of Culicoides varius Winn; later researches verified that they were of the same family Cecidomyidae.

In the mentioned work of Edwards, are described 7 new species: brunnicans, cubitalis, delta, fagineus, grisescens, simulator and truncarum.

In 1912, the wise Lutz (40) gave extensive and exact reports about the biology of these ceratopogonidae, and successively we copied textually in portuguese, a part of the Chapter "Morfolojia, Anatomia e Biolojia dos primeiras estados."

"Na descricao dos primeiros estádios das Ceratoponinae e principalmente das especies hematofagas nao me bazeio somente na literatura, que é bastante incompleta (sendo que os seus dados muitas vezes nao se aplicam ás nossas especies) mas, de preferencia, em observacoes proprias, feitas ora ocazionalmente (principalmente durante os longos estudos que realizei sobre as nossas culicidas), ora instituidas especialmente para a solucao das questoes pendentes."

"Os ovos sao olongados, em grao variavel; nos Culicoides tem a forma ovocilindrica alongada e um pouco incurvada que se pode comparar a das bananas; a casca de branco puro enegrece logo depois da expulsao, mas é tao fina, que a larva, e principalmente as manchas oculares desta, podem ser percebidas antes do dezalagamento. As larvas novas se distinguem das mais velhas, principalmente pelas dimensoes e sópodem ser percebidas a olho nú em condicoes muito favoraveis, visto nao serem sómente muito curtas, mas tamben extremamente finas e transparentes."

"As larvas das Ceratopogoninae manifestam certa tendencia a emanciparse das aguas correntes ou estagnadas, que, como para as outras Chrironomidae devem ser consideradas como habitat primitivo e normal; podem viver fóra da agua, mas, assim mesmo, precizam, sem duvida, de bastante humidade. Na Europa, algumas especies foram encontradas debaixo da casca de arvores, na madeira podre ou na seiva, que corre de certas arvores, o que pode ser considerado como uma tranzicao do meio humido para o ar. Estas observacaos nao devem ser consideradas como regra geral e, mesmo que se aplicassem a todas as especies europeas, o que me parece muito duvidozo, nao teriam o mesmo valor para as nossas especies indijenas. Estas, pelo menos em parte, sao francamente aquaticas, algumas sao hematofagas, vivem em agua doce corrente ou estagnada, sendo muitas vezes especialmente adatadas á agua contida em certas plantas, como bromeliaceas e bambuzacas."

"Uma das razoes porque estas larvas facilmente passam desapercibidas, é que nao gostam muito da luz. Se muitas Chironomidae fabricam tubos na lama, nos quaes se escondem, as Ceratopogoninae, muitas vezes se escondem, penetrando no fundo lodozo da agua. Sem duvida, aparecen, de vez em quando, na superficie, mas só com bastante esforco e com forte movimentos serpeantes e logo afundam-se outra vez, se nao acham um ponto de apoio. Neste ou no fundo, podem ficar imoveis durante muito tempo. Quando, em lugares humidos, saem da agua, o que ás vezes se observa, sao dificilmente percebidas, por cauza da sua transparencia. Mais facilmente encontram-se as pupas maduras que se demoram na superficie e os cazulos vazios que boiam, até achar um corpo solido no qual geralmente se prendem. Os cazulos maduros mostram as mesmas particularidades."

"As larvas de Culicoides, pedo menos as aquaticas, que nos interessam especialmente, tem todas o mesmo tipo, que se pode chamar vermicular o nematoide. O corpo cilindrico é sempre muito delgado com as extremidades afiladas, a cefalica um pouco menos do que a caudal. A baze da cabeca nao se destaca por maior grosura e a capsula cefalica, quitinoza, é delgada, e apenas lijeraimente amarelada. O corpo é formado por 12 segmentos, separados por constriccoes bastante profundas. A superficie, nos Culicoides, é quazi completamente glabra; em outros generos e munida de algunas cerdas finas de cor clara, sendo o numero, em cada segmento, pequeno. Ha outros com pelos ramificados. Culicoides tem tambem alguns pelos izolados, principalmente nas duas extremidades do corpo. As larvas ao principio, sao completamente transparentes; mais tarde, principalmente em alguns generos, tornam-se mais opacas pelo dezenvolvimento do corpo adiposo, mas sempre se distinguem facilmente os organs internos. Consistem no intestino com dois tubos de Malpighi muito contortos; o coracao e o sistema nervozo aparecem distintamente. Além disso, o corpo é percorrido por dois tubos traqueaes, adelgacados nas duas extremidades e tendo ramificacoes finas, formando um sistema fechado sem comunicacoes comestigmas. Ha, todavia, uns apendices branquiaes, mais ou menos dezenvolvidos que podem ser evertidos, aprezentando a forma de estrela, sendo formados de ramificaoes quazi conicas. A capsula cefalica é bastante longa um pouco dirijida para biaxo e munida de antenas e palpos muito reduzidos. Os olhos sao formados pɔr pequenas manchas de pigmento sinjelas o duplas; o olho composto só aparece depois da metamordoze".

"Correspondendo á cabeca delgada o orificio bucal é muito fino; sendo tambem os organs de mastigacao pouco dezenvolvidos, só poderao ser aproveitados para particulas alimentares muito miudas. O processo de nutricao parece puco ativo e o periodo larval pode durar bastante tempo".

"As ninfas, pouco moveis, parecem-se com as de culicidas sendo todavia mais finas e alongadas. Como nas pequenas culicidas, o periodo ninfal é muito curto e a ecdize parece realizar-se de modo perfeitamente analoio. As pupas aquaticas das ceratopogonidas terminam em duas pontas subconicas de direcao variavel, funcionando como orgam de propulsao. Sobre o dorso do cefalotorax da ninfa ha dois tubos respiratorios, cuja forma é o melhor distintivo das especies e, quica, tambem, dos generos".

"As larvas das Bromeliaceas, que fornecem geralmente especies de Ceratopogon S. str. e de Fórcipomyia, aproximamse mais do tipo das larvas de Chironomus, possuindo no ultimo e, ás vezes, tambem no primeiro anel do corpo dois pés truncados, nem sempre bem separados, mas tendo cada uma coroa terminal de ganchos. A cabeca com os seus apendices é menos reduzida, os segmentos mostram cerdas compridas simples ou compostas, em numero ora maior ora menor. Larvas analogas achao-se tambem nos bambús ao lado de larvas typicas de Culicoides. As especies marinhas de Ceratopogon tem o corpo quazi tao glabro como os Culicoides mas a cabeca é mais quitinizada e mais grossa".

"A morfolojia dos primeiros estádios nos varios generos e, talvez, mesmo nas especies dos mesmos, varia conforme o modo de viver, devendo-se evitar a generalizacao das poucas observacoes até hoje feitas".

"Das Coratoponinae observadas em zonas quentes e que atacam o homem e os grandes animaes domesticos, quazi todas as especies, principalmente as do mangue, pertenecem ao genero Culicoides Latreille que difere de Ceratopogon pelos empodios pouco dezenvolvidos dos adultos e pelas larvas. O dezenho e revestimento pilozo das azas parece constituir uma distincao adicional de percepcao mais facil. Pelo menos, as especies que eu conheco e que formam um grupo muito homojeneo nao mostram os pelos maiores tao egualmente espalhados sobre as azas como os tem a maior parte das especies de Ceratopogon e Forcipomyia, mas, a aza é caracterizada por uma particularidade que falta a estes ultimos. Quero falar da prezenca de manchas redondas, faxas ou zonas extensás de coloracao mas clara, já viziveis por transparencia, mas destacando-se muito mais á iluminacao latera, assumindo, entao, a aza aspeto muito esquizito. No interior, conheco uma ou duas especies hematofagas que, julgando sómente pelos caracteres das azas deviam ser clasificadas como Ceratopogon; todavía, reprezentam, induditavelmente, novo genero. As larvas destes, talvez se desenvolvam nas bromeliaceas que sao habitat predileto dos generos Ceratopogon e Forcipomyia; as taquaras parecem ser preferidas pelo genero Culicoides".

"Nao posso deixar de observar aqui que, provavelmente, as diferencas mais importantes entre os generos serao dadas pelos caracteres das partes bucais. Assim Culicoides, ao contrario do que se observa em Atrichopogon e Ceratopogon, tem sempre seis laminas quitinozas, mesmo, no macho, mas tambem toda a trompa tem uma forma diferente. Parece isso uma regra geral para todos os generos hematofagos; os outros tem um numero reduzido de partes bucais. O revestimento do corpo pode ter importancia, mostrando, as vezes, escamas distintas, embora estreitas. A forma dos ovos, que pode ser reconhecida na femea madira contribue ocazionalmente para distinguir os generos. Assim, achei-so muito compridos em Ceratopogon e Culicoides e curtos em Forcipomyia. As diferencas tiradas do tamanho do empodio nao podem sempre ser utilizadas, parecendo haver formas de tranzicao. O que Johannsen menciona como pequenas cerdas na baze das unhas nao me parece nada mais que as primeiras plumas do empodio e sem valor distintivo. Julgo, todavia, que Latreille foi muito bem inspirado, quando separou Culicoides e Ceratopogon, havendo diferencas nas azas, na tromba, nas larvas e ninfas e, finalmente, tambem, nos habitos''.

In 1926, Painter Reginald H. (41) gave reports of the life of five species; discovered evolutive stages and cause ecological data about larves, adults and control of them. Found larves and pupae of C. furens in swamps of salty water. In soil saturated with water specific gravity 1042, larves and pupae were obtained and also adults.

In inmaturo stages were found in rotten wood of mangrove trees in salty water. Observed that the larves eaten on diatoms and species of Leptoconops were obtained in similar conditions to those described for the genus Culicoides.

Lutz (42), en su trabajo, trae el género Ceratopogon Meigen, con los sub-géneros Atrichopogon (Kieffer), Ceratopogon (Mg.) i Forcipomyia (Mg.); el género Culicoides Latreille, i el género Alasión (Rondani), Sphaeromyia (Stephens) i Palpomyia (Megerle).

Theneman August (43) dice que las Cerotopogoninae están divididas en tres secciones, sobre la base de los caracteres larvarios i pupales. Trasladamos textualmente del inglés lo que sigue:

1.-Ceratoponinae genuine, body of larva with conspicuous setae or spines; anterior and posterior prolegs well developed; pupae with at least 1 pair of slender thoracic proceses, the prothoracic respiratory organs more or less piriform. 2.-C. intermediae, body of larva with inconspicuous setae; a retractile caudal proleg present; pupae without long thoracic tubular processes; prothoracic respiratory organ slender bandlike, or slender clavate. This section contains only Dasyhelea Kief. (Pseudoculicoides Mall., Prokempia Kief) with the species divided into the groups longipalpia, diplosis and halophila. 3.-C. vermiformes, body of larva slender with inconspicuous setae, no prolegs present; pupae lacking tubular processes, the prothoracic repiratory organ more or less piriform. The 1st group of this section comprises the genus Culicoides, the 2nd group, such genera as Bezzia, Proberzia, Palpomyia, Dicrobezzia, Johansenomyia and Xylocripta''.

da Costa Lima A. (44), examinando especímenes recolectados por Kumm en el Estado de Pará (Brasil), leyendo las célebres contribuciones de Lutz i Hoffmann sobre el asunto, i estudiando i revisando la colección del primero en el Instituto Oswaldo Cruz, llegó a confeccionar una clave para las especies brasileras descritas hasta esa fecha, tomando sobre todo en consideración los caracteres alares i sirviendo de comparación un ala de C. guttatus.

Textualmente tomamos de esta clave, lo que corresponde a especies citadas entre nosotros, así:

5' Proboscida mais longa que o diametro de un olho; 3° segmento do palpo nao consedravelmente entumescido e sem depressao sensorial; comprimento do corpo 1.75 mm; comprimento da aza, cerca de 1.4 mm.

maruim

Lutz 1913. 2° Mem. est. 7. fig. 1; est. 8, figs, 14, 16 e 19. Río de Janeiro.

8(7) Area hyalina, situada atraz do estigma, grande, quasi reniforme, por coalescer, com uma outra macula hyalina situada para atraz e para dentro de que limita o estigma para fóra; 3° segmento do palpo sem orgao sensorial cupuliforme.

acotylus

Lutz 1913. 2° Mem. est. 8. fig. 11. 21. Matto Grosso.

13' Para fóra da area hyalina que envolve o estigma ha, quasi tocando-a, uma pequena macula hyalina e, para fóra, pórem afastada do apice da cellula R5, uma grande macula hyalina reniforme, ás vezes dividida em duas pequenas celulas.

furens

(Poey 1853); Hoffmann 1925. est. 1. fig. 2; est. 2. fig. 7.(= maculithorax Willinston 1896; Lutz 1913. est. 7, fig. 5)); Cuba, México, Trinidad, Porto-Rico, Honduras, Florida, Panamá, Sao Vicente, Jamaica, Antilhas, Bahamas e Brazil.

13(11) Para fóra da area hyalina que envolve o estigma ha luma macula hyalina, afastada do apice, e, para fóra, uma outra menor, no apice da cellula R5; comprimento da aza 0.83 a 0.85 mm.

paraensis

(Goeldi 1905); Lutz 1913. 2° Mem. est. 6. fig. 10; est. 7. fig. 6; Pará e Bahia (Brasil) (? = undecimpunctatus Kieffer 1917. Rep. Argentina).

16(15) Cellula Ml, sem macula hyalina sobre o bordo da aza, entre o apice das nervuras Ml e M2.

insignis

Lutz 1913. 2° Mem. est. 7. fig. 3.; Bahia e Río de Janeiro (= guttatus Lutz 1913, nec Coquillet 1904).

18(14) Macrotrichia bem desenvolvidas; palpos como na figura 6. b.

debilipalpis

Lutz 1913. 2° Mem. est. 7. fig. 8; Paraná, Sao Paulo; Río de Janeiro e Pará (Ríos Maruarú-Curralinho).

Fox Irving (45) wrote about the proboscis respiratory of the pupae; shaping of the ends; number and implantation of the wings; seeing that the tubes with scaly appearence, it seems to be, in relation with the ambient, because it has been seen that they are characteristics of the species living in bromeliáceas or in holes of the trunks of trees.

In Venezuela, the first time that was described this type of insects, is in the book of Lutz A. and Núñez Tovar M. (46), where is cited the species paraensis.

Later, Ortiz C. Ignacio (47) (48), in 1942, did mention of the finding of Culicoides variipennis Coq. in the State Falcón, that after said to be the species C. arubae.

Fox and Hoffmann, according to Stone; at the same time appointed to Forcipomyia raleigh Macfie, F. sp. and Atrichopogon in dwellings, hemtophagous the first and possibly hematophagous the second. In those same communications appointed the finding of C. paraensis, done in the small village Los Dividivos, near Mene de Mauroa (State Falcón).

The following year, Iriarte David R. (49), found three species of culicoides: C. paraensis Goeldi, C. variipennis Coquillet and C. stellifer Coquillet; this last one was new for Venezuela. Besides, appointed other genus of Ceratopogonidae: Atrichopogon sp. and Lasiohelea sp., prickers, caught in several places and classified by Stone.

In 1946, Briceño Iragorry Leopoldo (50), said to have captured the specie C. debilipalpis Lutz, pricking, in Los Teques (State Miranda); sizing in the site C. paraensis Goeldi.

Ortiz C. Ignacio and Peña García Bernardo (51), in 1958, verified the presence of Culicoides furens Poey, in the District Bolívar of State Zulia.

At least, Briceño Iragorry Leopoldo (52) and Ortiz C. Ignacio in the present year, 1949, the first found the Culicoides marium Lutz in Higuerote (State Miranda), and the second one, found two new species: Culicoides insignis Lutz and Culicoides hoffmanni Fox; of the same manner, gives an account, of a species, whose characteristics, approach it to C. acotylus Lutz, classifications done for Stone. The seizures of these three last were made in Mene Mauroa (State Falcón).

Summarizing, up till today exist in the country 11 species of Ceratopogonidae, genus Culicoides, so:

C. paraensis Goeldi
C. variipennis Coquillet
C. stellifer Coquillet
C. arubae Fox i Hoffmann
C. heliconiae Fox i Hoffmann
C. hoffmanni Fox
C. furens Poey
C. debilipalpis Lutz
C. insignis Lutz
C. acotylus Lutz
C. maruim Lutz

ORIGINAL DESCRIPTIONS - COMMENTARIES AND GEOGRAPHICAL DISTRIBUTION OF THE ELEVEN SPECIES FOUND IN VENEZUELA

SECOND PART

Haematomyidium paraense nov. spec. Goeldi 1905. Vol. IV. pág. 137.
Goeldi E. 1905, Mem. Mus. Paraense. pág. 137.
Culicoides paraensis Lutz 1913.
Lutz A. 1913. Mem. do Inst. Osw. Cruz. Tomo V. Fasc. I. pág. 55.
Culicoides paraensis Lutz i Núñez Tovar 1928.
Lutz A. i Núñez Tovar M. 1928. Zool. i Paras. Venezolanos.
Culicoides paraensis Dunn, 1934.
Dunn. 1934. Psyche. Vol. XLI. pág. 178.
Culicoides paraensis da Costa Lima. 1937.
da Costa Lima A. Mem. do Ins. Osw. Cruz. Tomo 32. Fasc. 3. 1937.
Culicoides paraensis Martorell. 1939.
Martorell. 1939. Pto. Rico. Univ. Jour. Agriculture Vol. XXIII. pág. 210.
Culicoides paraensis Ortiz 1942.
Ortiz Ignacio C. Rev. de la Pol. Car. Vol. XI. No. 66. 258-260. 1942.
Culicoides paraensis Fairchild 1943.
Fairchild. Am. Jour. Trop. Med. Vol. XXIII. pág. 572.
Culicoides paraensis Iriarte 1943.
Iriarte David R. 1943. Bol. Lab. Cli. Raz. Año IV. No. 11.
Culicoides paraensis Briceño Iragorry 1946.
Briceño Iragorry Leop. 1946. Bol. Lab. Cli. Raz. Año VI. No. 19-20.
"Haematomyidium paraense nov. spec. Goeldi (1905).

Habitus geral da imago feminina (o) visivel na figura 143. Colorido em vida um azulado cinzento. A aza é atravessada de cima para bixo, por quatro series de grandes espacos claros redondos (janellas) em campo geral ligeiramente escuro. Estas conspicuas janellas disseminadas sobre os intervallos entre as veias da parte distal da aza conforme o schema 2, 3, 3, 3 (de fóra para dentro), enchendo quasi os respectivos vaos. Campo das azas crivado de pequenissimos cabellos curtos, entre os quaes se percebem algo maiores, regularmente acompanhando o percurso longitudinal das veias circumferencia guarnecida de cabellos um pouco mais fortes, os mais robustos encontrando-se na margen antero-medial. Fitas claras transversaes atravez das articulacoes trochanter-femur e femur-tibia dos dois pares de pernas anteriores (I e II) e uma fita clara atravez da parte medial da tibia do terceiro par (III), perto da articulacao tibio-femoral. Um forte espinho lanceolado pelo lado externo da tibia, na articulacao tibiotarsal. Dimensoes: Comprimento 1.54 mm.—Comprimento da antenna O.5 mm.—Largura do thorax 0.4 mm.—Comprimento do abdomen 0.93 mm. Maior largura do abdomen 0.48 mm.—Comprimento da aza 0.83 mm.—Largura da aza O.36 mm."

"Pequena mosca invadindo as casas, impertinentissima chupadora de sangue; picada dolorosa, produzindo regularmente uma zona circular inflamada bastante grande. Frequente na epocha das chuvas, sobretudo nas horas de maré baixa, o que parece apontar para uma creatura littoral. Pará e arredores".

Para Lutz esta especie se acerca mucho a C. stellifer Coq., sin embargo, en el dorso del abdomen de esta última existen dos series de puntos oscuros; mientras que en el paraensis, en el mismo sitio, pueden apreciarse manchas transversales rectangulares de color obscuro.

Distribución geográfica de esta especie

Fuera de Venezuela

Goeldi—Estado de Pará. Brasil.

Lutz—En Piedade. Tiété, en Estado de Sao Paulo, Brasil.

En Estado de Pará. Brasil.

En río Tocantiins.

En Venezuela

Lutz—Gonzalito, Turmero, Tucupido i cerca de la cuidad de Maracay.

Ortiz—Estado Falcón. (Caserío Los Dividives, cerca de Mene Mauroa).

Briceño Iragorry—En las urbanizaciones del Este de Caracas (La Florida, Los Palos Grandes, Los Chorros), en las inmediaciones de La Victoria (Edo. Aragua) i en Los Teques (Edo. Miranda).

Iriarte—En El Hatillo i Guarenas (Estado Miranda), Macuto (Dto. Federal) i en el Estado Barinas.

* * *

Ceratopogon variipennis Coquillet 1901.

Coquillet 1901. Proc. U.S. Nat. Museum. Vol. XXIII, pág. 602.

Culicoides variipennis Malloch 1915.

Malloch 1915. Bull. III. State. Lab. Nat. Hist. Vol. X. Art. VI. p. 297.

Culicoides variipennis Hoffmann 1925.

Hoffmann W.A. 1925. The Am. Journ. of Hyg. Vol. No. 3. pág. 274.

Culicoides variipennis Fox 1942.

Fox Irving. 1942. Pto. Rico J. Public H. and Trop. Med. Vol. 17. No 4.

Culicoides variipennis Ortiz 1942.

Ortiz Ignacio C. 1942. Rev. Pol. Caracas. Vol. XI. No. 66. p. 258-260.

Culicoides variipennis Iriarte 1943.

Iriarte David. R. 1943. Cont. a la Fau. Ven. Bol. Lab. Cli. Razetti. Año IV. No 11.

Culicoides variipennis Vargas 1945.

Vargas Luis. 1945. Rev. Inst. Salub. i Enf. Trop. Vol. VI.I pág. 45.

Type. Cat. No. 5463 U. S. N. M.

Apex of third vein near two-thirds or three-fourths length of wing, eye contiguous 12

Apex near middle of length of wing, fpruth forking beyond the small cross vein, empodia wanting...12

Wings not distinctly spotted, eyes contiguous........................13
Wings convered with whitish hyaline and dark gray spots. Head black, eyes rather widely separated, antennae black, base of flagellum yellowish, its joints except last two of nearly an equal length, noticeably longer than broad, mouth parts black, opaque, mesonotum gray pruinose and covered with brown spots, halteres and legs brown, tibiae bearing several rather long yellow hairs on outer side, a yellow ring before apices of front and middle femora and near bases of their tibiae, tarsis largely yellow; wings nearly wholly covered with brown hairs, third veins contiguous to the first and to the costal vein, apical portion of first and third veins and costal vein near them greatly dilated, forming a darker spot than any of the others, fourth posterior cell whitish hyaline except a central triangular gray spot extending to the outer angles; length nearly 2 mm... variipennis new species.
Three female specimens. Westville, New Jersey (july 2, C.W. Johnson); Richmond, Virginia (Mrs. A.T. Slosson)' and Mexico City (O.W. Barrett).

Fox, estudiando en Puerto Rico, material de Root i Hoffmann, da la descripción siguiente de la pupa:
"Trompa respiratoria—Mui larga i prominente, ancha en la base, disminuyendo gradualmente, ensanchándose ligeramente hacia el extremo distal. Región media, dividida en seudo-segmentos de aspecto no mui escamoso. Dos espiráculos de la base situados en un lado, uno de los cuales dirigido hacia afuera i el otro hacia arriba; en el vértice de la trompa hai una docena de espiráculos dispuestos en la forma en que aparecen en el grabado 18".

"Segmento anal—(Macho). Tiene una forma peculiar mas o menos cuadrada; los apéndices se implantan en ángulo recto en el segmento, con la punta negra i disminuyendo gradualmente hasta terminar en una punta mui afilada. Para más detalles, véase grabado 23".

"Material examinado—Piel de la pupa de un ejemplar macho procedente de Baltimore, Maryland, 1922".

"Notas—La pupa de esta especies se parece muchísimo a la de la especie Paleártica C. nubeculosus (Meig). El parecido ha sido también notado en los estudios sobre los machos adultos de la misma especie (Root i Hoffmann 13)".

Ortiz, en "Nota sobre nuevos Ceratopogónidos hematófagos para Venezuela", señala que la especie descrita por él como variipennis, posteriormente Stone la consideró como C. arubae Fox i Hoffmann. Somos nosotros, por tanto. los que hemos citado esta especie por primera vez en el país, determinación hecha por el mismo Stone.
Distribución geográfica de esta especie
Fuera de Venezuela
Coquillet—
Hoffmann—En West-ville. N.J., México City, Richmond, Va.; en localidades centrales i del Sur de Illinois; en Ithaca, N.J.; en Baltimore.

Vargas—San Jacinto D.F. 1931-32. A. Dampf.

Iguala, Gro. enero-julio 1936. R. Ruiz Soto.

Zumpango, Gro. marzo 1936. R. Ruiz Soto.

Chilpancingo, Gro. fbro-marzo 1936. R. Ruiz Soto.

Etla, Oax. junio 11, 1935. F. Reyes.

Sabinas, Hidalgo, N.L. octubre 6, 1943. B. Brookman.

En Venezuela

Iriarte—En Caracas. (D.F.)

* * *

Ceratopogon stellifer Coquillet 1901.

Coquillet 1901. Prc. U.S. Nat. Mus. Vol. XXIII. pág. 604.

Culicoides stellifer Malloch 1915.

Malloch 1915. Bull III. State Lab. Nat. Hist. Vol. X. Art. VI. pág. 300.

Culicoides stellifer Hoffmann 1925.

Hoffmann W.A. 1925. Am. J. of Hyg. Vol. V. No. 3.

Culicoides stellifer Fox 1942.

Fox Irving. 1942. P. R. J. P. H. and Trop. Med. Vol. XVII. No 4.

Culicoides stellifer Iriarte 1943.

Iriarte David R. 1943. Bol. Lab. Cli. Razetti. Año IV. No. 11.

Type.—Cat. No. 5469, U. S. N. M.

Upper branch of fourth vein destitute of a white mark. Same as the preceding species with the above and following differences: No dark spot near middle of costal cell, a large whitish spot in base of first posterior cell, one in each end of the send posterior cell, none on lower branch of fourth vein, the one in center of fourth posterior cell extended to margin of wing, only two in anal cell, situated near its apex along the fifth vein; lenght, near 1 mm. .... stellifer, new species.

A female specimen, collected June 6 by Mr. H.S. Barber. Washington, District of Columbia.

Fox, estudiando material de Root i Hoffmann, describe la pupa, como sigue:

"Trompa respiratoria—Corta i estrecha, semejante a la del furens, dividida en seudo-segmentos bien definidos, sobre todo en la porción media. Cuando se le examina en posición lateral obsérvanse tres ramas en cada una de las cuales se implanta un espiráculo. En el ápice hai un grupo de unos cuatro o cinco espiráculos i debajo de éstos otro más. (v. grabado 21).

Segmento anal—(femenino). Corto, con los procesos extendidos hacia los lados, moteados de negro i adelgazados hasta terminar en punta aguda. Un pequeño grupo de cerdas aparece en la superficie dorsal del segmento (grabado 15).

Material examinado—Cubiertas cutáneas de dos especies (masculina i femenina) procedentes de Middle River, Maryland. 8 de junio de 1932".

Fox, al describir el segmento anal masculino de C. furens, dice que se parece mucho al de stellifer, pero sin presentar las cerdas que caracterizan el segmento anal de éste.

Añade además, que las pupas de stellifer i phlebotomus, fuera de no tener aspecto escamoso, se separan de las trompas de otras especies, por el hecho de estar divididas en dos o mas segmentos, sin tomar en cuenta los seudo-segmentos.

Distribución geográfica de esta especie

Fuera de Venezuela

Coquillet—

Malloch—Las Vegas N.M. nov. 8 (H.S. Barber); Rock Creek, Washington, D.C. sept. 9 (H.S. Barber) "biting"; Urbana, III. junio 6-19; South Haven, Mich. julio 15.

Fox—Middle River, Maryland.

En Venezuela

Iriarte—Macuto (Dpto. Vargas) D.F.

* * *

Culicoides arubae Fox i Hoffman 1944.

Fox. I. i Hoffman W.A. 1944. P. R. J. P. H. T. M. Vol. XX. No. 1. p. 108.

Culicoides arubae Ortiz.

Ortiz Ignacio C. Apuntas Cintíficos.

"Culicoides arubae (n. sp.) fig. 3.

Female—Head and palpi dark brown, antennae lighter. Eyes narrowly separated; palpus with second segment shorter than third, the latter expanded beyond the middle. Mesonotum greyish, diffused with many dark brown punctations some of which, in certain specimens, almost unite to form a longitudinal median line in the pre-scutellum depression; scutellum greyish at the sides, brown medially. Legs brown, some of the joints with yellow annulations. For wing pattern, see fig. 3. Abdomen greyish brown. Total length, about 1.3. mm.

Male—Hypopygium with apico-lateral processes long and triangular. Claspers not bent. Aedeagus with a low arch and a broad truncate terminal portion. Harpes stout basally, sinuous, somewhat enlarged in the middle with slender curved tips ending in sharp points.

Type material—Described from the female holotype, male allotype, and female paratype collected at Aruba, Dutch West Indies, in August or September 1929.

Remarks—This species is very similar to C. furens Poey, particularly in possesing dark punctations on the mesonotum. It differs from that species, however, in the pattern of light and dark spots of the wing".

He aquí la descripción de la pupa, que ya dos años antes había sido hecha por Fox, utilizando material de Root i Hoffmann:

"Especies Culicoides
(Nota: esta es la ninfa de una especie no descrita aún)

Trompa respiratoria—Mui larga i ostensible, dividida en numerossos pseudo-segmentos, excepto en el extremo distal. Más ancha en la base, con dos ramas bien diferenciadas, cada una terminada en un espiráculo. En el ápice hai unos once espiráculos, dispuestos conforme grabado 5.

Segmento anal (Macho). En general se parece algo en la forma a la del furens, pero mucho más grande, i mas o menos cuadrada. Para más detalles, véase grabado 2.

Material examinado—Cubiertas de piel de una ninfa hembra i dos machos, i trozos de otros dos ejemplares recogidos en cuevas de cangrejos en las Antillas Holandesas, en agosto de 1929".

Distribución geográfica de esta especie.

Fuera de Venezuela

Fox i Hoffmann—Aruba, Dutch West Indies, agost-septiembre 1929.

En Venezuela

Ortiz—En el Distrito Bolívar del Estado Zulia i Mene de Mauroa (Estado Falcón).

* * *

Culicoides heliconiae Fox i Hoffmann 1944

Fox I. i Hoffmann. 1944. P. R. J. P. H. and T. Med. Vol. XX. No. 1. p. 108.

"Culicoides heliconiae (n. sp.)

Female—Head dark brown; antennal segments white basally, brown distally. Eyes distinctly separated; palpi with second segment shorter than third, the latter moderately expanded at about the middle. Mesonotum with a whitish and light brown design on a dark brown ground; anteriorly the design consists of an irregular transverse dirty white band with a more or less square light brown median area that expands posteriorly into a shield-shaped pattern of a dirty white ground color, having laterally a longitudinal brown band and an inner prominent brown spot on each side; scutellum a light brown. Legs brown, lighter at the joints. For wing pattern, see fig. 1. Dorsum of abdomen a light brown, sides and venter dark brown. Total length, about 2.00 mm.

Male—Hypopygium of the venustus type. Apicolateral processes small. Claspers bent. Aedeagus flask-shaped with ventral and lateral marginal bands, the tip spatula-or ball-like. Harpes robust and triangular at the base, distally long, slender and pointed.

Type material—Described from the female holotype, male allotype, and female paratype collected at Maracay, Venezuela, august 2, 1927.

Remarks—This species is similar in size and general structure to C. variipennis Coq., differing from that species, however, in the arrangement of the light and dark spots of the wings".

Ya Fox (1942), había descrito antes la pupa, de material de Root i Hoofmann, que es como sigue:
"Especies Culicoides (3)
(grabados 19 i 24)
(nota: esta es la pupa de una especie no descrita aún).

Trompa respiratoria—De forma general semejante a la del guttipennis, mas o menos parecida a una trompeta, dividida en seudo-segmentos de aspecto escamoso. El tronco traqueal principal de la trompa no tiene ramas en la base. En el vértice hay implantadas diecisiete espiráculos, distribuidos conforme al grabado 19.

Segmento anal (femenino)—Grande, con apéndices alargados hacia afuera. Los apéndices terminan en puntas mui delicadas, sin manchas negras (v. grabado 24).

Material examinado—Piel de dos pupas de sexo femenino i de cuatro de sexo masculino, procedentes de plantas bromeliáceas de Maracay, Venezuela (2 de agosto de 1927).

Notas—La pupa de esta especie es semejante a la de guttipennis, de la cual se distingue por tener la trompa respiratoria desprovista de ramas basales en el tronco traqueal. Difiere asimismo, por este carácter de las otras especies incluidas en este articulo".

Distribución geográfica de esta especie
Fuera de Venezuela
No ha sido citada
En Venezuela

Fox i Hoffmann. Macaray (Estado Aragua).

* * *

Culicoides hoffmanni Fox 1946.

Fox Irving 1946. Annals of the Entomological Society of America. Vol. XXXIX. No. 2. June.

Culicoides hoffmanni Fox 1949.

Fox Irving. 1949. Bulletin of the Brooklyn Entomological Society. Vol. XLIV. No. 1. págs. 29. 34.
29-30.
"Culicoides hoffmanni n. sp.

Diagnosis: a small species, the female of which is about 1.00 mm. long, brown in color with a distinctive mesonotal pattern conspicuosly banded legs, and definite wing markings. The mesonotal pattern is similar to castillae new species, but the markings and structure of the wing are very different.

Description: Female. Head dark brown. Eyes narrowly separated. Antennae not suitable for study. Third palpal segment markedly swollen at the middle bearing a large circular sensory pit. Third segment longer than second.

Mesonotum with two triangular brown markings between which is a grayish area, which broadens posteriorly and includes two prominent dark spots in the prescutellar depression. Scutellum dark in the medial area, light at the sides. For further details of the mesonotal pattern see fig. 6. Legs dark brown, conspicuously banded; femora I and II with subapical lighter annulations, femora III uniform dark brown; all the tibiae with subbasal annulations and tibiae III with subapical ones as well. Abdomen dark brown; spermathecae double, subpsherical, one slightly larger than the other.

Wing (fig. 9) about 80 mm. long and 34 mm. wide, provided with macrotrichia in the apical region. Cell R5 with three light spots. Cell M1 with two light spots. Vein M2 obliterated, replaced by horizontally directed macrotrichia. Cells M2 and Cul with one light spot each. Second radial cell included in a dark spot which extends posteriorly to include most of the first radial cell. Radio-median cross vein indistint, located in a light spot. Subcosta and posterior portion of the radius obliterated.

Type material: Female holotype (mounted in balsam on a slide) and female paratype (pinned specimen) from Camuto Village, Trinidad, April 11, 1941, biting, the types selected from a small series''.

Distribución geográfica de esta especie.

Fuera de Venezuela

Fox - Camuto Village - Trinidad.

En Venezuela

Ortiz. En Mene de Mauroa (Estado Falcón).

* * *

Oecacta furens Poey 1851-54.

Poey. 1851-54. Mem. sobre la Hist. de la Isla de Cuba. Tomo I. p. 236-242.

Ceratopogon maculithorax Williston 1896.

Williston. 1896. Trans. Ent. Soc. Londres. pag. 277.

Culicoides furens Lutz 1912.

Lutz A. 1912. Mem. do Ins. O. Cruz. Tomo IV, Fasc. I.

Culicoides furens (= maculithorax Williston?) Lutz 1913.

Lutz A. 1913. Mem. do Ins. O. Cruz. Tomo V. Fasc. I.

Culicoides furens Hoffmann 1925.

Hoffmann W.A. 1925. Am. J. of Hyg. Vol. V. No. 3. p. 274.

Culicoides furens Painter. 1926.

Painter 1926. Ann. Rpts. United Fruit Co. Med. Dept. pág. 255.

Culicoides furens Macfie 1937.

Macfie 1937. Ann. and Mag. Nat. Hist. Vol. XX. pág. 10.

Culicoides furens da Costa Lima 1937.

da Costa Lima 1937. Mem. do Inst. O. Cruz. Tomo XXXII. Fasc. III. p. 414.

Culicoides furens Fox 1942.
Fox Irving 1942. P.R. of P.H. and Trop. Med. Vol. 17. No. 4.
Culicoides furens Vargas 1945.
Vargas Luis. 1945. Rev. Inst. Salub. i Enf. Trop. Vol. VI. No. I.
Culicoides furens Ortiz 1948.
Ortiz Ignacio C. 1948. Apuntes Científicos. Vol. I. No. 2.

EL JEJEN *

Oecacta furens Poey

Insecto díptero, furibundo habitador de playas.

Lámina 27

1. Cualquiera que sea, para el navegante y el poblador de las costas cubanas, la molestia que recibe de las sanguinarias costumbres de los *Mosquitos,* todo es poco comparado con las crueles agresiones de unas mosquitas imperceptibles que el vulgo ha aprendido a conocer a pesar de su pequeñez, y que distingue con el nombre de *Jejenes.* Si los naturalistas no lo conocen bien todavía, echen la culpa a su desidia y no a la falta de instrucciones que hayan encontrado en el país habitado por estos diminutos y furiosos enemigos. No se ignora en Europa que hay en las Antillas algunas especies del género *Culex,* llamadas en Francia *Cousins,* que afigen a los hombres hasta el punto de obligarlos a encender hogueras en el campo para ahuyentarlas con humo, y de dormir al abrigo de cortinas transparentes que se llaman mosquiteros; entre ellos el que en la Habana se muestra con patas alternativamente anilladas de blanco y negro, y que el Sr. Robineau-Desvoisdy denominó *Culex Moquito;* pero no se sabe todavía a qué género, ni siquiera a que familia pertenecen los *Jejenes,* que los viajeros llaman confusamente en lengua francesa *Maringouins, Moustiques, Mosquilles, Mostiques,* corruptelas de la voz española *Mosquita* o mosca pequeña; correspondiente a la palabra inglesa *Gnat.* Unos creen que es una especie de *Culex,* de pequeñas dimensiones; y estos lo llaman *Maringouin,* nombre que también se aplica a los *Mosquitos;* otros lo indican con nombres genéricos que ni siquiera pertenecen a la división de los dípteros de antenas largas como los que sospechan que sea un *Empis.* El sabio Latreille, en el Nuevo Diccionario de historia natural, edición de Deterville, dice que abunda en la Luisiana y le fué comunicado por el botánico Michaux, habiéndole parecido una especie del género Simulium, que llaman vulgarmente Moustique. Veremos que este género es distinto del Jején; pues es de la familia Tipularias, y ofrece antenas de once artículos.

* Esta descripción original la debemos al Dr. Fox, quien a su vez la obtuvo del Profesor Carlos G. Aguayo, de La Habana.

El mismo Latreille parece conocerlo así, pues se lamenta de la incuria de los naturalistas viajeros, que solamente lo han indicado como perteneciendo a una especie de díptero distinto del Culex, mínimo de cuerpo, cuya presencia no se anuncia con zumbidos, plaga enojosa para el hombre y los animales. "Es muy extraordinario, dice aquel príncipe de los Entomologistas, que los viajeros no se empeñen con frecuencia en recoger los objetos que más merecen nuestra atención: los mosquitos y los jejenes (maringouins et moustiques), que atormentan los habitantes de las regiones de América, carecen de observadores científicos".

2. La pequeñez de este insecto, lejos de ser para mí un motivo de aversión, me ha empeñado con frecuencia en su estudio, deseoso de vencer la dificultad que presenta su anatomía externa a los ojos armados de aparatos microscópicos, y he creído que aficionados a la entomología, agradecerían mis esfuerzos, por el ahorro de tiempo y trabajo que traen consigo las figuras aumentadas de la lámina 27. Este ha sido un resultado obtenido con la inspección no de uno o de pocos individuos, sino de un número de ellos considerable, principalmente para la representación de la trompa, que por ser corta me pareció al principio propia de Tipularias, o compuesta de dos piezas córneas, y fuí descubriendo otras poco a poco, hasta verlas claramente como está en la fig. 7, esto es, compuesta de seis piezas, sin contar la inferior que las abraza todas: lo mismo diré del número de artículos de las antenas; pues la dificultad de ver la 1ª bien distinta de la 2ª, me ha hecho dudar mucho tiempo, si eran 14 en lugar de 15. Si queda alguna ambigüedad de algunos puntos, la indicaré escupulosamente en el párrafo 6, teniendo por costumbre dar lo seguro como

3. Llámanse *Dípteros* los insectos de dos alas, y de boca propia para chupar. Los naturalistas dividen primordialmente este órden en *Nemocera y Brachycera,* a saber: antenas largas, filiformes, i antenas cortas: el Jején pertenece a la primera división, como muestra la figura 5. Los Nemóceros se subdividen en dos familias: la de los *Culícidos,* en que está el Mosquito común, y que tiene por caracteres un sifón u horador de seis piezas, largo y delgado y palpos rectos; y la de las *Tipularias,* que son muy zancudas, y tienen por caracteres un sifón de dos piezas corto y grueso, palpos encorvados. El Jején no pertenece a ninguno de estos dos extremos, y forma una familia nueva, intermedia, que llamo las *Ecactanas,* y se distingue por un sifón de sies piezas, como los Culicidios, y de trompa corta, palpos corvos, como las Tipularias. Es al mismo tiempo el único género, única especie de dicha familia.

4. *Género Ecacta.* El género *Oecacta,* que aquí establezco, viene de la palabra griega *Oicactes* que significa *habitador de playas,* y que se escribe en latín *Oecactes,* habiendo preferido abandonar la terminación *es* para prohijarla en la lengua latina, conforme al consejo de Fabricio que dice en su Filosofía entomológica, *Sonos nominum, quantum fiere potest, facilitandus, ideoque nec graeca, nec barbara admittimus; et terminationen graecam in latinam mutamus; vg. Saperdes in Saperda.* Unicamente se me

ofreció una duda sobre hacer el nombre masculino o femenino, séase *Oecactus* o *Oecacta* (Ecacto o Ecacta); pareciéndome que puesto que en español *el Jején* es masculino, lo mismo que *el Mosquito,* debía conservarlo este género en latín. Pero mi amigo el Dr. Gundlach, a quien consulté seriamente sobre este particular, me ha dado con donaire una respuesta que no creo indigna de la seriedad de este artículo, y que tomo bajo mi responsabilidad ya que me he dejado convencer por ella, por más que las compañeras del género *Homo* se empeñan en desmentirla: y es que el modo de embestir del Jején, calladamente y con daga corta, es propio del sexo femenino; siendo al contrario la guerra del Mosquito varonilmente declarada con música, y sostenida con lanza o espada larga. Esta opinión de mi docto amigo es conforme con la del Entomologista citado, que muda la *es* en *a.*

El género Ecacta, además de los caracteres de la familia que trae el párrafo 3, presenta antenas de 15 artículos y palpos de 5, sin ocelos en la parte superior de la cabeza, ni espinas en las tibias, ni vesículas en los tarsos, alas con pocas nervaduras y en gran parte escamosas. Los dos sexos difieren poco.

5. *Oecacta furens,* la furibunda Ecacta. Longitud, 2 milímetros, desde la extremidad de la boca hasta la punta de las alas; thorax de un gris-cobrizo, pareciendo bronceado, con manchas oscuras por encima y por los lados, abdómen negro patas blanquecinas, con las articulaciones negruzcas y un anillo de este color en medio del fémur y de la tibia; alas apareciendo, sin reflejo, blancas con manchas negras: frente y antenas rubias.

6. La lámina 27, representa: fig. 1, el tamaño natural del insecto, 2, el mismo aumentado, visto por encima, 3, el mismo medio lado, 4, la cabeza de medio lado, con numerosos ojos, 5, la misma por encima, con las antenas, 6, la misma por debajo, 7, la boca, con las piezas separadas, e indicación de los palpos, 8, 9, el balancín. La cabeza se dirige hacia abajo: está cubierta casi del todo por los ojos compuestos o reticulados, cada cornéola luciendo con un cerco oscuro, y más numerosos en la cara inferior; no hay ocelos u ojos sueltos de los que los naturalistas llaman con más propiedad *Stemata.*

El epístome y la frente forman una sola pieza, con la estrangulación en el medio, donde está la base de las antenas; las mejillas parecen existir entre las antenas y la boca; los que no he visto con claridad; las demás piezas del epicráneo están soldadas; por debajo no pude distinguir las piezas basilares. La boca lleva generalmente el nombre de trompa o *proboscis,* bien que este último se aplica con más especialdad a la parte inferior que sirve de estuche o vaina al sifón siendo para Savingny el labio propiamente tal, o labio inferior, y yo creo que debe considerarse como formado por la reunión de los palpos labiales: es escamoso, forma codo en el medio, y lleva labios terminales; no pudiendo afirmar si la flexibilidad que se nota en este órgano pende de la articulación del medio o de mayor número. Las seis piezas córneas del sifón (*haustellum,* en francés *sucoir)* son lisas, lustrosas, rubias; la impar superior o labro, ancha y reforzada en la línea media, bastante comprimida y de punta aguda; la inferior o lígula, con las mismas dimensiones, correspondiendo al labio, las mandíbulas laminosos, formando un cuchillo de punta esmerada; las maxilas lineares y agudas; los palpos o maxilares tienen de longitud los dos tercios del sifón, son escamosos y velludos, arrancan de la parte inferior de la cabeza, y se componen de 5 artículos, los tres primeros largos y en línea recta, los dos últimos cortos, encorvados y con tendencia a descansar, como un dedo, sobre la parte anterior y más globulosa del artículo 3°, por lo que he sospechado que en el acto de chupar puedan servir con los labios terminales de la trompa para sujetar el sifón. Las antenas se componen de 15 artículos, habiendo visto constantemente la articulación del 1° con el 2° y aún me parece haber visto el tórulo que sirve de base. El primer artículo tiene la forma de una pirámide trunca; el 2° perfectamente esférico y muy grande, el 3° menor y subglobuloso; los siete que siguen son un poco más pequeños, iguales entre sí, un poco más prolongados; los cinco últimos largos, cónicos, con la mayor anchura en la base, el último es el más largo: todos tienen pelos cortos y largos: reunidos alcanzan hasta la parte posterior del thorax. El primero y el segundo artículo del thorax parecen soldados por encima, aunque distintos por debajo, el 2° es muy ancho, bombeado; el 3° delgado y levantado: no he visto bien las soldaduras laterales, pero sí la posición de las patas, estando las cuatro posteriores contiguas y separadas de las primeras; el trocánter de aquellas más largas: las anteriores algo menores, las posteriores mayores; el fémur de estos bastante largo, los tarsos también; el primer artículo de los tarsos es tan largo como todos los otros tomados juntamente, y lo mismo sucede en los demás, no hay espinas ni vesículas, pero hay pelos por todas partes. El abdomen se compone de 9 artículos, si contamos como segmento abdominal el que lleva los balancines; toma una dirección secundante hasta el fin del 3° que es el más desarrollado. Las alas son anchas, cubiertas de escamas menudas algunas más largas sobre las nervuras y en algunos pliegues, con una franja notable en los bordes. Tiene la nervura costal, la prebasilar, la basilar, la postbasilar, la abdominal incompleta y la axilar; y además una radial corta, una cubital, una discoidal, y la anal; algunas en la base tienden a formar células intertorácicas: no hay más que una sola trasversa, ya que es la recurrente basilar. Las células son la costal, la basilar, la postbasilar, la anal, la abdominal estrecha, confundida con la axilar; y además la radial incompleta, la cubital y discoidal; estas tres sin recurrentes, son al mismo tiempo apicales. La estimática existe bien pronunciada. El color es como se ha expresado en el párrafo anterior: pero en cuanto a las alas se nota que según la reflexión de la luz cambia de visos, apareciendo a veces de un bello azul de ultramar con espacios dorados, los que en otras luces parecen blancos sobre fondo pardo-oscuro. Los balancines son amarillos. A veces he visto los segmentos abdominales bordados de blanco en las articulaciones: el Dr. Gundlach ha visto esto mismo en base del abdómen del macho. Los sexos son iguales, salvo los apéndices abdominales del macho que no he podido reconocer: las antenas en este parecen un poco más velludas.

7. Las playas de las Antillas y de los estados meridionales de la Unión Americana están plagadas de pequeños dípteros, que tal vez pertenecen a diferentes géneros, como induce a creerlo el reconocimiento de la Simulia presentada por Michaux al Sr. Latreille: ignoro por lo tanto si la Ecacta furibunda o el Jején de Cuba es exclusivo en esta Isla. Solo podemos asegurar que entre todas las especies es de las más atormentadoras. ¿Quién podrá decir donde se cría la larva, y quien dará su descripción? Hay un dicho entre nosotros que expresa la dificultad de este descubrimiento; pues para ponderar el alcance de un hombre sabichoso, se dice que sabe donde el Jején puso el huevo. Lo único que sobre este capítulo podemos sospechar, es que la larva es acuática, y se cría en los focos de fermentación marina, a lo menos de agua salobre, porque solemos hallar los jejenes en las playas de la mar o en sus inmediaciones, aconteciendo rara vez encontrarlos en el interior de las tierras. Cuando más abundan es en los tiempos de calma y al acabarse el día: el viento los ahuyenta y los obliga a refugiarse en las malezas y a remontar los ríos; así es que en Cojímar, cuando no los hallaba en la playa, los iba a buscar con fruto a media legua de la boca, esto es, al pie de la loma que está enfrente a Guanabacoa. Acaso se cría en árboles marítimos. Pocos he encontrado en Cayoblanco, ensenada de Cárdenas, donde no hay más que arenas y mangles; y muchos en Cayo-Galindo que abunda en vegetación variada. Era allí tanta la abundancia en el mes de Agosto que anublaban el aire, se agolpaban a los ojos y se introducían por las fosas nasales hasta penetrar en la tráquea-arteria; yo fuí con ánimo de hacerles la lguerra, y me retiré vencido, consolándome con la fábula del león abatido por una mosca. Huyendo de esta playa, tienen las embarcaciones que mantenerse a una distancia de media legua del litoral, y los navegantes renuncian a la seguridad y placer de dormir en tierra, para no pasar la noche en compañia de aquellos habitantes inhospitalarios.

Cualquiera, al oír esta relación, pensará que la isla de Cuba es un país inhabitable, a lo menos en sus costas y riberas; pero afortunadamente no es así. Los puertos de mar, como son los de la Habana, Matanzas, Cárdenas & donde domina el trato y comercio de los hombres, no están invadidos por las legiones agrestes de Jejenes, como los cayos y costas solitarias, rodeadas de montes y espesuras: parece que los vegetales son necesarios a su existencia, no como criaderos de larvas, sino como abrigos seguros contra ventarrones y los excesivos ardores del sol a ciertas horas del día. Varias playas he recorrido inpunemente; y en las más afligidas por este linaje de insectos, hay meses, días y horas de descanso.

La picada del Jején es dolorosa, no menos que la del Mosquito; pero el Jején es más molesto, porque es más difícil de apartar. Invisible enemigo, y audaz, penetra por todas las aberturas que dejan el cuerpo indefenso; y cuando se viene a sentir su aguda lanceta, está enterrada hasta la base; por ser más corta que la del Mosquito, y más robusta. La actividad del veneno que vierte en la herida es mayor en proporción; siendo muy probable que si el insecto fuera más corpulento, causara efectos peligrosos, conspirando en nuestro daño la calidad y la cantidad del fluido derramado.

Para preservar sus cuerpos desnudos de las picadas de los mosquitos y jejenes, acostumbraban los Indios untar la piel de cuerpos aceitosos. Los autores indican el limón y el vinagre.

Mayo de 1853.

SUMARIUM

XIX—Oecacta furens, Poey.

1. 2. Dipterum vix hactenus a Culicibus distractum: vulgo nominatur Jejen.

3. Familiam Ecactanam costituere licet: hace inter Culicidam et Tipulariam, diptera Nemocera format; his characteribus sistens; haustellum breve, setae 6, palpi curvati.

4. Genus Oecacacta, graece Oicactes (littorens incola), recte terminationem latinam sumpsit: sit jubet Fabricius. Phil. entom: p. 114, 31. Articulis antennarum 15, palpi 5; stemmatibus, spinis tibiarum, vesiculis tarsalibus nullis; alis squamosis, numero cellularum parco: Sexus alter similis.
5. Species distinguitur longitudine maxima 2 mill.; Thorace aeneo, fusco punctato; abdomine fusco; pedibus albidis, annulo articulari fusco altero medio femorali et tibiali; fronte atque ante nis rufis; alisalbicans tibus, fusco muculatis; haltere fulvo. tab. 27.

6. Explicatio tabulae. Descriptio nimia. Infra vide.

7. Historia Infra vide.

ESTRAITS

6. La tete se dirige en bas; les corneoles offrent un cercle obscur; l'epistome et le front forment une seule piece; je crois que la joue existe separamente; je n'ai pu voir les pieces basilaires; toutes les sp es su sucoir sont cornees et nues; la trompe ou levre inferieure, qui les enveloppe, est ecailleuse. Si. Mr. Latreille a bien fait de donner le nom de ligule a la piece inferieure du sucoir (la lange de Savigny), on pourrait admettre que 1 (etui qu'on a nomme levre inferieure represente les palpes labiaux; cet etui forme un coude au milieu de la longueur, et peut-etre est-il compose de plusieurs articles. Les palpes maxillaires ont leur base au dessous de la tete; les deux derniers articles paraissent par leur courbure propes otnir le sucoir dans ses fonctions. Un des segments de l'abdomen le 3° si je ne me trompe, est beaucoup plus grand que les autres. Les nervures des ailes sont la costale, la prebasilaire, la basilaire, la postbasilaire, l'abdominaile incomplete et l'anale; il n'y a qu'une recurrente, c'est la basilaire. Les cella

basilaire, la postbasilaire, l'abdominale incomplete et l'abdominate etroite, qui se confond l'axillaire; de plus la radiale incomplete, la cubitale, et la discoidale que se prolongent jusqu'au bord apical; la cellule stigmatique est bien prononcee, les interthoraciques ne sont qu'ebauchee. La couleur des ailes est changeante; car la lumiere sons certains angles les colore de blu a taches doree.

7. Je laisee le nom vulgaire de Maringouins ou Cousins, ou especes du genre Culex, en espagnol Mosquito, que l'on trouve aux Antilles; et j'applique le nom de Moustique au Jejen de Cuba et autres dipteres du meme groupe. Il parait que Mr. Latreille l'a un momento sous les yeux, et l'a pris par une Simule, genre auquel il resemble par la trompe courte et ailes elargies. Ce beau des hommes et des animaux est plus a craindre que celui des maringouins; car les moustiques forment des nuees sur certainnes plages; et leur extreme petitesse leur permet de frapper les yeux, et de penetrer dans les fosses nasales: leur piqueurs n'est pas moins cruelle que celle des grands dipteres. Heureusement ou ne les trouve pas partout; et meme dans les lieux qu'ils frequentent le plus, il y a des mois, des jours et des heures de repit. Ils fuyent les coups de vent, et l'ardeur du soleil: aussi cherchent ils des cotes abritees et boisees. On ne les guere qu'aux embouchures des rivieres et au voisinage de la mer''.

Lutz sospecha que maculithorax Williston es sinónimo de furens. Copiamos un párrafo de su trabajo del año 13, que dice, refiriéndose a maculithorax:

''Esta especie foi descrita por Williston com o nome generico de Ceratopogon, servindo de tipo um unico exemplar proveniente de Sao Vicente (Antilhas). Examinei dois exemplares procedentes do Museu de Washington; foram determinados como Culicoides (Oecacta) furens Poey i llevam o rotulo Isl. de Pines, Columbia (E'a Isla dos Pinos perto de Cuba). Combinam tao bem com muitos exemplares colecionados aqui e caraterisados por varias particularidades que nao pode haver duvida sobre a identidade de especie''.

Hoffman se inclina en este mismo sentido i tomamos de su trabajo del año 25, lo que sigue:

''Maculithorax is undoubtedly a synonym of furens. While Poey's description is extremely faulty the wing diagram and account regarding its environment cause no uncertainty as to which form was under consideration. The specimens in the National Museum labeled furens and maculithorax show no differences. Mr. Malloch with whom the question was taken up, also inclines to this opinion''.

Fox, el año 42, hace una descripción de la pupa, como sigue:

''Trompa respiratoria—Corta, estrecha, perfectamente dividida en dos grandes segmentos, además de los seudo-segmentos. De los dos segmentos, el basal está más esclerotizado que el distal, i parece conformarse sobre el otro como si fuera una vaina. Dos ramas prominentes, provistas cada una con un espiráculo en el segmento basal i otro en el distal. En el ápice existen unos cuatro espiráculos dispuestos según aparecen en el grabado 9.

Segmento anal—(masculino). Semejante al del stellifer, pero sin los grupos de cerdas que caracterizan el segmento anal de esta especie.

Material examinado.—Piel de una pupa de un ejemplar macho, recogido en San Juan de Puerto Rico.

Notas—Las trompas respiratorias de estas especies stellifer i phlebotomus difieren de las trompas de otras especies en que están divididas perfectamente en dos o más segmentos, además de los seudo-segmentos. Las pupas de estas tres especies se caracterizan, además, por tener las trompas respiratorias sin aspecto escamoso''.

Distribución geográfica de esta especie

Fuera de Venezuela

Poey—

Lutz—En la Costa del Brasil.

Hoffmann—Havana, Cuba (J.R. Taylor); Cárdenas, Cuba. June (E.A. Schwarz); Laguna del Carmen, Mex., June 26, 1903 (Dr. A. Duges); Perihueta, Mex. (Dr. A. Duges); Port of Spain, Trinidad (F.W. Urich); Río Piedras, Porto Rico, July and Sept. 1921 (Dr. F.M. Root); Aguirre, P.R. August 1921 (Dr. Root); Palm Beach, Fla. (E.P. Sedgewick); Gatum, Canal zone, Panamá, May 15, 1914 (Dr. S.T. Darling). También ha sido citado en St. Vincent (Willistón); Jamaica (Edwards), (Townsend); en State Vera Cruz, Mex. (Townsend); Costa del Brasil (Lutz); San Salvador del grupo Bahamas, verano de 1923 (Dr. P. Barrtrch). Por último, Hoffmann revisando ejemplares del National Museum de Washington ha encontrado ejemplares capturados en Santiago, en la Costa mexicana del Pacífico.

Vargas—Costa del Golfo de México (Root i Hoffmann 1937)

En Venezuela—

Ortiz—Distrito Bolívar (Estado Zulia)

Briceño Iragorry—Laguna de la Reina en Higuerote (Estado Miranda).

* * *

Culicoides debilipalpis Lutz 1913.

Lutz A. 1913. Mem. do Inst. O. Cruz. Tomo V. Fasc. I.

Culicoides debilipalpis da Rocha Lima 1937.

da Rocha Lima A. 1937. Mem. do Inst. O. Cruz. Tomo XXXII. Fasc. III.

Culicoides debilipalpis Vargas 1945.

Vargas Luis. 1945. Rev. Inst. Salub. i Enf. Trop. Vol. VI. No. 1.

Culicoides debilipalpis Briceño Iragorry 1946.

Briceño Iragorry Leopoldo. 1946. Bol. Lab. C. Razetti. Año VI. No. 19-20.

"Culicoides debilipalpis n. sp.

O: Comprimento do corpo e da aza ca. de 1 mm., largura desta 0.36-0.38 mm. Cor geral parda.

Antenas com pelos de brilho branco; palpos com pequeno segmento basal, o segundo bastante comprido, o terceiro um pouco espessado com abertura subterminal do pequeno orgam palpal, quarto e quinto como de costume. Occiput mais escuro do que os apendices.

Escudo mais escuro do que o resto de torax.

Abdome pardo um pouco amarelado.

Pernas com os joelho escuros, os primeiros pares com anel claro de cada lado, o ultimo com anel branco-amarelado só na base e no apice a tibia. Esporao do primeiro par claro.

Azas com costa terminada no fim dos 3/5 basais, com muitas manchas claras e uma bastante escura no estigma; costa e subcosta marcadas com riscos escuros. Alguns pelos enabertura do orgam palpal no meio da metade apical e dirijida para diante. Tromba castanha, do comprimento dos palpos.

Torax pardacento, em cima trez estrias escuras, formando un fechado por diante.

Abdome pardo, mais escuro em cima e com pelos maiores no apice.

Pernas pardo-amarelas, as tibias e o ultimo femur mais escuros; os pares anteriores com os joelhos mais claros, amarelados, a tibia de atraz nas duas extremidades com zona bastante larga de cor amarela; unhas simples com angulo um pouco saliente. Tibia I com esporao comprido e escuro; II inerme, III um pouco alargado no apice com um espinho curto e escuro seguido de alguns mais compridos e claros.

Azas em geral bastante escuras com desenho muito caracteristico; as zonas claras em forma de manchas ou estrias. Na costa trez man chas escuras. Nervuras normais e espurias marcadas de escuro, a veia transversal obliqua e em parte largamente marcada de preto.

Halteres pardo-amarelados, a base mais clara.

O macho se distingue pelos caracteres de costume, a parte basal da pinca anal mui grossa.

A especie se reconhece facilmente a olho nú pelo tamanho maior e as azas muito variegadas. As femeas picam o homem, mas nao com muita frequencia e atacam tambem os bovinos; ambos os sexos sao apanhados á luz com bastante facilidade. Podem tambem ser obtenidos em aparelhos que cobrem o fundo do mar, a seco nas marés pequenas. Ocorrem no Rio de Janeiro e na Bahía, onde pareciam mais abundantes.

As ninfas sao maiores que as ninfas das outras especies; as pontas terminais sao dirijidas para atraz e tem a extremidade preta. A rejiao do clipeo com espinhos finos e curtos".

Tomamos de da Rocha Lima, lo que sigue:

"No material de C. insignis Lutz, ao lado de exemplares desta especie apanhados em Angra dos Reis (Edo. Rio, XII 1913) pelo Dr. L. Travassos e montados em laminas por Lutz, tres a marjem da aza e as nervuras que sao lijeiramente tarjadas de pardo sepia.

Recebi esta especie de Anhemby no Estado de Sao Paulo e apanhei outras femeas em Formoso (Serra de Bocaina), em cavalos, na hora do crepusculo. Parece atacar tambem as pessoas".

da Rocha Lima, examinando los Culicoides recogidos por Kumm en Pará, encontró C. debilipalpis, etiquetados como ejemplares capturados en el río Maruará (Curralinho).

Distribución geográfica de esta especie

Fuera de Venezuela

Lutz A. en Anhemby (Estado de Sao Paulo); en Formoso (Serra de Bocaina).

da Rocha Lima—en Río Maruarú (Estado de Pará).

En Venezuela

Briceño Iragorry—En Los Teques (Edo. Miranda) i en las inmediaciones de La Victoria (Edo. Aragua).

Culicoides insignis Lutz 1913.

Lutz A. 1913. Mem. do Inst. O. Cruz. Tomo V. Fasc. I.

Culicoides insignis da Rocha Lima 1937.

da Rocha Lima. 1937. Mem. do Inst. O. Cruz. Tomo XXXII. Fasc. III.

Culicoides insignis Vargas 1945.

Vargas Luis. 1945. Rev. Inst. Salub. i Enf. Trop. Vol. VI. No. I.

Culicoides insignis Ortiz 1949.

Ortiz Ignacio C. 1949. Bol. Lab. Cli. Razetti. Año IX. No. 29-30.

"Culicoides insignis n. sp.

o: Cor geral pardo-enegrecida; comprimento do corpo puoco menos de 2, da aza 1.5 mm. Antenas pardo-acinzentadas; o toro pardo avermelhado, de tamanho regular, a base dos segmentos um mais clara. Palpos castanhos, o primeiro segmento curto, como tambem o quarto e quinto; o segundo e terceiro mais compridos, este ultimo um tanto dilatado, a ha alguns especimens de um outro Culicoides. Nos rotulos dessa lamina le-se a indicacao: "Culicoides flavivenula Lutz e Culicoides insignis Lutz. Tapuhyba, Angra dos Reis XII-13, Dr. Travassos".

Os exemplares dessa outra especie C. flavivenula, provavelmente por esquecimento, nao foram descriptos por Lutz em seu trabalho. Creio que elle adoptou o nome flavivenula porque nos azas nao se ve, somo em insignis, as nervuras r-m e R4 ÷ 5 enfuscadas.

Alem dos caracteres já indicados na chave, Culicoides flavivenula Lutz distingue-se de Culicoides insignis Lutz pelo aspecto do 3° segmento do palpo, como se pode ver comparando com as figuras.

Nos demais caracteres as duas especies sao extremamente semelhantes".

Distribución geográfica de esta especie

Fuera de Venezuela

Lutz—En Río de Janairo i Bahía (Brasil)
da Rocha Lima—Angra dos Reis (Edo. de Río); Bahía (Brasil).

En Venezuela

Ortiz—en Mene de Mauroa (Estado Falcón).

* * *

Culicoides acotylus Lutz 1913.

Lutz A. 1913. Mem. do Inst. O. Cruz. i Tomo V. Fasc. I. p. 69.

C. acotylus? Ortiz 1949.

Ortiz Ignacio C. 1949. Bol. Lab. Cli. Razetti. Año IX. No. 29-30.

"Culicoides acotylus n. sp

o Cor geral parda, em grandes exemplares o comprimento do corpo ca. de 1.6, da aza de 1.5 e a largura aza de 0.6 m.m.

Cabeca chocolate, o occiput com brilho esbranquicado e alguns pelos mais claros; tromba cilindrica de 0.25 mm. de comprimento; palpos pouco mais longos, com 5 segmentos distintos, os ultimos quatro progressivamente mais compridos na ordem seguinte: 4, 5, 2, 3, o terceiro articulo entumecido toro fusiforme, mas sem orgam cupuliforme. Antenas: O toro castanho, o flajelo pardo-acinzentado, tendo os oito primeiros segmentos bastante curtos, os outros pouco mais compridos com excecao do ultimo que é mais de 11/2 vezes mais comprido do que o penultimo, sem prolongamento, mas com cerda sub-apical bastante comprida.

Torax chocolate, o escudo com pelos claros espacados e densamente pontilhado de papilas microscopicas transparentes que macroscopicamente aparecem como incrustacao de brilho branco, formando manchas ovalares cujos contornos mudam conforme a posicao; no escudo sao lonjitudinais, no escutelo e no metatorax transversais.

Abdome com poucos pelos, pardo, as membranas laterais enegrecidas com dobras e puntuacoes elevadas escuras, muito densas.

Pernas de pardo de sepia, mais ou menos, carregado; a base de todos os femures mais clara, como tambem a das tibias, principalmente das quatro posteriores, e a do maior numero dos tarsos. A ultima tibia tem tambem o apice branco, porem um tanto amarelado. Tibias I e III com esporoes pardos. Unhas sem particularidades.

Azas: Terceira nervura separada da subcostal em toda e sua extensao, espessada e enfuscada na sua parte apical, a quarta e quinta enforquilhada; todas elas, incluindo a transversal, marcadas de pardo. Pelos mais compridos, em fileiras paralelas ás nervuras e espalhados, principalmente no terco apical.

O desenho apparece na fig. 1 da estampa 8.

Halteres bastante claros, apenas a face apical mais escura".

Distribución geográfica de esta especie

Fuera de Venezuela

Lutz—En Salto Augusto, Río Tapajoz (Brasil)

En Venezuela

Ortiz—En Mene de Mauroa (Estado Falcón).

* * *

Culicoides maruim Lutz 1913.

Lutz A. 1913. Mem. do Inst. O. Cruz. Tomo V. Fasc. I. pág. 48.

Culicoides maruim Vargas 1945.

Vargas Luis, 1945. Rev. Inst. Salub. i Enf. Trop. Vol. VI. No. I.

Culicoides maruim Briceño Iragorry 1949.

Briceño Iragorry. 1949. Bol. Lab. Cli. Razetti. Año IV. No. 29-30.

Culicoides maruim n. sp.

o: Cor geral enegrecida; comprimento do corpo ca. de 1.75; das azas ca de 1.4 mm. por 0.65 de largura.

Trompa castanha; palpos pardo acinzentados, o articulo basal curto, o segundo comprido, subcilindrico, o terceiro em forma de fuso truncado nas extremidades, sem depressao apreciavel, os ultimos relativamente curtos, cilindricos ou ovoides. Antenas pardo-acinzentadas, o tóro pardo-ocraceo, segundo e ultimo segmento mais compridos do que os visinhos, o ultimo com pequena cerda apical. Occiput com pelos maiores. Olhos escuros com pigmento vermelho.

Torax pardo (na preparacao microscopica cor de mogno); o escudo, com duas faixas lonjitudinais indistintas e o matanoto um pouco mais escuros, o escutelo um pouco mais claro.

Abdome pardo, com indicacao duma faixa dorsal, formada de manchas mais escuras.

Pernas, inteiramente pardo-ocraceas nas preparacaes e enegrecidas nos exemplares secos. Esporoes das tibias anteriores pardo-amarelos, tibias no meio com apice hialino, inermes; as posteriores tem no apice pouco dilatado um ou dois espinhos curtos e escuros, sucedidos por um pente de espinhos claros, primeiramente compridos e torando-se gradualmente mais curtos.

Azas pontilhadas de pelos microscopicos pretos, um pouco mais claros nas zonas hialinas; os pelos maiores, distribuidos entre as nervuras; muito caducos e deixando no cair um resto que aparece como escamula microscopica. A costa, que ocupa 5/7 da marjem anterior, as nervuras lonjitudinais e transversal obliquas marcadas de cor escura. As manchas hialinas de precepcao menos facil do que em outras especies. Perto do apice ha uma mancha parda com direcao obliqua.

Halteres claros na base, tornando-se pardo-acinzentados, na estremidade.

O macho se distingue apenas pelos caracteres sexuais e pelas dimensoes menores. Pode ser apanhado á luz ou nas janelas dos quartos''.

Esta especie é o verdadeiro mariim dos Estados Rio de Janeiro e Sao Paulo, mas a sua zona estende-se mui mais lonje. Na Bahia é comum na zona do mangue. Recebi de Washington exemplares de TRINIDAD determinados como C. phlebotomus Will., o que certamente é um erro. E'sempre periodico e proprio da vizinhanca do mangue, aparecendo ás vezes com tanta abundancia, que as outras especies parecem raras, comparadas com ela. Pica indiferentemente pessoas e animais maiores, cavalos, mulas, bois e caes, atacando tambem passaros e animais menores.

As larvas sao dificeis de achar; vivem sem duvida no mar, mas muito escondidas no lodo; os casulos sao encontrados vasios e, ás vezes, a inda cheios na superficie do lodo ou boiando; deitadas sobre areia humida, dao a imajem carateristica. Todavia a sua procura dá muito trabalho e o resultado nao está em relacao com a grande abundancia com a qual os adultos aparecem nas mesmas ocaioes. Obtive a postura in vitro mas nunca a observei no mangue. Os ovos de forma de banana sao postos isoladamente e torna-se completamente negros. O casulo na sua forma geral, se parece com os das outras especies.

A imajem se carateriza pela cor enegrecida, as pernas escuras, o desenho das azas, e principalmente, a falta dum orgam palpal distinto''.

Distribución geográfica de esta especie.

Fuera de Venezuela.

Lutz—en los Estados de Río de Janeiro i Sao Paulo (Brasil).

En Venezuela.

Briceño Iragorry—en un manglar cercano a Higuerote (Edo. Miranda), llamado Los Totumos.

* * *

Listas de las especies de Culicoides encontradas en América (Norte, Centro i Sur)

C. acotylus Lutz 1913.
C. albomacula Root i Hoffman 1937
C. amazonicus Macfie 1935
C. arboricola Root i Hoffmann 1937
C. arubae Fox i Hoffmann 1944
C. bambusicola Lutz 1913
C. baueri Hoffmann 1925
C. biguttatus Coquillet 1901
C. borinqueni Fox i Hoffmann 1944
C. canithorax Hoffmann 1925
C. chiopterus Meigen 1830
C. cockerelli Coquillet 1901
C. cockerelli var. tristriatulus Hoffmann 1925
C. columbianis Kieffer 1917
C. copiosus Root i Hoffmann 1937
C. crepuscularis Malloch 1915
C. dampfi Root i Hoffmann 1937

C. dasyophrus Macfie 1940
C. debilipalpis Lutz 1913
C. debilipalpis var. glabior Macfie 1940
C. decor Williston 1896
C. diabolicus Hoffmann 1925
C. flavivenula Lutz 1937 (da Rocha Lima)
C. fluvialis Macfie 1940
C. germanus Macfie 1940
C. gigas Root i Hoffmann 1937
C. guttatus Coquillet 1904
C. guttipennis Coquillet 1901
C. haematopotus Malloch 1915
C. hoffmani Fox
C. heliconiae Fox i Hoffmann 1944
C. hieroglyphicus Malloch 1915
C. hirtipes Kieffer 1917
C. hirtulus Coquillet 1900
C. hollensis Melander i Brues 1903
C. horticola Lutz 1913
C. hylas Macfie 1940
C. inamollae Fox i Hoffmann 1944
C. indianus Macfie 1932
C. insignis Lutz 1913
C. loughnani Edwards 1922
C. loughnani var. jamaicensis Hoffmann 1925
C. luteovenus Root i Hoffmann 1937
C. lutzi da Costa Lima 1937
C. maruim Lutz 1913
C. melleus Coquillet 1901
C. mississipiensis Hoffmann 1926
C. multipunctatus Malloch 1915
C. nanus Root i Hoffmann
C. niger Root i Hoffmann 1937
C. nocivum Harris 1862
C. obsoletus Meigen 1818
C. oliveri Fox i Hoffmann 1944
C. pachimerus Lutz 1914
C. palmerae James 1943
C. paraensis Goeldi 1905
C. phlebotomus Williston 1896
C. pictipennis Philippi 1865
C. piliferus Root i Hoffmann 1937
C. pulchripennis Macfie 1939
C. pulimus Winnertz 1852
C. pusillus Lutz 1913

C. recifensis Simoes Barbosa 1943
C. reticulatus Lutz 1913
C. riethi Kieffer 1914
C. sanctae-martae Kieffer 1917
C. scopus Root i Hoffmann 1937
C. setifer Lutz 1913
C. simulans Root i Hoffmann 1937
C. sordidellus Zetterstedt 1828
C. spinosus Root i Hoffmann 1937
C. stellifer Coquillet 1901
C. stonei James 1943
C. stylifer Lutz 1913
C. trinidadensis Hoffmann 1925
C. undecimpunctatus Kieffer 1917
C. unicolor Coquillet 1901
C. venustus Hoffmann 1925
C. variipennis Coquillet 1901
C. villosipennis Root i Hoffmann 1927
C. villosipes Kieffer 1917
C. yukonensis Hoffmann 1925

* * *

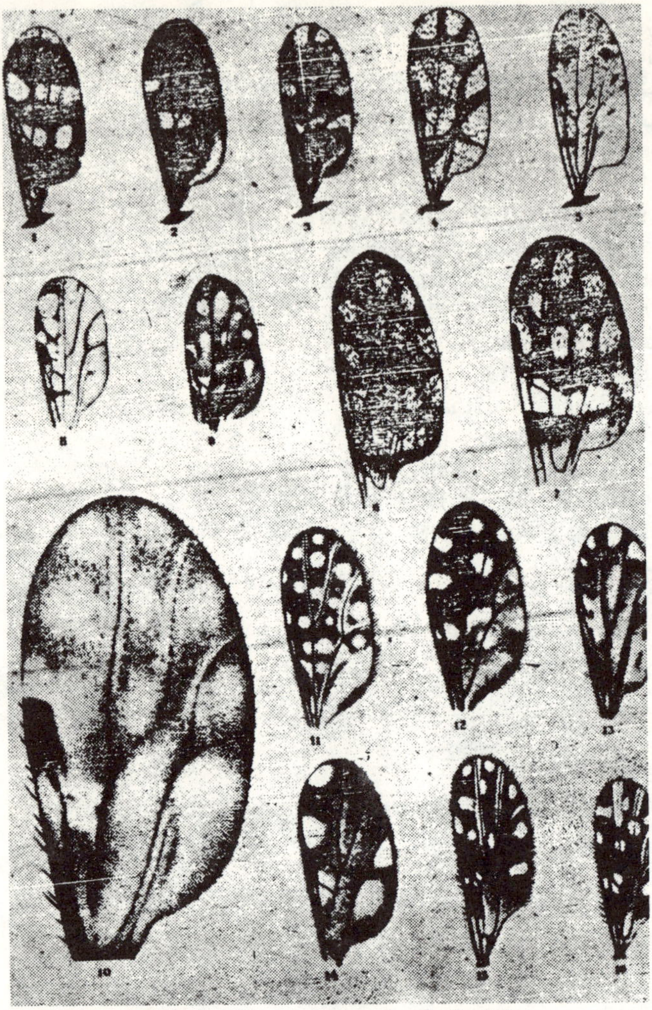

Plancha No. 1 (tomada de Lutz)

fig. 1. Ala de hembra de C. varius Winnertz.
fig. 2. Ala de hembra de C. fascipennis Staeg.
fig. 3. Ala de hembra de C. pictipennis Staeg.
fig. 4. Ala de hembra de C. arcuatus Winnertz.
fig. 5. Ala de hembra de C. pulicaris L.
fig. 6. Ala de hembra de C. marmoratus Skuse.
fig. 7. Ala de hembra de molestus Skuse.
fig. 8. Ala de hembra de C. maculithorax Williston.
fig. 9. Ala de hembra de C. phlebotomus.
fig. 10. Ala de hembra de C. paraense G.
fig. 11. Ala de hembra de C. pictipennis Philippi.
fig. 12. Ala de hembra de C. milnei Austen.
fig. 13. Ala de hembra de C. brucei Austen.

fig. 14. Ala de hembra de C. grahami Austen.
fig. 15. Ala de hembra de C. stellifer Coquillet.
fig. 16. Ala de hembra de C. guttipennis Coquillet.

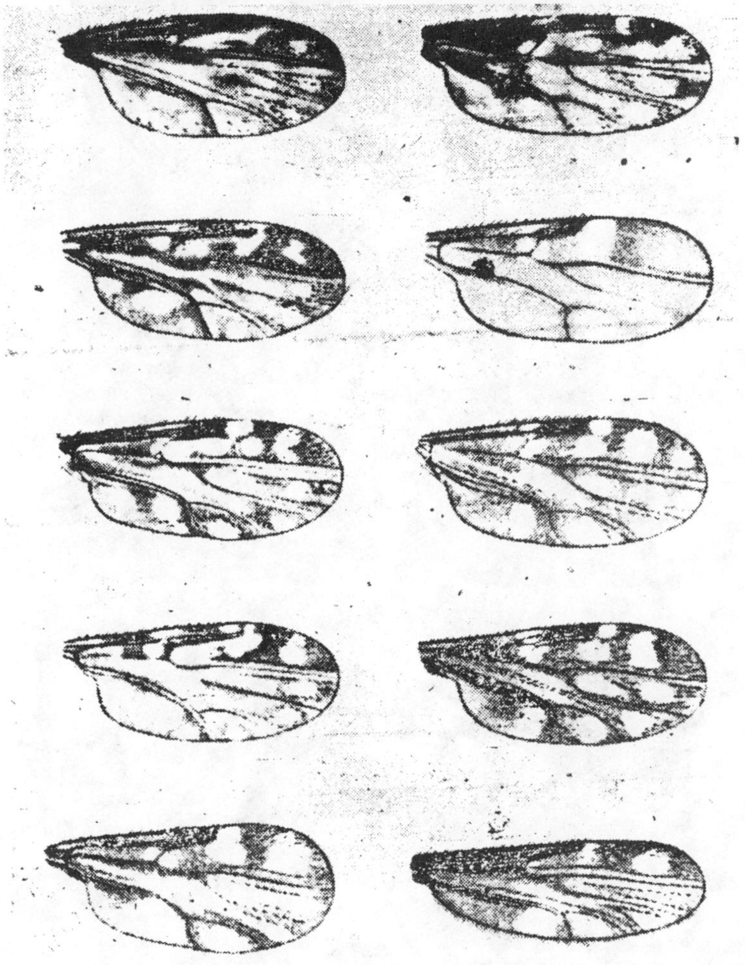

Plancha No. 2 (tomada de Lutz)

fig. 1. Ala de hembra de C. maruim L.
fig. 2. Ala de hembra de C. reticulatus.
fig. 3. Ala de hembra de C. insignis L.
fig. 4. Ala de hembra de C. pusillus.
fig. 5. Ala de hembra de C. maculithorax.
fig. 6. Ala de hembra de C. paraensis.
fig. 7. Ala de hembra de C. guttatus.
fig. 8. Ala de hembra de C. debilipalpis.
fig. 9. Ala de hembra de C. horticola.
fig. 10. Ala de hembra de C. bambusicola.

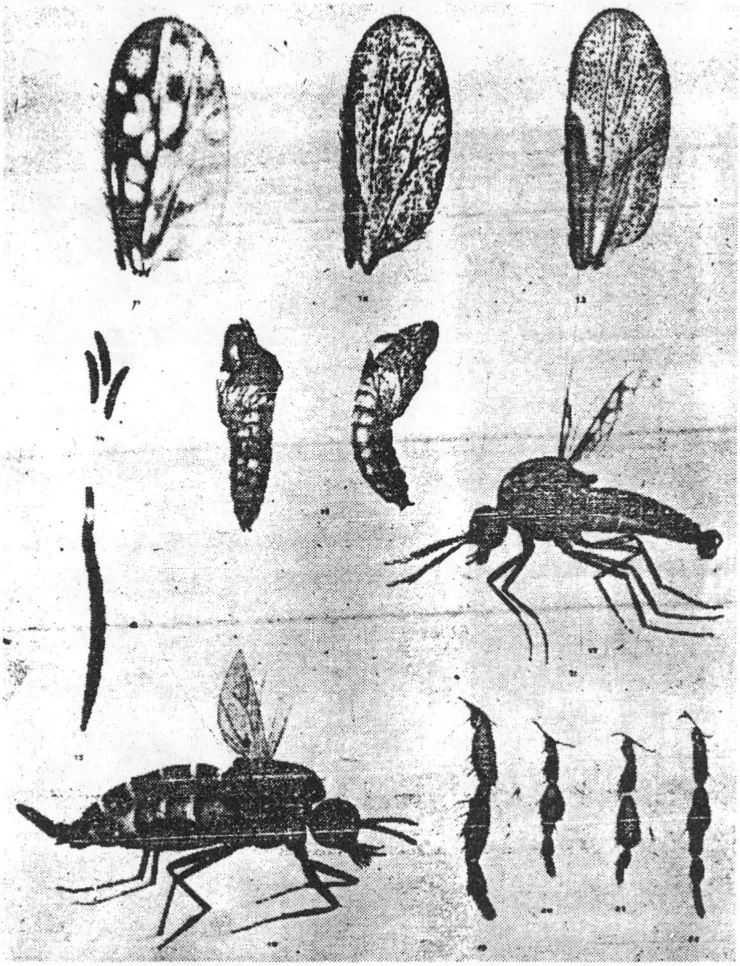

Plancha No. 3 (tomada de Lutz)

fig. 11. Ala de C. acotylus.
fig. 12. Ala de C. stylifer.
fig. 13. Ala de C. setifer.
fig. 14. Huevos de C. maruim.
fig. 15. Larva De C. reticulatus.
fig. 16. Ninfa de C. maruim.
fig. 17. Macho de C. reticulatus.
fig. 18. Tersesthes brasiliensis. hembra.
fig. 19. Palpo C. maruim.
fig. 20. Palpo C. reticulatus.
fig. 21. Palpo C. acotylus.
fig. 22. Palpo C. stylifer.

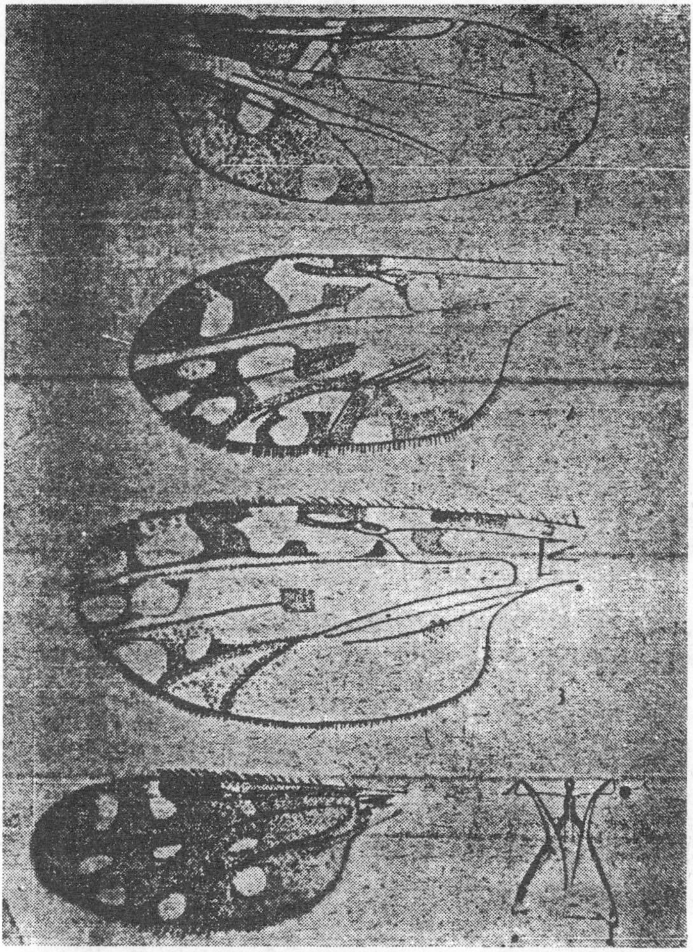

Plancha No. 4 (tomada de Fox i Hoffmann)

fig. 1. Ala de hembra de C. heliconiae.
fig. 2. Ala de hembra de C. inamollae.
fig. 3. Ala de hembra de C. arubae.
fig. 4. Ala de hembra de C. borinqueni.
fig. 5. Aedeagus i harpes de C. olivieri.

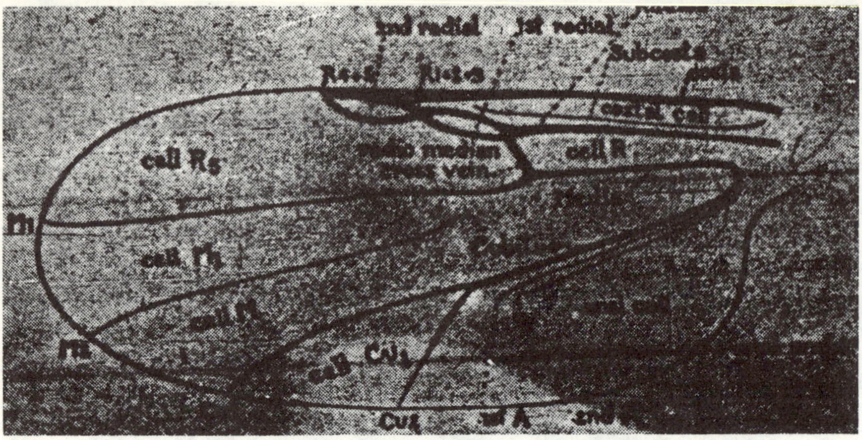

Plancha No. 5. (tomada de Hoffmann)

fig. 1. Terminología adoptada para las células i nervaduras del ala de un Culicoides.

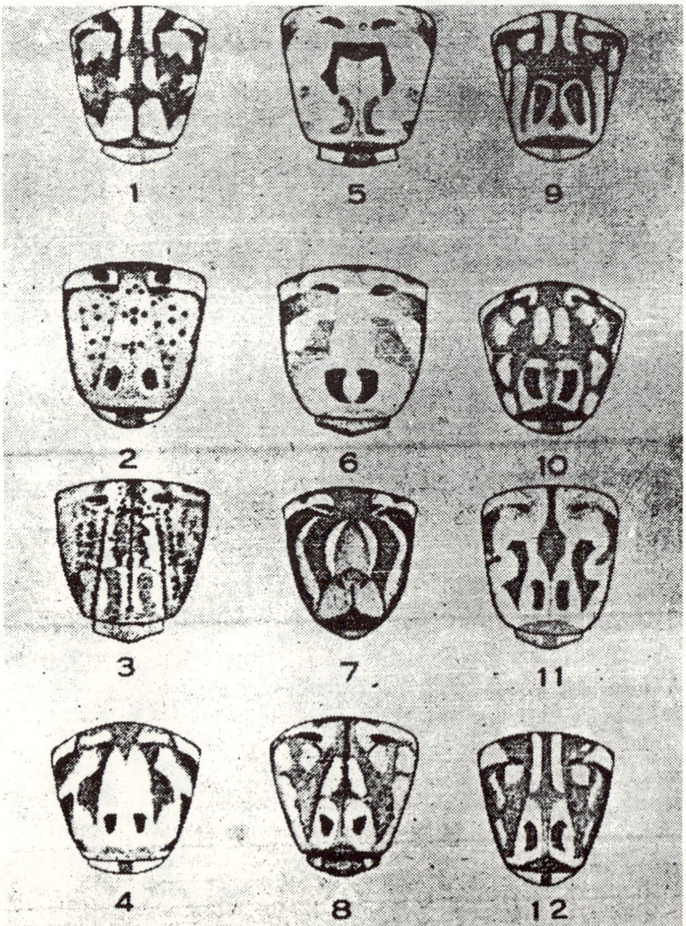

Plancha No. 6 (tomada de Hoffmann)

Diagrama de dibujos torácicos de varias especies.

fig. 1. C. hieroglyphicus Mall.
fig. 2. C. furens Poey.
fig. 3. C. variipennis Coq.
fig. 4. C. venustus Hoffmann.
fig. 5. C. yukonensis Hoffmann.
fig. 6. C. cockerelli Coq.
fig. 7. C. diabolicus Hoffmann.
fig. 8. C. stellifer Coq.
fig. 9. C. guttipennis Coq.
fig. 10. C. baueri Hoffmann.
fig. 11. C. crepuscularis Mall.
fig. 12. C. haematopotus Mall.

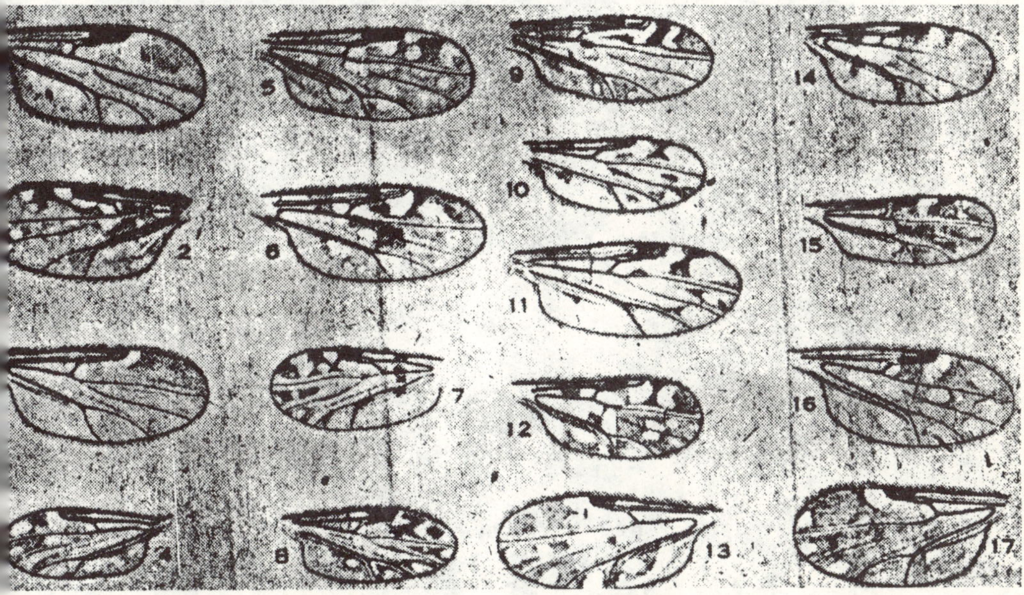

Plancha No. 7 (tomada de Hoffmann)

fig. 1. Ala de hembra de C. sanguisugus Coq.
fig. 2. Ala de hembra de C. loughnani var. jamaicense Edw.
fig. 3. Ala de hembra de C. biguttatus Coq.
fig. 4. Ala de hembra de C. canithorax Hoffmann.
fig. 5. Ala de hembra de C. phlebotomus Will.
fig. 6. Ala de hembra de C. trinidadensis Hoffmann.
fig. 7. Ala de hembra de C. furens Poey.
fig. 8. Ala de hembra de C. variipennis Coq.
fig. 9. Ala de hembra de C. venustus Hoffmann.

fig. 10. Ala de hembra de C. yukonensis Hoffmann.
fig. 11. Ala de hembra de C. cockerelli Coq.
fig. 12. Ala de hembra de C. diabolicus Hoffmann.
fig. 13. Ala de hembra de C. stellifer Coq.
fig. 14. Ala de hembra de C. guttipennis Coq.
fig. 15. Ala de macho de C. baueri Hoffmann.
fig. 16. Ala de hembra de C. crepuscularis Mall.
fig. 17. Ala de hembra de C. haematopotus Mall.

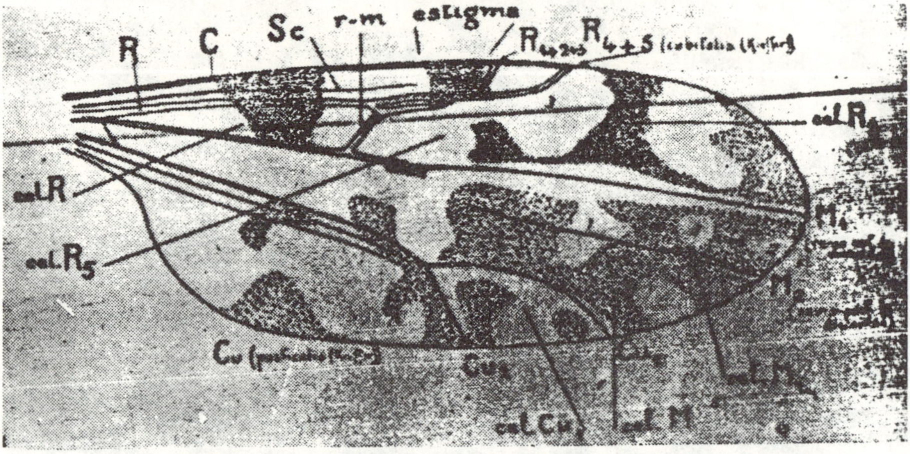

Plancha No. 8 (tomada de da Costa Lima)

fig. 1. Ala de Culicoides guttatus Coquillet.

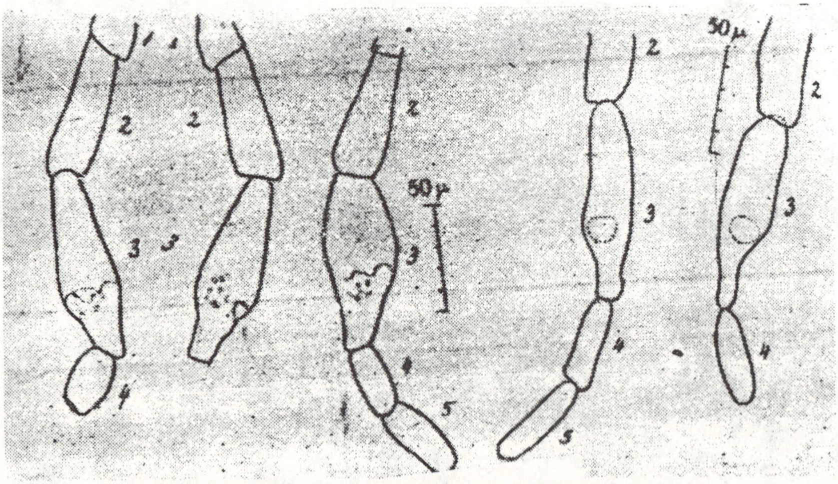

Plancha No. 9 (tomada de da Costa Lima)

fig. 3. Palpos de Culicoides insignis Lutz.
fig. 4. Palpos de Culicoides flavivenula (Costa Lima).

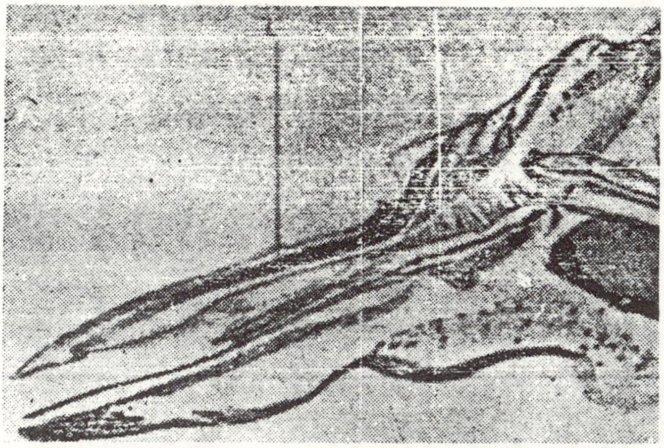

Plancha No. 10 (tomado de Sharp)

fig. 7. Larva de F. perstans atrevesando la trompa de C. austeni.

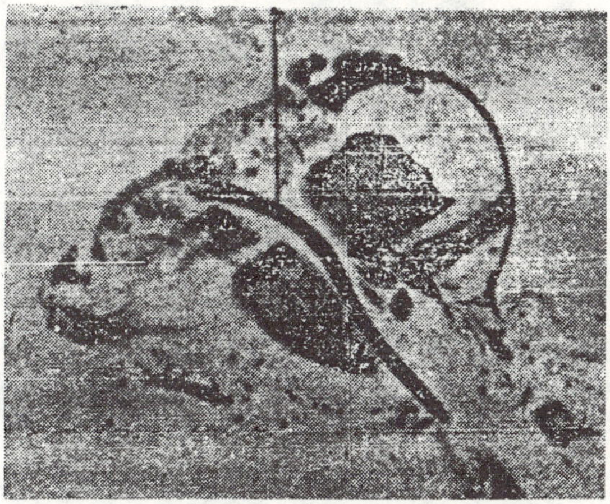

Plancha No. 11 (tomado de Sharp)

fig. 6. Larva de F. perstans en cerebro de C. austeni.

fig. 1. Trompeta respiratoria de C. phlebotomus Will.
fig. 2. Segmento anal macho de C. sp.
fig. 3. Segmento anal hembra de C. guttipennis Coq.
fig. 4. Trompeta respiratoria de C. sp.
fig. 5. Trompa respiratoria de C. sp.
fig. 6. Trompa respiratoria de C. crepuscularis Mall.
fig. 7. Trompa respiratoria de C. villosipennis Root i Hoffmann.
fig. 8. Trompa respiratoria de C. guttipennis Coq.

fig. 9. Trompa respiratoria de C. furens Poey.
fig. 10. Segmento anal hembra de C. villosipennis Root i Hoffmann.
fig. 11. Segmento anal hembra de C. crepuscularis Mall.
fig. 12. Segmento anal macho de C. furens Poey.

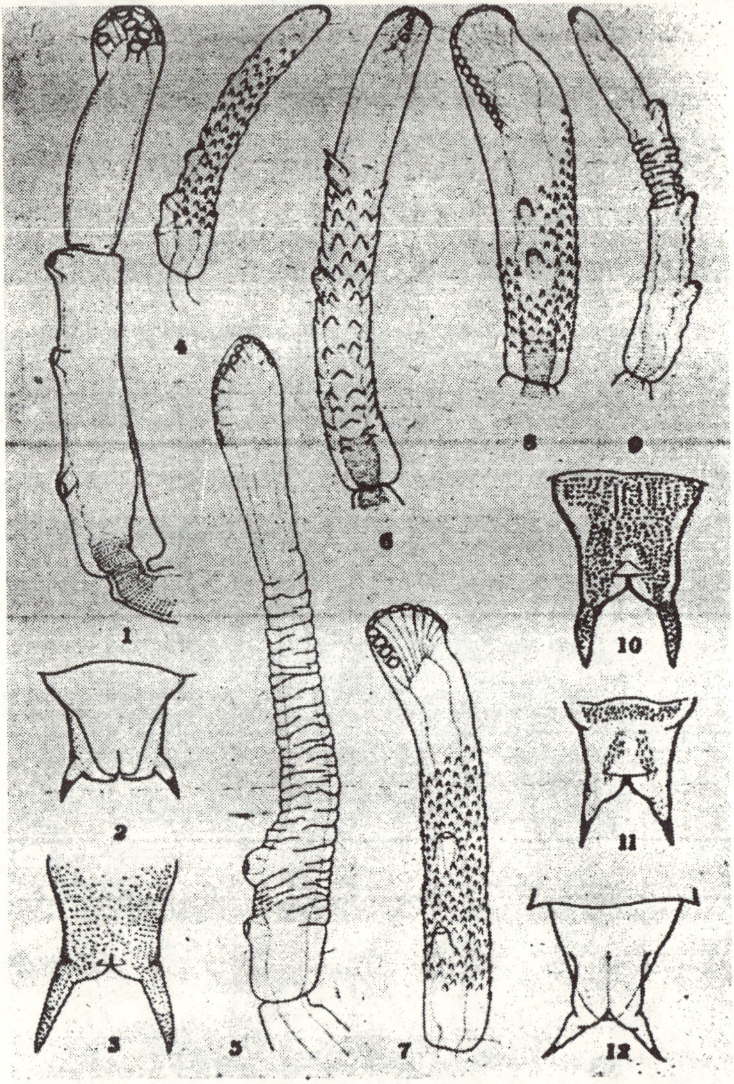

Plancha No. 12 (tomada de Fox)

fig. 13. Trompa respiratoria de C. nanus Root i Hoffmann.
fig. 14. Segmento anal hembra de C. nanus Root i Hoffmann.
fig. 15. Segmento anal hembra de C. stellifer Coq.
fig. 16. Segmento anal macho de C. arboricola Root i Hoffmann.

fig. 17. Trompa respiratoria de C. arboricola Root i Hoffmann.
fig. 18. Trompa respiratoria de C. variipennis Coq.
fig. 19. Trompa respiratoria de C. sp.
fig. 20. Trompa respiratoria de C. niger Root i Hoffmann.
fig. 21. Trompa respiratoria de C. stellifer Coq.
fig. 22. Segmento anal hembra dc C. niger Root i Hoffmann.
fig. 23. Segmento anal macho de C. variipennis Coq.
fig. 24. Segmento anal hembra de C. sp.

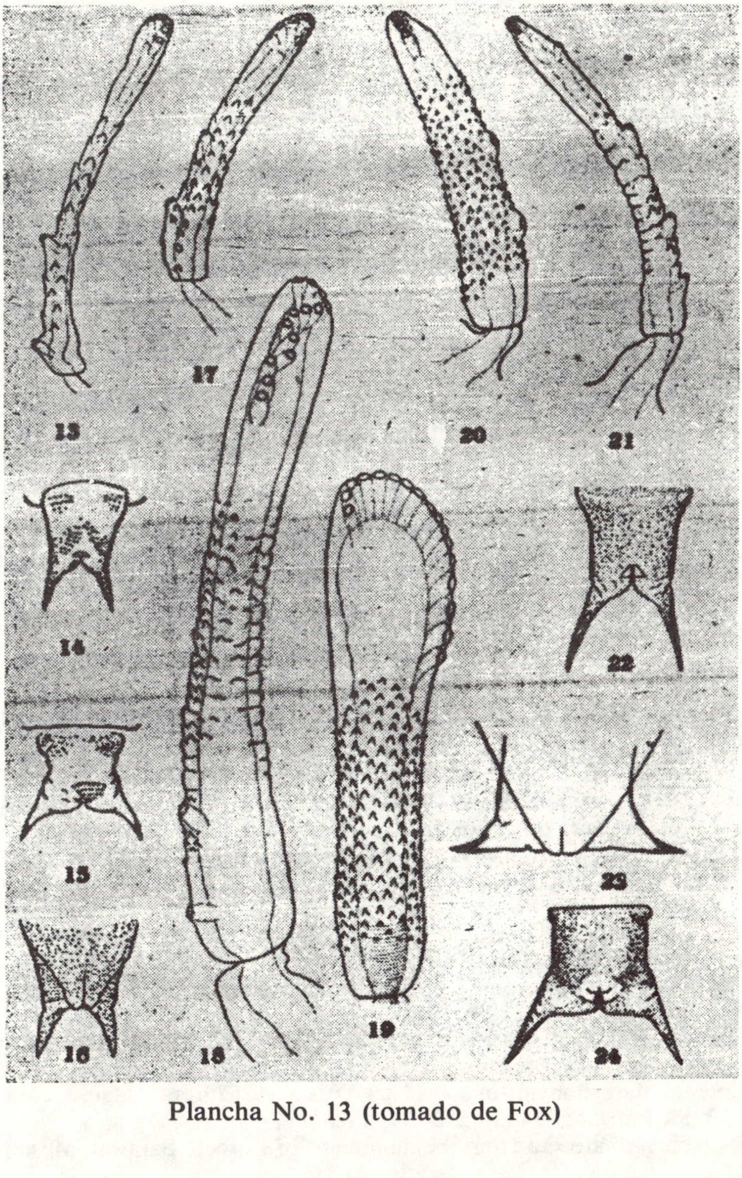

Plancha No. 13 (tomado de Fox)

BIBLIOGRAPHY

(1) Iliger's Mag. Ins. Vol. 2. 1803.

(2) Genera crustaceorum et insectorum secundum Ordenem naturalem in Familias disposita, etc. Vol. IV. 1809.

(3) Beitrag zur Kenniniss der Gattung Ceratopogon. Stett. ent. Zeit. Vol. 44. pag. 1-80. 1852.

(4) Fauna austriaca. Diptera. Vol. I. Viena. 1862.

(5) Diptera. Fam. Chironomidae. Genera insectorum. 1906.

(6) Observations on the Ceratoponinae midges of the Gold Coast, with descriptions of new species. Annals of Trop. Med. and Paras. XIV. pag. 187, 210; 211, 274; 309, 331. XV. pag. 177, 212. 1920-21.

(7) Filaria perstans; its development in Culicoides austeni. Trans. Royal Soc. of Trop. Med. and Hyg. XXI. 371-96. 1928.

(8) Development of Microfilaria perstans in Culicoides grahami; a preliminary note. Trans. of Roy. Soc. of Trop. Med. and Hyg. Vol. XXI.I. 1927.

(9) On the development in Culicoides furens Poey of Filaria (Mansonella) ozzardi Manson 1897. Journal Helminthology. XII. 1934.

(10) Preparations illustrating the life history of the filarial worm Onchocerca cervicalis of the thorax. Trans. Roy. Soc. of Trop. Med. and Hyg. Vol. XXVII. I. 1933-34.

(11) Onchocerca cervicalis (Raillet and Henry 1910) and its development in Culicoides nuberculosus Mg. Rpts. University Cambridge. Inst. Animal Path. III. 272-284. Cambridge.

(12) On culicoides as a vector of Onchocerca gibsoni Cleland and Johnston 1910. Journal Helminthology. 16. 121-158. 1938.

(13) Culicoides filariferus. Biol. Abstracts. Vol. 15, 2. 172. 1939.

(14) Boletín Oficina Sanitaria Panamericana. Vol. 23. 12. 1944.

(15) Los ceratopogónidos o jejénes como trasmisores de filarias. VII. Cong. Cient. Americano. 7 pags. Méjico. 1934.

(16) The causation of Pellagra. Trans. Roy. Soc. Trop. Med. and Hyg. 21-70. 1913.

(17) Notes on some insects found in Egypt of Medical and Veterinary Interest. Bull. Soc. Ent. d'Egypt. 10. 19-90. 1917.

(18) The insect vector of Uta. Peruvian disease. Journal of Parasitology. 2-67. 1915.

(19) Notes et reflexions sur les Toxoplasmes et toxoplasmose du Gundi. Arch. Inst. Pasteur de Tunisie. 10. 1-40. 1917.

(20) Quelques observations sur la biologie des Ceratopogonines d'Algerie. Cong. Intern. d'Ent. 2. 743-49. 1933.

(21) Observations sur la biologie des ceratopogindés et des similudés du Bas Congo. Ann. Soc. Belge. Med. Trop. 19. 97-112. 1939.

(22) Contribuicao para o estudo das "Ceratopogoninas" hematofagas encontradas no Brasil. Mem. do Inst. O. Cruz. Tomo IV. Fasc. I. 1912.

(23) Nota sobre Ceratopogónidos i Culicoides. Rev. del Inst. de Salub. i Enf. Trop. Tomo VI. N° 1. 1945.

(24) Contribuicao para o estudo das Ceratopogoninas hematofagas do Brasil. Mem. do Inst. O. Cruz. Tomo V. Fasc. I. 1913.

(25) Contribuicao para o conhocimento das Ceratopogoninas do Brasil. Mem. do Inst. O. Cruz. Tomo VI. 81-89. 1914.

(26) A review of the species of Culicoides of North and Central America and the West Indies. The Am. J. of Hyg. Vol. V. 2. 1925.

(27) Notes on the synonymy of some New York State Chironomidae. J. New York. J. New York Ent. Soc. 34 (3). 273-277. 1926.

(28) Diptera. Nematocera from the mountains of Borneo. Sarawak Mus. Jour. 3

(3). 243-278. 1926.
(29) Un nouveau diptere piqueur de la region bordelaise. J. Med. Bordeaux. 103 (12). 511. 1926.
(30) Neue Species aus der Unterfamilien Ceratopogoninae (from the Bodenheimer collection). Shornick ent. Oddél. Nar, Mus. Praga. 10. (79) 130-144. 1932.
(31) Ceratopogonidae from the Society Islands. Bernice P. Bishop Mus. Bull. 113. 75-80. 3 figs. 1935.
(32) Ceratopogonidae from the Marquesas Islands. Bernice P. Bishop Mus. Bull. 114. 93-103. 3 figs. 1935.
(33) Ceratopogonidae (Dipt.) from the River Amazon. Stylops 4 (3). 49-56. 3 figs. 1935.
(34) Culicoides of Siam with descriptions of new species. Am. J. Hyg. 27 (2). 399-415. 8 pls. 1938.
(35) Observations on biting sandflies (Ceratopogonidae) in Trinidad. British West Indies Trop. Agric. (Trinidad) 16 (4). 79-81. 1939.
(36) Sur quelques moucherons piqueurs de la region lyonnaise appartenant au genre Culicoides (Dipt-Ceratopogonidae). Bull. Mens. Soc. Linn. Lyon. 10 (3). 38-39. 1941.
(37) A generic synopsis of the Ceratopogonidae (Heleidae) of the Americas, a bibliography, and a list of the North American species.
(38) Loc. cit.
(39) British blood-sucking flies. British Museum (Natural History). Londres. 1939.
(40) Loc. cit.
(41) The biology, inmature states and control of the sandflies (biting Ceratoponinae) at Puerto Castilla (Honduras) Ann. Reports Med. Dept. United Fruit Co. 15. 245-262. 1 pl. 1926.
(42) Loc. cit.
(43) Chironomiden. Metamorphosen en 1. Arch. Hydrobiol. 19 (4) 585-623. 32 figs. 1928.
(44) Chave das especies de Culicoides da regiao neotropica (Diptera-Ceratopogonidae). Mem. do Inst. O. Cruz. 32 (3). 411. 6 figs. 1937.
(45) The respiratory trumpet and anal segment of the pupae of some species of Culicoides (Diptera-Ceratopogonidae) Pto. Rico-Journal Public Health 17 (4) 1942.
(49) Contribución a la Fauna Venezolana. Bol. del Lab. Clínica Razetti Año IV. No. 11. 1943.
(50) Nota acerca de Culicoides (Diptera-Ceratopogonidae). Descripción de una nueva especie para el país. Bol. del Lab. de la Clínica Razetti. Año VI. No. 19-20. 1946.

THE SIMULIIDAE FAMILY IN VENEZUELA

(Work of incorporation to the National Academy of Medicine as Member of Number).

(Dedicated to the memory of Dr. M. Núñez Tovar admirer of the Natural Sciences).

INTRODUCTION

The publication today of the present work is owed to the help of two persons: To Dr. Alan Stone, clever entomologist of the Department of Agriculture of Washington, and to Dr. Pablo J. Anduze, in charge of the Section of Entomology of our Institute of Hygiene, who has given us some material and good advise. For both our acknowledgment.

Long time ago we have been working in researches about the disease called *carate* and then we have had the opportunity of handling this kind of insects, because since the last century have been appointed by the colombian investigators as transmissors of that sickness. In that way, in the year 1929, in "Observaciones sobre el Carate en el Distrito Perijá del Estado Zulia", presented some specimens of Simuliidae, classified in United States, but without arrive to the species, insects caught to on the border of the Apon river; after that, in 1934, in trip to the State of Barinas, always in the same researches, caught in the river Socopó, specimens of the same family, classified in Washington, not giving the species.

We are very glad to know, that our Surcouf and González Rincones and after Professor Lutz, accompanied by Núñez Tovar, during his stay among us, researches published in the book "Zoología y Parasitología Venezolanas", appointing eight species (six news for Venezuela and two for the world), is to the labor of "Laboratorio de la Clínica Razetti" (Briceño Iragorry and us) that has continued and completed the studies about this Arthropoda.

This contribution, probably, will have errors, because we have chosen a family of insects very complicated, and also will be incomplete, but there are no specialists, entomologycal collections and bibliography. Besides, the world war had all the members of science incomunicated of both continents.

CHAPTER I

History - Biologycal Observations

The Simuliidae are called in english *Black flies* or *Buffalo gnats;* some authors say *Sand flies,* but this name brings confusion, because this word is used commonly to denominate the psychodidae (flebotomus) and the ceratopogonidae (culicoides).

In Guatemala, according to Bequaert, are called *Mosquito negrito* the species metallicum and *Mosquito alazan,* the species ochraceum and callidum or mooseri. Lutz shows for Brazil the names *Pium* and *Borrachudos.* In French Congo call the S. damnosum *fourou,* and in Luganda and Lutero (Africa) call them *mbwa,* taking in account the aggressivety and ferocity.

In Venezuela the name used by the people is *mosquitos,* as we have observed in trips all over the country; only in the region of the coast, in the villages of Naiguatá and Anare listened *Barrigón.* The name of *Jejen,* given by Phillippe for these insects in Chile is not correct, because it is used referring to culicoides, family which we have found three species for Venezuela: *paraensis,* cited before by Lutz and that we have captured in El Hatillo and Guarenas (State Miranda), Macuto (Department Vargas), District Federal and San Mateo (State Aragua); *variipennis* (Los Caobos Park - Caracas) and *stellifer* (Macuto - Department Vargas - District Federal), as has been assured by Knab for that country and has been verified by us here, in Venezuela. The venezuelan people say when there is abundance of insects, either culicidae, ceratopogonidae, simuliidae, psychodidae, etc: *plaga.*

The simuliidae have narrow relation with the human pathology; in the year 1930 were known 330 species, and are an important chapter of the medical entomology. Was an english man, Blacklock, the first accusing the simulium, in Africa, as transmissor of the onchocerca volvulus Leuckart in Sierra Leona.

Robles in Guatemala (Central America) on 1919, thought that the simuliidae could transmit the onchocercosis and appointed the S. *samboni* and S. *dinelli.* Hoffmann and Dampf in Mexico and Strong and his coworkers in the States of Oaxaca and Chiapas and later in Guerrero (Mexico - 1931), started researches about Onchocerca caecutiens, verifying for the first time the complete cycle of the filarial in the thoracic muscles of three species *(Mooseri, ochraceum* and *metallicum),* details published in New Englands Journ. of Med. of April, of the same year. Bequaert, on 1931, of 2.088 simuliidae caught stinging, 430 of them on patients with onchocercosic nodules, finding 11% of infection in them and 5% in simuliidae taken to the hazard.

Marchoux and Bourret thought the leprosy could be transmitted by these insects. Equally, Sambon, considered them as transmissors of pellagra, denial by Jennings. The brazilians appointed the simuliidae as transmitting the tropical penfigus.

It seems to be these arthropoda have produced deaths in animals in States, chiefly the cattle, and in Europe, in certain countries as Hungary, Rumania, Bulgaria, Yugoslavia human deaths. So great is the abundance that are true clouds invading the respiravías and asphyxia. In those regions there is a specie S. *columbaczense* Schiner very dangerous having a toxic

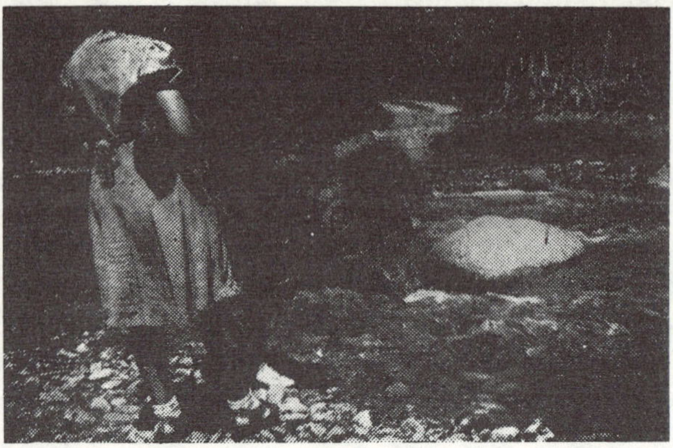

*Catching simuliidae at eleven in the morning on the border of river Guarenas. We caught in this site scarce specimens of S. **metallicum.***

spittle. This simuliidae or fly of Goloubatz produced in 1923, 16.000 deaths, in accord to J. Ciurea and G. Dinulescu. (Ravages causés par la mouche de Goloubatz in Rumania; ses attaques contre les animaux et contre l'homme Ann. of Trop. Med. and Paras. 1924).

Lutz and Neiva speak about the abundance of these animals in Isla Grande and in a place of State Sao Paulo in Brazil. Alcock in 1920 says of deaths in the mountains of Himalaya in Asia. In Venezuela, Anduze refers of true clouds in his trips to Gran Sabana, and us, without seeing that excessive amount, but numerous in the borders of the river Socopó and others in State Barinas, being impossible to be quiet.

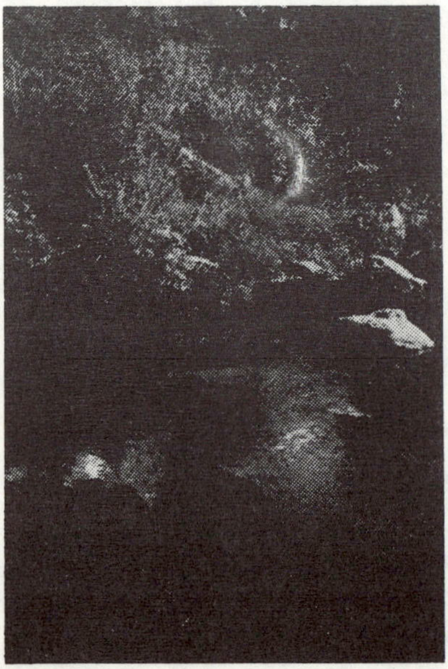

Small river near the village of Caraballeda (Department Vargas) D. F. where we have caught rare exemplaires of S. metallicum.

These dipterous are a great importance among us, because they are considered as transmissors of the *Carate.* In the mycological epoch, was on believed, that the insects carried the fungi as ectoparásites and we did cultures employing material from States Zulia and Barinas with negative results. When the discovery of Professor González Herrojon finding a spirochete after having been stinging *caratosos,* utilizing dark field, but before had been found spirochetes living as parasites in these arthropoda. In simuliidae, examined by us, from Guarenas and Los Teques, we never found flagellates, nematodes, nor ciliated.

H. W. Bates in the book "The naturalist on the river Amazon", describes the abundance of simuliidae as small clouds of the smoke of cigarettes.

Referring to the transmission of this sickness, in our book "Estudios de Patología Tropical", we give details about the species *exiguum,* appointed by us in Guarenas, either collected in Alto Sarare by Geay and classified by Roubaud in 1906. We did essays submitting a patient with spirochete positive, but the rearing of the simuliidae is very difficult and so: 43 specimens caught in the morning at eleven o'clock, the following day only nine were alive. In a special dispositive with humid atmosphere we have maintained them alive for 72 hours.

Bequaert in researches in Santa Emilia (Guatemala) made two dispositives: one, by obtaining adults at the side of the river, and the other, by pricking on the patient. This last one, was a box covered with mosquito net where the ill could introduce head, neck and shoulders, however, only one time did the specimen sting. This explains how hard it is to verify the transmission of *carate.*

Lastly, the S. *venustum* Say 1823 in Canada and United States produce a high mortality among the ducks, transmitting the Leucocytozoon anatis. This specie attacks the cattle in Denmark and other countries.

Skidmore, 1931, accused the S. *occidentale* Townsend 1891, as transmissor of Leucocytozoon smithi, in States.

Up till today, the simuliidae have been appointed of transmitting the following parasites of human and animal diseases.

Human	Onchocerca volvulus Onchocerca caecutiens Treponema carateum ?
Animal	Leucocytozoon anatis Leucocytozoon smithi

We have captures these insects in any month of the year. Our trips to Perijá (State Zulia) were in the raining season (July, August, September and October); the trip to Barinas was in May beginning of the rains; the travel to Ciudad Bolívar, in December; the journey to Choroní, in March, and our last researches was during the whole year of 1942. We can not say if the abundance of the insects change with the months; we were in Choroní after a strong drought, and in Barinas starting the rains, but always the same abundance.

In the Department Vargas did caught in the small river of Caraballeda and catch four specimens in July; in another journey in September to the same places it was impossible to see these kind of insects. This observation possibly demonstates that the simuliidae are not numerous in these zones. The rains, we believed, do not have a big influence; notwithstanding the long drought 1938-1941, the quantity of these animals are always very numerous.

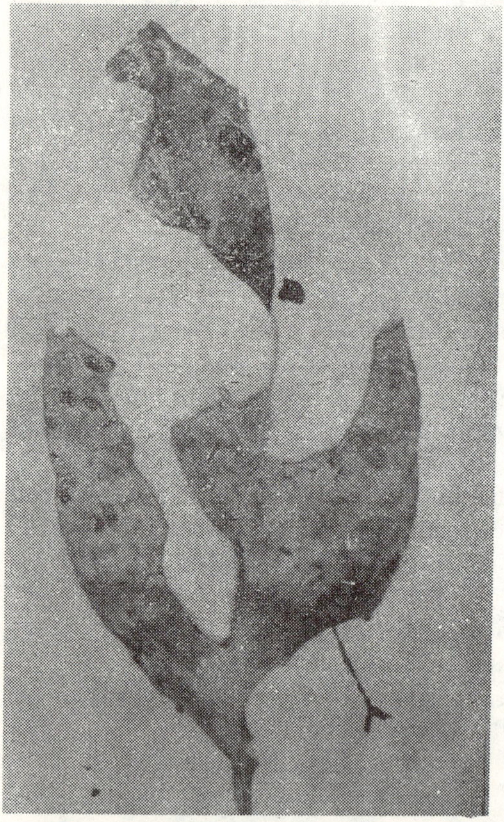

Pupae, glued to a leaf of a rubiácea, possible genus Borreria, found in the stream running throught the Los Teques park.

The temperature it seems has no effect. In Barinas with 27° c. the simuliidae were numerous; the same abundance in Caracas 21° c.; in Tabay, according to Anduze, with 17.7° c. The water of the river Chama is very cold, where we have done catchs.

The altitude it seems also has no effect, and so, we have collected since sites as Macuto to the level of sea; in the way to Choroní to 300 m.; in Caracas to 900 m.; in Los Teques to 1.169 m. still Tabay to 1.710.

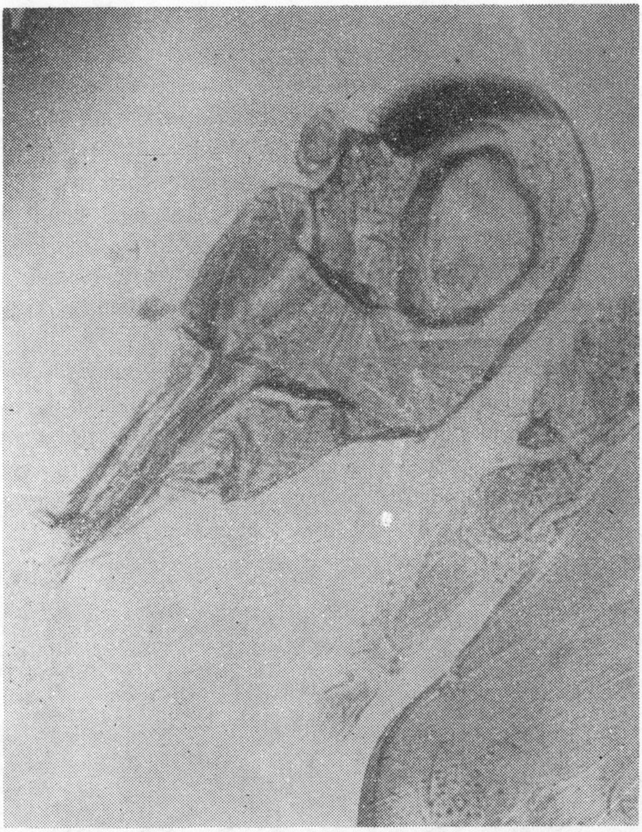

Section of head of simuliidae showing clearly muscles ana glands salivaries. Microphoto made of material given kindly by Dr. Luis Vargas.

The larves we have caught were living on vegetable parts: dry branches, garbage submerged, green and fresh leaves sunk or dry leaves, equally, submerged. The larves are very numerous and we have found still 40 or 50 in a space of 2 cm. Among the vegetables we have seen aquatic plants, gramineous (Panicum maximum Jacq.) and others as a rubiácea, possibly genus Borreria (classified by Pittier). We have not found larves living on the stones, but Anduze says that in the Gran Sabana, where waterfalls are common, they form a slippery layer on the suface of the stone.

Sometimes we have not caught insects on the borders of the rivers of great volumen, as Caroní, but easy in small rivers; sometimes rivers of impetuous current or small streams of little speed.

In some places the larves and pupae are abundant and in others, scarce or none. So, in Guarenas, in the site (photo 1) where we had captured the *exiguum,* whose pupae is unknown, we were fifteen minutes in an extension of 50 meters, getting only one pupae. However, in the same river, in the place Ahuyamita o Paso del Encantado, ten km. farther, we got numerous larves and pupae of several species.

In leaves sunk, besides larves de simuliidae, we have found larves of the families leptoceridae and hydropsychidae, classified by Townes. There are streams or rivers that we could call ''simulidosos'', and so in a recent trip to State Barinas, we observed the following: in the river Trincheras (State Carabobo), very numerous; in El Salao and other small rivers, between Morón and San Felipe, not any; in State Barinas, very irrigated, at side of Guanare, where we need to blow avoiding the introduction throught mouth and nostrils, or Boconó, without the need to go out of the car to make the catch, exist the Mazparro and Camaguan with few specimens.

In the beginning we thought as all the persons that have studied the simuliidae, that they need pure water and current in order to develop. Notwithstanding, we have caught these animals in the garden home situated in front of the Parque Los Caobos, and where the only place to develop is in the stream El Guaire, running 500 meters away and this small river received all the sewage of Caracas; the same, near Barquisimeto, in the site

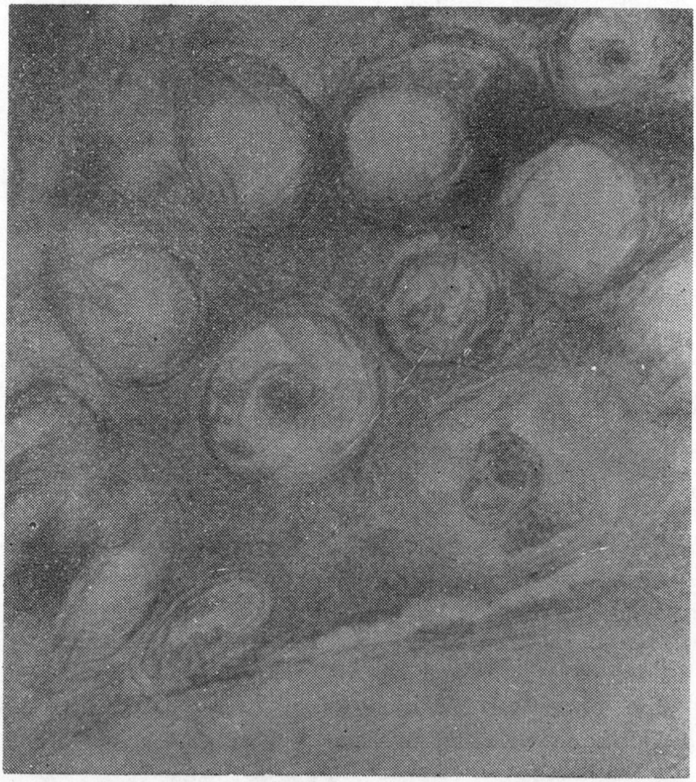

Section of a cyst having inside an adult of Onchocerca caecutiens. As the filaria is rolled is possible to see several sections and in some eggs. Microphoto of material sent to us kindly by Dr. Luis Vargas.

Macuto, with muddy water, we have collected exemplaires. Referring to the current, we have done captures in ''caños'' (dirty and stagnant waters) as in the Quebrada del Padre in State Barinas.

The simuliidae are very voraceous (the females are the prickers) choose chiefly the legs, but may attack other places. They are attracted to the soft and not hairy skin and can sting through the stockings, but there is fleshy skin, and so, while my wife and us were not disturbed much, a relative that accompanied us was surprisingly attacked (photo 1).

When arriving to a stream of water, at the beginning it is often rare; it is necessary to wait for a while.

The captures have been made almost always on the borders of streams of water, but sometimes to long distances. In Choroní, around 100 meters from the river, and in Macuto, in the court yard of a house, around 1000 meters from the stream running to the entrance of the village.

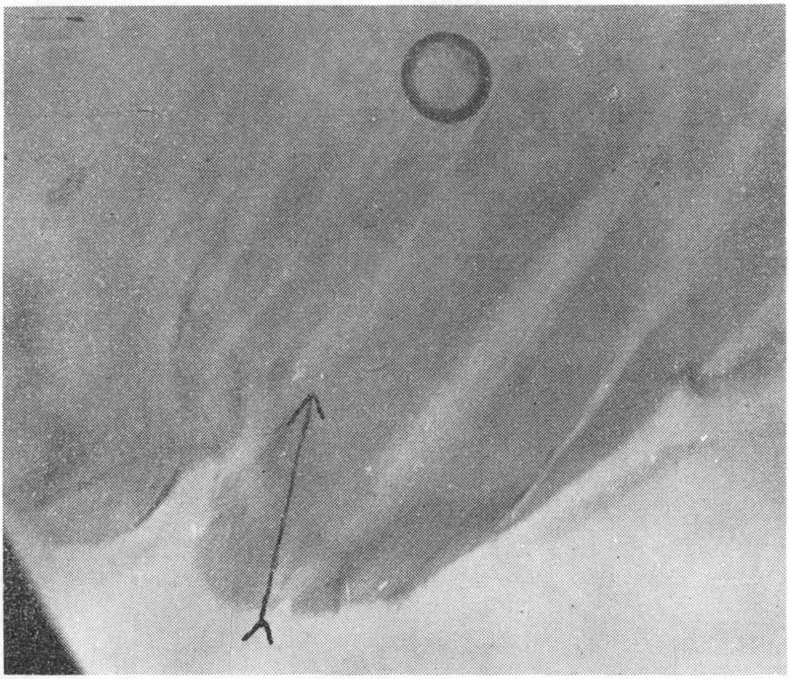

Section of thorax of S. ochraceum showing with the arrow a microfilaria of Onchocerca caecutiens. Microphoto of material sent to us kindly by Dr. Luis Vargas.

The vehicles possibly will help the spreading of many arthropoda land we have seen that numerous simuliidae come to the glass of the car, glue to the glass from Pedrazas to Barinas and from different rivers (Boconó, Portuguesa, etc.) to Barquisimeto, final of the journey.

The simuliidae do not sting immediately, they begin flying around the legs, and for the catching it is good to wait half or one minute. After two or three minutes is enjoying the food and it is very easy and sure the capture, and being inside the tube it is necessary to detach it. We have caught 18 of these insects in 15 minutes, and sometimes, 2 or 3, when they are very near to each other, stinging.

The simuliidae sting from sunrise to nightfall. Our ferryman tells: "during the day the simuliidae, during the night the mosquitos".

The simuliidae never fall to the soil. They can be full of blood after the meal, but they are always apt to start to fly.

The sting is slightly painful and produce a point that gives a small drop of blood, later appears a papule, very visible in some persons and also some itching. To the papule continue a light pigmentation and a dark point that remains two or three weeks or more, and so we have in a finger of the right hand one of these, after the come back of one of these trips to Barinas.

To obtain adults from the pupae we put inside the small tubes a piece of wet cotton. The rearing has 2 or 3 days, as maximum 5. After this period concluded this test.

Our captures have been done in ten States and District Federal, since 1929 catching simuliidae in Perijá (State Zulia) still now in December 1942 in State Barinas. The States are: Zulia, Miranda, Aragua, Carabobo, Yaracuy, Portuguesa, Mérida, Barinas, Bolívar, and Lara. Staying in Caracas the material has been more abundant in District Federal and State Miranda.

In all this territory explored up today we have found ten species: seven either described and three new for Venezuela. In the specimens of Perijá not arrived to the species, and probably had more than one, because Perijá is a far region, near the border with Colombia, not much explored and our last abundant material from five States is yet without classification. We have material in Boston, Panama and Rio de Janeiro. We hope later to present new contributions about so wide a family that must be rich in a country so large and diverse.

CAPITULO II

Clasificación de los Simulidos

La clasificación de los simulidos es bastante complicada i se ha tratado de hacerla sirviéndose de larvas, pupas i adultos.

Dyar i Shannon en su trabajo The North American two-winged flies of the family Simuliidae reconocen cuatro géneros i no los 17 aceptados por Enderlein. Los autores citados se expresan del modo siguiente: "We have found Enderlein's classification entirely unsuited to the American fauna". "We have found that the genera he proposed are too finely drawn and of no practical value".

Mas adelante traen el cuadro siguiente:

Table of ge: :era of Simuliidae

Radius setose on its entire length.

Radius joining costa at middle of coastal vein; radial sector forked; antenna 10—jointed..... *Parasimulium Malloch*

Radius joining coastal vein far beyond its middle

Radial sector with long fork; hind basitarsus not produced apically; second hind tarsus without dorsal incision and much longer than width of basitarsus, front usually broad..... *Prosimulium Roubaud*

Radial sector simple; hind basitarsus produced or not produced apically, second hind tarsus with or without dorsal incision and less than twice the width of the basitarsus; front narrowed..... *Eusimulium Roubaud*

Radius bare between the stem vein and base of radial sector; radial sector simple; hind basitarsus produced apically; the second hind tarsus with dorsal incision and less than twice the width of basitarsus..... *Simulium Latreille*

Malloch en su trabajo del año 1941, en la pág. 24 trae tres géneros: Simulium Latreille, Prosimulium Roubaud, que fue originalmente propuesto como subgénero, separádolo del género Simulium por el hind tarsus i la formación de los capullos i del Parasimulium Malloch, del cual dice: "this genus differs in the female from Prosimulium Roubaud in having the eyes much more widely separated al vertex, in having the frons much higher than highest level of eyes when viewed from the side, in having the face linear, in having the eye facets gradually enlarged as they descend, and in the absence of the closed cell in the wing. The male is unknown".

M.E. Roubaud en Comptes rendus de l'Academie des Sc. pag. 519, divide el género Simulium en dos subgéneros basados en la formación del segundo tarso posterior i otros caracteres. He aquí a Roubaud: "el segundo artículo de los tarsos posteriores en los dos sexos, alargado, lineal, sin escotadura de la base. Capullos pupales, agrupados, imperfectos. Un gran número de filamentos ninfales.....*Prosimulium*".

"el segundo artículo de los tarsos posteriores corto, arqueado, escotado dorsalmente en su base, en los dos sexos. Capullos pupales solitarios perfectos. Filamentos ninfales en general poco numerosos..... *Eusimulium*''.

Lutz en su libro Estudios sobre Zoología i Parasitologìa Venezolanas dice en un párrafo: ''Todos los simulidos, como ya lo hemos dicho, están comprendidos en un solo género que es mui homogéneo i que no debe subdividirse, antes de que el aumento de las especies sea mas perfecto de los que es en los momentos actuales. Cuando mas, las subdivisiones, hechas por los autores, pueden considerarse como subgéneros i aún así no satisfacen''.

Clave que hemos confeccionado para la clasificación de las especies de simulidos hallados hasta hoi en el país. Esta clasificación está basada en los tubos branquiales de las pupas. Figuran solamente 12 especies, porque las pupas de las otras cinco especies, creemos se desconocen.

Tubos branquiales gruesos *

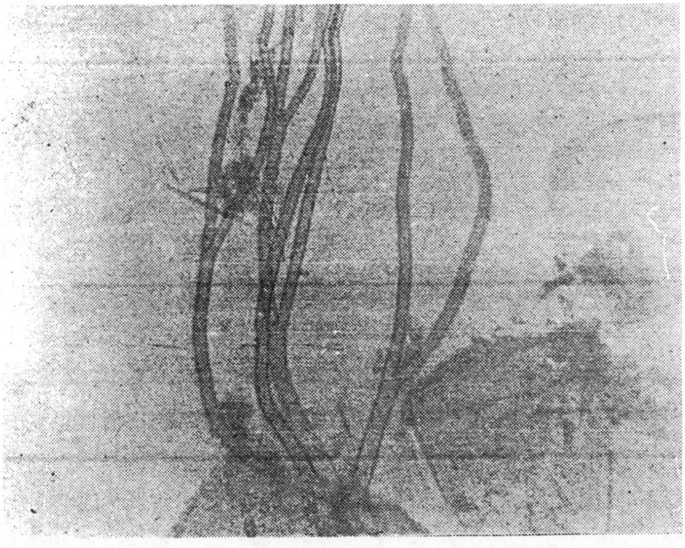

(Fig. 7) Ramillete de ocho tubos branquiales de S. metallicum, según la descripción de Pinto. Material de Guarenas. (Edo. Miranda)

Tubos branquiales finos
Con 6 tubos branquiales de cada lado
Con más de 6 tubos branquiales de cada lado
Tubos branquiales cortos
Tubos branquiales largos
Con 6 tubos branquiales cortos

tubos branquiales cortos, longitud mediana, con una bifurcación próxima a la base i las otras dos mas lejos, éstas últimas a diferentes alturas. Trico-

* Anduze i Briceño Iragorry han encontrado pupas con tubos cortos, posiblemente Auristriatum o Botulibranchium.

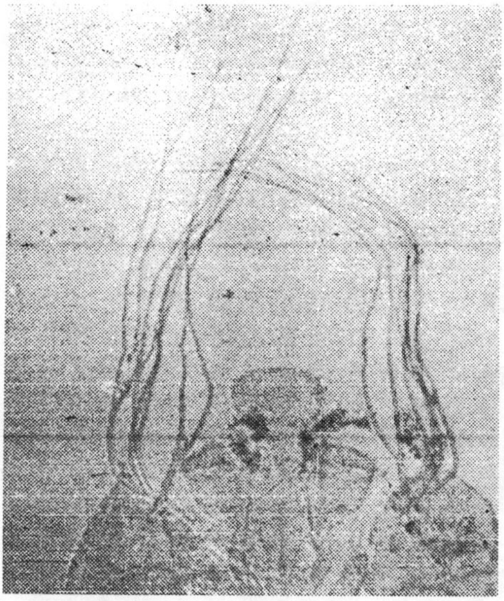

(Fig. 8) Se ven los dos mechones respiratorios de ocho tubos, cada uno. S. metallicum según Pinto. Material de Guarenas. (Edo. Miranda)

mas bífidos.

S. incrustatum Lutz.

Con mas de 6 tubos branquiales cortos.

con 10 de medio mm. de largo. Todos los ramos bastante juntos i bifurcaciones cercanas a la base.

S. pulverulentum Knab.

Con 6 tubos branquiales largos

con 6 tubos branquiales largos, con las bifurcaciones pegadas a la base. Capullo cónico i con tejido amplio.

S. metallicum Bell. según Fairchild

con 6 tubos branquiales de 3.3 mm. de largo, naciendo de tres troncos, produciéndose las bifurcaciones cerca de la base i a igual distancia de ella. Capullo cónico de 2.8 mm. de longitud, con margen de abertura grueso i textura abierta y poco visible.

S. clarki Fairchild

Con tubos branquiales con ensanchamiento en los extremos.

Con tubos branquiales sin ensanchamiento en los extremos.

Con tubos branquiales

Con más de 6 tubos branquiales

tubos branquiales que salen de dos troncos principales, bifurcándose uno lejos de la base i el otro mui cerca de ella en cuatro tubos.

S. amazonicum Goeldi

tubos branquiales con dos bifurcaciones lejos de la base al mismo nivel, la otra mui próxima a la base.

S. vericolor Lutz i Núñez Tovar

tubos branquiales con las tres bifurcaciones a un mismo nivel i próximas a la base.

S. subnigrum Lutz

Con 8 tubos branquiales

Con más de 8 tubos branquiales

tubos branquiales naciendo de tres troncos, dos con tres tubos i el otro con dos. Todas las divisiones cercanas a la base.

E. paraguayense Schrottky

tubos branquiales que salen de tres troncos uno de ellos se bifurca lejos de la base, en los otros dos uno de ellos da una primera bifurcación mui cerca de la base i la segunda un poco mas lejos, pero en tercer tronco, tanto la primera, como la segunda bifurcación se hacen un poco mas lejos que en el tubo anterior.

S. metallicum Bell. según Pinto.

tubos branquiales con un tronco de dos tubos i los otros dos de tres. Todos los tubos saliendo de la base.

S. rubrithorax Lutz

tubos branquiales de tres troncos: uno da cuatro tubos, otro simple i el tercero da dos bifurcaciones a alturas diferentes.

S. ochraceum Walker

tubos branquiales originarios de tres troncos: uno de dos tubos con bifurcación lejos de la base, los otros dos dando cada uno tres tubos con la segunda bifurcación lejos de la base.

S. lutzianus Pinto

Con 12 tubos branquiales de cada lado

tubos branquiales que nacen de cuatro troncos: uno da cinco tubos, uno tres i dos de dos tubos cada uno, naciendo todos mui, cerca de la base.

S. lugubre Lutz i Núñez Tovar.

CAPITULO III

Descripciones originales de las 11 especies encontradas por nosotros en el País. Anotaciones. Distribución Geográfica.

Simulium haematopotum Malloch 1914

Malloch J.R. 1914. U.S. Depart. Agric. Bur. Ent. Tech. Serv. No. 26. págs. 61-2.

Simulium haematopotum Dyar i Shannon 1917

Dyar i Shannon 1927...Proc. U.S. Nat. Mus. vol. 69—art. 10—pág. 38. Est. 6—figs. 86-87.

Simulium haematopotum Dampf 1927

Dampf A. 1927. Revista Mexicana de Biol. vol. VII.

Simulium pseudo-haematopotum C.C. Hoffmann 1930

Hoffmann C.C. 1930. An Inst. Biol. Univ. México. T. I—No. 4—págs. 293-306. The Rev. of Appl. Entomol. (Serie C) vol. 19—parte 6—pag. 113 (junio de 1931).

Simulium haematopotum Fairchild 1940

G.B. Fairchild. 1940. Ann. Ent. Soc. of Amer. Vol. XXXIII. No. 4—dcbre.

Simulium Haematopotum new species

Female: Black. Frons and face with shining pearlaceous pollinosity. Antennae yellow, browned from fourth joint to tip; palpi brown, paler at base. Scutum velvety black, with broad perlaceous stripes, which are broader at anterior ends than the black space between them, taper slightly posteriorly, but are uncurved; posterior and lateral margins similarly pollino se; pleaurae shining black, with more or less distinct pearlaceous pollinosity; scutellum brown. postscutum with pearlaceous pollinosity. Abdomen brownish; opaque en basal four segments, each of which has a rounded, opaque, black dorsal, and a less distinct lateral spot, posterior margins of these setments whitish dusted; apical four segments with dorsal portions shining; the fifth segment with a rounded dorsal spot, the others almost entirely black. Legs yellow, black as follows: mid and hind coxae; fore tarsi; apices of first four and all apical joints of mid tarsi; femora except bases, apica 1 half of tibiae, apical halves of joints 1-3, and all last two joints of tarsi of hinds legs. Wings clear, basal and thick veins yellow. Halteres yellow, stalk blackened.

Frons slighlty divergent-sided, less than one-third the head width at upper angle of eyes, surface hairs weak, brownish yellow; face as long as frons and one-half longer than broad, haired as frons; hairs en palpi brown. postocular cilia brown. Scutum with close-lying, golden-yellow, hairlike pilosity; pleural tuft brownish yellow; scutellum with closely placed yellow pilosity, and brownish, upright, longer hairs. Abdominal basal fringe short, yellow; segments of abdomen with short, sparse, yellow hairs, and longer, dark hairs at apex. Legs with pale yellowish pilosity, which is whitish at bases of tibiae and on basal joint of hind tarsi; dorsal surfaces with longer, blackish, upright hairs, fore tarsi slightly dilated, the paired apical hair present on joints 1 and 3; claws simple. Wings with brown hairs at base and brown surface hairs on thick veins; cross-vein at two fifths from and of subcosta.

Length: 1.5-2 mm

Type. Cat. No. 15. 414 U.S. National Museum

Locality. Santa Lucrecia, Vera Cruz, Mexico (F.W. Urich)

There is also a specimen from Cayamas, Cuba (E.A. Schwarz) which evidently belongs to this species.

The series taken by F.W. Urich is labeled "Bloodsucking, man, October, 1911."

The early stages and male are unknown.

(descripción original tomada del trabajo American black flies or buffalo gnats por J.R. Malloch, April 6, 1914—U.S. Dept. of Agric. Bur. of Entom)

Copiamos a continuación lo que dice Fairchild sobre esta especie en su trabajo: "Notes on the Simuliidae of Panamá (Dipt. Nematocera) Annals of the Entomological Society of América. vol. No. 4. dcbre. 1940. pag. 714.

"My material does not agree in certain respects, with Dyar and Shannon's figures of this species (I was unable to consult Malloch's original description), as a comparison of our figures of the o genital fork will show. S. pseudohaematopotum of C.C. Hoffmann seems close also, but the genital fork is still different and the tarsal claws are unarmed. S. quadrivittatum of Loew seems to be the name under which Dunn (1934, Psyche XLI, 3, pp. 177-178) listed the present species, but no description of Loew's species is available to me here. It was described from Cuba, where haematopotum is stated to occur also Bradt (1 c.) lists both species from Puerto Rico, but gives no description. It is probable that there are a number of similarly marked species in this group, but their elucidation will have to wait until further material accumulates".

"This is the only species which seems to bite man at all readily at lower elevations on the Isthmus. During the latter part of the rainy season it becomes quite annoying at the Laboratory's station at Juan Mina on the Chagres River above Gamboa. The early stages have been taken on grass and dead leaves in small stream which feeds the lily ponds al Summit Gardens, Canal Zone".

S. haematopotum Malloch 1914, algunos lo consideran distinto a S. pseudohaematopotum C.C. Hoffmann 1930, sobre todo en que este último no tiene "tarsal claws". Vargas en 1942 a su paso por Panamá examinando el material de S. haematopotum de Fairchild, llegó a la conclusión de que se trataba de otra especie, i verbalmente nos comunicó pensaba llamarla S. fairchildii.

A este respecto Stone nos dice en carta de 22 de octubre de 1942, lo que sigue: the species, which I determined as S. haematopotum Mall., I still believe to be that species or a very closely related one. Dr. Vargas, who is with me now, has found S. pseudohaematopotum Hoffm. to be the same as haematopotum. However, the species which Fairchild determined as haemapotum is another species to be described by Dr. Vargas. Your specimens are quite different from Fairchild's haematopotum''.

Distibución geográfica de esta especie.

Fuera de Venezuela.

Malloch: Santa Lucrecia. Vera Cruz, México, Cayamas, Cuba Dyar and Shannon: México, Guatemala, Cuba, Puerto Rico.

(ref. de Fairchild).

Dampf: México, Vera Cruz, Ver., Sta. Lucrecia. Ver., Chiapa de Corzo, Chiapas. (ref. de Pinto).

Hoffmann: Chiapas (ref. Pinto).

Fairchild: México, Guatemala, Cuba, Puerto Rico, Panamá, también recibió especímenes de British Honduras. Las capturas de Panamá fueron hechas en los siguientes sitios: Summit C. Z., San Juan Mina Station, Río Chagres, C. Z., Canal Zone Forest Reserve, Las Guacas, R. P., Guayabalito, R. P., Chilibre, R. P.

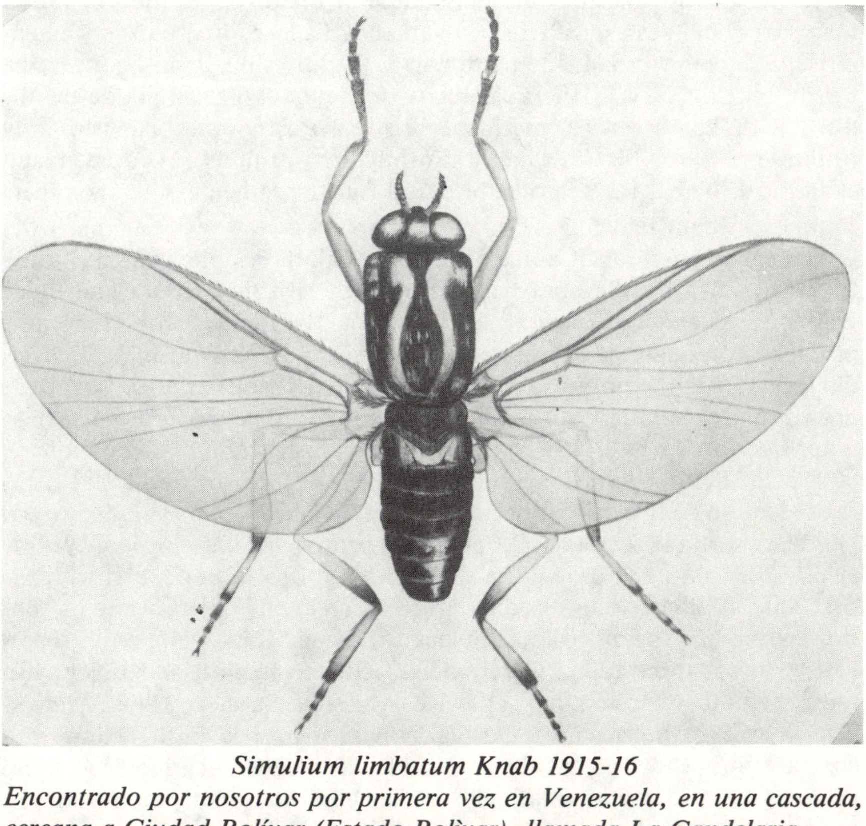

Simulium limbatum Knab 1915-16
Encontrado por nosotros por primera vez en Venezuela, en una cascada, cercana a Ciudad Bolívar (Estado Bolìvar), llamada La Candelaria.

En Venezuela

Iriarte: en Moitaco, en el bajo Orinoco, Estado Bolívar.

Simulium limbatum Knab 1915-16

Knab Frederick. Bull. of Ent. Research. vol. VI., Pt. III, p. 280-1.

Simulium limbatum Knab 1915-16

Pinto César. Simuliidae da America Central e do Sul (Diptera) 1931

Simulium limbatum Knab 1915-16

Iriarte David R. Boletín del Laboratorio de la Clínica Luis Razetti Año III, No. 8. Vol. II, junio 1942.

Simulium limbatum, sp. nov.

Female—Head blackish, both frons and face with strong metallic blue and pearly lustre; frons broad above and distinctly narrowing toward the antennae. Antennae blut, the first two joints yellow, the following ones luteous brown, slightly pruinose and with delicate white pubescence. Scutum deep chocolate brown, pearly, pale blue ornamentation consisting of broad lateral margins involving the humeri and a narrower posterior margin, as well as two large wedge-shaped spots on the anterior fourth, their blunt ends resting on the anterior margen and their sharp end continued as narrow lines beyond the middle of the disk; vestiture of rather long silvery hairscales, rather sparse and not disposed in groups or regular series. Scutellum broad, the hind margin slightly sinuate and converging nearly rectangulary to the apex, dark ferruginous brown, nude on the disk, with coarse black marginal bristles. Postnotum blackish, gray pruinose. Pleurae blackish and uniformly gray pruinose. Abdomen suncylindrical, black, the second, third and fourth segments dull, the others shining, without markings, the apical margins of the segments narrowly pale. Legs slender; coxae and trochanters of all three apirs ochreous, tinged with brown on the hind pair. Front legs with the femora and tibiae ochreous yellow, the former paler apically, the tibiae with silvery mite pruinosity on outer side except at base; tarsi wholly brownish black. Middle legs with the femora brown, broadly pale ochreous at apex, the tibiae brown in the middle, both base and apex broadly pale ochraceous, their outer sides on the basal half with a white pruinosity terminating obliquely; tarsi with the first joint long and slender, whitish, brown on distal fifth, the second joint broadly white at base, the last three joints wholly brown. Hind legs with the femora and tibiae dark brown, the latter broadly yellow at base, their outer sides with a white sheen on basal half; tarsi with the first joint slender, compressed, nearly as long as the tibiae, white its ventral margin and the distal fourth blackish, second joint white on the basal half, the last three joints wholly black. All the femora and tibiae with long, recumbent, shinning yellowish white hair-scales. Claws simple. Wings broad, the venation normal; thick veins brownish yellow, the coastal spines short, stout, dense and black; integument iridescent, more pronounced and predominatingly red on basal half, but not forming a pronounced spot. Halteres white, brownish at base.

Length: Body about 1.3 mm; wing 1.7 mm.

British Guiana: Rupununi River, ix. 1913 (Dr. K.S. Wise) a series preserved in spirits received together with a larger number of S. amazonicum Goeldi.

This species belongs to the same group as S. amazonicum and shows its relationship by the close agreement in structural and other details, it differs strikingly in the absence of the pair of thoracic dorsal stripes. The two species were preserved together in the same vial, so evidently occur together.

(descripción original tomada del trabajo Some new neotropical Simuliidae por Frederick Knab, Bureau of Entomology, U.S. Department of Agriculture. Bull. of Ent. Resch. Vol. VI. Pt. III, diciembre de 1915, pag. 280)

Distibución geográfica de esta especie

Fuera de Venezuela

Knab: Río Rupununi, Guayana Inglesa

En Venezuela

Iriarte: Cascada llamada La Candelaria, a mas o menos 50 km. de distancia de Ciudad Bolívar, Estado Bolívar. (captura de ocho hembras picando)

Simulium bicoloratum Malloch 1912

Malloch J.R. U.S. National Museum. Vol. XLIII. No. 1945. pags. 649-50.

Odagmia bicolorata Enderlein 1925

Enderlein G. Zool. Anz. T. LXIII. pag. 208. 1925.

Simulium bicoloratum Malloch 1913.

Pinto César. Simuliidae da America Central e do Sul (Diptera)—7th Reun. Soc. Arg. de Pat. Reg. Norte. 1931.

Simulium bicoloratum Malloch, new species.

Female—Frons black, shining, with slight whitish dusting, raised in center slightly tuberculate at lower angle, side very slightly divergent toward vertex, width at upper angle of eyes about one-fourth the breadth of the head; face (see fig. 6) distinctly white dusted, especially on upper portion, the dusting below the bifid raised portions yellowish, very few hairs on either face of frons, antennae broken, but the two basal joints still left are black; palpi black, postocular cilia pale, with an admixture of much longer black hairs. Prescutum bright yellow, scutum concolorous, opaque, with opaque deep black markings as in figure 7, pilosity sparse and hair like, yellow, some upright black hairs on posterior margin, middle part of extreme lateral margin deep black, pleurae brownish, yellowish posteriorly, on center with silkly white pollinosity, pleural hair tuft brown; scutellum clear, with numerous upright black hairs which are most conspicuous on anterior lateral angles: postnotum deep black with a silvery sheen. Abdominal basal scale yellow, fringe long, yellow, first segment yellow darkened at apex, next three opaque, velvety black, apical four segments shining brown-black, sides of fifth yellow, apical four segments with scattered pale, and numerous longer, black hairs. Legs black, fore

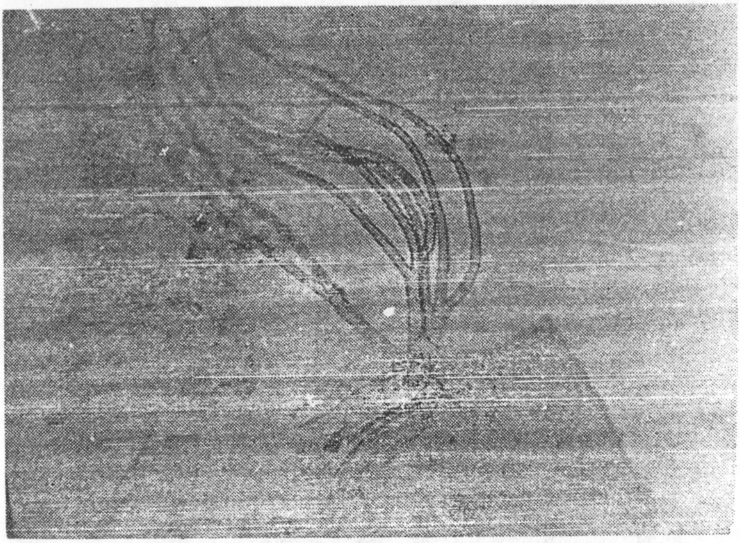

(Fig. 9) Conjunto de tubos branquiales pupales de S. paraguayense, según descripción y figuras de Pinto. Material del sitio El Samán (Edo. Miranda).

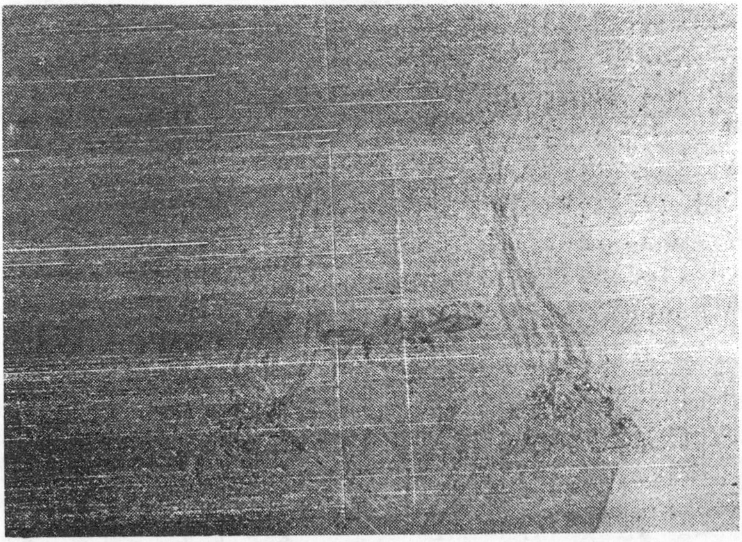

(Fig. 10) Ramilletes de ocho tubos respiratorios pupales de S. paraguayense según Pinto. Material del sitio El Samán.

coxae, bases of all femora, and all tibiae except apices yellow; all pale portions of legs with silvery, very short pilosity, the black parts with black pilosity, the usual scattered, long black, upright hairs on all legs, basal joint of hind tarsus with prolonged apical flaplike process posteriorly, second joint of same tarsus with scale like basal process and dorsal constriction, claws with minute tooth in addition to the basal tubercule. Wings clear, with a slight indication of grayish color at apex, costal vein black-brown at base, becoming black shortly beyond base, subcostal vein yellowish, apical portions of first vein and radial vein black, costal vein with short spinelike bristles and soft hairs, first and radial veins joining the costa very close together and forming a conspicuous black thickening of the costa at about midway from end of subcosta to end of costa which tapers off to end of costa, venation normal. Halteres yellow with base of stalk darkened.

Length—2.5 mm.

Type—Cat. No. 15.304 U. S. N. M.

One female, Río Charape, Perú, September 13, 1911 (C.H.T. Townsend)

This species is readily distinguishable from any other in the genus by the remarkable coloration of the thorax and abdomen. I know of no closely allied species already described.

(descripción original tomada de J.R. Malloch, del Bureau of Entomology, U.S. Department of Agriculture. Procedings U.S. National Museum, Vol. 43, n. 1945, publicado en diciembre 31 de 1912, pags. 649-650).

Distribución geográfica de esta especie

Fuera de Venezuela.

Malloch: Río Charape, Perú (C. H. T. Townsend col. 1911)

En Venezuela:

Iriarte: En Tabay, a orillas del Río Chama, Estado Mérida (captura de hembras picando).

Simulium sanguineum Knab, 1915-16 *

Knab Frederick. 1915-16. Bull. Ent. Research. Vol. VI. pags. 279-280.

Simulium sanquineum Knab 1915-6

Pinto César. 1931. Simuliidae da America Central e do Sul (Diptera).

Simulium sanguineum Knab 1915-6

Fairchild G. B. 1940. Annals of the Entomological Soc. of America, pag. 701.

Simulium sanguineum Knab, sp. nov.

Female—Occiput, frons and face black, with strong blue and green pearly pruinosity and with scattered short black hairs; frons broad, above nearly one-third the width of head, narrowing slightly towards antennae. Antennae with the three proximal joints ferruginous, the others dull blackish and with fine, appressed pale pubescence. Scutum velvet black, with four broad, pruinose, strongly iridescent, metallic blue stripes, visible only in certain lights; outer stripes very broad, leaden gray in some lights, on lateral margins and continued along posterior margin; submedian stripes broad, nearer to each other than to lateral stripes, slightly sinuate and very slighty narrowed beyond the middle. In some lights the subme-

* Esta especie fue citada simultáneamente con nosotros por mi compañero Briceño Iragorry, en el No. 11 de nuestra revista "Boletín del Laboratorio de la Clínica Luis Razetti". Briceño la señala en el río Neverí (Edo. Anzoátegui).

dian stripes nearly disappear and a pair of similarly coloured wedge shaped spots appear anteriorly in their place, the base of the wedge on anterior margin, its point terminating at about the middle of the disk; vestiture of long golden hair scales, evenly distributed and not arranged in rows or groups. Scutellum narrow, subtriangular, velvet-black, with long golden transverse hair-scales and black bristles on the margin. Postnotum short, black, with pruinosity like that on margins of scutum.

Pleurae and coxae black, gray pruinose. Abdomen black, elongate, somewhat constricted beyond base, thickened beyond middle; first segment dorsally strongly iridescent, the four following ones dull velvet-black and with the flexible basal portion gray; segments 5 to 8 shining black, highly polished and with a few scattered black bristles. Front legs with the femora luteous and with a brownish shade dorsally; tibiae luteous; with silvery lustre, the apex very slightly darkened; tarsi black. Middle legs with the femora and tibiae brownish black, the knees narrowly and the apices of the tibiae yellowish; tarsi with the first joint whitish except at extreme apex, second joint whitish with dark apical ring, the others wholly dark. Hind legs with the femora brownish black, the tibiae white on basal third, black beyond; tarsi with the first joint white, black on apical fourth, the second joint white, black on apical third, the last three black. Claws simple. Wings hyaline, without iridescent spot in anal field; coarse veins pale yellow. Halteres pale yellow, black basally.

Length: Body about 1.2 mm. wing 1.5 mm.

Columbia: Boca de Arquia, Atrato River, v. 1914, attacking man (Dr. A. Balfour).

The species is closely related to S. amazonicum, Goeldi, and shows very similar thoracic ornamentation. It differs in the absence of the iridescent green-blue bands, present in that species at the apices of some of the abdominal segments. There are also less appreciable differences in the coloration of the legs and in other details.

(descripción original tomada del trabajo Some new neotropical Simuliidae por Frederick Knab, Bureau of Entomology, U.S. Department of Agriculture. Bulletin of Entomological Research, Vol. VI, pl. III (diciembre 1915) pags. 279-280.

Distribución geográfica de esta especie

Fuera de Venezuela

Knab: Boca de Arquia, Río Atrato, Colombia.

En Venezuela:

Iriarte: En Tabay, a orillas del Río Chama, Estado Mérida.

En el río Orinoco, en Puerto Ayacucho, Territorio Amazonas.

En el río Sananariapo, Territorio Amazonas.

Simulium ochraceum Walker 1860.

Walker Francis. 1860. Trans. Ent. Soc. of London (n. ser.) v. pag. 332.

Simulium ochraceum Ost-Sack 1878.

Osten Sacken 1878. Cat. Dipt. N. Amer. ed. II. 14 (ref. Pinto).

Simulium ochraceum Coquillet 1898.

Coquillet 1898—Bull U.S. Dep. Agric. Ent. (n. ser.) Bull. No. 10. pag. 68 (ref. Pinto).

Simulium ochraceum Kertész 1902.

Kertész C. 1902. Catalogus Dipterorum. vo. I, pag. 289.

Simulium ochraceum Surcouf i González Rincones 1911.

Surcouf y González Rincones. 1911. Essai. Dipt. Vuln. Ven. Pt. I. pag. 291.

Simulium ochraceum Malloch 1914.

Malloch J.R. 1914. U.S. Dept. Agric. Bur. Ent. Tech. Serv. No. 26, pag. 30-31.

Odagmia ochracea Enderlein 1925.

Enderlein G. 1925. Zool. Anz. t. LXII, pag. 208.

Eusimulium ochraceum Dyar i Shannon 1927.

Dyar and Shannon. 1927. Proc. U.S. Nat. Mus. vol. LXIX, art. 10, pag. 16.

Eusimulium ochraceum Dampf 1927.

Dampf A. 1927. Rev. Mexicana de Biol. vol. VII.

Simulium ochraceum Lutz i Núñez Tovar 1928.

Lutz i Núñez Tovar. 1928. Est. de Zool. i Paras. Ven. pags. 45-6. Est. 4. fig. 4. Est. 6. fig. 3.

Simulium ochraceum Walker 1934.

Strong, Bequaert, Sandground, Muñoz Ochoa. 1934—Onchocerciasis. pag. 210.

Simulium ochraceum Walker 1940.

Fairchild G.B. 1940. Annals of the Ent. Soc. of Ame. pag. 706.

Simulium ochraceum Walker 1943.

Iriarte David R. 1943. Cont. a la Fauna Ven.—Bol. del Lab. Cli. Raz.—No. 11.

Simulium ochraceum.

Foem. Testaceum, albo-témentosum, capite albo, thorace ochraceo vittis duabus albis, abdomine nigricante basi testace, femoribus, tibiisque apice nigris, tarsis nigris basi testaceis, alis vitreis pallido-venosis.

Female. Testaceous, with white tomentum; head white; antennae testaceous; thorax ochraceous, with two white stripes; abdomen blackish, testaceous at base; femora and tibiae with black tips; tarsi black, testaceous towards the base; wings vitreous; veins pale testaceous.

Length: of the body I line; of the wings 2.5 linears.

México.

This species can hardly be the female of S. metallicum Bellardi.

(descripción original de The Transactions of the Entomological Society of London, new series, vol. V, part. VII, nov. 1860. —XXIII. Characters of underscribed Diptera in the Collection of W.W. Sanders, Esq., F.R.S., etc. by Francis Walker. Esq., F.L.S., etc. (leído el 2 de febrero de 1857) pags. 332-335).

Sobre la especie ochraceum Walker 1861, dice Malloch J.R. en su trabajo American black flies or buffalo gnats en 1914, lo siguiente: "the records of the ocurrence of this species in the United States which I have had the opportunity of examining are erroneous and refer to notatum Adams".

Referente a Simulium ochraceum Walker, dice Fairchild en su trabajo Notes on the Simuliidae of Panamá (Dipt. Nematocera), 1940, lo que sigue. "My material agrees well with Bequaert's and Hoffmann's descriptions and figures, except that the pupal filaments branch somewhat more basally than shown in Hoffmann's figure. S. ochraceum of Lutz and Núñez Tovar (1928. Est. Zool. Parasit. Venezolanas pag. 45, Pt. 4, Fig. 4 (o) Pl. 6, Fig. 3 respiratory filament), and of Pinto (1931, 7th Reun. Soc. Argentina Pat. Reg. Norte, pp. 739, 752, Fig. 10) seems to be different, as the arrangement of the pupal filaments is not the same, the size is larger, the abdomen entirely dark, and the legs extensively light colored. Recently, J. Lane and C.E. Porto (Bol. Biol. Sao Paulo, (N. s.) IV, 2, p. 171 1939) mention specimens (as Eusimulium ochraceum) from Bolivia, but they give no description".

"The species has been bred from pupae on dead leaves in a small stream on the Atlantic side of the Isthmus, and a single pupa secured at El Valle on the Pacific side. It has no been seen to bite man".

Distribución geográfica de esta especie

Fuera de Venezuela.

Walker: México.

Pinto: En Méjico, Tuxtla Gutiérrez, Chiapas (A.L. Herrera) Simojonel, Chiapas (A.L. Herrera).

Fairchild: Panamá records: El Valle, Coclé Prov., (pupa solamente) Cerro Sta. Rita, Colón Prov., Río Puente, R.P.

Bequaert: Sta. Emilia, Mocá, Finca Helvetia i Mezeval, Guatemala.

Dampf: El Zapote, Chiapas, Méjico.

En Venezuela:

Lutz i Núñez Tovar: obtuvimos larvas i ninfas en el río de El Limón.

Iriarte. 1° en Tabay, a orillas del río Chama, Estado Mérida 2° En el riachuelo que corre al lado de la carretera que va de Caracas a Guarenas, en el sitio llamado El Samán, Estado Miranda.

Simulium exiguum Roubaud 1906.

Roubaud M.E. 1906. Bull. Mus. Hist. Nat. No. 2. pag. 107-108.

Simulium exiguum Roubaud 1906.

Malloch J.R. 1914—U.S. Depart. Agric. Bur. Ent. Tech. Serv.

Simulium exiguum Roubaud 1906.

Strong, Bequaert, Sandground i Muñoz Ochoa. 1934 Onchocerciasis, pag. 210.

Simulium exiguum Roubaud 1906.

Fairchild G.B. 1940. Annals of Ent. Soc. of Amer. No. 4

Simulium exiguum Roubaud 1906.

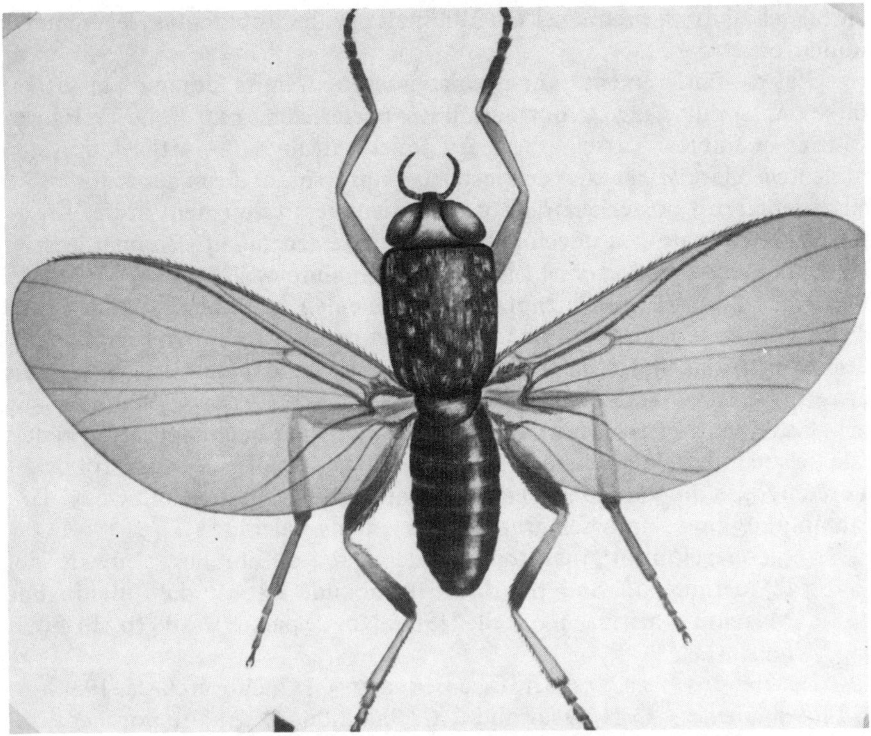

Simulium exiguum Roubaud 1906

Encontrado por nosotros por segunda vez en el país, ya que Geay lo capturó en 1889 en el Alto Sarare. Esta pequeña especie, además de tener una repartición amplia en Venezuela, en caso de que el carate fuera trasmitido por estos dípteros, la especie ***exiguum*** *desempeñaría un gran papel, porque casi el 100% de los simúlidos que hemos capturado en el Estado Barinas, sede del gran foco de esta endemia, pertenecen a esta especie.*

Iriarte David R. 1942. Estudios de Patología Tropical. (obra).
Simulium exiguum Roubaud 1942.

Iriarte David R. 1942. Bol. del Lab. Cli. Luis Razetti. No. 8. junio.
Simulium exiguum nov. sp.
o Inconnu.

° Gris bleu, pruineux; condensée, globuleuse, à membres courts entièrement jaune clair. Trés petite espèce variant de 1 millimétre à 1 millim: 5; rarement 2 millimétres. Ailes courtes, blanchâtres, de la longuéur du corps.

Tete.—Large, sphérique. Yeux roussâtres, à reflets verts. Face et front gris verdatre, antennes, palpes e piéces buccales brun jaunatre, les premieres jaune clair à la base.

Thorax.—Fortement convexe, lisse, globuleux, entiérement d'un gris pruineux; quelques traces de poils courts jaune d'or. Ecusson gris, jaunissant a la pointe. Balanciers blancs. Ailes blanchậtres, laiteuses. Nervure costale et les trois premières longitudinales seules apparentes, légèrement jaunâtres.

Patte—Entièrement jaune clair, nues; extrémite des métatarses et tarses anterieurs, des fémurs et tibias postérieurs, plus foncée. Pattes courtes et faibles. Tarses antérieurs greles, enfumés, les articles moyens nullement élargis. Métatarses postérieurs présentant deux ou trois longs cils à leur bord postérieur; le bord anterieur tres faiblement armé. L'expansion terminale peu développée, mais nette cependent. Premier article tarsien sublinéaire, fortement incisé. Griffes simples.

Abdomen.—Brun clair, glabre, extrêmement volumineux, tout é fait disproportionnê chez certains individus; la portion tout à fait superieure des segments basilaires, la majeure partie des segments terminaux, légèrement bronze brilliant.

Cette petite espèce, tout á fait remarquable par la condensation générale de son corps, la brièveté et la débilité de ses pattes, son allure robuste, a été envoyée du Vénézuela (Haute Sarare) en 1899, par M.F. Geay. Un examplaire piqué; un assez grand nombre dans l'alcol.

(descripción original tomada del trabajo Simulies nouvelle de l'Amérique du Sud por M.E. Roubaud. Extrait du Bulletin du Museum d'histiore naturelle. 1906. No. 2. pag. 107-108 (p. 3 i 4 del reprint).

Refiriéndose a esta especie dice Bequaert, en Onchocerciasis, 1934, p. 212 los siguiente: "G.H. Dyar and R.C. Shannon (1927 a) do not mention this species which thus far was recorded from Guatemala, Venezuela, and Perú. I have recently seen specimens obtained by Mr. Sam Clark at Provincia, on the Río San Pedro, State of Tabasco, Mexico (August 18, 1933)." "In the coffee-growing region of Guatemala S. exiguum is probably widely distributed, although apparently less abundant than the three Onchoccerca-carrying black-flies. I have observed it only once, at the Finca Sa. Adelaida, a few miles from Mocá, where it was biting man on April 11, 1931. It was also brought to us at Sa. Emilia, from a neighboring cafetal where it was annoying horses as well as people. Finally a number of specimens were taken by D.M. Bates in March, 1931, at Antigua (altitude about 5.000 ft.) while biting man, being the only species observed at the time".

"S. exiguum is one of the smallest species of black-flies, the living females varying in length from 1.5 to 1.8 mm. The body is black, the mesonotum covered with scales. There are no iridescent spots on the thorax, nor pruinose bands on the abdomen, in fresh individuals. Antennae and legs are extensively yellowish; but the hind femora are brownish and the apical half of the hind tibiae, as well as some of the tarsal segments, are black. Male, larva, cocoon, pupa and breeding places are unknown".

"In the female, S. exiguum is characterized as follows: Frons and face wide. Antennae eleven-segmented, more slender than usual, equally wide throughout, all the segments except the last of about same width and most of them nearly square, the last very broadly rounded off. Front tarsi slender. Hind tarsus with distinct pedisulcus and large calcipala; the sector of radius (R 2-3) unbranched, reaching the costa close basal heel, apparently without sub-basal tooth. Wings with sector of radius (R 23) unbranched, reaching the costa close to the tip of the radius (R1), setose over its apical portion; radius setose over its apical portion only, the basal section bare; cubitus (Cu2) with conspicuous double bend; anal vein (An) curved upward apically; no basal cell. Tip of abdomen shiny".

"In F.W. Edward's (1931b) key to the subgenera, this species would run to Simulium, proper".

Este simulido señalado la primera vez por Roubaud, proveniente del Alto Sarare, que suponemos sea un sitio del Estado Lara, lo hemos citado nosotros por segunda vez en Venezuela, en capturas hechas en el río de Guarenas, Estado Miranda (v. Est. de Pat. Trop.)

Si el carate tiene un vector i si este es un simulido como se ha sospechado hace tanto tiempo i como ha tratado de demostrarlo González Herrejón con el S. haematopotum en Méjico, el exiguum desempeñaría posiblemente igual papel entre nosotros, porque casi el 100% de los simulidos que hemos capturado en el Estado Barinas, en el propio gran foco de esta endemia, son de la especie mencionada. Sin embargo, nuestras últimas experiencias a orillas del río Canaguá en las inmediaciones de la ciudad de Barinas, poniendo a picar especímenes de S. exiguum sobre lesiones caratosas con treponemas positivo, sacrificándolos corto tiempo después i examinando el contenido de ellos en fondo obscuro, la búsqueda de treponemas ha sido negativa.

Distribución geográfica de esta especie.

Fuera de Venezuela.

Pinto: en Guatemala, Cacao, Trece Aguas en Malloch 1914 i abordo a 4 millas de Livingston en Malloch. 1914.

Bequaert: en la finca Sa. Adelaida, cerca de Mocá, en Sa. Emilia i en Antigua, (a 5.000 pies de altura), sitios todos de Guatemala.

En Venezuela:

Roubaud: Haut Sarare.

Iriate: En Tabay, a orillas del río Chama, Estado Mérida.

En riachuelo Curucurumbo, a 16 km. de Maracay i a una altura de 550 metros, Estado Aragua.

En el río Guarenas, Guarenas, Estado Miranda.

Acequias El Salao i Canuabita, Estado Yaracuy

Río Yurubí, piscina de San Felipe, Estado Yaracuy

Río Aguascalientes, cercano a Las Trincheras, Estado Carabobo.

Río Trincheras, Hotel Trincheras, Estado Carabobo.

Riachuelo de los baños de Duaca, Estado Lara.

Riachuelo de la piscina de Macuto, cerca de Barquisimeto, Estado Lara.

Quebrada Aguascalientes, Estado Barinas.

Ríos Mazparro, Boconó, Tucupido, Canaguá i quebrada La Parángula, Estado Barinas.

En el río Sananariapo, cerca de Pto. Ayacucho, Territorio Amazonas.

En el río Orinoco, en Puerto Ayacucho, Territorio Amazonas.

Simulium rubrithorax Lutz 1909.

Lutz Adolfo. 1909. Mem. Inst. Osw. Cruz. t. I. fasc. II. pag. 132-3.

Simulium rubrithorax Lutz 1910.

Lutz A. 1910—Mem. Ins. Osw. Cruz. t. II. fasc. 2. pag. 222.

Simulium rubrithorax Surcouf i González Rincones 1911.

Surcouf i González Rincones. 1911. Essai. Dipt. Vuln. Ven. Pt. I, pag. 285-6.

Simulium rubrithorax Lutz, Araujo e Fonseca 1918.

Lutz, Araujo, e Fonseca. 1918. Mem. Inst. Isw. Cruz. t. X. fasc. I. pag. 165.

Simulium rubrithorax Pinto 1931.

Pinto César. 1931. Simuliidae da Amer. Cent. e do Sul. 7th Reu. Pat. Reg. Norte.

Simulium rubrithorax Lutz 1928.

Lutz A. 1928. Estud. de Zool. i Paras. Venez. pag. 42.

Simulium rubrithorax Iriarte 1942.

Iriarte David R. 1942. Bol. Lab. Cli. Razetti. No. 8. vol. II. junio.

Simulium rubrithorax Lutz 1909 n. sp.

Côr geral preta e vermelha, comprimento 3 a 4 mm.

Cabeça, preta com brilho prateado, tromba e palpos pardo-ferrujinozos; occiput com pelos bastante compridos.

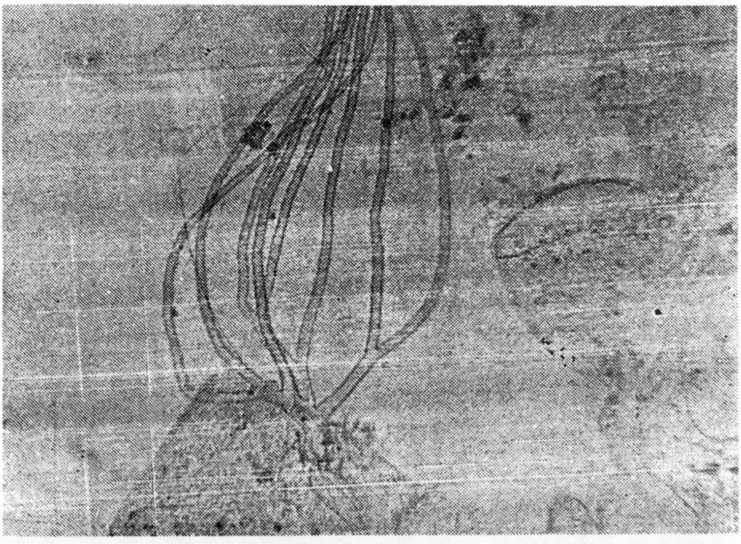

(Fig. 11) Filamentos branquiales de S. paraguayense, si nos atenemos a la descripción y figura de Pinto. Material de Tabay (Edo. Mérida).

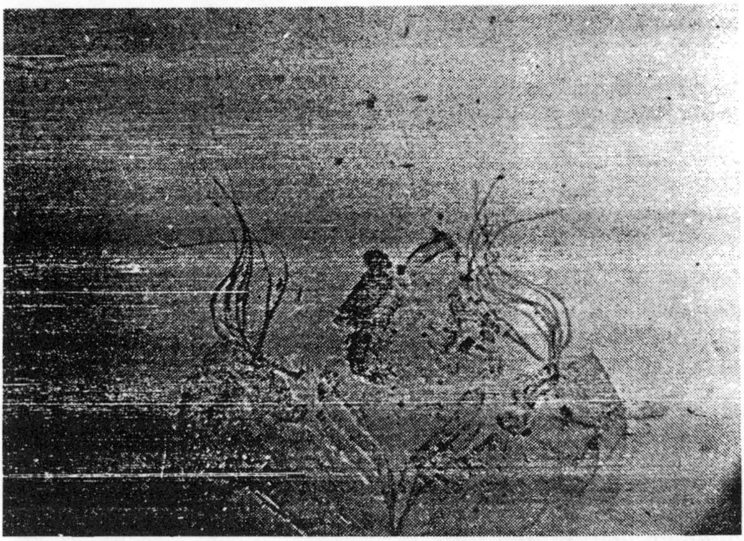

(Fig. 12) Mechones branquiales pupales de S. paraguayense, según Pinto, proveniencia Tabay (Edo. Mérida).

Torax: escudo vermelho escuro, alaranjado ou pardacento, com escamas piliformes douradas; escutelo como escudo, com pelos escuros na marjem livre; pleuras côr de chocolate, as vezes um puco avermelhada, com brillo cinzento.

Abdome, em cima enfuscado, com brilho cinzento; dos lados e em baixo com cintas claras e escuras.

Pernas: primeiro par ocraceo até os ojelhos com pelos e escamas finas, ora claras ora escuras, tibias, na parte anterior, com pó claro e escamas piliformes brancas, o resto ocraceo ou pardacento, o pé quazi preto. Segundo par como o primeiro, mas o metatarso, nos terços posteriores, de côr clara, como tambem a tibia com exceçao das extremidades.

Terceiro par: coxas escuras, trocanteres e fumures ocraceos, como tambem a baze das tibias que no restante sao enegrecidas, mas cobertas de escamas estreitas claras; metatarsos na metade bazal é na maior parte da sua circumferencia claros o resto escuro, apenas a baze do segundo articulo do pé um pouco mais claro. Unhas com un dente.

Azas como de cotume, apenas na baze da costa com uns pelos mais compridos, protejados na celula costal; halteres com o capitulo de côr palida de cera, tornando-se escura em direcao á baze.

Descrito de algunas femeas apanhadas na serra da Bocaina a 1.500 m. de altura e em Batataes.

(descripción original tomada del trabajo Contribuicao para o conhocimento das especies brazileiras do gnero "Simulium" por A. Lutz. en Memorias do Instituto Oswaldo Cruz, t. I. fasc. II. 1909. agosto. pag. 132)

Distribución geográfica de esta especie.

Fuera de Venezuela.

Lutz: Sierra de Bocaina a 1.500 m. i Batataes, Brasil (1909). cerca de Lassance, Estado de Minas Geraes (Lutz 1910) Brasil.

Lutz i Machado: Sierra de Guacuhy (1915) Brasil.

Lutz, Araujo e Fonseca: Bonplan. Missoes. (1918) Brasil.

Pinto: En Argentina.

En Venezuela.

Lutz: lo encontramos formando colonias de larvas i de ninfas sobre las piedras de un afluente del río de Ocumare de la Costa. El adulto, que ocasionalmente ataca al hombre, no fue posible capturarlo en condiciones naturales.

Iriarte: en riachuelo cercano al pueblo de Choroní, Estado Aragua. Este riachuelo lo llaman río Choroní; la captura fue hecha en el sitio El Parnaso.

Pifano: En el Estado Yaracuy.

Simulium incrustatum Lutz 1910

Lutz A. 1910. Mem. do Ins. Osw. Cruz. t. II. fasc. 2. pag. 243-5 i 263-4.

Simulium incrustatum Surcouf i González Rincones 1911

Surcouf i González Rincones. 1911. Essai. Dipt. Vuln. Ven. Pt. I. pag. 288.

Simulium incrustatum Lutz i Machado 1915

Lutz i Machado. 1915. Mem. Ins. Osw. Cruz. t. VII. pag. 46.

Simulium incrustatum Lutz i Núñez Tovar 1928

Lutz i Núñez Tovar en Lutz A. 1928. Est. do Zool. i Paras. Ven. pag. 44-5. Est. 6. fig. I.

Simulium incrustatum Pinto 1931

Pinto César. 1931. Simuliidae da Amer. Cent. e do Sul. 7th Reu. Pat. Reg. del Norte.

Simulium incrustatum Iriarte 1942

Iriarte David R. 1942. Bol. del Lab. Cli. Razetti. No. 8. vol. II. junio.

Simulium incrustatum Lutz 1910-n. sp.

Tamanho: cerca de 2-3 mm.; côr geral preto

Macho: antenas inteiramente de côr chocolate escura com pouca pubecencia esbranquicada, apenas o tóro avermelhado; palpos da mesma côr chocolate, como tamben a tromba e a face; esta ultima com alguns pêlos dourados; olhos confluentes e muito grandes, na parte de cima, com as grandes facetas, de côr chocolate, na de baixo, de facetas pequenas, e com brilho verde-dourado; o occiput parece escuro.

Torax, em cima de preto aveludado, menos nos lugares seguintes: duas estrias em forma de virgula ou cuneiformes, partindo da marjem anterior, a distancia quazi egual das marjens e da linha mediana e correspondendo ao terço do comprimento do escudo, duas faxas largas tarjando os lados do escudo e outra ocupando a marjem posterior adiante do escutelo; aqui, o fundo tem a côr de chumbo velho com lijeiro brilho nacarado. Ha escamas curtas, estreitas e pouco densas de uma côr de latão bastante brilhant que se tornam mais compridas por cima de faxa posterior e no escutelo têm direção transversal; as pleuras e a face inferior do torax tem of fundo parecido com o das faxas descritas, mas memos brilhante.

Abdomen preto, do quinto anel para tranz com algunas manchas prateadas dos lados e em baixo, uma mancha branca de cada lado do segundo segmento e uma franja de pelos escuros e bastante compridos na marjem posterior do primeiro anel.

Azas iriantes em vermelho, alaranjado e amarelo, as nervuras grossas amarelo dourado, as finas quazi sem côr; a base pardacenta de pèlos da mesma côr; halteres com o capitulo de côr de canario (do reino), assaz brilhante.

Pernas: primeiro par ocraceo, mais ou menos enegrecido, até aos joelhos, as tibias pretas com a fac anterior clara. o resto completamente preto; na coxa e no femur ha pêlos compridos escuros e escamas douradas obovais, compridas, muito conspicuas; na tibia ha outras, de côr branca, como o fundo; segundo par na sua totalidade pardacento, na coxa com muitas escamas douradas e algumas mais claras, o péquazi preto; terceiro par pardo-acinzentado até ao apice da tibia, com pelos bastante compridos; o metatarso é branco, menos ñas extremidades a na face posterior que são pretas; o resto do pé é preto; as unhas têm a forma do costume.

A femea tem os trez primeiros articulos das antenas avermelhadas; a côr das pernas varia, podendo sêr mais clara ou mais escura, geralmente, porém, parece-se com a descrição acima, mostrando distintamente as escamas.

Os pêlos no primeiro anel abdominal e na perna de traz são mais curtos do que no macho, o lado inferior do abdome é distintamente canelado em baixo e as unhas têm um dente pequeno.

A larva, de côr encarnada diluida, é bastante pequena; transforma-se em pupa muito pequena com tubos branquiais compridos e finos terminados por ponta subcónica. Logo na base nacem tres troncos por duas divizões secessivas, bifurcando-se sômente muito mais acima, primeiro o impar e depois os dois pares. Os tricomas são simples ou bifidos, a pele.

As larvas e pupas, mais raramente o mosquito perfeito, foram obtidos em muitos lugares, por exemplo em Petropolis, Mendes e na Serra da Bocaina, em São Paulo (rios Pacaembú e Anhangabahú); o mosquito foi tambem colecionado em Alfenas pelo Dr. Gurgel do Amaral e no interior de Pernambuco pelo Dr. David Madeira. Ataca aos cavalos mas não persegue o homem.

(descripción original tomada del trabajo Segunda contribuicão para o conhocimento das especies brazileiras do genero "Simulium" en Mem. do Inst. Osw. Cruz. t. II. fasc. II. 1910. pag. 243).

Distribución geográfica de esta especie
Fuera de Venezuela.

Lutz: en Estado de Río de Janeiro, Petropolis i Mendes.
en Estado São Paulo, Serra de Bocaina, rios Pacaembú i Anhangabahú.
en Estado de Minas Geraes, Alfenas
en Estado de Pernambuco, en el interior (col. Dr. Madeira) Lutz 1910
Lutz i Machado: en Estado de Minas Geraes, corriente de Jatobá
en Estado de Bahía, Ribeirao i rio Ondas i Vila Nova.

En Venezuela:

Lutz i Núñez Tovar: observado en sus tres estados cerca de Maracay i en Guayabita, hacienda que está próxima a la población de Turmero. Ataca al hombre, pero tiene marcada predilección por los equídeos.

Iriarte: en riachuelo llamado La Quebrada que pasa en las afueras del pueblo Choroní, Estado Aragua.
a orillas del río Choroní, en el sitio El Parnaso, cercano al pueblo Choroní, Estado Aragua.
en riachuelo que corre al lado de la carretera que va de Caracas al pueblo de Guarenas, en el sitio llamado El Samán, Estado Miranda.
en quebrada llamada Pavía, Estado Yaracuy.
a orillas de la quebrada llamada Aguascalientes i a orillas del río Canaguá, Estado Barinas (capturas de hembras picando).

Simulium lugubre Lutz i Núñez Tovar 1928

Lutz i Núñez Tovar en Lutz A. 1928. Est. de Zool. i Paras. Ven.

Simulium lugubre Pinto 1931

Pinto César. 1931. Simuliidae da America Central e do Sul. 7th Reu. de Pat. Reg. Norte.

Simulium lugubre Fairchild 1940

Fairchild G.B. 1940. Ann. Ent. Soc. of Amer. vol. XXXIII. pag. 708.
Simulium lugubre nobis
Est. 4. fig. 2. Est. 6. fig. 6.

Hembra. Longitud total de 3 a 4 mm. Color general negro, mas o menos brillante, con reflejos color de nácar i plateados.

Antenas con base ferruginosa oscura; el resto de estos apéndices revestido de pelos cortos i blancos. Clipeo i frente con brillo blanquecino, principalmente en los bordes. Cuello i torax marrón oscuro. Escudo i escudete de aspecto escarchado, debido a numerosos grupos de escamas lineales de color dorado pálido.

Abdomen profundamente anillado; por su cara dorsal es negro lustroso como antracita con reflejos plateados sobre todo en la conjunción de los anillos; inferiormente sin brillo, con los primeros segmentos ocráceos, cenicientos o verdes. Lóbulos genitales subcilíndricos i largos.

Patas: Primer par ocráceo hasta la rodilla, con pelillos i escamas blanquecinas; lo demás negro. Los pares posteriores son negros, con la base de los tres primeros tarsos mas o menos blanca. Todas las tibias están guarnecidas, por su lado externo, con pelos níveos. Uñas con diente.

Alas con brillo irisado. Balancines con pedículo oscuro i oliva casi blanca.

Macho: Se distingue de la hembra por los caracteres sexuales comunes que siguen: tamaño menor, uñas, reflejos plateados mas vivos i ojos confluentes, con el segmento superior de facetas mayores anaranjado. Nuestro único ejemplar muestra en el escudo, en donde se han desprendido las escamas lineales, una línea oscura mediana i dos laterales mas claras. Los órganos genitales son recogidos.

Larva: La larva busca los sitios en donde la corriente de las aguas es mui fuerte, allí vive en soportes vegetales o adherida directamente a las piedras. Puede alcanzar hasta ocho milímetros de longitud i no tiene espinas en la piel. El color es claro, con muchas manchas negras.

Ninfa. La cápsula exterior con un vestíbulo corto i saliente, tiene la forma de un zapato alto. La ninfa es de cuatro milímetros de longitud i de color ceniciento oscuro en el segmento anterior, en donde hai muchos gránulos de una coloración más subida. Los tricomas, raros i finos, son simple o bifidos. Tiene doce tubos branquiales bastante largos que disminuyen de ancho en dirección a la punta. Las dos terceras partes de la bifurcaciones se hallan cerca de la base. Colocada en una cámara húmeda, los adultos salen durante los primeros dos días. En muchas ocasiones las ninfas se encuentran adheridas a la cara inferior de las piedras, aún cuando éstas están colocadas en corrientes de agua de curso fuerte.

Nota: Esta especie se parece mucho al Simulium orbitale (Lutz 1910) del cual se diferencia por la piel lisa de la larva, por el sistema branquial de la ninfa i por la uñas del adulto con 2 puntas en la hembra i 3 en el macho. Lugar de captura: río de Maracay i en las inmediaciones de La Trinidad.

(descripción original tomada del trabajo de Lutz i Núñez Tovar, en A. Lutz. 1928. Estudios de Zoología i Parasitología Venezolanas. Río de Janeiro, diciembre, pág. 46).

En su trabajo Notes on the Simuliidae of Panamá (Dipt. Nematocera) del año 1940, Fairchild trae entre las sinonimias de Simulium mexicanum Bellardi a la presente especie i a este respecto dice: ''My material agrees quite well with Bequaert's description. Lutz and Tovar's descriptions and figures of the adult and the pupal filaments seem to fit the present species closely, though they do not mention the hairy base of the radius''. In the text the length is given as 3-4 mm. which would be about right for this species, but the figure indicates a species considerably less than 2 mm. in length. However, the part of this work dealing with Simuliidae apparently was not checked, and the text and figures do not agree in many instances''

Distribución geográfica de esta especie

Fuera de Venezuela:

Fairchild: si se acepta la posibilidad de que mexicanum Bellardi sea igual a lúgubre Lutz, Fairchild trae la siguiente distribución: México, Guatemala, Panamá, Venezuela.

Sitios de captura en Panamá: El Valle, Coclé Prov. adultos i pupas.

En Venezuela:

Lutz i Núñez Tovar: río de Maracay i en las inmediaciones de La Trinidad.

Iriarte: río que corre al lado de la carretera que va de Caracas a la población de Guarenas, en el sitio llamado El Samán, mui cerca de Petare, Estado Miranda.

Simulium lutzianus Pinto 1931

Pinto César—1931. Simuliidae da Ame. Cent. e do Sul. 7th. R. Pat. Reg. Norte pags. 748-751. figs. 39 i 40.

Simulium rubrithorax Lutz i Núñez Tovar 1928

Lutz i Núñez Tovar en Lutz A. 1928. Est. de Zool. i Paras. Ven. Est. 6. fig. 2 (en parte, no S. rubrithorax Lutz 1909).

Simulium lutzianus Smart 1940

Smart. 1940. Transactions Royal Ent. Soc. of London. XC. pag. 7.

Simulium lutzianus Fairchild i Briceño Iragorry 1943

Fairchild G.B. i L. Briceño Iragorry. 1943. Bol. Lab. Cli. Razetti. No. 10. vol. III. mayo.

Simulium lutzianus (descripción del adulto).

Hembra.—Cabeza negra, frente ancha, de aspecto nacarado pulverulento. Fronto-clipeus amarillo pulverulento. Antena con el primer segmento i base del segundo rojizo, el resto negro. Longitud del mesonotum i scutellum, 0-8 mm. Mesonotum de un amarillo anaranjado intenso, con escasos pelos dorados, márgenes laterales con pulverulento plateado. Scutellum de un amarilo pálido, con pelos erectos en el margen posterior. Pleura negra, escasamente gris pulverulento. Patas negras con pelos negros, con escepción de la tibia anterior, i los basitarsos medianos i poste

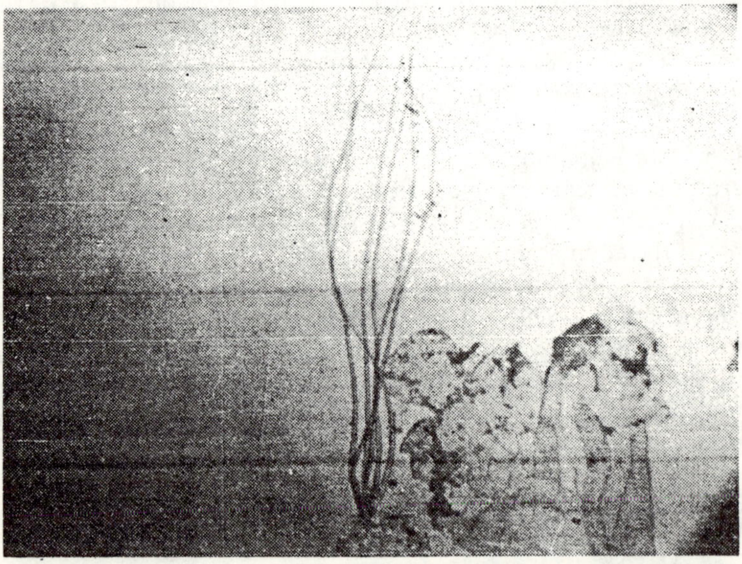

(Fig. 13) Manojo de seis tubos respiratorios que pensamos pueda tratarse de S. metallicum o clarki según Fairchild, o bien de S. subnigrum, según Pinto. Material colectado en la acequia del Parque Knoop en Los Teques.

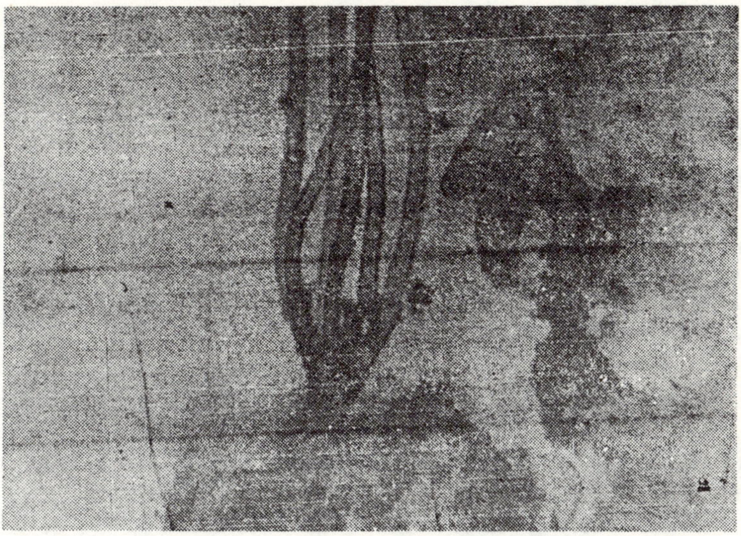

(Fig. 14) Ramillete de tubos branquiales en número de seis, que creemos pueda ser de S. clarki o metallicum según Fairchild, o bien de S. subnigrum según Pinto. Material capturado en acequia del Parque Knoop de Los Teques.

rior que son en parte blanquecinos con pelos del mismo color. Alas con la costa i el radius cerdosos, subcostal casi desnuda o con mui pocas espinas; sección basal del radius con una simple hilera de espinas o pelos. Halteras amarillo pálidas. Abdomen enteramente negro i lustroso con un pequeño mechón de pelos amarillos i largos a los lados del primer segmento. Calcipala i pedisulcus bien desarrolados, garras tarsales con pequeño diente sub-basal.

Macho.—Semejante a la hembra en coloración, ojos con los dos tercios superiores i facetas mui grandes. Los genitales no fueron estudiados. Capullo ninfal de contextura densa con escasa rutilancia lateral. Pupa con 8 filamentos branquiales largos i delgados, naciendo de dos troncos principales; el primer tronco se divide casi a un 1/4 de su largura de la base, el segundo lo hace mui cerca de la base, las ramas resultantes se dividen a su vez a corta distancia i una de cada de estos pares de ramos divídese una vez más cerca de un 1/4 de su largura de la base.

Los pelos en el sector basal de radius colocan esta especie en el sub-género Eusimulium. Se distingue de samboni Jennings por las garras tarsales i el abdomen completamente negro, del panamense Fairchild por no tener el tórax rayado, del ochraceum Walk, por tener el abdomen enteramente negro, del antillarum Jennings por la fémora negra, del dinelli Joan por la negrura del abdomen i pleura, del perflavum Roub. por la fémora negra i del rubrithorax Lutz por su pequeñez, ausencia de rayas en el mesonotum i caracteres de la pupa.

(descripción original tomada del trabajo Nota sobre Simulium lutzianus (descripcíon del adulto) por G.B. Fairchild i L. Briceño Iragorry. 1943. Bol. del Lab. de la Clí. Razetti. Año IV. No. 10. vol. III. pag. 189).

Este especie fue individualizada por Pinto en 1931, sirviéndose de material llevado por el Profesor A. Lutz en su viaje hecho a nuestro país. Esta especie estaba englobada en dicho material en la especie rubrithorax. Pinto había descrito solamente la pupa.

Distribución geográfica de esta especie.

En Venezuela.

Pinto: río Castaño, Estado Aragua (pupa).

Fairchild i Briceño Iragorry: Los Chorros, cerca de Caracas al estado de pupa i de adulto atacando al hombre.

Iriarte: En Tabay, a orillas del río Chama, Estado Mérida. En el sitio El Samán, al lado de la carretera que conduce a la población de Guarenas, Estado Miranda.

Nota: con material que enviamos a Alan Stone con fecha 5 de octubre de 1942, colectado a orillas del río Chama, en el pueblo de Tabay, Estado Mérida, nos decía en carta lo siguiente: "Eusimulium sp. ♂. ♀. With orange scutum. This is probably the same as Simulium rubrithorax, as determined by Smart, but is, I believe, quite different from the rubrithorax described by Lutz. We have two specimens of the latter, determined by Lutx, and it is a true Simulium and very different".

Luego en carta marzo 13 de 1943, clasificándome material colectado en el riachuelo que corre a lo largo de la carretera que conduce de Caracas a Guarenas, Estado Miranda, en el sitio llamado El Samán, nos dice en carta lo que sigue: "Eusimulium lutzianus (Pinto), adult and pupal skin. This is the same as the Eusimulium sp. of my letter of October 22. I overlooked Pinto's description of this species because he called it a Simulium rather than a Eusimulium".

Simulium metallicum Bellardi 1859

Bellardi Luigi. 1859. Saggio di ditterología Messicana. Pt. I. pag. 13-4. Torino.

Simulium metallicum Kertesz 1902

Kertesz C. 1902. Cat. Dipterorum. vol. I. pag. 288.

Simulium metallicum Roubaud 1906

Roubaud E. 1906. Bull. Mus. Hist. Nat. París. t. XII. No. 7. nvbre. pag. 518.

Simulium metallicum Sourcouf i González Rincones 1911

Surcouf i González Rincones 1911. Essai. Dipt. Vuln. Ven. pag. 381-2.

Simulium metallicum Malloch 1914

Malloch J.R. 1914. U.S. Dept. Agric. Bur. Ent. Tech. Serv. Serie 26. pags. 48-9.

Odagmia metallica Enderlein 1925

Enderlein 1925. Zool. Anzeiger. LXII. pag. 208.

Simulium metallicum Dyar i Shannon 1927

Dyar i Shannon—1927. Proc. U.S. Nat. Mus. vol. LXIX, pag. 41. figs. 72-3.

Simulium metallicum Dampf 1927

Dampf A. 1927. Rev. Mex. de Biol. vol. VII.

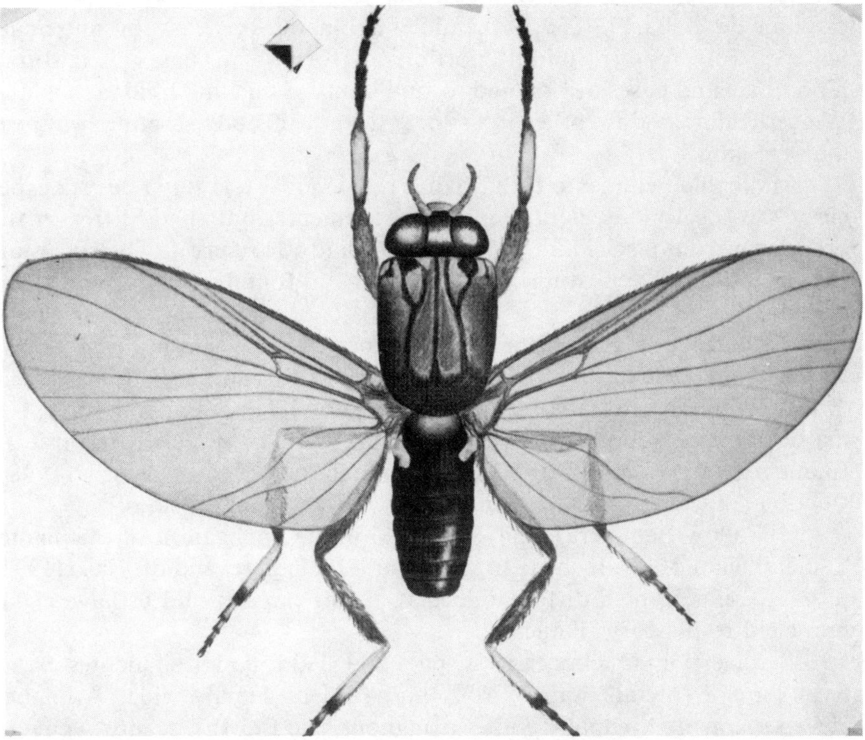

Simulium metallicum Bellardi 1859

Hallado por primera vez en Venezuela por Briceño Iragorry y seguidamente citado por nosotros. Es la especie más repartida en el país, encontrándola hasta ahora nosotros en el Distrito Federal, donde es la especie corriente, y en siete Estados, el último de ellos ha sido el Estado Zulia (orillas del río Apón, Distrito Perijá).

Simulium metallicum Pinto 1931

Pinto César. 1931. Simuliidae da Amer. Cent. e do Sul. 7th Reu. Pat. Reg. del Norte.

Simulium metallicum Strong, Bequaert, Sandground, Muñoz Ochoa 1934

Strong, Bequaert, Sandground, Muñoz Ochoa. 1934. Onchocerciasis. pag. 208.

Simulium metallicum Fairchild 1940

G.B. Fairchild. 1940. Ann. Ent. Soc. of Amer. vol. XXXIII. pag. 712.

Simulium metallicum Briceño Iragorry 1941

Briceño Iragorry L. 1941. Bol. Lab. Cli. Razetti. vol. II. No. 6. pag. 114.

Simulium metallicum Iriarte 1942

Iriarte David R. 1942. Bol. Lab. Cli. Razetti. vol. II. No. 8. junio.

Damos una traslación en inglés del macho de S. metallicum, tomando del trabajo de Malloch J. R. U. S. Dep. Agri. Bur. Ent. Tech. Serv. del original de Bellardi 1859. "metallicum blue-black. Base of antennae, halteres, fore femora, middle portions of fore tibiae, bases of mid and hind tibiae and bases of first and second joints of mid and hind tarsi white. Wings hyaline, veins rather indistinct. Length of body, 2 mm.. wing expanse, 5 mm".

Malloch en el mismo trabajo dice refiriéndose a la pupa de esta especie: "the species has eight respiratory filaments, but these differ in the branching from piscicidum, as shown in Plate VI, figure 4. The cocoon is similar to that of venustum, closely woven and found on leaves and stems of plants".

"The foregoing details are drawn from material sent in by Mr. F.W. Urich, from Trinidad, along with imagines of this species". (pag. 49).

Fairchild, en su trabajo Notes on the Simuliidae of Panamá (dipt. Nematocera) dice sobre este especie: "Pupa with six-branched respiratory filaments, the filaments long and the branches close to the base (fig. 38). Cocoon conical, of rather open weave, and with flaring sides".

"I follow Bequaert (1934, pag. 208) in the application of this name. S. metallicum of Malloch (1914, p. 28) at least in part, and of Pinto (1931, p. 676) seems to be a different species, as the pupa is said to have eight-branched respiratory filaments".

Bequaert, en Onchocerciasis, pag. 209, 1934, da los siguientes caracteres para S. metallicum: "Frons and face of female wide. Antennae eleven-segmented, equally wide throughout, the fourth to tenth segments wider than long. Front tarsi distinctly flattened. Hind tarsus with distinct pedisulcus and a long and broad calcipala; the second segment pale at base. Claws without strong basal tooth, with a minute sub-basal tooth. Wings with sector of radius (R2-3) unbranched, reaching the costa close to the tip of the radius (R1), covered with setae over nearly its entire length; radius setosa inapical portion only, the basal section bare; cubitus (Cu2) with a conspicuous double bend. anal vein (An) curved upward apically; no basal cell. Tip. of abdomen of female shinny".

El mismo Bequaert respecto a la pupa escribe: "This is characterized by the few, very long thread-like respiratory filaments, which reach 4 mm. in length, being longer than the pupa. There are on each side 6 filaments, arranged in three pairs, three short common stalks of each pair branching off from the main stem in close succesion. The respiratory filaments are figured by C.C. Hoffmann (1931b, p. 216, fig. 17)".

Malloch i Pinto traen 8 tubos branquiales para las pupas de esta especie: Fairchild i lo mismo Bequaert traen 6 tubos branquiales para el metallicum. Es un punto que es necesario dilucidar i nosotros creemos que en el grupo metallicum debe haber más de una especie. Si aceptamos lo de Malloch asignable a la descripción primera de Bellardi, lo de Bequaert i Fairchild, mui posiblemente corresponderá a una nueva especie.

Con respecto a esto, copiamos párrafos de dos cartas de Stone: "the filamentary pupa agrees with that of metallicum as described by Pinto, but not as described by Fairchild. This will require further material and study". (julio 28 de 1942).

"Simulium sp. three pupal skins. These were associated with the adult metallicum so that this adult there were two, or possibly three different species represented by pupal skins. No three of the pupal skins agreed exactly with either the figures of Pinto of Fairchild, although one was close to that of Pinto and two were close to that of Fairchild. This complex is very puzzling, and we will not solve the problem until we have a considerably larger amount of material".

Este es el simulido mas repartido i abundante en el país según mis determinaciones hasta ahora. Esta especie, lo mismo que S. ochraceum son acusados de trasmitir en Méjico la O. caecutiens.

Distribución geográfica de esta especie.

Fuera de Venezuela.

Malloch: Trinidad, West Indies (F.W. Urich); Arroyo di los Nogales, Chihuahua, Mex. (C.H.T. Townsend); San José, Costa Rica; Córdoba i Orizaba, Mex. (F. Knab); Livingston i Alta Vera Paz, Guatemala (Schwarz i Barbar).

Dyar i Shannon: Cacao, Trece Aguas, Guatemala. Ref. Pinto 1931.

Dampf: Nogales, Son.; Córdoba, Ver. México. San José, Costa Rica, según (F. Knab col.) Ref. Pinto 1931.

Pinto: en Trinidad.

Bequaert: México (Nogales, Córdoba; Orizaba; Chiapas; Oaxaca), Guatemala, Trinidad i la isla de Trinidad. En Guatemala, en la finca Las Sabanetas cerca de Barberena (50 km. de la ciudad de Guatemala); cerca de Pochuta (Finca Pacayal i Finca Sa. Emilia); en las estribaciones del volcán Atitlán (Finca Mocá; Finca Sa. Adelaida); en las estribaciones del volcán Sa. María (Finca Helvetia i sus anexas Suiza, Acultazingo i Nil). Los hallazgos han sido hechos entre 1.100 i 1.300 m. de altura, poniendo Bequaert en duda la captura en Linvingston, en la misma Guatemala, dada por Malloch, por ser hecha casi a nivel del mar.

Fairchild: México, Guatemala, Costa Rica, Panamá. En este último país en El Valle, Provincia Coclé, R.P.

En Venezuela.

Briceño Iragorry: haciendo Altamira, jurisdicción de Güigüe, Estado Carabobo i en Los Teques, San Diego, San Antonio, Baruta i El Encantado, todos estos lagares pertenecen al Estado Miranda.

Iriarte: En Caracas, en el jardín de mi casa de habitación situada fte. al Parque Los Caobos. En la región de la Costa, a orillas del mar, desde Macuto hasta Anare, así: En el río de Macuto; en el río de Caraballeda; en los ríos Cerro Grande i Uria. En el río Naiguatá escasos. En el río Anare mas

numerosos. Hacia la región de Catia la Mar no hemos hallado simulidos. Todos estos sitios corresponden al Distrito Federal.
En el sitio llamado El Samán, al lado de la carretera que va de Caracas a la población de Guarenas, Estado Miranda.
A orillas del río Auyamita, en el Paso del Encantado, al lado de la carretera que conduce a Guarenas, Estado Miranda.
En los Chorros i El Hatilo, Estado Miranda.
En la quebrada Curucurumbo, a 16 km. de distancia de Maracay, a 550 m. de altura, Estado Aragua.
En el riachuelo La Quebrada, cerca del pueblo de Choroní, Estado Aragua.
En el río Choroní, en el sitio llamado Los Cerritos, Estado Aragua.
En el río Trincheras, cerca del pueblo Las Trincheras, Estado Carabobo.
En el río Aguascalientes, Estado Carabobo.
En la quebrada Pavia, Estado Yaracuy.
En las quebradas Salao i Canuabita, Estado Yaracuy.
En los baños de la población de Duaca, Estado Lara.
En el riachuelo de la piscina de Macuto, cerca de Barquisimeto, Estado Lara.
En Tabay, a orillas del río Chama, Estado Mérida.

* * *

CAPITULO IV

* * *

DESCRIPCIONES ORIGINALES DE LAS ESPECIES NO ENCONTRADAS POR NOSOTROS. ANOTACIONES. DISTRIBUCION GEOGRAFICA

* * *

Simulium clarki Fairchild 1940

Fairchild G.B. 1940. Annals Ent. Society of Amér. vol. XXXIII.

Simulium clarki Briceño Iragorry 1942

Briceño Iragorry L. 1942. Bol. del. Lab. Cli. Razetti. vol. II. No. 9. pag. 161.

Simulium clarki n. sp.

Female.—Length of mesonotum and scutellum 0.9 mm., of wing 1.9 mm. Frons subtriangular, narrow at antennae, broad at vertex, excision of eye margin opposite antennal base as deep or deeper than wide. Clypeus longer than broad, broadest at apex, narrow at antennal insertion. Frons and clypeus pale silvery grey pollinose, the former with a few, the latter with many silvery hairs. Antennae suncylindrical, of 11 segments, yellowish at base, darkening to a black apex, grey pollinose and pubescent. Palpi and proboscis dusky.

Mesonotum (viewed from above) uniformly silvery grey pollinose, rather evenly beset with well spaced silvery to pale brassy hairs, which are longer and denser on the margins than on the disc. On the posterior fourth and posterior lateral margin to as far forward as the level of the wing bases, these hairs point towards the anterior end of the insect, while those on the rest of the mesonotum point backward, and a ridge of upstanding hairs is formed where the two types join. Scutellum silvery grey with dense, long, curved, silvery hairs. Pleura and sides of mesonotum silvery grey pollisose.

Legs: Fore coxae and femora yellow with yellow pubescence, the latter very slightly dusky at apex. Tibiae yellow, with dense silvery pollinosity on the outer side and yellow pubescence on the inner; apex dusky. Tarsi black, slightly inflated, black pubescent. Mid coxae dusky, femora yellow, dusky at apex and with yellow pubescence. Basal third of tibiae white, silvery pubescent, apical two thirds black, with mixed yellow and black pubescence. Basitarsis basally two-thirds white, rest and remaining tarsal segments black. Hind legs as figured (fig. 10) Calcipala and pedisulcus well developed. Claws of mid tarsi with a minute tooth, (fig. 18).

Wings with stem vein hairy, R2 simple. Halteres white.

Abdomen dusky with scattered pale hairs, the last five segments rather well chitinized, shiny.

Male.—Essentially like the female but mesonotum (from above) deep velvety black, more densely covered with rich golden hairs. With light of suitable incidence, a broad continuous marginal band of silvery pollinosity encircling the mesonotum can be made out, the scutellum is much less hairy, the abdomen, less highly chitinized, is velvety black, with patches of bright silvery pollinosity on the sides of tergites two and five.

Pupa.—with six-branched filaments 3.3 mm. long. (fig. 30). Cocoon 2.8 mm. long. subconic. The aperture at about 90° to the long axis, the aperture sides flaring and produced beyond the aperture on the substratum. About half floored. Margin of aperture thickened. Texture quite loose and open, net-like laterally.

Holotype ♀, Allotype ♂, 1 ♀ 3 ♂ Paratypes bred from pupae on grass blades in a small stream feeding lily ponds at Summit Experiment Gardens, Summit, C. Z., January 9, 1940. 5 ♀ 4 ♂ Paratypes bred from water weeds in a small stream at El Valle, Coclé Prov., R.P. December 10, 1939.

(descripción original tomada del trabajo Notes on the Simuliidae of Panamá (Dipt. Nematocera) por G.B. Fairchild, en Annals Entomological Society of America. vol. XXXIII, No. 4. diciembre 1940. pag. 710).

Distribución geográfica de esta especie.

Fuera de Venezuela.

Fairchild: en Panamá, en los sitios Summit Experiment Gardens, Summit, C. Z. i El Valle, Coclé, Provincia Coclé. R.P.

En Venezuela.

Briceño Iragorry: Los Teques, Estado Miranda.

Simulium pulverulentum Knab 1914

Knab Frederick. 1914. Insecutor Inscitiae Menstruus. vol. II. No. 12.

Simulium pulverulentum Fairchild 1940

Fairchild G.B. 1940. Ann. Ent. Soc. of Amer. vol. XXXIII. pag. 734.

Simulium pulverulentum Pinto 1931

Pinto César. 1931. Simuliidae da Amer. Cent. e do Sul. pag. 734.

Simulium pulverulentum Briceño Iragorry 1942

Briceño Iragorry L. 1942. Bol. Lab. Cli. Razetti. vol. II. No. 7.

Simulium pulverulentum new species.

Female. Occiput, frons, and face gray pruinose; frons broad above, greatly narrowed to near the antennae. Antennae ahort, the two basal joints dull ferruginous yellow, the others blackish, clothed with pale pubescence, the tip pointed. Scutum almost uniformly blackish with gray pruinosity, an ill-defined, straight, median black line extending the entire length, and outwardly broader, hardly perceptible, situate stripes of the usual conformation; vestiture of small, hair like silvery scales, rather dense and nearly uniformly distributed. Scutellum broad short, bluntly rounded, concolorous with the mesonotum and with longer, transversaly directed, silvery hair-like scales. Postnotum blackish.

Pleurae dark gray pruinose, the pteropleurae paler. Abdomen subcylindral, dull black, without marked plications, the basal segment paler. Legs black and white, the small, appressed hair-scales en femora and tibiae pale and shining; anterior coxae, trochanters, and bases of all the femora dull ferruginous yellow; anterior tibiae white on the basal two-thirds, a blackish ring close to base, the tarsi wholly black and with the first joint long and rather slender; middle tibiae whitish at base and with a whitish ring at basal third, the first tarsal joint white on the basal two-thirds; hind tibiae broadly whitish at base, a whitish ring before the middle, the first tarsal joint white on the basal two-thirds, the second with a white ring at base. Claws with a miute acute toothlose at base. Wings hyaline, a predominatingly reddish iridescent spot in the anal field; venation normal, the thick veins yellowish brown, spines and setulae black. Halteres with dark stem and white knob.

Length: Body about 1.8 mm., wing 2.8 mm.

Punta Gorda. British Honduras (J.D. Norton).

Type. Cat. No. 19111, U.S. Nat. Mus.

Described from a series of 35 specimens poor preservation. The species is remarkable for the peculiar double annulation at the bases of the tibiae the almost uniformly gray mesonotum rather densely clothed with evenly distributed hair-like scales.

(descripción original tomada del trabajo New date and Species in Simuliidae (Diptera) por Frederick Knab en Insecutor Inscitiae Menstruus, vol. II. No. 12. diciembre de 1914).

Fairchild en su trabajo Notes on the Simuliidae of Panamá del año 1940 refiriéndose al macho de esta especie dice: Male.—Essentially the same as female, but mesonotum with stripes obsolescent, either entirely black with a few grey patches anteriorly (viewed from above), or entirely grey with small black streaks anteriorly (viewed from the side). Shiny hairs much sparser than in female and brassy instead of silvery".

La descripción de la pupa la hace el mismo autor como sigue: "Pupa.—Branchial filaments 10, about 1/2 mm. long. All branches quite close together and to the base (fig. 36). Cocoon subconical, about 2 mm. long, slipper shaped, the aperture at about 60° to the long axis. Margin not thickened, but continuous all the way around opening. Close woven, no visible openings".

Fairchild continúa: "the only other described Neotropical species known to me with 10 respiratory filaments is S. hirtipupa Lutz, described from a single pupal skin from Minas Geraes, Brazil. Pulverulentum differs in having much longer filaments which are strongly annulated, and in lacking the numerous trichomes of hirtipupa. The inmature stages of this species fairly swarm in some of the swifter and clearer streams of the Pacific, slope, being partial to those with a heavy growth of Marathrum schiedeanum Cham., on whose finely divided leaved the pupae are often massed in incredible numbers. I have not observed this species biting".

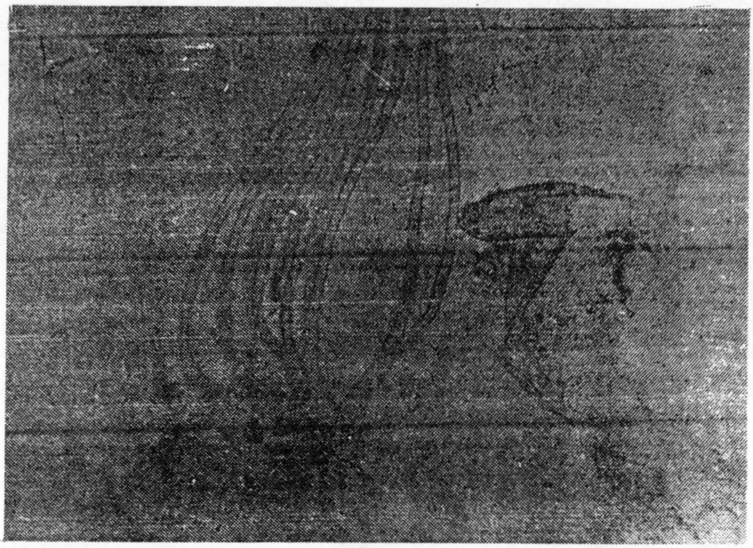

(Fig. 15) Mechón de tubos branquiales que bien pueden ser de S. pulverulentum, de hirtipupa o de jenningsi. Material colectado en el Estado Mérida. El ramillete tiene 10 tubos.

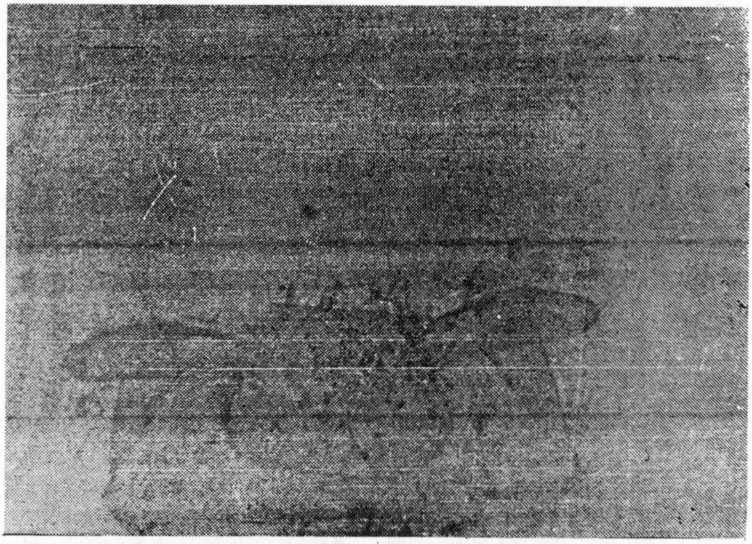

(Fig. 16) Pupa de S.? donde se aprecia muy bien los tricomas. Material colectado en Tabay, Estado Mérida.

Distribución geográfica de esta especie.
Fuera de Venezuela.
Knab: Punta Gorda, British Honduras (J.D. Norton).
Fairchild: Punta Gorda, British Honduras.
Panamá: en los siguientes sitios: Río Las Lajas, Panamá Prov., R.P.;

Chorrera Falls, Chorrera, R.P.; Quebrada Mañanita, cerca Pedregal, Panamá Prov., R.P., Río Paloma, cerca de Juan Díaz, Panamá Prov., R.P.

En Venezuela.

Briceño Iragorry: en Los Teques, Estado Miranda, a 1.169 mts. (captura de hembras picando).

Simulium versicolor Lutz i Núñez Tovar 1928

Lutz i Núñez Tovar en Lutz A. 1928. Est. de Zool. i Paras. Ven.

Simulium versicolor Pinto 1931

Pinto César. 1931. Simuliidae da América Cent. e do Sul.
Simulium versicolor nobis.
(Est. 4. fig. 2; Est. 6, fig. 3).

Hembra: Longitud de 2 a 3 mm. Color general negro.

Antenas con la base marrón oscuro, lo demás negro, con pelos cortos plateados. Clipeo i frente con brillo color da nácar.

Tórax: escudo con un dibujo que, a cambiantes de luz, muda de aspecto. Con iluminación de frente aparecen tres estrías longitudinales oscuras; una mediana i dos laterales que no llegan al margen anterior. Las mismas se observan claras con iluminación posterior, al paso que las dos estrías incluidas i las regiones laterales vuelven al color negro. En la parte anterior las estrías laterales se dilatan en triángulos oscuros que también se pueden observar plateados o blanco nacarados haciendo girar la luz. El occipucio toma parte en estas alteraciones de los colores.

Escudete, pleuras i región esternal de color negro, con reflejos blanco-plata i balancines con la oliva amarillenta.

Abdomen con reflejos nacarados en el borde de los segmentos; vientre negro.

Patas negras: los pares posteriores con tres tarsos blancos en la base i en una extensión mas o menos variable; todas las tibias plateadas del lado anterior i externo. Las pequeñas escamas son negras i doradas. Uñas con pequeño diente poco visible.

Los ejemplares frescos son extremadamente característicos i bellos. En los conservados los colores vivos se apagan, debido a una costra pulverulenta que hace entonces la determinación mas difícil. Esta especie se parece mucho al pium del Amazonas (Simulium amazonicum), al S. incrustatum, i en un grado menor al S. paraguayense.

Ninfa: La cápsula exterior es de forma chata, sin vestibulo, i formada de seda gruesa. La ninfa no muestra tricomas i tiene de cada lado seis tubos respiratorios largos i finos que nacen de tres bifurcaciones cerca de la base, lo cual no se observa en ninguna otra especie de Venezuela.

(descripción original tomada de la obra Estudios de Zoología i Parasitología Venezolanas, 1928, por A. Lutz, pag. 47. ed. en Río Janeiro).

Distribución geográfica de esta especie.

Fuera de Venezuela.

Desconocida.

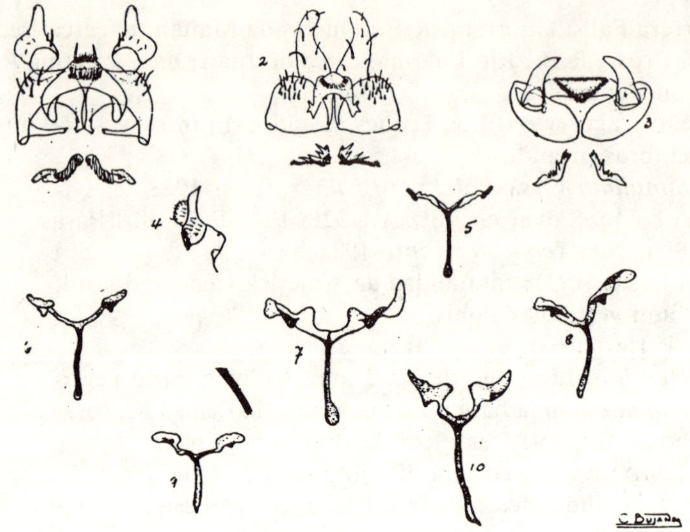

Plancha 1

En Venezuela.

No señala Lutz el sitio donde él i Núñez Tovar encontraron esta especie.

Simulium subnigrum Lutz 1910.

Lutz A. 1910. Mem. do Ins. Osw. Cruz. t. III. fac. II. pag. 239.

Simulium subnigrum Surcouf i González Rincones 1911

Surcouf i González Rincones 1911. Essai Dipt. Vul. Ven. pag. 293.

Simulium subnigrum Pinto 1931

Pinto César. 1931. Simuliidae da Amer. Cent. e do Sul. 7th Reu. Soc. Pat. Reg. Norte.

Simulium subnigrum Lutz i Núñez Tovar 1928

Lutz i Núñez Tovar en Lutz A. 1928. Est. de Zool. i Paras. Ven. pag. 43.

Simulium subnigrum n. sp.

Cõr geral enegrecida; comprimento cerca de 2 1/2 a 3 mm.

Tromba e palpos enegrecidos, estes ultimos con cinco segmentos; antenas com os segmentos bazaes pardo-amarelados; o resto pardo con pubecencia esbranquiçada, o articulo terminal pouco pontudo; olhos chocolate com reflexos esverdeados e avermelhados; fronte e clipeo com induto prateado, finamente granulozo, sobre fundo escuro e pêlos curtos de cõr clara.

Escudo: o fundo escuro com faxa tranversal anterior e trez estrias lonjitudinais, nem sempre distintas, de cõr escura; nas marjens lateraes e posterior de cõr acinzentada mais clara e com brilho de prata. As escamas piliformes bastante caducas não são dispostas em feixes ou estrias; na parte central do escudo são côr de ouro, sobre o fundo claro das marjens mais palidas, quazi côr de crême; na estremidade do escutelo seguem direção transversal. Pleuras com brilho claro sobre fundo escuro.

Abdome preto ou pardo-amarelado, em geral distintamente canelado, pelo menos no meio da face ventral; na marjem do primeiro segmento ha pelos claros mais compridos; outros ha, mais curtos, disseminados em grande numero sobre toda a face dorsal.

Pernas: o primeiro par pardo-amarelado até ao apice preto da tibia e, muitas vezes, mais ou menos enegrecido, com escamas piliformes de côr clara; face anterior de tibia com pó o pêlos niveos, o resto da perna preto; segundo par acima do joelho, pardo-ocraceo até quazi preto com escamas de amarelo palido, tibia na metade bazal (mais por diente que por traz) e metarso nos dois tercos superiores com fundo e escamas claras; terceiro par acima de joelho enegrecido, apenas com a baze do femur clara, a haste do mesmo com escamas côr ouro; tibia na baze até perto do meio de cór clara, com escama brancas, metarso nos dois tercos superiores pardo-ocraceo com escamas brancas, os tar. ɔs vizinhos com a baze mais claras, o resto enegrecido.

Azas sem particularidades; halteres com a haste escura e o capitulo variando de amarelo palido até quazi branco.

No macho, os olhos acima parecem castanho-vermelhos, em baixo verdes, com reflexos dourados; o escudo e preto aveludado, atraz, dos lados e nas partes laterais da marjem anterior com larga tarjeta nacarada; as escamas piliformes (não formando feixes nem estrias) com brilho dourado claro sobre o fundo escuro, mais palidas e mates sobre as partes claras, são mais abundantes perto das marjems do que no meio; nas pleuras, no metanoto e no dorso dos segmentos abdominais 1, 3 e 5 ha manchas de brilho prateado e nacarado que na femea flatam ou são menos brilhantes. As unhas correspondem ao tipo comom dos machos.

Esta especie varia bastante em tamanho e côr sendo isto talvez em parte devido a uma absorção anterior de sangue. Para distinguila de outras, mais ou menos similhantes, observe-se principalmente o dezenho e revestimento do escudo e as numerozas escamas claras sobre o fundo escuro das pernas que, pelo maior parte, são compridas e estreitas, quazi lineares, e mal se distinguem de formas de tranzição; ha tambem outras mais curtas, mas nunca são tão largas, que a forma de escamas seja bem evidente. Os mosquitos não perseguem ao homem, mas são apanhados em cavalos com alguma frequencia; todavia sómente pelo estudo das larvas e pupas se conhoce tratar-se de especie muito comum e espalhad. São encontradas, em todas as elevacaos, em pequenos regatos, frequentemente em companhia do S. perflavum e do S. incrustatum se deixam criar com bastante facilidade; principalmente as pupas não precizam de muito arejamento da agua, de modo que os dous sexos podem ser obtidos com facilidade. Criei-os em São Paudo de larvas dos rios Pacaembú e Anhangabahúeno Rio de pupas de Mendes e Petropolis, sem que sofressem durante horas necesarias para o transporte. (Todavia e preferivel conservar os fragmento vejetais, nos quais se suportam, apenas humidos, a nao transportal-as dentro de agua).

O tronco principal dos apendices branquiais de cada lado divide-se em trez ramos, dos quais um se bifurca inmediatamente e os dois autros sómente assaz mais para cima, de modo que por algum espaco se vêm quatro ramos grandes, correndo paralelos. Os tubos são terminados em ponta conica que parece sobreposta. A pele da pupa aprezenta granulos finos no parte anterior e tricomas com quatro e mais ramos.

Na extremidade posterior existem apenas duas pontinhas não formando ganchos tipicos.

(descripción original tomada del trabajo Segunda contribuicao para o conhecimento das especies brazileiras do genero "Simulium" en Mem. do Inst. Osw. Cruz. T. II. Fac. II. 1910. pags. 239-241).

Distribución geográfica de esta especie.

Fuera de Venezuela.

Lutz: En Estado de Sao Paulo, Brasil, en los ríos Pacaembú i Anhangabahú.

En el Estado de Río de Janeiro, Brasil, en Mendes i Petropolis.

Pinto: En Anhembi, Estado de Sao Paulo, Brasil (mat. de Lutz).

En Angra dos Reis, Estado de Río de Janeiro, Brasil (material de Travassos).

En Venezuela.

Lutz i Núñez Tovar: las ninfas características las encontramos en un afluente del río Guaire; dieron nacimiento a varios adultos.

Simulium amazonicum Goeldi 1905

Goeldi E. 1905. Os mosquitos do Pará. IV. Simulium amazonicum nov. sp. Goeldi (1905) pag. 138-9.

Simulium exiguum Lutz 1909 *nec Roubaud* 1906

Lutz A. 1909. Mem. do Inst. Osw. Cruz. t. I. No. 2. pag. 141.

Simulium minusculum Lutz 1910

Lutz A. 1910. Mem. do Inst. Osw. Cruz. t. II. fasc. II. pag. 253-6.

Eusimulium minusculum Surc. i González Rincones 1911

Simulium amazonicum Surcouf i González Rincones 1911

Surcouf i González Rincones. 1911. Essai. Dipt. Vuln. Ven. Pt. I. pags. 282-3.

Simulium lutzi Knab 1913

Knab Frederick. 1913. Insec. Insc. Menstruus. vol. I. pag. 155. dcbre.

Simulium nitidum Malloch 1913

Malloch J.R. 1913. Proc. U.S. Nat. Museum. vol. XLIII. No. 1945. pag. 652.

Simulium lutzi Malloch 1914—*S. exiguum Lutz 1909 nec. Roubaud 1906.*

Malloch J.R. 1914. U.S. Depto. Agric. Bur. Ent. Tech. Serv. No. 24. pag. 14.

Simulium amazonicum Neiva 1916

Neiva A. 1916. Mem. do Ins. Osw. Cruz. t. VIII. fac. III, pag. 93.

Simulium amazonicum Lutz 1917

Lutz A. 1917. Mem. Inst. Osw. Cruz. t. IX. fac. I. pags. 63-66. Est. 25. figs. 1-10.

Simulium amazonicum Lutz, Araujo i Fonseca 1918

Lutz, Araujo i Fonseca. 1918. Mem. do Inst. Osw. Cruz. t. X. fac. II. pag. 165.

Simulium amazonense Lutz 1922

Lutz A. 1922. Folha medica. Año III. pags. 90-92. dcbre.

Odagmia nitida Enderlein 1925

Enderlein G. 1925. Zool. Anz. t. 62. pag. 208.

Simulium amazonicum Strong. Bequaert, Shattuck i Wheeler 1926

Strong, Shattuck, Bequaert i Wheeler. 1926. Medical Report of the Ham. Rice Exp. Parte II. pags. 221-214.

Simulium amazonicum Lutz i Núñez Tovar 1928

Lutz i Núñez Tovar en A. Lutz. 1928. Est. de Zool. i Paras. Ven. pag. 48. Est. 5. figs. 1-10.

Lo que sigue es la descripción que hace Lutz en 1910, en la página 253, de Memorias de Instituto Oswaldo Cruz, Tomo II. Fac. II.

S. minusculum n. sp. (¿amazonicum Goeldi?).

Côr geral preta, tamanho, cerca de 1-1 1/4 mm.

Antenas pretas com pubecencia clara, apenas o articulo bazal pardo-ocraceo; tromba preta, palpos escuros, o segundo artículo fuziforme. Fronte, clipeo e occiput com fundo preto e induto granulozo de forte brilho prateado ou nacarado, com escamas piliformes claras e pelos mais escuros.

Torax em cima com tres faxas lonjitudinais (uma mediana inteira e duas laterais um pouco abreviadas em frente), cujo fundo aparece preto aveludado; entre estas e as marjens laterais e posterior e n'uma linha em frente das faxas laterais o fundo é mais claro, finamente granulado, com brilho nacarado muito intenso, si a luz fôr favoravel e o exemplar bem conservado; dos dous lados da linha mediana e bem perto da marjem anterior existe uma mancha triangular com apice virado para traz que, vista de frente, parece pretae de traz, branca; as faxas laterais têm a forma um tanto irregular; a faxa mediana é alargada no meio e arredondada nas extremioades; a pleura e o esterno são pretos, com brilho claro; sobre o escudo ha escamas piliformes comparativamente largas, um tanto curvadas, de dourado palido tornandose transversais sobre o escutelo de côr preta.

Abdome preto, muito canelado, com pêlos claros pouco numerozos.

Azas: A baze e as nervuras mais grossas de ocraceo diluido; na raiz una pêlos de brilho dourado, nas costas pelos cuartos e espinchos bastante disante entre si; halteres com a haste muito ecura e o capitulo amarelo palido.

Pernas em geral pardacentas, o metatarso e os tarsos vizinhos dos ultimos pares com apice escuro; o primeiro com espinhos escuros e uma linha preta, formada por aculeos finos, na face posterior, metatarso do ultimo par com palheta distinta, o tarso vizinho bastante comprido, mas com

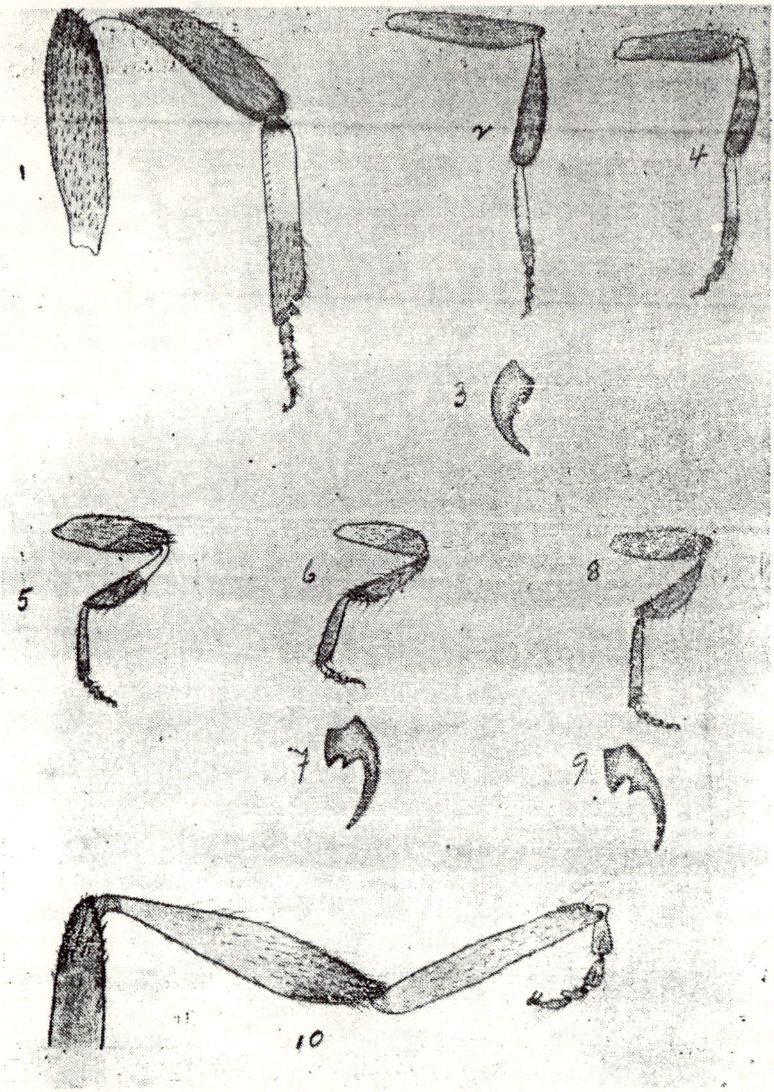

Plancha 2

a incizura dorsal distinta; unhas generalmente sem um dente distinto, apenas com o angulo saliente, mas excecionalmente parece existir; tibia anterior ocracea, a face anterior com escamas branco-nacaradas; tibia do meio ocracea nas duas extremidades, a ultima com a metade bazal clara; nas partes claras ha escamas branco nacaradas bastante densas, nos outros lugares escamas e pelos de dourado palido; as escamas sao espatuladas com extremidades arredondadas e especialmente conspicuas nos femures, onde prevalece uma forma curta.

As femeas adultas atacam tanto o homem, como os cavalos e parecem muito avidas de sangue. Da maior parte das especies distinguem-se já pedo seu tamanho pequeno; daquelas que sao menores e mais parecidas podem facilmente ser discriminadas pelas faxas do escudo; todavia é somente em bons exemplares e com incidencia correta da luz que as manchas nacaradas se acentuam em sua belleza toda. As femeas que serviram de baze a decricao foram colecionadas em marco e abril deste anno em Lassance (Minas) pelo Dr. Carlos Chagas''.

Mas tarde en 1917, refiriéndose a esta misma especie, dice Lutz en Memorias do Instituto Oswaldo Cruz, en trabajo titulado Terceira contribuicão para o conhecimento das especies brazileiras do genero Simulium. O piúm do norte (Simulium amazonicum) t. IX. fac. I. pag. lo siguiente: ''O nome ''pium'' pode ser aplicado a todas as especies de Simulium, mas designa de preferencia uma pequena especie comum e espalhada no sistema fluvial do Amazonas, que foi descripta por Goeldi sob o nome Simulium amazonicum. Num trabalho anterior, publicado nestas memorias em 1910, descrevi uma especie encontrada em Lassance cujas aguas vao para o rio de S. Francisco, e dei-lhe o nome S. minusculum. Discuti a possiblilidade de tratar-se do S. amazonicum, nao obstante certas divergencias, notadas nas descricoes.

Desde então recebi abundante material de varios lugares e cheguei ao resultado que se trata de uma sóespecie, muito espalhada. Não parece variar muito, mas, devido a certas particularidades da imajem, a sua aparencia modifica-se extraordinariamente com a incidencia da luz e o estado de conservacao. Nota-se tambem um fenomeno que já descrevi em varias ocasioes. Tratase de uma alteracçâo da côr do corpo, principalmente nas partes que recebem muito sangue. Ocorre em exemplares que tiverem occasiaõ de absorver, uma ou mais vezes, grande copia de sangue ingerido.

Assim na minha descrição, alias correta e minuciosa, as pernas forao dadas como pardacentas, quando, em exemplares novos, sao muito claras e o abdome, que em exemplares frescas mostra no dorso um desenho muito carateristico, foi dado como preto.

As larvas, fora do seu tamanho reduzido, não tem nada de carateristico. Dos casulos damos boas figuras com aumento de 20 vezes. O coção, de ca. 2.5 mm. de comprimento, tem a forma de um cartucho, achatado sobre o plano de suporte, onde a parede só tem a metade da altura. A boca, um pouco espessada, inclina-se para fora em fórma de anel, faltando um segmento do lado achatado. Os fios de seda pardecenta sao claramente visiveis. O casulo tem a pêle pouco grossa, finamente granulosa na parte anterior e semeada de trichomas curtos e finos, geralmente bifurcados. O sistema respiratorio, mais curto do que o cocao, tem o comprimento mais ou menos igual ao do casulo. Comeca de cada lado com um tubo grosso, bifurcado quasi imediatamente. O ramo posterior bifurca-se logo e cada um dos galhos tambem, o dorsal um pouco mais acima do que o do meio. O ramo ventral bifurca-se bastante mais acima. Os ramos e galhos afilam-se gradualmente; os seis galhos terminam em ponta subconica, um pouco destacada, de côr clara.

Distribución geográfica de esta especie.

Fuera de Venezuela.

Goeldi: En Teffé, en los ríos Purús i Acre. Brasil.

Lutz: de Lassance, Estado de Minas Geraes, Brasil, provenían según este autor los ejemplares hembras que le sirvieron de base para describir el S. minusculum.

Neiva: En el río Tocantins, Estado de Goyaz, Brasil.

En Peri-Peri, alrededores de Joazeiro, Estado de Bahia, Brasil.

Lutz i Machado: En Lassance, Estado Minas Geraes, Brasil.

En río Ondas, en Río Grande i en el río San Francisco, cerca de Barrenas, Brasil. (1915).

Lutz: En río Madeira (col. O. Cruz).

En el Alto Amazonas, en río Tocantins, en río Paranapanema i Río Grande. (1917).

Pinto: En Paraguay, en Porto Bertoni (seg. Lutz, Araujo i Fonseca, 1918, pag. 165).

En el Perú, en Huancabamba (2 hembras col. por C.H. Townsend. 1911).

Bequaert: en el bajo Río Negro, en el bajo Río Branco, Brasil.

En Venezuela.

Lutz: lo cita para Venezuela en su obra Est. de Zool. i Paras. Venezolanas, pero no señala el sitio de hallazgo.

Eusimilium paraguayense (Schrottky 1909).

Simulium paraguayense Schrottky 1909

Schrottky C. 1909. Zeitschr. Wiss. Insektenbiol. t. V. Heft. 2. pag. 63.

Eusimulium paraguayense Lutz 1909

Lutz A. 1909. Mem. do Inst. Osw. Cruz. t. I. No. 2. pag. 146.

Simulium paraguayense Lutz 1910

Lutz A. 1910. Mem. do Inst. Osw. Cruz. t. II. Fac. 2. pags. 235 i 263.

Simulium paraguayense Surcouf i González Rincones 1911

Surcouf i González Rincones. 1911. Essai Dipt. Vuln. Ven. pag. 291.

Simulium paraguayense Lutz, Araujo i Fonseca 1918

Lutz, Araujo i Fonseca. 1918. Mem. do Ins. Osw. Cruz. t. X. fac. I. pag. 165.

Simulium paraguayense Lutz i Núñez Tovar 1928

Lutz i Núñez Tovar en Lutz A. 1928. Est. de Zool. i Paras. Ven. pag. 43. Est. 4, fig. 5. Est. 6. fig. 8.

S. paraguayense n. sp.

In der Farbüng ännlich S. inexorabile, von dieser jedoch ausser durch die geringere Grösse sofort durch das nicht geriefte Abdomen, sowie das letzte Antennenglied zu unterscheiden, welches bei S. paraguayense nicht spitz, sondern viereckig, auch im Verhältniss bedeutend grösser ist. Die Augen sind (beim lebenden Tiere) kupferrotgrün schillernd. Der Thorax ist mit goldiggrünen Härchen besetzt; die Flügel sind hyalin, die Halteren weissliche; Beine; I. Femur und Tibie gelbbraun Tarsus schwarz, II. gelbbraun mit helleren Tarsen, III. Femur und Tibie gelbbraun mit dunkelbraunnem Apex, Tarsen weisslich, die Endglieder dunkler. Länge 2 mm.

Paraguay, Argentinien am Alto Paraná, nur in nächster Nãhe des Flusses.

(descripción original tomada del trabajo de Lutz Mem. do Inst. Osw. Cruz. t. I, Fac. II. pag. 145. titulado Contribuicao para e conhecimento das especies brazileiras do genero ''Simulium'').

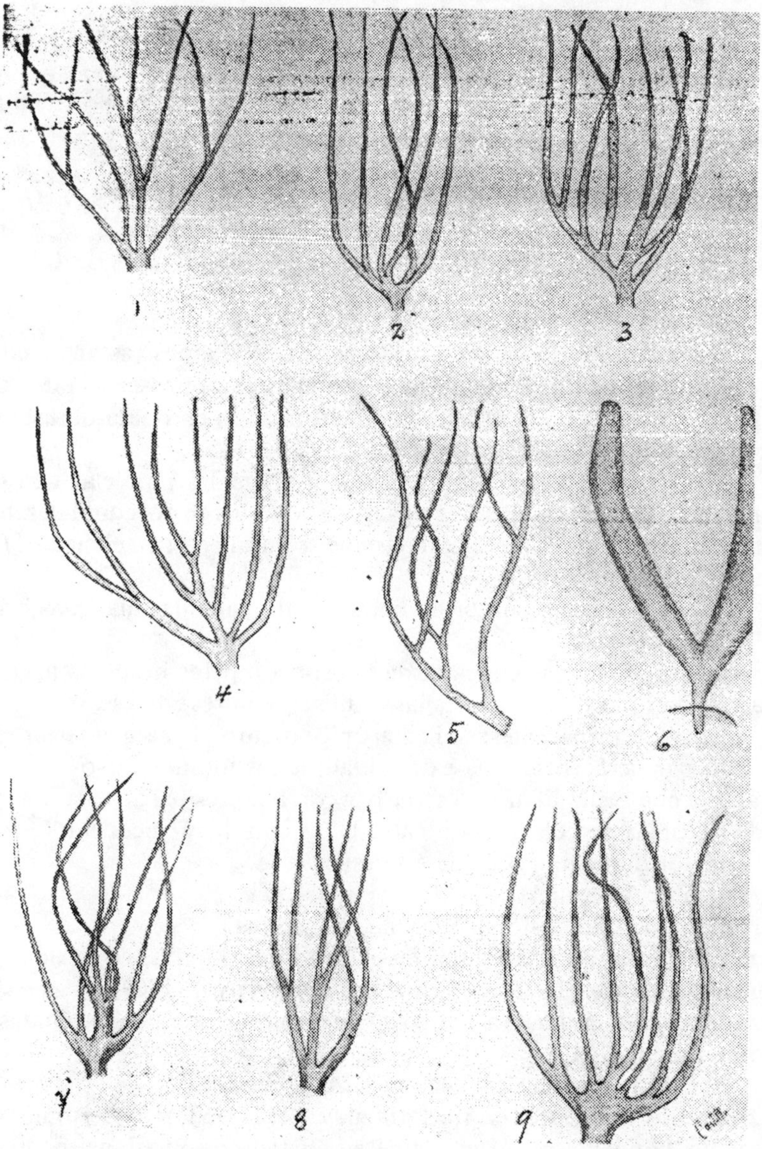

Plancha 3

Lutz, en su obra Estudios de Zoología i Parasitología Venezolanas, del año 1928, trae lo siguiente para esta especie: "Hembra: color general oscuro. Longitud 1 1/2—2 mm.

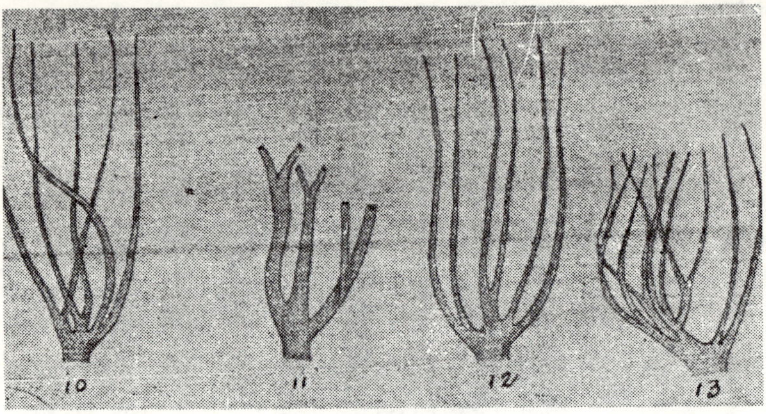

Plancha 4

Cabeza con fondo oscuro i brillo nacarado. Palpos castaños, con los dos últimos segmentos blanquecinos. Antenas con pubescencia casi blanca; base vermeja i con el último anillo terminando en punta obtusa. Ojos color de cobre.

Tórax: escudo negro, con líneas longitudinales paralelas que están formadas de escamas angostas i cortas, de color verde dorado; lateralmente el escudo presenta fajas nacaradas que se ensanchan en el medio. Escudete negro i sin escamas.

Abdomen oscuro, con brillo blanco mate i algunas manchas brillantes.

Alas irisadas; base ennegrecida i costa con pelos i espinas negras. Patas: primer par ocráceo hasta las rodillas; fémures con escamas nacaradas, anchas i transparentes; tibia con ápice oscuro i la cara anterior nívea. Segundo par ocráceo, con la extremidad de los últimos tarsos parduzca, metatarso con brillo blanco. Tercer par con fémures pardos i la mitad basal de las tibias de color amarillento. Uñas con diente pequeño".

Distribución geográfica de esta especie.

Fuera de Venezuela.

Schrottky: en el Salto del río Paraná, Argentina.

Lutz: En Estado de Sao Paulo, en el Salto del Itapura, cerca de la confluencia de los ríos Tieté con el Paraná (col. Neiva) (1909).

Lutz i Machado: en Lassance, Estado de Minas Geraes i en río Ondas, Estado de Bahía. (1915)

Lutz, Araujo i Fonseca: en Tucumán, Argentina.

Lutz, Araujo i Fonseca: en río Paraguay, cerca de Porto Bertoni. (1918)

Pinto: En Trapicheiro i Angra dos Reis, Estado de Río Janeiro, Brasil.

En Venezuela.

Lutz: "En Venezuela lo observamos atacando al hombre i también lo habemos criado de material procedente de Caracas i de los alrededores de la cuidad de Maracay".

CAPITULO V

DISTRIBUCION POR ESTADOS DE LAS 11 ESPECIES DE SIMULIDOS ENCONTRADAS POR NOSOTROS EN EL PAIS

* * *

Distrito Federal . . . Simulium metallicum.
Estado Miranda . . S. ochraceum, exiguum, incrustatum, lúgubre, lutzianus i metallicum.
Estado Aragua . . . S. exiguum, metallicum i rubrithorax.
Estado Carabobo . S. metallicum, exiguum e incrustatum.
Estado Yaracuy . . . S. incrustatum, exiguum i metallicum.
Estado Lara . . . . . . S. metallicum i exiguum.
Estado Mérida . . . . S. metallicum, lutzianus, bicoloratum, sanguineum, ochraceum i exiguum.
Estado Barinas . . . S. incrustatum i exiguum.
Estado Bolivar . . . . S. limbatum i haematopotum.

* * *

Las especies más repartidas son: metallicum i exiguum.

Los Estados que presentan mayor número de especies son: Miranda i Mérida con seis especies.

* * *

CAPITULO VI

SIMULIDOS EN CENTRO Y SUR AMERICA

Damos el número de especies por países para junio de 1931, añadiendo a la cifra de 10 que estaba asignada a Venezuela, 7 especies más señaladas posteriormente, 4 de ellas citadas por primera vez por nosotros. La cifra de 17 sólo la iguala Méjico i la sobrepasa Brasil.

En Norte América esta familia ha sido motivo de grandes comunicaciones: Say (1823), Riley (1870-1888), L.O. Howard (1887-1911), Coquillet (1898-1902), Forbes (1912), F. Knab (1913-1914), Malloch

(1913-14), W.J. Pomeroy (1916), hasta la monografía de H. Dyar i Shannon en 1927 donde hacen una clara revisión de 53 especies de América del Norte.

PAIS	NUMERO DE ESPECIE
Argentina	11 especies
América Meridional	1 especie
Brasil	37 especies
Bolivia	1 especie
Colombia	1 especie
Costa Rica	2 especies
Chile	14 especies
Ecuador	2 especies
Guatemala	3 especies
Guayana Inglesa	2 especies
Honduras	1 especie
Isla St. Vincent	1 especie
Isla de Jamaica	1 especie
Isla de Trinidad	2 especies
Méjico	17 especies
Perú	11 especies
Paraguay	6 especies
Panamá	1 especie
Patria ignorada	1 especie
Venezuela	17 especies

* * *

ARGENTINA

S. antarcticum	Bigot	1888
S. anthracinum	Bigot	1888
S. delpontei	Paterson i Shannon	1927
S. jujuyense	Paterson i Shannon	1927
S. rubrithorax	Lutz	1910
S. wolfhügeli	Enderlein	1922
E. dinelli	Joan	1913
S. inaegualis	Paterson i Shannon	1927
E. lahillei	Paterson i Shannon	1927
E. paraguayense	Schrottky	1927
E. pertinax	Kollar	1832

AMERICA MERIDIONAL

S. tarsatum	Macquart	1846

BRASIL

S. aequifurcatum	Lutz	1910
S. amazonicum	Goeldi	1905
S. angrensis	Pinto	1931
S. auristriatum	Lutz	1910
S. baiensis	Pinto	1931
S. botulibranchium	Lutz	1910
S. brachycladum	Pinto	1931
S. brevifurcatum	Lutz	1910
S. catarinensis	Pinto	1931
S. clavibranchium	Lutz	1910
S. distinctum	Lutz	1910
S. diversibranchium	Lutz	1910
S. diversifurcatum	Lutz	1910
S. flavopubescens	Lutz	1910
S. hirticosta	Lutz	1910
S. hirtipupa	Lutz	1910
S. incertum	Lutz	1910
S. incrustatum	Lutz	1910
S. infuscatum	Lutz	1910
S. lutzi	Knab	1913
S. nigrimanum	Macquart	1837
S. orbitale	Lutz	1910
S. pernigrum	Lutz	1910
S. pruinosum	Lutz	1910
S. quadrifidum	Lutz	1917
S. rubrithorax	Lutz	1909
S. scutistriatum	Lutz	1909
S. simplicicolor	Lutz	1910
S. subclavibranchium	Lutz	1910
S. subnigrum	Lutz	1910
S. subpallidum	Lutz	1910
S. varians	Lutz	1909
S. paraguayense	Schrottky	1909
E. perflavum	Roubaud	1906
E. pertinax	Kollar	1832
S. flavifemur	Enderlein	1921

BOLIVIA

S. bolivianus	Enderlein	1925

COLOMBIA

S. sanguineum	Knab	1915-6

COSTA RICA

S. metallicum	Bellardi	1859
S. quadrivittatum	Loew	1862

CHILE

S. annulatum	Philippi	1865
S. antarcticum	Bigot	1888
S. anthracinum	Bigot	1888
S. chilense	Philippi	1865
S. chilianum	Rondani	1865
S. fulvescens	Blanchard	1852
S. montanum	Philippi	1865
S. philippianus nov. nom. S. tarsatum Philippi 1865 nec. Macquart 1846		
S. pulchrum	Philippi	1865
S. simile	Figueroa	1917
S. tenuipes	Knab	1914
S. varipes	Philippi	1865
E. escomeli	Roubaud	1909

ECUADOR

S. ignescens	Roubaud	1906
S. riveti	Roubaud	1906

GUATEMALA

S. aureopunctatum	Malloch	1914
S. metallicum	Bellardi	1859
E. exiguum	Roubaud	1906

GUAYANA INGLESA

S. guianense	Wiese	1911
S. limbatum	Knab	1915-6

HONDURAS (parte británica)

S. pulverulentum	Knab	1914

ISLA ST. VICENT

S. tarsale	Williston	1896

ISLA JAMAICA

S. antillarum	Jennings	1915

ISLA DE TRINIDAD

S. metallicum	Bellardi	1859
S. placidum	Knab	1915-6

MEJICO

S. avidum	Hoffmann	1930
S. haematopotum	Malloch	1914
S. metallicum	Bellardi	1859
S. occidentale	Townsend	1891
S. pseudo-haematopotum	Hoffmann	1930
S. tephrodes	Speiser	1904
S. trivittatum	Malloch	1914
S. virgatum	Coquillet	1903
S. virgatum var. chapanense	Hoffmann	1930
S. vittatum	Zetterstedt	1838
S. falculata	Enderlein	1929
E. alticolum	Dyar i Shannon	1927
E. callidum	Dyar i Shannon	1927
E. mexicanum	Dyar i Shannon	1927
E. mooseri	Dampf	1927
E. ochraceum	Walker	1860
E. turgidum	Hoffmann	1930

PERU

S. amazonicum	Goeldi	1905
S. bicoloratum	Malloch	1913
S. chalcocoma	Knab	1914
S. flavopictum	Knab	1914
S. gandeatum	Knab	1914
S. glaucophathalmus	Knab	1914
S. seriatum	Knab	1914
S. spinifer	Knab	1914
S. townsendi	Malloch	1913
E. dinelli	Joan	1913
E. escomelli	Roubaud	1909

PARAGUAY

S. amazonicum	Goeldi	1905
S. orbitale	Lutz	1910
S. paranense	Schrottky	1909
S. subpallidum	Lutz	1910
E. paraguayense	Schrottky	1909
E. pertinax	Kollar	1832

PANAMA

S. samboni	Jennings	1915

PATRIA IGNORADA

S. pubescens	Macquart	1834

VENEZUELA

S. amazonicum	Goeldi	1905
S. incrustatum	Lutz	1910
S. lugubre	Lutz i Núñez Tovar	1928
S. lutzianus	Pinto	1931
S. rubrithorax	Lutz	1909
S. subnigrum	Lutz	1910
S. versicolor	Lutz i Núñez Tovar	1928
S. exiguum	Roubaud	1906
E. ochraceum	Walker	1860
E. paraguayense	Schrottky	1909
E. bicoloratum	Malloch	1913
S. metallicum	Bellardi	1859
S. pulverulentum	Knab	1914
S. limbatum	Knab	1915-6
S. clarki	Fairchild	1940
S. sanguineum	Knab	1915
S. haematopotum	Malloch	1914

NOM NUDA

S. brevibranchium	Lutz i Machado	1915
S. subviride	Lutz	1922
S. obesum	Lutz	1922
S. amazonense	Lutz	1917-1922(*)

(*) Posteriormente el número de especies ha aumentado notablemente en países como Méjico i Guatemala, debido a la obra sobre todo, de investigadores como Luis Vargas i Romeo de León.

CAPITULO VII

RESUMEN

1° Se hace un recuento de la historia de la familia Simuliidae.
Se citan las experiencias de Blacklock, Robles, Hoffmann, Dampf, Strong, Bequaert; los estragos causados por estos animales i las relaciones de esta familia con la trasmisión del carate.
2° Se aportan numerosos datos sobre la vida de estos dípteros: sus capturas en las diferentes épocas del año, la influencia de la altura, temperatura, volumen de la corriente de agua, velocidad de ésta. Como importante se da cuenta de sospechas del desarrollo de simúlidos en aguas estancadas i sucias.
3° Las capturas han sido hechas en el Distrito Federal i en 10 Estados del país: Zulia, Miranda, Aragua, Carabobo, Yaracuy, Portuguesa, Mérida, Barinas, Bolívar i Lara.
4° Se dedica un capítulo a la clasificación de estos insectos, citando los trabajos al respecto de Dyar i Shannon, Malloch, Roubaud i Lutz. Se presenta una clave para las especies señaladas hasta hoi en el país.
5° Se dan las descripciones originales de las 11 especies halladas hasta hoi por el autor en Venezuela, citándose los sitios de captura.
6° Se presentan las descripciones originales de las 6 especies no halladas por el autor i se dan datos sobre los lugares de hallazgos.
7° Suminístrase un mapa de Venezuela con la distribución por Estados de las 11 especies encontradas por el autor.
8° Se suministra otro mapa con la distribución de las 6 especies no halladas por el autor.
9° Se da una lista con los simúlidos de Centro i Sur América i una bibliografía con 38 fichas consultadas.

SUMMARY

1st A review of the history of the family of Simuliidae is made. The experiences of Blacklock, Robles, Hoffmann, Dampf, Strong and Bequaert; the havoc caused by these animals and the connection of this family with the transmission of carate are cited.
2nd Numerous data are given on the life of these dipterae, their capture at different times of the year, the influence of altitude, temperature, volume and speed of the current of water. As an important fact the suspects of the development of simulium in stagnant and dirty water is cited.
3rd Captures have been made in the Federal District and in 10 States of the Republic: Zulia, Miranda, Aragua, Carabobo, Yaracuy, Portuguesa, Mérida, Barinas, Bolívar and Lara.
4th A chapter is devoted to the classification of these insects, quoting the works of Dyar and Shannon, Malloch, Roubaud and Lutz. A key is given

for the species found up to the present in the country.

5th The original descriptions of the 11 species found up to now in Venezuela by the author, and the places of capture are given.

6th The original descriptions are given of the 6 species not found by the author, and data relating to the places where they were found.

7th A map of Venezuela is supplied with the distribution of the 11 species found by the author.

8th Another map is supplied with the distribution of the 6 species not found by the author.

9th A list is given of Simuliidae of Central and South America. Thirty nine treatises and books which have been consulted are enumerated.

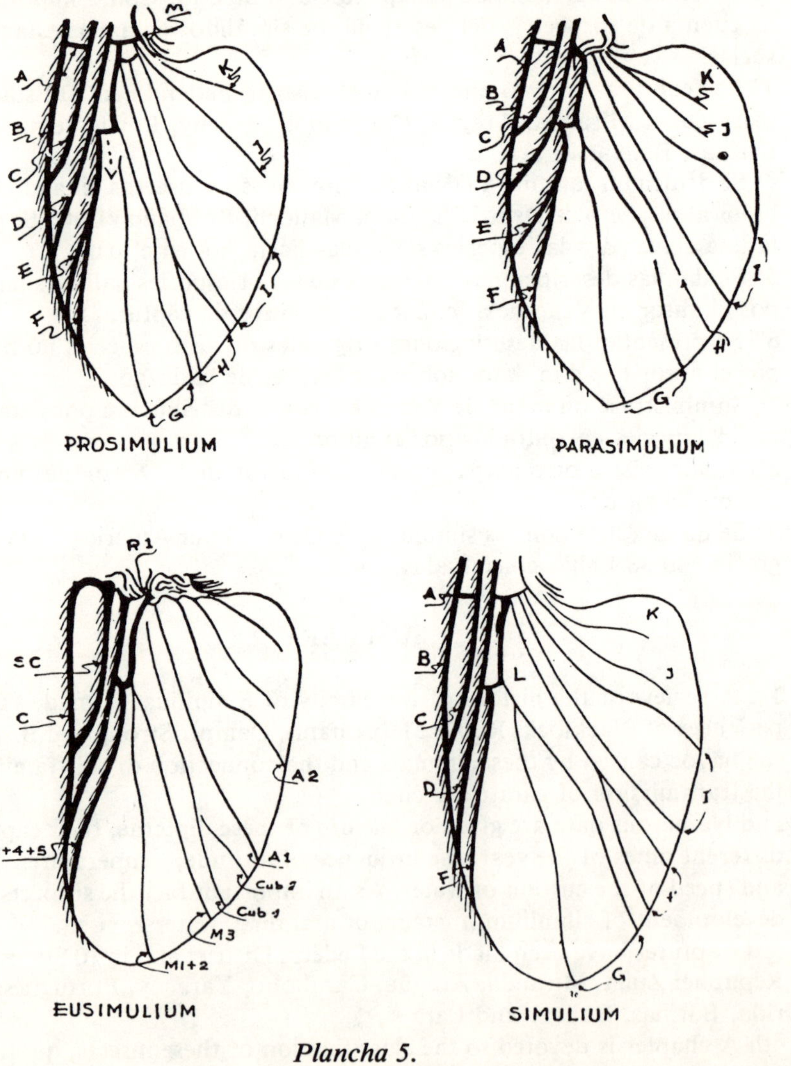

Plancha 5.

CAPITULO VIII

BIBLIOGRAFIA CONSULTADA

1936 Brumpt Emile—Precis de Parasitologie—1936.

1938 2 Bequaert Joseph C.—The black-flies, or Simuliidae of The Belgian Congo. The American Journal of Tropical Medicine. January—1938.

1941 3 Briceño Iragorry L.—Nota sobre Simuliidae (Diptera) con citación de una nueva especie para el país i lista de las conocidas en Venezuela. Boletín del Laboratorio de la Clínica Razetti. Año II - Vol. II - No. 6 - 1941.

1942 4 Briceño Iragorry.—Nota sobre Simulium pulverulentum Knab.—1914—Boletín del Laboratorio de la Clínica Razetti. Año III - Vol. II - No. 7 - 1942.

1938 6 Carbonell Diego.—La Parasitología en Venezuela i los trabajos del Dr. Núñez Tovar.—1938.

1934 7 Curran C.H.—The Diptera of Kartabo, Bartica District, British Guiana. Bulletin of The American Museum of Natural History—Vol. LXVI - 1934.

1940 8 Fairchild G.B.—Notes on the Simuliidae of Panama (Dipt. Nematocera) Annals of the Entomological Society of America. Vol. XXXIII, No. 4 - 1940.

1942 9 Fairchild G.B. i Briceño Iragorry L.—Nota sobre Simulium lutzianus (Descripción del adulto)—Boletín del Laboratorio de la Clínica Razetti. Año III - Vol. II - No. 9 - 1942.

1932 10 Gibbins E.G.—Studies on Etiopian Simuliidae. Simulium damnosum Theo. - 1932.

1916 11 Jobbins-Pomeroy Arthur W.—Notes on five North American buffalo gnats of the genus simulium. 1916.

1942 12 Iriarte David R.—Nota sobre una nueva especie de simulido en el país. (Simulium limbatum Knab 1915-6)—Boletín del Laboratorio de la Clínica Razetti. Año III. Vol. II No. 8. 1942.

1942 13 Iriarte David R.—Estudios de Patología Tropical. 1942.

1909 14 Lutz A. Contribuicao para o conhecimento das especies brazileiras do genero Simulium. Mem. do Inst. Oswaldo Cruz. Tomo I. Fac. II. 1909.

1910 15 Lutz A. Segunda contribuicao para o conhecimento das espeies brazileiras do genero Simulium. Mem. do Inst. Oswaldo Cruz. Tomo II. Fac. II - 1910.

1917 16 Lutz A. Terceira contribuicao para o conhecimento das especies brazileiras do genero Simulium. Mem. do Inst. Oswaldo Cruz. Tomo IX. Fac. I. 1917.

1918 17 Lutz, Souza Araujo i O. da Fonseca filho—Viagem scientifica no Rio Paraná e a Assuncion com volta por Buenos Aires, Montevideo e Río Grande. Mem. do Inst. Oswaldo Cruz. Tomo X. Fac. II - 1918.

1928 18 Lutz A. i Núñez Tovar M.—Estudios de Zoología i Parasitología Venezolanas. 1928.

1932 19 Metcalf C.L.—Black flies and other biting flies of the Adirondacks. New York State Museum Bulletin. No. 189. 1932.

1939 21 Orfila.—Simuliidae (Diptera) de la República Argentina.—IX Reunión de la Sociedad Argentina de Patología Tropical. Tomo III. 1939.

1931 22 Pinto César.—Simuliidae da America Central e do Sul (Diptera) VII Reunión de la Sociedad Argentina de Patología Regional del Norte. 1931.

1938 23 Pinto César.—Zoo-parasitos do Interesse Médico e Veterinario. 1938.

1940 24 Patiño Camargo Luis.—Artrópodos hematófagos de la Fauna Colombiana. Revista de la Facultad de Medicina. Vol. IX. No. I. 1940.

1941 25 Romeo de León J.—Nuevo tipo de Insectario para el cultivo de simulidos. Boletín Sanitario de Guatemala. 1941.

1934 26 Strong, Sandground, Bequaert, Ochoa.—Onchocerciasis. Harvard University Press. 1934.

1926 27 Strong, Bequaert, Shattuck, Wheeler.—Medical Report of the Hamilton Rice Seventh Expedition to the Amazon. 1924-1925. Año 1926.

1942-1943 28 Stone Alan.—Varias cartas.

1935 29 Shiraki Tokuichi.—Simuliidae of the Japanese Empire. Memoirs of the Faculty of Science and Agriculture. Vol. XVI. No. I. 1935.

1942 30 Vargas Luis.—Notas sobre la terminalia de algunos simulidos de México. Revista del Inst. de Salubridad i Enf. Tropicales. Tomo III. No. 3. 1942.

1910 31 Surcouf i González Rincones.—Les diptéres vulnérants du Venezuela. Primera parte. 1910.

1941 32 Vargas Luis.—Nota sobre el papel de algunos artrópodos en la trasmisión de la Onchocerca volvulus. Revista del Inst. de Salubridad i Enfermedades Tropicales. Dcbre. 1941.

1914 33 Malloch J.R.—American black flies or buffalo gnats. U.S. Department of Agriculture—Technical Series No. 16 - 1914.

1914 34 Knab Frederick.—New data and species in Simuliidae—(Diptera). Insecutor Inscitiae Menstruus. Vol. II. No. 12. 1914.

1938 35 S. González Herrejon i Dra. M. del C. Ortiz Lombardini. ¿Es el Simulium haematopotum (Malloch) trasmisor del Mal del Pinto? Medicina. México. No. 330-Dcbre.

1888 36 Skuse Frederick A.A.—The Simuliidae and Biblionidae. Proceedings of the Linnean Society of New South Wales. vol. III. Ser. 2nd. Octubre.

1927 37 Dyar Harrison G. and Shannon Raymond C. The North American two winged flies of the family Simuliidae. Proceedings of the United States.

1942 5 Briceño Iragorry L.—Notas sobre Simulium clarki Fairchild 1940 (Nueva especie para Venezuela.—Boletín del Laboratorio de la Clínica "Luis Razetti"—Año III. Vol. II, N° 9 -1942.

1939 38 Edwards F.W. Oldroyd H. and Smart J.—British bloodsucking flies. Simuliidae. pag. 50. Dept. of Ent. British Museum.

1938 39 Neveu Lemaire M.—Traité d'Entomologie Médicale. - 1938.

BIBLIOGRAFIA CONSULTADA DESPUES DE TERMINADO ESTE TRABAJO

Iriarte David R.—Contribución a la Fauna Venezolana. Boletín del Laboratorio de la Clínica Razetti. Año IV. No. 11.

Briceño Iragorry L.—Nota sobre simulidos del Estado Anzoátegui con citación de una especie nueva para el País. Boletín del Laboratorio de la Clínica Razetti. Año IV. No. 11.

Vargas Luis, Díaz Najera A. i Martínez P.A. Tres simulidos nuevos para Méjico—Rev. del Inst. de Salubridad i Enf. Tropicales. Vol. IV - No. 3. 1943.

Vargas Luis.—Nuevos datos sobre simulidos mexicanos (Dipt. Simuliidae) Rev. del Inst. de Salubridad i Enfermedades Tropicales. Vol IV. No. 4. 1943.

Romeo de León J.—Preliminares sobre la descripción de cinco nuevas especies de simúlidos en Guatemala. Boletín Sanitario de Guatemala. Año XIV. No. 51. 1943.

Vargas Luis.—Nombres i datos nuevos de Simulidos del nuevo mundo.—Rev. de la Soc. Mexicana de Historia Natural—Tomo IV. Nos. 3-4. 1943.

* * *

Nota: gran parte de los dibujos de estas planchas han sido tomados de los trabajos de Pinto, Fairchild, Vargas, Malloch, Lutz, etc. Las microfotos fueron hechas en el Instituto de Higiene bajo la dirección de Anduze.

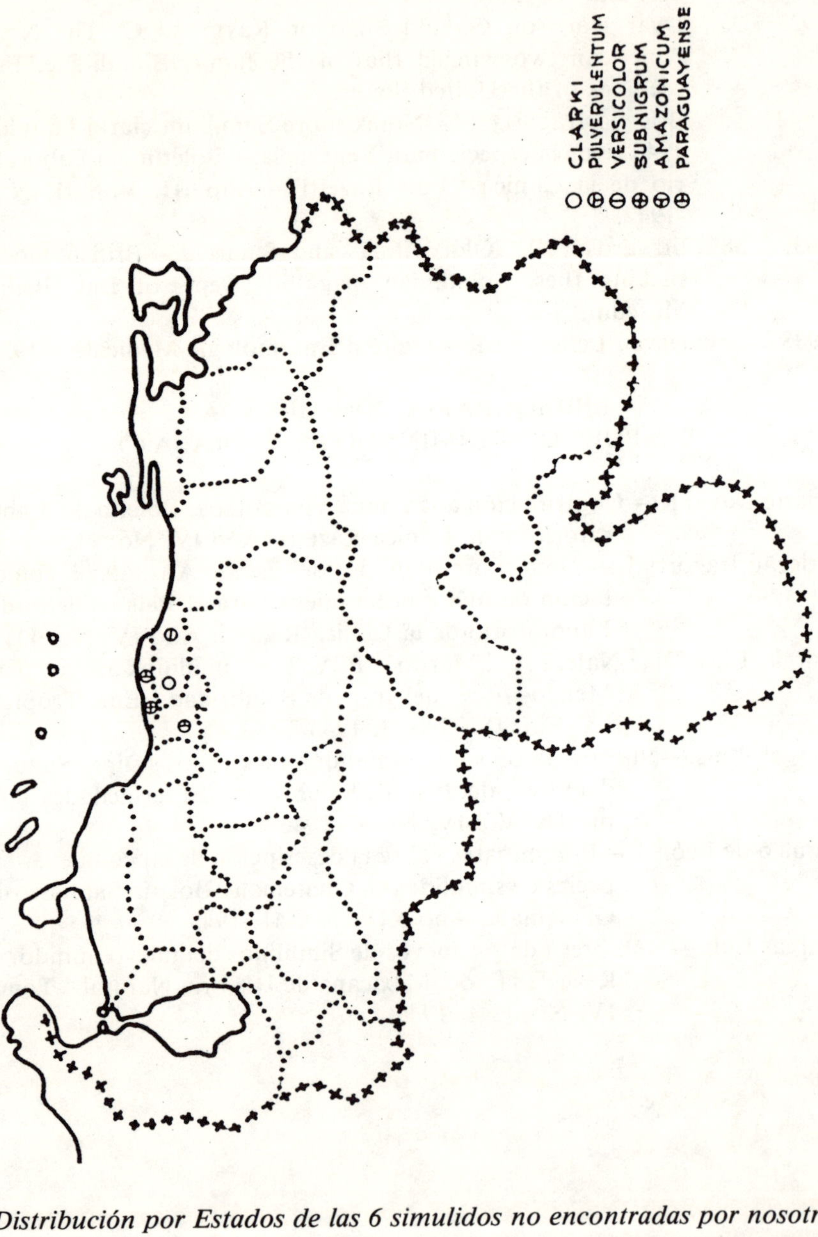

Distribución por Estados de las 6 simulidos no encontradas por nosotros en el país.

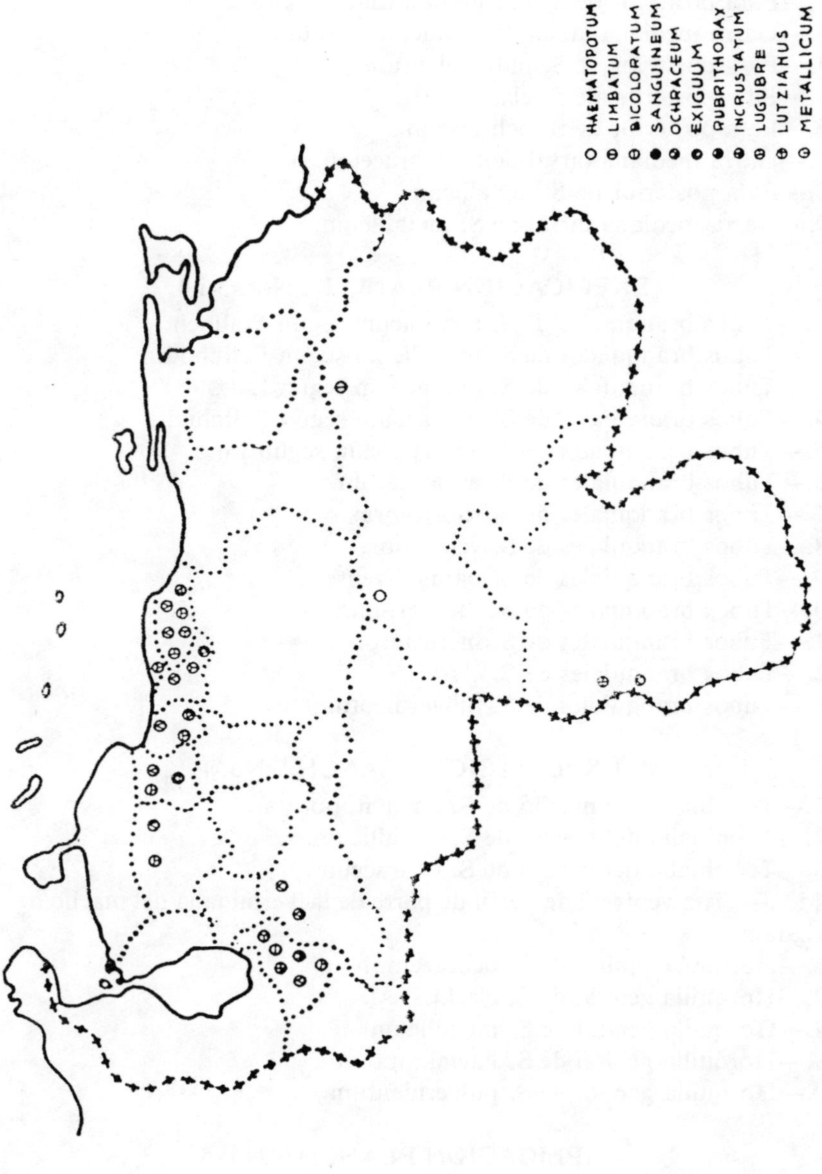

Distribución por Estados de las 11 especies de simulidos encontradas por nosotros en el país.

EXPLICACION PLANCHA No. 2

1.—Pata posterior de S. mexicanum.
2.—Pata posterior de S. haematopotum.
3.—Garra mediana tarsal de S. haematopotum.
4.—Pata posterior de S. pulverulentum.
5.—Pata posterior de S. clarki.
6.—Pata posterior de S. ochraceum.
7.—Garra mediana tarsal de S. ochraceum.
8.—Pata posterior de S. metallicum.
9.—Garra mediana tarsal de S. metallicum.

EXPLICACION PLANCHA Nos. 3 i 4

1.—Tubos branquiales de S. metallicum según Malloch.
2.—Tubos branquiales de S. metallicum según Fairchild.
3.—Tubos branquiales de S. ochraceum según Lutz.
4.—Tubos branquiales de S. ochraceum según Fairchild.
5.—Tubos branquiales de S. amazonicum según Lutz.
6.—Tubos branquiales de S. auristriatum.
7.—Tubos branquiales de S. rubrithorax.
8.—Tubos branquiales de S. versicolor.
9.—Tubos branquiales de S. paraguayense.
10.—Tubos branquiales de S. subnigrum.
11.—Tubos branquiales de S. incrustatum.
12.—Tubos branquiales de S. clarki.
13.—Tubos branquiales de S. pulverulentum.

EXPLICACION PLANCHA No. I

1.—Terminalia del macho de S. haematopotum.
2.—Terminalia del macho de S. metallicum.
3.—Terminalia del macho de S. ochraceum.
4 i 5.—Vista ventral i de perfil de parte de la Terminalia del macho de S. exiguum.
6.—Horquilla genital de S. ochraceum.
7.—Horquilla genital de S. clarki.
8.—Horquilla genital de S. metallicum.
9.—Horquilla genital de S. haematopotum.
10.—Horquilla genital de S. pulverulentum.

EXPLICACION PLANCHA No. 5

1.—Ala de prosimulium.
2.—Ala de parasimulium.
3.—Ala de eusimulium.
4.—Ala de simulium.

DETAILS AND CLASSIFICATION ABOUT THE VORACIOUS CATERPILLAR THAT SCOURGED THE VALLEY OF CARACAS, DURING THE MONTHS OF JULY AND AUGUST (1940) *

At the half of this year, July and August, the Valley of Caracas was scourged for the abundance of a caterpillar very voracious, that brought commentaries in the journals of the city, and whose ravages were extended to the States Aragua and Carabobo.

We had the opportunity to observe these worms, because the pasture brought from places near of our Laboratory of Clínica Razetti, for feeding the animals of experimentation, came attacked with numerous worms similar to those that Ballou, entomologist to Service of Ministry of Agriculture had showed us in his Laboratory of Valle Abajo.

The worms had of 2 to 3 c.m. of length and sometimes a little more, of a greenish dark color, more clear in the center, looking it on back.

Observing the evolution of this lepidopterous, we saw that worms of 1 c.m. placed in test tubes on 15-6-40, feeding greedily with grass *gamelote* (Panicum maximum Jacq.) Sometimes, not having this gramineous, we gave cabbage (Brassica oleracea capitata) and *pira brava* (Amarantus spinosus L.), eating equally, but with less avidity. These worms arrived the pupae stage the days 23-7-40 and 24-7-40, remaining the pupae stage till 3-8-40, going out a small butterfly, of 1.5 c.m. of length, of ash color red.

Specimens sent to Department of Agriculture in Washington were classified for the specialist in lepidopterous, Dr. Clark, as Laphygma frugiperda S. A. telling us that in the United States, sometimes, this species has been a problem to the agriculture.

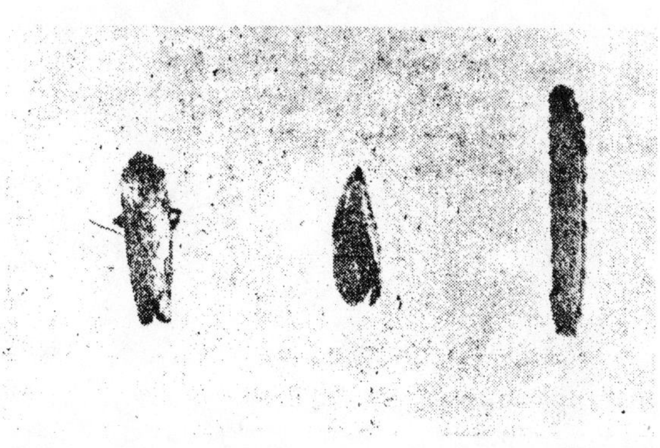

Adult, pupae and larve reared in our Laboratory.

(*) Reprinted from "Boletín del Laboratorio de la Clínica Luis Razetti". Año I. No. 2. 1940.

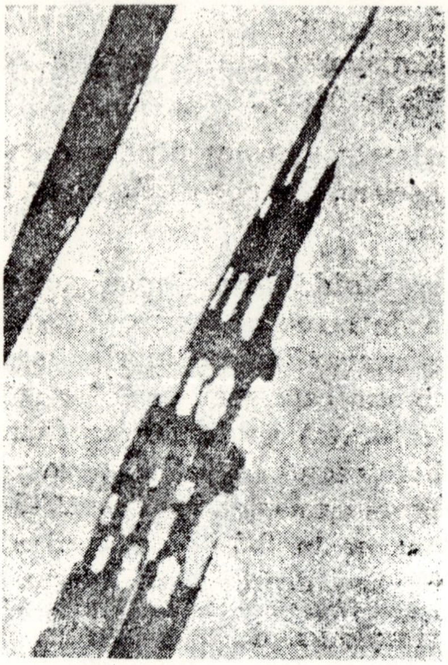

Leaf of grass gamelote (Panicum maximum Jacq.) brought from a place near our Laboratory, attacked for the worms.

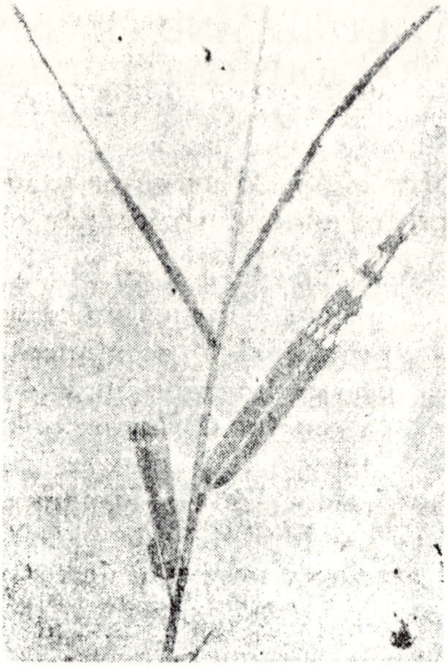

Branch of gamelote where is easy to appreciate the voracity of these caterpillars.

COPROLOGICAL STATISTICS *

(with the collaboration of Briceño Iragorry)

We publish a parasitological statistic having as base 2.941 examinations of feces in persons of different ages, staying the majority in the zone of Caracas, during a time among 1934-1944 (ten years). The value that we gave to our results was because they were obtained with material coming from high social class and we believed it is the first time between us. Up till today our statistics have been made working with feces from hospital patients, health departments and surveys in the interior populations. This explains that our percentages are low in comparison with other former publications.

Our tests were made always ıʋr direct examination; rarely we used concentration methods and we never did the investigation of oxyuris employing swabs.

NUMBER OF TESTS 2.945

Positive 1.459 Parasites found	Negative 1.482 Percentage found
Ascaris	6.05%
Anguilulas	0.65%
Amiba Disenterica	10.60%
Amiba Coli	11.90%
Bilharzia	0.68%
Blastocistis	14.00%
Chilomastix	5.95%
Enteromonas	2.51%
Embadomonas	0.61%
Endolimax	0.27%
Lamblias	3.77%
Levaduras	8.81%
Necator	1.02%
Oxiuros	0.20%
Quistes de Flagelados	9.28%
Tricocefalos	8.84%
Tenia Nana	0.01%
Tenia Saginata	0.24%
Tenia Solium	0.03%
Trichomonas	3.98%

* Reprinted from "Boletín del Laboratorio de la Clínica Luis Razetti". Año VI. Vol. XIII. No. 17. 1945.

STATISTIC OF COPROLOGICAL TESTS MADE IN THE "LABORATORIO DE LA CLINICA LUIS RAZETTI", DURING THE YEARS: 1935 - 1949. *

COMMENTARIES

We expose here a scatologic statistic referring to 4. 638 examinations of feces done during fifteen years, from 1935 to 1949. The samples arising from patients of the zone of Caracas and some of them coming from the interior of the country. They are persons with good social and econimic position. Our statistic is relatively low, demonstrating that the digestive troubles of the wealthy persons, often, have no parasitie origin.

When we were students occupying the job in charge of the Section of Coprology of the Laboratory of the Vargas Hospital, and published statistics made in the Hospital. Something of this material was studied with the help of Briceño Iragorry.

In rare occasions we used the swab to search oxyuris. Almost always we practice the direct examination. In scarce cases, we realized concentration methods, to request.

YEAR 1935

Parasites	Number of Tests	Percentages
Amiba disentérica y sus quistes:	10	17.85%
Amiba coli y sus quistes:	3	5.35%
Endolimax:	1	1.78%
Chilomastix:	4	7.14%
Trichomonas:	11	19.64%
Embadomonas:	0	0%
Enteromonas:	0	0%
Quistes de flagelados:	17	30.35%
Lamblias y sus quistes:	4	7.14%
Espiroquetas:	0	0%
Ascaris:	8	14.28%
Tricocéfalos:	16	28.57%
Oxiuros:	0	0%
Anguílulas:	1	1.78%
Necator y Anquilostomo:	3	5.35%

* Reprinted from "Boletín del Laboratorio de la Clínica Luis Razetti". Año XI. Vol. XVI. No. 33-34. 1951.

Bilharzia:	2	3.57%
Tenia saginata:	0	0%
Tenia solium:	0	0%
Tenia nana:	1	1.78%
Blastocistis:	17	30.35%
Levaduras:	18	32.03%
Total de exámenes practicados durante el año:		56
Positivos:		47
Negativos:		9

YEAR 1936

Parasites	Number of Tests	Percentages
Amiba disentérica y sus quistes:	26	28.57%
Amiba coli y sus quistes:	5	5.49%
Endolimax:	0	0%
Chilomastix:	0	0%
Trichomonas:	0	0%
Embadomonas:	0	0%
Enteromonas:	0	0%
Quistes de flagelados:	16	17.58%
Lamblias y sus quistes:	4	4.39%
Espiroquetas:	0	0%
Ascaris:	11	21.08%
Tricocéfalos:	15	16.48%
Oxiuros:	0	0%
Anguílulas:	0	0%
Necator y Anquilostomo:	1	1.08%
Bilharzia:	0	0%
Tenia saginata:	0	0%
Tenia solium:	0	0%
Tenia nana:	3	3.29%
Blastocistis:	25	27.47%
Levaduras:	25	27.47%
Total de exámenes practicados durante el año:		91
Positivos:		78
Negativos:		13

YEAR 1937

Parasites	Number of Tests	Percentages
Amiba disentérica y sus quistes:	32	21.33%
Amiba coli y sus quistes:	11	7.33%
Endolimax:	0	0%
Chilomastix:	3	2%
Trichomonas:	10	6.66%
Embadomonas:	0	0%
Enteromonas:	0	0%
Quistes de flagelados:	31	20.66%
Lamblias y sus quistes:	7	4.66%
Espiroquetas:	0	0%
Ascaris:	9	6%
Tricocéfalos:	19	12.70%
Oxiuros:	0	0%
Anguílulas:	1	0.66%
Necator y Anquilostomo:	1	0.66%
Bilharzia:	2	1.33%
Tenia saginata:	1	0.66%
Tenia solium:	0	0%
Tenia nana:	1	0.66%
Blastocistis:	48	32%
Levaduras:	58	38.66%
Total de exámenes practicados durante el año:		150
Positivos:		122
Negativos:		28

YEAR 1938

Parasites	Number of Tests	Percentages
Amiba disentérica y sus quistes:	52	16.34%
Amiba coli y sus quistes:	52	16.34%
Endolimax:	0	0%
Chilomastix:	19	6.08%
Trichomonas:	24	7.69%
Embadomonas:	0	0%
Enteromonas:	15	4.80%
Quistes de flagelados:	60	19.20%
Lamblias y sus quistes:	11	3.52%
Espiroquetas:	2	0.64%

Ascaris:	39	12.50%
Tricocéfalos:	47	15.06%
Oxiuros:	0	0%
Anguílulas:	4	1.25%
Necator y Anquilostomo:	6	1.92%
Bilharzia:	2	0.64%
Tenia saginata:	2	0.64%
Tenia solium:	0	0%
Blastocistis:	122	39.10%
Levaduras:	55	17.62%
Total de exámenes practicados durante el año:		312
Positivos:		245
Negativos:		67

YEAR 1939

Parasites	Number of Tests	Percentages
Amiba disentérica y sus quistes:	58	15.50%
Amiba coli y sus quistes:	56	14.97%
Endolimax:	0	0%
Chilomastix:	98	26.20%
Trichomonas:	13	3.47%
Embadomonas:	21	5.61%
Enteromonas:	82	21.92%
Quistes de flagelados:	125	33.42%
Lamblias y sus quistes:	11	2.94%
Espiroquetas:	5	1.33%
Ascaris:	49	13.10%
Tricocéfalos:	53	14.17%
Oxiuros:	2	0.53%
Anguílulas:	3	0.80%
Necator y Anquilostomo:	10	2.66%
Bilharzia:	4	1.07%
Tenia saginata:	1	0.26%
Tenia solium:	0	0%
Tenia nana:	1	0.26%
Blastocistis:	127	33.95%
Levaduras:	44	11.83%
Total de exámenes practicados durante el año:		374
Positivos:		285
Negativos:		89

YEAR 1940

Parasites	Number of Tests	Percentages
Amiba disentérica y sus quistes:	73	16.78%
Amiba coli y sus quistes:	62	14.25%
Endolimax:	0	0%
Chilomastix:	160	36.78%
Trichomonas:	36	8.27%
Embadomonas:	135	31.03%
Enteromonas:	147	33.79%
Quistes de flagelados:	168	38.62%
Lamblias y sus quistes:	30	6.89%
Espiroquetas:	10	2.28%
Ascaris:	23	5.28%
Tricocéfalos:	51	11.70%
Oxiuros:	1	0.23%
Anguílulas:	5	1.14%
Necator y Anquilostomo:	4	0.92%
Bilharzia:	8	1.83%
Tenia saginata:	2	0.42%
Tenia solium:	0	0%
Tenia nana:	1	0.23%
Blastocistis:	193	44.36%
Levaduras:	81	18.62%
Total de exámenes practicados durante el año:		435
Positivos:		361
Negativos:		74

YEAR 1941

Parasites	Number of Tests	Percentages
Amiba disentérica y sus quistes:	30	9.67%
Amiba coli y sus quistes:	13	4.19%
Endolimax:	0	0%
Chilomastix:	77	24.83%
Trichomonas:	11	3.54%
Embadomonas:	1	0.32%

Enteromonas:	22	7.09%
Quistes de flagelados:	54	17.41%
Lamblias y sus quistes:	12	3.87%
Espiroquetas:	2	0.64%
Ascaris:	22	7.09%
Tricocéfalos:	31	.10%
Oxiuros:	0	0%
Anguílulas:	0	0%
Necator y Anquilostomo:	0	0%
Bilharzia:	1	0.32%
Tenia saginata:	0	0%
Tenia solium:	0	0%
Tenia nana:	1	0.32%
Blastocistis:	98	31.61%
Levaduras:	50	16.12%
Total de exámenes practicados durante el año:		310
Positivos:		220
Negativos:		90

YEAR 1942

Parasites	Number of Tests	Percentages
Amiba disentérica y sus quistes:	65	14.94%
Amiba coli y sus quistes:	55	12.44%
Endolimax:	0	0%
Chilomastix:	157	39.64%
Trichomonas:	10	2.50%
Embadomonas:	98	24.74%
Enteromonas:	117	29.54%
Quistes de flagelados:	153	38.61%
Lamblias y sus quistes:	37	9.34%
Espiroquetas:	11	2.75%
Ascaris:	21	5.30%
Tricocéfalos:	48	12.12%
Oxiuros:	0	0%
Anguílulas:	2	0.50%
Necator y Anquilostomo:	3	0.75%
Bilharzia:	3	0.75%
Tenia saginata:	1	0.25%

Tenia solium:	0	0%
Tenia nana:	0	0%
Blastocistis:	172	40.90%
Levaduras:	88	22.22%
Total de exámenes practicados durante el año:		396
Positivos:		307
Negativos:		89

YEAR 1943

Parasites	Number of Tests	Percentages
Amiba disentérica y sus quistes:	44	11.85%
Amiba coli y sus quistes:	40	10.78%
Endolimax:	0	0%
Chilomastix:	103	27.77%
Trichomonas:	16	4.31%
Embadomonas:	0	0%
Enteromonas:	7	1.88%
Quistes de flagelados:	96	25.87%
Lamblias y sus quistes:	24	6.46%
Espiroquetas:	4	1.06%
Ascaris:	24	6.46%
Tricocéfalos:	16	4.31%
Oxiuros:	0	0%
Anguílulas:	1	0.27%
Necator y Anquilostomo:	3	0.80%
Bilharzia:	2	0.53%
Tenia saginata:	0	0%
Tenia solium:	0	0%
Tenia nana:	1	0.87%
Blastocistis:	111	29.93%
Levaduras:	78	21.02%
Total de exámenes practicados durante el año:		371
Positivos:		270
Negativos:		101

YEAR 1944

Parasites	Number of Tests	Percentages
Amiba disentérica y sus quistes:	30	9.86%
Amiba coli y sus quistes:	32	10.52%
Chilomastix:	74	24.34%
Trichomonas:	7	2.30%
Embadomonas:	0	0%
Enteromonas:	3	0.98%
Quistes de flagelados:	50	16.44%
Lamblias y sus quistes:	9	2.96%
Espiroquetas:	0	0%
Ascaris:	20	6.57%
Tricocéfalos:	25	8.22%
Oxiuros:	0	0%
Anguílulas:	3	0.98%
Necator y Anquilostomo:	1	0.32%
Bilharzia:	2	0.65%
Tenia saginata:	0	0%
Tenia solium:	0	0%
Tenia nana:	0	0%
Blastocistis:	75	24.67%
Levaduras:	69	22.69%
Total de exámenes practicados durante el año:		304
Positivos:		197
Negativos:		107

YEAR 1945

Parasites	Number of Tests	Percentages
Amiba disentérica y sus quistes:	31	6.05%
Amiba coli y sus quistes:	51	9.96%
Endolimax:	0	0%
Chilomastix:	84	16.40%
Trichomonas:	6	1.17%

Embadomonas:	0	0%
Enteromonas:	0	0%
Quistes de flagelados:	57	11.13%
Lamblias y sus quistes:	13	2.53%
Espiroquetas:	0	0%
Ascaris:	37	7.22%
Tricocéfalos:	34	6.64%
Oxiuros:	0	0%
Anguílulas:	1	0.19%
Necator y Anquilostomo:	2	0.39%
Bilharzia:	1	0.19%
Tenia saginata:	0	0%
Tenia solium:	0	0%
Tenia nana:	2	0.39%
Blastocistis:	51	9.96%
Levaduras:	85	16.60%
Total de exámenes practicados durante el año:		512
Positivos:		268
Negativos:		244

YEAR 1946

Parasites	Number of Tests	Percentages
Amiba disentérica y sus quistes:	20	4.81%
Amiba coli y sus quistes:	30	7.20%
Endolimax:	0	0%
Chilomastix:	91	21.92%
Trichomonas:	10	2.40%
Embadomonas:	0	0%
Enteromonas:	2	0.48%
Quistes de flagelados:	60	14.45%
Lamblias y sus quistes:	11	2.65%
Espiroquetas:	0	0%
Ascaris:	21	5.06%
Tricocéfalos:	14	3.37%
Oxiuros:	0	0%
Anguílulas:	1	0.24%
Necator y Anquilostomo:	2	0.48%

Bilharzia:	3	0.72%
Tenia saginata:	0	0%
Tenia solium:	0	0%
Tenia nana:	0	0%
Blastocistis:	50	12.04%
Levaduras:	47	11.08%
Total de exámenes practicados durante el año:		415
Positivos:		218
Negativos:		197

YEAR 1947

Parasites	Number of Tests	Percentages
Amiba disentérica y sus quistes:	4	1.51%
Amiba coli y sus quistes:	20	7.57%
Endolimax:	0	0%
Chilomastix:	58	22%
Trichomonas:	10	3.78%
Embadomonas:	0	0%
Enteromonas:	0	0%
Quistes de flagelados:	31	11.62%
Lamblias y sus quistes:	13	4.92%
Espiroquetas:	3	1.12%
Ascaris:	20	7.57%
Tricocéfalos:	15	5.68%
Oxiuros:	0	0%
Anguílulas:	0	0%
Necator y Anquilostomo:	1	0.37%
Bilharzia:	0	0%
Tenia saginata:	0	0%
Tenia solium:	0	0%
Tenia nana:	0	0%
Blastocistis:	58	22%
Levaduras:	35	13.25%
Total de exámenes practicados durante el año:		264
Positivos:		133
Negativos:		131

YEAR 1948

Parasites	Number of Tests	Percentages
Amiba disentérica y sus quistes:	10	3.24%
Amiba coli y sus quistes:	40	12.98%
Endolimax:	1	0.32%
Chilomastix:	65	21.10%
Trichomonas:	6	1.94%
Embadomonas:	0	0%
Enteromonas:	3	0.97%
Quistes de flagelados:	32	10.38%
Lamblias y sus quistes:	17	5.51%
Espiroquetas:	1	0.32%
Ascaris:	21	6.81%
Tricocéfalos:	25	8.11%
Oxiuros:	0	0%
Anguílulas:	1	0.32%
Necator y Anquilostomo:	3	0.97%
Bilharzia:	1	0.32%
Tenia saginata:	0	0%
Tenia solium:	0	0%
Tenia nana:	0	0%
Blastocistis:	27	8.76%
Levaduras:	58	18.83%
Total de exámenes practicados durante el año:		308
Positivos:		174
Negativos:		134

YEAR 1949

Parasites	Number of Tests	Percentages
Amiba disentérica y sus quistes:	10	2.94%
Amiba coli y sus quistes:	27	7.94%
Endolimax:	0	0%
Chilomastix:	55	16.17%

Trichomonas:	7	2.05%
Embadomonas:	1	0.29%
Enteromonas:	2	0.58%
Quistes de flagelados:	36	10.58%
Lamblias y sus quistes:	28	8.23%
Espiroquetas:	0	0%
Ascaris:	20	5.58%
Tricocéfalos:	20	5.58%
Oxiuros:	0	0%
Anguílulas:	2	0.58%
Necator y Anquilostomo:	2	0.58%
Bilharzia:	0	0%
Tenia saginata:	1	0.29%
Tenia solium:	0	0%
Tenia nana:	1	0.29%
Blastocistis:	35	16.17%
Levaduras:	87	25.58%
Total de exámenes practicados durante el año:		340
Positivos:		194
Negativos:		146

STATISTIC OF SEROLOGICAL TESTS MADE IN THE "LABORATORIO DE LA CLINICA LUIS RAZETTI", DURING THE YEARS: 1935 - 1949. *

COMMENTARIES

This percentage seems a little high. They are figures obtained in a private laboratory, with good clientele, the majority of patients reported by physicians, existing, possibly, suspicions of positivity.

The test used has been Kahn standard, utilizing, almost always, the antigen Difco. Some of these results have been obtained with the micro-reaction (technique Briceño Rossi), chiefly in children and in some persons who are very fat.

The average of annual tests, during the fifteen years that we present, is of 250.53. The year with the greatest abundance of tests corresponded to 1945, with 378, and that one with largest positivity, 1939, with 109.

Thanks to Misses Rondón and Muñoz, assistants, for their collaboration.

YEAR	TOTAL	POSITIVE	PERCENTAGE	NEGATIVE
1935	73	17	23.28%	56
1936	145	45	31.03%	100
1937	159	45	28.30%	100
1938	238	78	32.77%	160
1939	288	109	37.84%	179
1940	276	78	28.26%	198
1941	276	79	28.62%	197
1942	228	45	19.73%	183
1943	295	42	14.23%	253
1944	229	36	15.69%	193
1945	378	48	12.69%	330
1946	349	53	15.18%	296
1947	275	45	16.35%	230
1948	267	52	19.47%	215
1949	282	51	18.08%	231
Total:	3.758	823	21.89%	2.935

* Reprinted from "Boletín del Laboratorio de la Clínica Luis Razetti". Año XI. Vol. XVI. No. 33-34. 1951.

THE PARASITOLOGY IN VENEZUELA *

(Work presented to the VI Venezuelan Congress of Medical Sciences, with the close collaboration of Drs. Gutiérrez Alfaro and Díaz Ungría)

CAPITULO I

Breve Resumen Histórico sobre los fundadores e investigadores sobresalientes en el campo de la Parasitología en Venezuela. Relación cronológica de los hechos más destacados en el período 1926-1955.

CAPITULO II

Especies de Parásitos señaladas en Venezuela desde 1926, con indicación de año, autor, hospedero y nota bibliográfica relativa a su descripción.

CAPITULO III

Especies de Protozoarios señaladas en Venezuela hasta 1930 (Gabaldón). 1930-1955 (Gutiérrez Alfaro, Iriarte, Díaz Ungría).

CAPITULO IV

Tesis Doctorales sobre Parasitología presentadas ante la Universidad Central para obtener el Título de Doctor en Ciencias Médicas.

CAPITULO V

Bibliografía Parasitológica Venezolana que se ha podido obtener desde 1926 hasta la fecha, montante en 1.370 fichas, ordenadas alfabéticamente por los autores.

CAPITULO VI

Bibliografía.

* Reprinted from the "Boletín del Laboratorio de la Clínica Luis Razetti". Año XV. Vol. XVI. Nos. 45-46. noviembre 1955.

CAPITULO I

Breve Resumen Histórico sobre los fundadores e investigadores sobresalientes en la Parasitología Venezolana. Relación Cronológica de los hechos más destacados en el período de 1926 hasta 1955.

Venezuela por su posición geográfica, es un país comprendido en la zona tropical, y su desarrollo está en relación directa con múltiples problemas de importancia práctica e higiénica, cuya gravedad no se puede juzgar, sino en el mismo ambiente, sitio y condiciones. Por eso el trópico ha sido eternamente un atractivo para investigadores y parasitólogos.

La Economía mundial es hoy de primer orden. Los destructores de plantas y animales, principalmente los parásitos del hombre, requieren la atención científica. Se ha intensificado la lucha contra esos enemigos, por medio de la investigación botánica, zoológica y médica, buscando solución a la explotación agrícola-industrial. Ecología, fisiología, nutrición, reproducción, son bases para esa compaña. Por consiguiente, la labor de investigación no ha sido sólo desde el punto de vista especulativo, sino eminentemente práctica, porque para lograr el éxito se hace imprescindible el conocimiento profundo de la biología del parásito.

El empirismo indígena con su piache, mezcla de sibilismo, religíon, hechicería y medicina, tuvo acción igualmente sobre la mentalidad de los primeros españoles invasores, de tanta ignorancia como los indios, y adoptaron sus prácticas. Un herbolario consumado era el "piache": sabía distinguir entre una hierba venenosa o no, estaba en cuenta de sus propiedades revulsivas, eméticas, purgativas, depurantes, hemostáticas y sudoríficas; por sus manos pasaban hojas, flores, frutos, raíces, semillas, tubérculos y resinas.

El precursor Luis Daniel Beauperthuy en 1838 por conducto de Roseville, presentaba ante la Academia de Ciencias de París, anticipándose a Ross, a Grassi, Bastianelli y Bignami, sus conceptos sobre las enfermedades palúdicas y la fiebre amarilla, resumiendo en éstas sus palabras: "No atribuyo a la acción de las emanaciones telúricas, ni a los efluvios pútridos, la producción de la grave enfermedad que nos ocupa (la epidemia sobrevenida después del terremoto de Cumaná, el 15 de julio de 1853). Esa enfermedad proviene, después de mis investigaciones, de la inoculación en la economía humana de un germen séptico destructor, sea esta inoculación confiada a los nematoceros tipulares, como sucede en los actos de fiebre palúdica o del tifus icteriodes, como sucede en las afecciones pestilenciales".

"Cada enfermedad específica tiene su agente específico denominado *virus.* La inoculación del producto alterado produce siempre una enfermedad idéntica a la que suministra". Así el sabio de Cumaná se adelantaba al descubrimiento trascendental de Remlinser y los postulados fundamentales del gran Koch.

José Gregorio Hernández, fundador de los estudios experimentales en Venezuela y de las Cátedras de Bacteriología (según Ovalles la Primera en América), de Fisiología Experimental, de Histología Normal y Patológica, regentó la cátedra de Bacteriología desde el 6 de noviembre de 1891 hasta junio de 1908. En 1910 publica "De la Bilharziosis en Caracas", según Dominici "el primer grito de alarma por lo frecuente de la tremenda infección entre nosotros" y que vio luz pública en momentos que era negada por los representantes del País a la Cuarta Conferencia Sanitaria Internacional. Sobre este trabajo de Hernández dice Briceño Iragorry: "fuera de llamar la atención por primera vez acerca de la importancia de la enfermedad en nuestro medio, lo destaca como descubridor, pues propone casi al mismo tiempo que Piraja da Silva en el Brasil, el nombre de americanum para la especie en cuestión por haber observado algunas diferencias en las descripciones que de los huevos se conocían entonces; y es bajo su dirección que uno de sus discípulos descubre, años más tarde, el vermes adulto."

En 1895 se funda el Instituto Pasteur, con Dominici, Acosta Ortíz, Guardia hijo, Elías Rodríguez y Meier Flegel. El establecimiento del Instituto Pasteur y la fundación de las cátedras por José Gregorio Hernández,

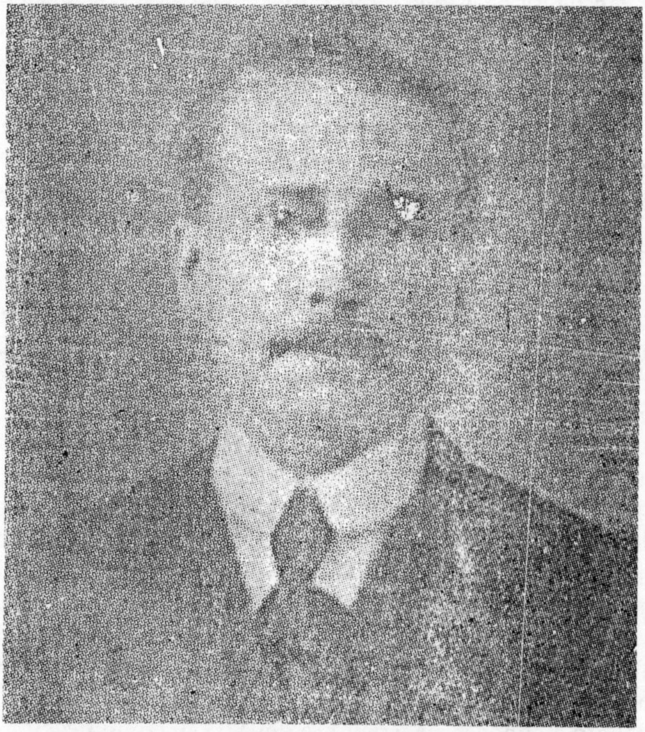

José Gregorio Hernández

ejercieron una gran influencia para que aparecieran trabajos de Rangel sobre Paludismo, de González Rincones, sobre "Culicidos del Estado Monagas"; de González Rincones y Surcouf, la célebre obra sobre los "Dípteros Vulnerantes de Venezuela"; de Guevara Rojas, sobre "Malaria"; de Rísquez viejo y Velásquez sobre el mismo tema; de Romero Sierra sobre los mosquitos de Caracas, etc.

Dominici al frente del Instituto Pasteur preparó por primera vez en el país la vacuna antivariólica por inoculación del virus vaccígeno en la ternera; creó una Sección para el diagnóstico y tratamiento de la lepra e hizo los primeros diagnósticos bacteriológicos, al mismo tiempo que clasificaba zancudos del Valle de Caracas y estudiaba la relación del Anquilostoma duodenal con la anemia tropical. Dominici fue el iniciador de la aplicación del Laboratorio a la Clínica en su doble condición de hombre de laboratorio y clínico eminente.

En 1896, Mosquera ve por primera vez la Amiba disentérica en Caracas; Guevara Rojas en su tesis doctoral de 1904 asienta que la Amiba coli fue encontrada por Dominici y Meier Flegel; Rísquez Francisco Antonio, Mosquera, Machado y Herrera Tovar a partir de 1896 sospechan que muchos procesos febriles (fiebres largas de Caracas) no son debidos a los Hematozoarios y sugieren la existencia de la fiebre tifoidea y pseudo tíficas (antes de la descripción de las paratíficas por Achard Bensaude).

Sobre Hernández y Rangel, escribió Rísquez hijo, en su clase inaugural del curso de Bacteriología y Parasitología de 1925: "Hernández y sus discípulos penetraron por todos los senderos trillados por los especialistas en la materia, estudiaron la mayor parte de los gérmenes morbíficos en el país e hicieron a la Escuela Venezolana, marchar al unísono con las conquistas de la nueva ciencia. Más tarde, cuando la era de los microbios —como dijo Patrick Manson- había llegado a su apogeo y la de los protozoarios comenzaba, un discípulo de Hernández marcó época en los anales de nuestra medicina y empieza entonces la era de la Parasitología en Venezuela con los trabajos de Rafael Rangel." En efecto, funda el Laboratorio del Hospital Vargas, el 18 de febrero de 1902, dando un paso de avance de largo alcance, en el desarrollo de la Parasitología en Venezuela. De allí salieron sus magníficos trabajos sobre la Uncinaria, los de Soto sobre "Disentería en Caracas" que lo llevaron al descubrimiento del S. mansoni (25-10-1905) y de todos los interesados en los estudios de Laboratorio de las sub-siguientes generaciones médicas, quienes han tenido sus primeros contactos con la investigación parasitológica en los salones de esa venerable casa de aspecto conventual en su arquitectura, verdadero templo de enseñanzas prácticas, con el óbolo desprendido de los que, purificados por el dolor, legan sus productos patológicos a nuestra curiosidad de investigación, iluminando nuestras pupilas con la refringencia de los treponemas sobre el fondo oscuro o la policromía maravillosa de los hematozoarios coloreados.

Rangel dio a conocer en setiembre de 1903 su comunicación sobre las anemias de Guarenas, Guatire y Santa Lucía producidas por la Uncinaria stenocefala, y en 1904, comprobó que el Tripanosoma venezuelensis era el productor de la derrengadera de los caballos. Trabajó sobre bronquitis verminosa de los bovinos, sobre las lesiones cutáneas de la Dermatobia

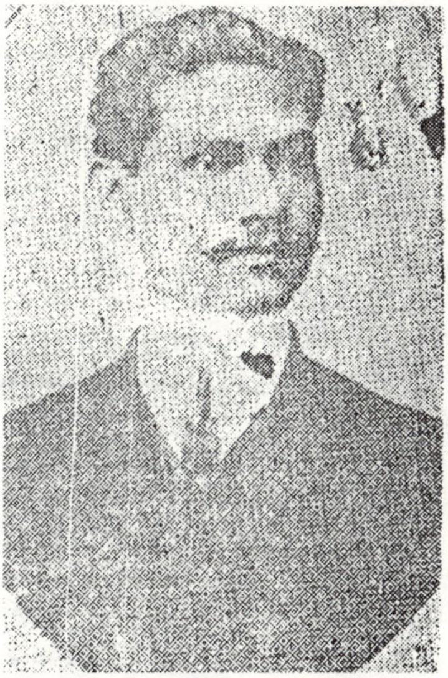

Rafael Rangel

cyaniventris, sobre la Bacteridia carbonosa y sobre el "grito de los chivos" de Coro.

Rafael Rangel, el Padre de la Parasitología Venezolana, representa la historia de la parasitología vernácula, un hito luminoso e imperecedero que divide el período de su evolución en: pre-Rangeliano y post-Rangeliano.

Entusiasmados por los trabajos de Rangel, se acrecienta el interés por la investigación científica y aparecen trabajos de Ascanio Rodríguez, Rivas, González Rincones, Carvallo, Luciani y otros.

En los últimos tiempos cuatro hombres aparecen en escena y han influído considerablemente en el desarrollo de la Parasitología en Venezuela: Iturbe con su eficiente colaborador Eudoro González, Tejera, Rísquez hijo y Núñez Tovar.

Sobre Manuel Núñez Tovar, uno de los autores le dedicó una semblanza publicada hace algún tiempo. Se le puede considerar como el Padre de la Entomología Médica Venezolana. Sus comunicaciones sobre "Insectos venezolanos trasmisores de enfermedades", "Presencia de dos anofelinos", "Nota de Historia Natural", "Mosquitos y Flebotomos de Venezuela" y los "Dípteros Hematófagos de Venezuela" en compañía de Lutz, son algunos de sus trabajos más destacados.

Rísquez, Jesús Rafael, desempeñó por muchos años la Cátedra de Bacteriología y Parasitología, en la cual tuvimos el honor de colaborar por varios años, estimulándonos en nuestra vocación docente. Su tesis doctoral trata sobre "Estado Actual de la Parasitología en Venezuela". Descubrió las Distomatosis Humanas en 1912. En 1916 y siguientes, en una serie de publicaciones, estudió la anatomía patológica de la bilharziosis, (invasión de ganglios linfáticos, bilharziosis apendicular, bilharziosis pulmonar, modificaciones hepáticas, etc.). En 1918 obtuvo el Premio Vargas con su trabajo "La Bilharziosis mansoni en Venezuela" y en 1923, el Premio José Gregorio Hernández, con su trabajo "La Espiroquetosis bronquial en Venezuela."

De Iturbe ha hecho uno de nosotros, un claro bosquejo sobre su personalidad. Hace trabajos sobre bacteriología, lo mismo que sobre protozoología: leishmanias, tripanosomas, flagelados de las plantas. Su labor irradia desde su célebre "Laboratorio Iturbe."

Tejera, tesoneramente trabaja e investiga, y en 1918 obtiene el premio Vargas de la Academia Nacional de Medicina con sus trabajos sobre Leishmania; descubre la enfermedad de Chagas en Venezuela y estudia el Ornithodorus venezuelensis, los blátidos, etc.

Desempeña transitoriamente la cátedra de Patología Tropical, y actualmente se dedica intensamente al estudio de los hongos venezolanos, especialmente en relación con la producción de sustancias antibióticas.

Recientemente una pléyade de estudiosos han seguido las huellas de Hernández y Rangel y de tantos otros investigadores, que la brevedad de este resumen impide evocar hoy por su contribución a la Parasitología en nuestra Patria, pero su recuerdo estará siempre presente y es semilla fértil que hoy se transforma en óptimo fruto en los trabajos de los investigadores actuales: Barnola, Briceño Iragorri, Briceño Rossi, del Corral, Iriarte, O'Daly, Pifano, Torrealba, Cuenca, etc., en el aspecto parasitológico puro; O'Daly, Jaffé, Potenza y la Escuela del Hospital Vargas, en sus aspectos anatomo-patológicos; Dominici, Ruíz Rodríguez, Benaim Pinto, Gil Yépez y otros, en la parte clínica; Guerra, O'Daly, Montemayor, Barnola, Potenza, Campins, Borelli y Feo en la parte relativa a la micología; Gabaldón, González Rincones, Cova-García, Anduze, Ortíz, Mirsa, etc., en la entomología vernácula; Vogelsang, Díaz Ungría, Gallo, Baumeister y demás investigadores en la parasitología animal; y aquellos otros que debido al espacio limitado de este bosquejo hemos silenciado, pero como aquéllos dignos del reconocimiento de sus compatriotas.

He aquí una lista cronológica de los hehos más importantes, acaecidos en la etapa parasitológica motivo de este relato, es decir desde 1926 hasta la fecha:

1926.— Se señala al A. darlingi como el principal vector del Paludismo en Venezuela, por Root.

1927.— Se clasifican las ratas de Caracas por el Dr. Bello.
Se instala en Maracay la Comisión Rockefeller para el estudio del Paludismo.
Se prepara personal venezolano: Benarroch, Cova-García, etc.

1927 Se estudian en Maracay por disección los anofeles venezolanos,
1928.— verificándose infecciones experimentales y pruebas de precipitinas. Se comprueba el A. albitarsis como vector por R.B. Hill y colaboradores.

1929.— Se crea la dirección de Salubridad y Asistencia Pública en el Ministerio de Relaciones Interiores.

1930.— Se reune la Conferencia Sanitaria Nacional.
Se crean Laboratorios en la Oficina de Sanidad de La Guaira, Puerto Cabello y Maracaibo.
Es señalado el A. pseudopunctipennis como vector de malaria por Cova García.

1932.— Se señala la moniliasis por Rísquez, hijo.

1934.— Se usa la atebrina por primera vez en el mundo por vía endovenosa, por del Corral.
Se describe el Trichosporum venezuelensis por del Corral. Clasificación de anofelinos venezolanos por Gabaldón y Cova García.

1935.— Primer caso de Esporotricosis en Venezuela por Vegas.
Se estudia la Piedraía y se encuentra Piedraía hostai, por Briceño Iragorri.

1936.— Se funda la División de Malariología (28 de julio de 1936).
Se inicia en Venezuela con gran éxito la Ingeniería Antimalárica.

1936.— Se sanea, eliminando el A. darlingi, por obras de Ingeniería Sanitaria, la ciudad de Acarigua.
Se estudia la fauna Anofelina, aumentando el número de especies de 18 a 30, y se describen 4 nuevas especies para el mundo: vargas, rangeli, benarrochi y núñez-tovari.
Es descrito el primer caso de Rhinoclaudiosis schencki, por Briceño Iragorry.

1937.— Se diferencian las llamadas blastomicosis, identificando perfectamente los agentes etiológicos, por O'Daly.

1938.— Es encontrado el Actinomyces madurae de un micetoma de la mano por O'Daly.
Primer caso de Quiste hidático del pulmón, por Gómez López y Luna.

1938.— Hormodendrum pedrosoi, por Briceño Iragorri.

1938.— Se describe como vector de Trypanosoma cruzi el Psammolestes arthuri y el Eutriatoma nigromaculata por Pifano.

1938.— Se describen las cromoblastomicosis, señalando el Hormodendrum communis, por O'Daly, n. sp. para el mundo.

1939.— Se encuentra el Phlebotomus panamensis (Shannon 1926) infestado con leishmanias, por Pifano.

1939.— Se comprueba el agente etiológico del carate por Iriarte y Briceño Rossi.

1939.— Primer caso de sodokú, Iriarte.

1939.— Paracoccidiosis en el vivo por Iriarte y Rodríguez.

1940.— Se comprueba la presencia de leishmania en ulceraciones de perros en zonas de endemia humana, por Pifano.

1940.— Reacciones cutáneas-alérgicas en bilharziosis, Rísquez hijo y Vélez Boza.

1940.— Se encuentra en Venezuela el Plasmodium ovale por Hernán Méndez.

1940.— Se comprueba la existencia del granuloma paracoccidioidico y su importancia en la patología pulmonar por Guerra.

1941.— Se describe el Microsporum felineum por Briceño Iragorri.

1941.— Se describe el primer caso de Kala-azar por Martínez Niochet y Pons en un paciente proveniente de Las Mercedes, Edo. Guárico.

1941.— Se emplea la intradermorreacción a la leishmanina como método de diagnóstico por Mayer i Pifano.

1941.— Se utiliza la reacción Fairley para el diagnóstico de la bilharziosis por Mayer y Pifano.

1941.— Se comprueban casos de mielitis por S. mansoni con el hallazgo de huevos en cortes de la médula por Espin.

1942.— Se describe el primer caso humano de coccidiosis por Isospora hominis por Briceño Rossi.

1943.— Se describe un nuevo método de investigación de huevos de bilharzia por transparencia por Ottolina y Atencio.

1943.— Se describe la Histoplasmosis por Briceño Maaz.

1945.— Se utiliza por primera vez en Venezuela el D.D.T. el 2 de diciembre en la población de Morón, Estado Carabobo.

1946.— Se describe el primer caso de Favus aviarius por Montemayor.

1947.— Se describe una nueva especie de hongos para el mundo Madurella grisea por Mackinson, Montemayor y Herrera Ursúa.

1947.— Se aisla por primera vez por cultivo de sangre humana el Tripanosoma rangeli por Pifano, Mayer, Benaím y Medina.

1947.— Se describe el primer caso de Rhinosporidiosis nasal por Potenza y Célis Pérez.

1947.— Se señala el segundo caso en Venezuela de Hymenolepis diminuta por Rísquez y Ortíz.

1948.— Se señala parasitismo humano por Dypilidium caninum por Vogelsang y Gallo.

1949.— Se describe la coccidiomicosis por Campins, Schariff y Gluck.

1949.— Se señala a una región de Venezuela como nuevo foco en el mundo de Oncocercosis humana por Potenza, Febres Cordero y Anduze. Dto. Montes (Edo. Sucre), Dtos. Cordero y Andueza. Dto. Montes (Edo. Sucre), Dtos. Acosta, Caripe y Piar (Edo. Monagas).

1949.— Se describe el primer caso por Mansonella ozardi por Briceño Rossi.

1949.— Se encuentra el Cryptococus neoformans en el sistema nervioso central por Potenza y Benaím.

1950.— Se comprueba la Toxoplasmosis y se describen tres casos congénitos por Gavaller.
1950.— Se comprueba la sensibilidad cutánea a la Histoplasmina por Campins y Shariff.
1951.— Se diagnostica en Caracas el primer caso de Onchocerca volvulus por Guerrero.
1951.— Primer caso agudo de Tripanosomosis rangeli, por Torrealba.
1951.— Se encuentran por primera vez, formas evolutivas de microfilarias en el tórax de culicoides (C. pifanoi Ortíz 1951), por A. Mirsa, M. Mirsa y Ortíz.
1951.— Se describe la Torulopsis por Rodríguez, Potenza, Feo.
1951.— Se emplea en el diagnóstico de la bilharziosis la prueba de la inmovilización de Mining-Voggel.
1951.— Se describe un caso de actinomicosis abdominal primitiva por Velutini.
1951.— Primera comunicación sobre paradentosis paracoccidioidica por Barros.
1951.— Paracoccidiosis esplénica primitiva por Díaz.
1952.— Se estudia la Wuchereria brancrofti por Briceño Rossi.
1953.— Se presenta el primer caso de tiña causado por M. ardouini por Velutini.
1953.— Señalada la Paracoccidiosis infantil por Potenza y Feo.
1954.— Se señala una nueva zona de onchocercosis en una región del Edo. Aragua por Arends, Rondón y González Mijares.
1954.— Se encuentran microfilarias de Dipetalonema perstans en la sangre periférica de los indios uiniquinas del Delta del Orinoco por Díaz Ungría.
1954.— Se señala el Trypanosoma rangeli como causante de una tripanosomiasis neotropical por Pifano.
1954.— Se describen las reacciones cutáneas en enfermos de pinta, buba o sífilis por inoculación del T. pertenue, y su aplicación al diagnóstico de curación de estas enfermedades por Medina.
1954.— Se encuentra la histoplasmosis pulmonar por Campins.
1955.— Se comprueba la enfermedad de Gilchrist en Venezuela por Montemayor y se describe el primer caso clínico por Brass, Pelo y Montemayor.
1955.— Se describe el tercer caso en el mundo por Chladosporium trichoides por Barnola.
1955.— Se señala un caso de histoplasmosis cutánea de la boca en sujeto vivo por Velutini.
1955.— Se separa la Parasitología de la Bacteriología en las Cátedras Universitarias (Facultad de Medicina).
1955.— Se señala nuevo foco filariano entre indios Uiniquinas y Guaraúnos causado Mansonella ozardi, por Hernández Pieretti.
1955.— Se señala entre los indios Uiniquinas y Guaraúnos los primeros

casos de Acanthocheilonemiasis encontrados en Venezuela.

Esta época de la Parasitología Venezolana podemos resumirla así:

1.—Creacíon de Laboratorios en las Oficinas Sanitarias.

2.—Preparación de Personal para Laboratorios.

3.—Fundación de la Escuela Malariológica Venezolana, cuyo rendimiento sanitario, económico y científico es de todos conocido.

4.—Estudios profundos llevados a cabo sobre nuestras endemias, especialmente Bilharziosis, Tripanosomiasis, Leishmaniasis, etc., en sus aspectos: parasitológico, clínico, histopatológico, sus transmisores y hospederos, su tratamiento.

5.-Descripción de nuemerosas especies nuevas para el País, algunas para el mundo, en las diversas ramas de la Parasitología. Desde 1926 hasta la fecha han sido descritas:

Setenta y siete especies de Protozoarios	77
Setenta y tres de Trematodes	73
Trece de Cestodes	13
Setenta y nueve de Nematodes	79
Cuatro de Acantocéfalos	4
Veinte de Hongos	20
	226

En los Artrópodos se han descrito muchas especies nuevas y varias para el mundo, pero no hemos tenido tiempo para su completa revisión. El interesado en estos asuntos puede consultar la nómina aparecida en el Boletín de Entomología Venezolana.

6.—Nacimiento de la Micología científica, con auge creciente en estos últimos tiempos y con resultados científicos positivos.

7.—Separacíon de la Parasitología de la Bacteriología en las Cátedras Universitarias de Venezuela, a la cual se la mantenía tradicionalmente unida. Esto, sin duda, dará mayor auge al desarrollo de la Parasitología Médica en nuestro medio.

8.—El descubrimiento de nuevas especies parasitológicas, crea consecuencialmente nuevas entidades clínicas, sobre las cuales debe estar alerta el médico, para utilizar los métodos adecuados a cada caso.

Queremos agradecer muy sinceramente el honor que se nos confirió al habernos escogido para la elaboración del relato sobre la Parasitología en Venezuela desde 1926. Dentro del tiempo y las dificultades del medio, hemos tratado de llenar nuestro cometido con nuestra mejor voluntad y esfuerzo; sabemos que no está completo, que seguramente faltaron muchos hechos notables que no hemos relatado y muchas fichas bibliográficas ignoradas, por lo cual pedimos la indulgencia de nuestros auditores. Está abierto el camino, para que, como es nuestro deseo, algún colega interesado llene los vacíos, y sea en el futuro una obra de ayuda a los estudiosos sobre la materia.

Nuestro sincero agradecimiento para el Dr. Carlos Díaz Ungría, quien en gesto caballeroso y desprendido, nos cedió parte de su trabajo inédito, permitiéndonos la consulta libre y amplia de sus ficheros; a nuestras secretarias Srta. Franci Billi Ghio, Angela Galea y Angela Ruiz Gómez, por la copia paciente de los manuscritos.

Señores Congresantes:

Para terminar este rápido recuento sobre la Parasitología Venezolana actual, permitidnos una vez, que hagamos un apostolado de las palabras que nuestro maestro Jesús Rafael Rísquez pronunció en la lección inaugural del Curso de 1919: "Mañana cuando lejos de estas aulas, oigáis el nombre de la Patria señalada justicieramente entre las demás Naciones que han vibrado en el concierto mundial, recordad que esos hechos, son una de los mejores oraciones que pueden llegar hasta los manes de José Gregorio Hernández y Rafael Rangel. Dos hombres que por capricho del destino me toca enlazar hoy con arco de inmortalidad, y que la historia contemporánea señalará como las dos columnas que han de sostener el edificio de la Bacteriología y la Parasitología nacionales".....

Nada más estimulante y vigorizante hemos encontrado que esas palabras de nuestro Profesor para llevarlas a la consideración de las presentes y futuras generaciones médicas venezolanas, responsables de la conservación de ese edificio, el cual debemos custodiar y guardar celosamente, legándolo a nuestros sucesores, intacto, aumentado, y decorado con nuestra producción científica, en una secuela ininterrumpida en el tiempo y en el espacio: LA ESCUELA PARASITOLOGICA VENEZOLANA.

BIBLIOGRAFIA

1.— *Archila, Ricardo Dr.:* Bibliografía Médica Venezolana. Publicaciones de la Fundación Biogen. Número 4 1946.—Caracas.

2.— *Berti, Dr. Arturo Luis:* Almanaque de la Lucha Antimalárica en Venezuela.—M.S.A.S. Septiembre.—Diciembre 1951.—Volumen XVI N° 5 y 6.

3.— *Díaz Ungría, Dr. Carlos:* La Parasitología en Venezuela.—Comunicación personal inédita.

4.— *Carbonell, Dr. Diego:* La Parasitología en Venezuela y los Trabajos del Dr. M. Núñez Tovar.—Caracas, 1938.

5.— *Carvallo, Dr. Temistocles:* Sinopsis de la Obra científica del Dr. José Gregorio Hernández.

6.— *Risquez, Dr. Jesus Rafael:* Folletos sobre sus Bòdas de Oro Profesionales.—Tipografía Americana, Caracas, 1936.

7.— *Vergani, Dr. Franco y Díaz Ungría, Dr. Carlos:* Boletìn del Instituto- de Investigaciones Veterinarias Vol. V.—April de 1953.—N° 21.

Revistas: Gaceta Médica de Caracas (G.M. de C.).
Revista del Ministerio de Sanidad y Asistencia Social (M.S.A.S.).
Revista de Gastro-Enterología y Nutrición (G.E.N.).
Revista de Medicina Veterinaria y Parasitología (R.M.V. y P.).
Revista Policlínica Caracas (R.P.C.).
Archivos Venezolanos de Patología Tropical y Parasitología Médica (A.V. de P.T. y P.M.).
Archivos Venezolanos de Puericultura y Pediatría (A.V. de P.P.).
Cuadernos Amarillos (Conferencia Panamericana de Caracas 1946).

* * *

ESPECIES DE PROTOZOARIOS SEÑALADAS EN VENEZUELA

HASTA 1930: GABALDON

Babesia bigemina
Balantidium coli
Bodo edax
Carchesium sp. del agua dulce
Chilomastix cuniculi
Chilomastix intestinalis
Chilomastix mesnili
Chilomastix sp. de Bufo marinus
Chilomonas sp. del agua dulce
Copromonas subtilis
Craigia hominis
Crithidia liturae
Crithidia nalipi
Crithidia sp. de Apiomerus elatus
Crithia sp. de Hammatocerus cinctipes
Crithidia sp. de Pselliopus zebra
Crithidia sp. de Zelus janus
Eimeria nieschulzi
Eimeria perforans
Eimeria stidae
Endaboeba blattae
Endolimax nana
Embadomonas intestinalis
Entamoeba cobayae
Entamoeba cuniculi
Entamoeba gingivalis
Entamoeba histolytica
Entamoeba muris
Enteromonas hominis
Enteromonas intestinalis
Euglena sp. del agua dulce
Eutrichomastix sp. (¿lacertae?)
Giardia caviae
Giardia duodenalis
Giardia intestinalis
Giardia muris
Haemogregarina sp. de Crotalus terrificus
Haemogregarina sp. de Tropidorus torquatus

1930-1955: GUTIERREZ ALFARO, IRIARTE, DIAZ UNGRIA

Anaplasma marginale (45)
Babesia argentina (3)
Babesia bovis (2)
Babesia caballi (4)
Babesis caballi (4)
Babesia canis (4)
Bartonella canis (5)
Bartonella baciliformis (6)
Bodo edax Klebs (1)
Chilomastix bittencourti da Fonseca (1)
Chilomastix cuniculi da Fonseca (1)
Chilomastix intestinalis Ruczynski (1)
Chilomastix sp. (1)
Copromonas subtilis Debell (1)
Castia necatrix Henneguy (8)
Eimeria avium (4)
Eimeria debliecki (9)
Eimeria faurei (4)
Eimeria nieschulzi Dieben (1)
Eimeria perforans (1)
Eimeria travassosi (48)
Eimeria zürni (4)
Endolimax nana Wenyon & O'Connor (1)
Entamoeba cuniculi Brug (1)
Entamoeba muris (1)
Enteromonas intestinalis da Fonseca (1)
Epherytrozoon coccoides Schilling (10)
Epherythrozoon sp. (2)
Eutrochomastix batrachorum (1)
Eutrichomastix sp.
Giardia canis (4)
Giardia caviae Hegner (1)
Giardia duodenalis (1)
Giardia muris (1)
Globidium besnoiti (11)

Haemoproteus columbae
Haemoproteus danilewsky
Haemoproteus sp. de Cardinalis phoeniceus
Helkesimastix faecicola
Herpetomonas muscarum
Herpetomonas sp. de Hiranetis braconiformis
Herpetomas sp. (¿Luciliae?) de Lucilia sp.
Herpetomonas sp. (sarcophagae?) de Sarcophaga sp.
Iodamoeba butschlii
Leishmania brasiliense
Leptomonas culicis
Leptomonas foveati
Leptomonas sp. de Amblyomma sp.
Leptomonas sp. de Zeulus janus
Leptomonas blattarum
Noctiluca miliaris
Nyctotherus cordiforme
Nyctotherus ovalis
Nyctotherus sp. de Hyla (Hylelia)
Oikomonas sp. de cultivos de heces del hombre
Opalina ranarum
Phytomonas davidi
Plasmodium falciparum
Plasmodium gonzalezi
Plasmodium malariae
Plasmodium praecox
Plasmodium rangeli
Plasmodium vivax
Plasmodium sp. de Anopheles (Nyssorhynchus albimanus)
Protoopalina intestinalis
Protoopalina sp. de Hyla (Hylella) sp.
Schizotrypanum cruzi
Telohania sp. de Culex pipiens
Tricercomonas intestinalis
Trichomonas (Pentatrichomonas) ardindelteili
Trichomonas (Tritrichomonas) batrachorum

Grahamania sp. (2)
Grahamella muris Carini (38)
Gregarina ctenocephalus canis (17)
Haemogregarina sp. (1)
Haemoproteus columbae & Sanfelice (1)
Helkesimastix faeciola Woodcock & Lepage
Herpetomonas floresi Scorza & Dagert
Histomonas meleagrides (4)
Iodamoeba bütschlü (1)
Isospora bigemina (4)
Isospora felis (4)
Isospora hominis (37)
Leishmanis donovani (31)
Leptomonas culicis (1)
Leptospira canicola (35)
Nuttalia equi (4)
Nyctotherus sp. (1)
Oikomonas sp. (1)
Opalina renarum (1)
Phytomonas davidi (1)
Plasmodium sp. (1)
Protoopalina intestinalis (1)
Protoopalina sp. (1)
Sarcocystis blanchardi (48)
Sarcocystis iturbei (4)
Sarcocystis miescheriana (4)
Schizotrypanum sp. (24)
Spirochaeta gallinarum (22)
Treponema anserinum (4)
Tricercomonas intestinalis Wenyon & O'Connor (1)
Trichomonas (Pentatrichomonas) (1)
Trichomonas (Tritrichomonas) (1)
Trichomonas (Tritrichomonas) caviae (1)
Trichomonas (Tritrichomonas) elongata (1)
Trichomonas fetus (4)
Trichomonas (Trichomonas) macacovaginae (Hegner & Ratcliffe) (1)

CONCLUSION (*)

1955.— Se dicta un curso de Zimología Médica en el I.N.H. por gestiones de Gutiérrez Alfaro y Montemayor y patrocinio del M.S.A.S. Se obtiene el ofrecimiento de la UNESCO y del Instituto de Higiene de Montevideo por medio de su representante Dr. Ricardo Artagaveytía Allende para la fundación en Caracas de una Micoteca con las cepas de la Sección de Micología del I.N.H. de Montevideo. Se presenta un proyecto al Despacho de Sanidad por Gutiérrez Alfaro y Montemayor.

1955.— Campins y Col, describen una epidemia de Histoplasmosis en una región del Estado Lara y sugieren la investigación en zonas similares del País.

CAPITULO II

Este capítulo nos ha sido cedido gentilmente por el Dr. Carlos Díaz Ungría, de su obra inédita "La Parasitología en Venezuela".

PARTE I
PROTOZOOS

PARTE II
TREMATODES

PARTE III
CESTODES

PARTE IV
NEMATODES

PARTE V
ACANTOCEFALOS

* * *

(*) Reprinted from the "Boletín del Laboratorio de la Clínica Luis Razetti". Año XVII - Julio 1957 - Nos. 47-49.

PARTE I
PROTOZOOS

Anaplasma marginale (Ziemann, 1905).
A.J. FERNANDEZ, 1931. Sangre Bos taurus (45).
Babesia argentina (Ligniéres, 1903).
E.G. VOGELSANG y col., 1939, en sangre y cerebro de Bos taurus (3).
Babesia bovis (Babes 1888).
PIERO GALLO Y E.G. VOGELSANG, 1940, en sangre de Bos taurus (2).
Babesia caballi (Guglielmi, 1895).
E.G. VOGELSANG Y PIERO GALLO, 1951, en sangre de Equus caballus (4).
Babesia canis (Pianna y Galli Valerio, 1895).
E.G. VOGELSANG Y PIERO GALLO, 1950, en sangre de Canis familiaris (4).
Bartonella canis (Kikuth, 1982).
E.G. VOGELSANG Y JOSE ESPIN, 1949, en sangre de Canis familiaris (5).
Bartonella baciliformis (Mayer, 1921).
E.G. VOGELSANG Y L. POTENZA, en sangre de Rattus norvegicus, 1945 (6).
Bodo edax Klebs, 1892.
A. GABALDON, en heces humanas, 1930 (1).
Chilomastix bittencourti da Fonseca, 1915.
A. GABALDON, en ciego de Rattus norvegicus, 1930 (1).
Chilomastix cuniculi da Fonseca, 1915.
A. GABALDON, en ciego de oryctolagus, 1930 (1).
Chilomastix intestinalis Kuczynski, 1941.
A. GABALDON, en ciego de Cavia porcellus, 1930 (1).
Chilomastix sp.
A. GABALDON, en intestino Bufo marinus, probablemente es Chilomastix caulleryi (Alexeieft, 1909), 1930 (1).
Copromonas subtilis Dobell, 1908.
A. GABALDON, en heces humanas, 1930 (1).
Costia necatrix Henneguy.
E.G. VOGELSANG, en Plecostomus, 1937 (8).
Eimeria avium (Rivolta y Silvestrini 1873).
E.G. VOGELSANG Y P. GALLO, en intestino de Gallus gallus y Meleagris gallopavo, 1951 (4).
Eimeria debliecki, Douwes 1921.
NOVISZKY, en intestino de Sus scrofa, 1945 (9).
Eimeria faurei (Moussu y Marotel, 1901).
E.G. VOGELSANG Y PIERO GALLO, en intestino de Capra hircur, 1950 (4).
Eimeria nieschulzi Dieben 1942.
A. GABALDON, intestino Rattus norvegicus, 1930 (1).
Eimeria perforans (Leuckart. 1872).
A. GABALDON, intestino Oryctolagus cuniculus, 1930 (1).
Eimeria travassosi (Reichenow y Carini, 1937).
E.G. VOGELSANG Y C. RODRIGUEZ C., 1952, en intestino de oso melero (Tamadua tetradactyla) (48).
Eimera zürni (Rivolta, 1878).
E.G. VOGELSANG Y P. GALLO, intestino Bos taurus, 1950 (4).
Endolimax nana Wenyon & O'Connor, 1917.
A. GABALDON, intestino humano, 1930 (1).
Entamoeba covayae Walker, 1908.
A. GABALDON, ciego Cavia porcellus, 1930 (1).
Entamoeba cuniculi Brug. 1918.

A. GABALDON, intestino Oryctolagus cuniculus, 1930 (1).

Entamoeba muris (Grassi, 1879).

A. GABALDON, ciego Rattus norvegicus, 1930 (1).

Enteromonas intestinalis da Fonseca, 1918.

A. GABALDON, ciego Oryctolagus cuniculus, 1930 (1).

Epherytrozoon coccoides Schilling, 1928.

ORTIZ, en sangre Rattus norvegicus, 1940 (10).

Epherythrozoon sp.

P. GALLO Y E.G. VOGELSANG, sangre Bos taurus, 1940 (2).

Eutrochomastix batrachorum (Dobell, 1909).

A. GABALDON, intestino renacuajo, 1930 (1).

Eutrichomastix sp.

A. GABALDON, intestino "mato real", 1930 (1). Quizás se trate de Eutrichomastix lacertae (Bütsichli, 1884).

Giardia canis (Heguer, 1922).

A. GABALDON, intestino Cavia porcellus, 1930 (1).

Giardia caviae (Hegner, 1923).

E.G. VOGELSANG Y PIERO GALLO, intestino del canis familiaris, 1950 (4).

Giardia duodenalis (Davanis, 1875).

A. GABALDON, intestino Oryctolagus cuniculus, 1930 (1).

Giardia muris (Grassi, 1879).

A. GABALDON, intestino Rattus norvegicus, 1930 (1).

Globidium besnoiti (Marotal, 1912).

E.G. VOGELSANG Y PIERO GALLO, intestino Bos taurus, 1914 (11).

Grahamia sp.

P. GALLO Y E. VOGELSANG, en Bos taurus, 1940 (2).

Grahamella muris Carini 1915.

M. MAYER e I. ORTIZ, en Rattus norvegicus, 1914 (38).

Gregarina ctenocephalus canis.

MARIE MIRSA, estómago Ctenocephalides sp., 1950 (17).

Haemogregarina sp.

A. GABALDON, sangre y órganos Crotalus terrificus, 1930 (1).

Haemoproteus columbae (Sanfelice, 1891).

A. GABALDON, sangre Columba livia doméstica, 1930 (1).

Helkesimastix fasciola Woodcok & Lepage, 1915.

A. GABALDON, heces humanas, 1930 (1).

Herpetomonas floresi Scorza & Dagert, 1954.

SCORZA Y DAGERT, digestivo de Conicera sp. (Díptera), 1954 (18).

Histomonas meleagridis (Theobald Smith, 1895).

E.G. VOGELSANG Y P. GALLO en el Meleagris gallopavo, 1951 (4).

Iodamoeba bütschlii (Prowasek, 1952).

A. GABALDON, intestino humano, 1929 (1).

Isospora bigemina (Stiles, 1891).

E.G. VOGELSANG Y P. GALLO, en intestino Canis familiaris, 1951 (4).

Isospora felis (Wenyon, 1923).

E.G. VOGELSANG Y P. GALLO, en Canis familiaris y Felis catus, 1951 (4).

Isospora hominis.

A.L. BRICEÑO ROSSI, intestino humano, 1945 (37).

Leishmania donovani.

PONS Y MARTINEZ, casos humanos, 1941 (31).

Leptomonas culicis (Patton, 1912).

A. GABALDON, intestino Culex quinquefasciatus (fatigans), 1928 (1).

Leptospira canicola.

C. GOLDMAN Y J. ESPIN, en Canis familiaris, 1951 (35).

Nuttalia equi (Laveran, 1901).
E.G. VOGELSANG Y P. GALLO, en sangre de Equus caballus, 1951 (4).
Nyctotherus cordiforme (Ehrenberg, 1838).
A. GABALDON, intestino renacuajos, 1930 (1).
Nyctotherus sp.
A. GABALDON, intestino Hyla (Hylella) sp. 1930 (1).
Oikomonas sp.
A. GABALDON, heces humanas, 1930 (1).
Opalina ranarum (Purkinje & Valin 1835).
A. GABALDON, intestino renacuajos, 1930 (1).
Phytomonas davidi (Lafont, 1909).
D.R. IRIARTE, intestino Corizus sidae, 1928 (1).
Plasmodium sp.
HILL, intestino Anopheles (Nyssorhynchus) albimanus, 1928 (1).
Protoopalina intestinalis (Stein, 1956).
A. GABALDON, intestino renacuajo, 1930 (1).
Prottopalina sp.
A. GABALDON, intestino Hyla (Hyella) sp. 1930 (1).
Sarcocystis blanchardi (Doflein).
E.G. VOGELSANG Y C. RODRIGUES C., 1952, en miocardio de Bos taurus (48).
Sarcocystis iturbei, Vogelsang 1938.
E.G. VOGELSANG, en Bos taurus, 1938 (16).
Sarcocystis miescheriana (Kühn, 1865).
E.G. VOGELSANG Y P. GALLO, en sus scrofa, 1951 (4).
Schizotrypanum sp.
E. DIAZ Y F. PIFANO, sangre de Carollia perspillata, 1940 (24).
Spirochaeta gallinarum.
A.L. BRICEÑO ROSSI Y D.R. IRIARTE, en Gallus gallus L., 1942 (22).
Treponema anserinum (Sakharov, 1891).
E.G. VOGELSANG Y P. GALLO, en sangre de Meleagris gallopavo, 1951 (4).
Tricercomonas intestinalis Wenyon & O'Connor 1917.
A. GABALDON, intestino humano, 1929 (1).
Trichomonas (Pentatrichomonas) ardindenteili (Derrieu & Raynaud 1914).
A. GABALDON, intestino humano, 1930 (1).
Trichomonas (Tritrichomonas batrachorum Perty 1852).
A. GABALDON, intestino renacuajos, 1930 (1).
Trichomonas (Tritrichomonas) elongata Steinberg, 1862.
A. GABALDON, boca del hombre, 1930 (1).
Trichomonas fetus (Wenrich & Emmerson 1933).
E.G. VOGELSANG Y P. GALLO, en Bos taurus, 1951 (4).
Trichomonas (Tritrichomonas) macacovaginae Hegner & Ratyliffe 1927).
A. GABALDON, intestino Macacus rhesus, 1930 (1).
Trichomonas (Tritrichomonas) muris (Grassi, 1879).
A. GABALDON, ciego de Rattus norvegicus, 1929 (1).
Trichomonas (Tritrichomonas) ruminantium Braune, 1913.
A. GABALDON, intestino Bos taurus, 1930 (1).
Trichomonas (Tritrichomonas) trichomonas, Wenyon, 1926; en Gabaldón, 1930.
A. GABALDON, intestino humano, 1930 (1).
Trypanosoma equiperdum, Doflein 1901.
RIVAS LARRALDE, en Equus caballus, 1939 (14).
Trypanosoma megalodermal Wenyon 1919.
F. PIFANO Y BUSTAMANTE, sangre de Miotis nigrans (Wied). 1939 (29).
Trypanosoma barnolai n. sp.
Torrealba, J.F., Ricardi, B., Ramos, I., Díaz Vázquez y Torrealba P.A. En Cebus nigrivittatus (300).

PARTE II
TREMATODES

Alaria compacta Lutz, 1928.
A. LUTZ, 1928, en Carbo brasiliensis (52).
Alaria elongata Lutz, 1928.
A. LUTZ, 1928, en pato (Podiceps dominicus L.) (52).
Allassostoma venezuelensis, Cordero & Vogelsang, 1940.
E.H. CORDERO Y E.G. VOGELSANG, estómago Podocnemis sp., 1940 (42).
Apatemon gracilis (Rud., 1819) Szidat, 1928.
E. CABALLERO Y E.G. VOGELSANG, en intestino de Cathartes urubu, 1949 (40).
Athesmia attilae.
A. LUTZ, 1928, en Parra jacana y Nerrion brasiliense (52).
Balarnorchis anastrophus (Fischoeder, 1901).
E.G. VOGELSANG Y C. RODRIGUEZ C., estómago de venado (Odocoileus gymnotis) 1952 (48).
Calatropis appendiculata Lutz 1928.
A. LUTZ, 1928, en pato (Nettion brasiliense) (52).
Chaunocephalus paduriformis (Travassos, 1923).
E.G. VOGELSANG Y C. RODRIGUEZ C., en quistes intestinales en Euxenura maguari, 1952 (48).
Cladorchis heteroxenus, Cordero & Vogelsang, 1940.
E.H. CORDERO Y E.G. VOGELSANG, estómago de Podocnemis sp. 1940 (42).
Clinostomum detruncatum (Braun, 1899),
E.G. VOGELSANG Y C. RODRIGUEZ C., en esófago y boca de la garza común (Casmerodius albus), 1952 (48).
Clinostomum heluans Braun.
A. LUTZ, 1928, en garzas (52).
Clinostomum pusillum Lutz, 1928.
A. LUTZ, 1928, en Podiceps dominicus (52).
Conchogaster ellipticus (Brandes).
A. LUTZ, 1928, en Crotophaga, ani y Piaya cayana (52).
Conchogaster obesus Lutz, 1928.
A. LUTZ, 1928, en Martín pescador (Ceryle sp.) (52).
Cotylophoron cotylophorum (Fischoeder, 1901).
E.G. VOGELSANG, 1940, en panza de Bos taurus (43).
Cyclocoelium brasilianum Stossich.
A. LUTZ, 1928, sacos aéreos de Charadriidas (52).
Cyclocoelium brasiliense.
A. LUTZ, intestino aves acuáticas, 1928 (52).
Cyclocoelium sp.
A. LUTZ, 1928, en Aniscalis mayor (52).
Diplodiscus pygmaeus, Lutz 1928.
A. LUTZ, recto de una Pseudis, 1928 (52).
Distomum repandum Rudolphi.
A. LUTZ, 1928 (52).
Drepanocephalus spathans Dietz.
A. LUTZ, 1928, en cotúa (Phalacrocorax brasiliensis) (52).
Duboisiella proloba Baer, 1938.
E. CABALLERO Y E.G. VOGELSANG, en intestino de Didelphis marsupialis, 1949 (40).
Echinostoma revolutum (Frohlich, 1802) Looss 1899.
E. CABALLERO, E.G. VOGELSANG Y M.C. ZERECERO, en intestino de Didelphis marsupialis, 1953 (49).

Echinostomum alepidotum Dietz.
A. LUTZ, Porphyrio martinica y Gallinula galeata, 1928 (52).
Echinostomum aphylactum Dietz.
A. LUTZ en Porphyrio martinica y Gallinula galeata, 1928 (52).
Echinostomum mendax Dietz.
A. LUTZ, intestino de pato (Nettion brasiliense), 1928 (52).
Echinostomum nephrocystis Lutz.
A. LUTZ, 1928 (52).
Echinostomum parcespinosum Lutz.
A. LUTZ, en varias especies de Aramides, 1928 (52).
Echinostomum parvum Lutz, 1928.
A. LUTZ, en paloma doméstica, 1928 (52).
Echinostomum uncatum Dietz.
A. LUTZ, intestino Crotopraga ani y Piaya cayana, 1928 (52).
Echinostomum sp.
A. LUTZ, en cloaca de gavilán bermejo, 1928 (52).
Eumagacetes perodiosus Travassos.
A. LUTZ, 1928, en Piaya cayana (52).
Fasciola sp.
I. ORTIZ, hígado Rattus norvegicus, 1948 (39).
Glypthelmins palmipedis (Lutz, 1928) Travassos, 1930.
E. CABALLERO, E.G. VOGELSANG Y ZERECERO, M.C., 1953, en intestino delgado de Rana palmipes Spix. (49).
Gorgoderina diaster.
A. LUTZ, 1928, en vejiga urinaria de batracios (52).
Haematoloechus lutzi Freitas y Lent, 1939.
E. CABALLERO. E.G. VOGELSANG Y ZERECERO, M.C., 1953, en pulmones de Rana palmipes Spix. (49).
Haplometra palmipedis Lutz, 1928.
A. LUTZ, 1928, en Rana palmipes (52).
Hippocrepis hippocrepis (Diesing, 1851).
E.G. VOGELSANG Y C. RODRIGUEZ C., intestino grueso de chigüire (Hydrochoerus hydrochoeris), 1952 (48).
Leucochloridium holostomum.
A. LUTZ, 1928, en gallitos de agua (Gallinula sp. y Parra sp.) (52).
Mesorchis conciliatus Dietz.
A. LUTZ, en 1928, en Butorides stristus (52).
Monniliever pitangi Lutz.
A. LUTZ, 1928, en Cristofué (Pitangus sulfureus) (52).
Nematophila ovalis, Cordero & Vogelsang, 1940.
E.H. CORDERO Y E.G. VOGELSANG, estómago de Podocnemis sp., 1940 (42).
Neodiplostomum branchiocystis Lutz, 1928.
A. LUTZ, 1928, en gavilán bermejo (52).
Neodiplostomum nephrocystis Lutz, 1928.
A. LUTZ, 1928, en gavilán bermejo (52).
Ochetosoma miladelarocai, Caballero & Vogelsang, 1947.
E. CABALLERO Y E.G. VOGELSANG, en esófago de Bothrops atrox, 1947 (44).
Opistorchis interruptus Braun.
A. LUTZ, 1928, en garzas (52).
Paramphistomum cervi (Zeder, 1790).
E.G. VOGELSANG, 1935, en panza de bovino (54).
Paramonostomum ionorne.
A. LUTZ, Intestino gallito de agua (Porphyrio martinica) 1928 (52).
Parastrigea cineta (Brandes, 1838) Szidat, 1929.
E. CABALLERO Y E.G. VOGELSANG, en intestino de Jabiru mycteria (Tantalus locu-

latur), Gabán, 1949 (40).

Paryphostomum segregatum Dietz.

A. LUTZ, zamuros (Cathartes aura y C. atrata), 1928 (52).

Petasiger novemdecim Lutz 1928.

A. LUTZ, 1928, en pato (Podiceps dominicus) (52).

Plagiorchis hepaticus.

A. LUTZ, 1928, en Bufo marinus (52).

Pneumonoeces iturbei, Cordero & Vogelsang, 1939.

E.H. CORDERO Y E.G. VOGELSANG, en pulmón de rana palmipes Spix. 1939 (41).

Pneumonoeces neivai.

A. LUTZ, 1928, lo citó como Pn. pseudis. Pasó a sinonimia con Pn. neivai por Travassos & Darriba (53).

Pneumonoeces planorbinus.

A. LUTZ, 1928, en rana (52).

Pneumonoeces tejerae, Cordero & Vogelsang, 1939.

E.H. CORDERO Y E.G. VOGELSANG, en pulmón de rana palmipes Spix. 1939 (41).

Prionosoma serratum Dietz.

A. LUTZ, 1928, en carrao (Aramus scolopaceus) (52).

Prosthogonimus cuneatus Rudolphi.

A. LUTZ, 1928, en Carbo brasiliensis y Rhynchops nigra (52).

Pulchrosoma pulchrosoma Travassos.

A. LUTZ, 1928, en sacos aéreos de Ceryle amazoica (52).

Rhopalias coronata.

A. LUTZ, 1928, en Didelphis nudicaudata (52).

Rhopalias coronatus (Rudolphi, 1819).

E. CABALLERO Y E.G. VOGELSANG, en intestino de Didelphis marsupialis, 1949 (40).

Rhopalias horridus (Diesing, 1850).

E. CABALLARO Y E.G. VOGELSANG, en intestino de Didelphis marsupialis, 1949 (40).

Stichorchis giganteus (Diesing, 1835).

E.G. VOGELSANG, ciego cerdo doméstico, 1935 (54).

Stichorchis giganteus (Fischoeder, 1901).

E.G. VOGELSANG, Y G. RODRIGUEZ C., ciego de váquiro (Tagassu tajacu), 1952 (48).

Strigea ardearum Lutz, 1928.

A. LUTZ, 1928, en garzas (52).

Strigea gallinulae Lutz, 1928.

A. LUTZ, 1928, en gallitos de agua (52).

Strigea ophiocystis Lutz.

A. LUTZ, 1928, duodeno de zamuro y gavilán (52).

Strigea ornithocystis Lutz.

A. LUTZ, 1928, en aves (52).

Strigea sphaerocephala Westrumb.

A. LUTZ, 1928, en patos (Nettion brasiliense) (1952).

Strigea tarda Steenstrup.

A. LUTZ, 1928, en patos (Nettion sp.) (52).

Strigea theriocystis Lutz.

A. LUTZ, 1928, en aves (52).

Tylodelphys elongata (Lutz, 1928) Dubois, 1937.

E. CABALLERO Y E. VOGELSANG, en intestinos de Jabiru mycteria (Tantalus loculatur), 1940 (40).

PARTE III
CESTODES

Anoplocephala magna Abild., 1789.
Citada por GALLO y VOGELSANG, 1951, en intestino de Equus caballus (4).

Cysticercus acostaii Vogelsang, 1935.
Citado por FERNANDEZ y VOGELSANG, 1935, en conejo (Sylvilagus nigronuchalis nigronuchalis) (116).

Cysticercus ernsti, Fernández y Vogelsang, 1935.
Citado por FERNANDEZ y VOGELSANG, 1935, en venado (Odocoileus gymnotis gymnotis) (116).

Dyphyllobothrium decipiens (Diesing, 1850).
Citado por VOGELSANG, 1848, en intestino de Canis familiaris (51).
Citado por VOGELSANG Y RODRIGUEZ, 1952, en intestino de zorro (Cerdocyon thous) (48).
GALLO y VOGELSANG en (4) dicen que el Diphyllobothrium reptans fue hallado en caninos y zorros. Creemos que debe referirse al Sparganum reptans, estado larvario del Diphyllobothrium decipiens.

Raillietina demerariensis. (Daniels, 1895).
HORACE W. STUNKARD, 1953, en Proechinus cayenesis trinitatus (61).

Inermicapsifer cubensis (Kouri, 1939).
ORTIZ, 1945, en intestino humano (56).

Meniezia benedeni (Moniez, 1879).
GALLO y VOGELSANG, 1951, intestino Bos taurus (4).

Sparganum ameivai, Vogelsang y Gallo, 1949.
VOGELSANG Y GALLO, 1949, en Ameiva a. a., cavidad general (67).

Taenia hydatigena (Pallas, 1766).
FERNANDEZ Y VOGELSANG, 1935, Cysticercus tenuicollis en Sus scrofa (116).
VOGELSANG, 1948, Cysticercus tenuicollis, peritoneo venado (Odocoileus sp.) (51).
VOGELSANG Y RODRIGUEZ, 1952, adulto intestino Canis familiaris (48).

Taenia taeniformis (Batsch, 1786).
VOGELSANG Y POTENZA, 1945, Cysticercus fasciolaris en Mus norvegicus (6).
VOGELSANG Y RODRIGUEZ, 1952, adulto en Felis catus (48).
VOGELSANG Y RODRIGUEZ, 1952, larva en Mus (E) rattus (48).

Thysanosoma actinoides (Diesing, 1836).
VOGELSANG Y RODRIGUEZ, 1952, colédoco de Capra hircus (48).

Adición:

Citottaenia pectinata (Goeze).
DIAZ UNGRIA, 1955, intestino de conejo (Sylvilagus margaritae) "Mem. S. C. N. La Salle", 1955.

PARTE IV.
NEMATODES

Agamospirura sp.
VOGELSANG, 1950, larva en nódulos sobre Astyanax essequibensis (97).

Aleurostrongylus abstrusus (Raillet 1898) Cameron 1927.
VOGELSANG y RODRIGUEZ, 1952, Pulmón gato doméstico (Felis dom.) (48).

Ancylostoma caninum Ercolani, 1859.
VOGELSANG, 1939. Canis familiaris (81), Felis catus dom. (81), Gato montés (Felis yaguarandi) (81).

VOGELSANG y RODRIGUEZ, 1952. Cunaguaro (Felis tigrina) (48) y en zorro (Cerdocyon thous thous).

Ancylostoma duodenale.

RANGEL, 1903, en el hombre (7).

Ascaridia lineate (Schneider, 1866).

VOGELSANG y RODRIGUEZ, 1952, intestino faisán (Phasanius colchicus) (48).

Ascaris vitulorum (Goeze, 1782).

VOGELSANG y MAYAUDON, 1952, intestino Bos taurus (10?).

Bunostomum phlebotomum (Railliet, 1900).

VOGELSANG y MAYAUDON, 1952, intestino Bos taurus (102).

Bunostomum trigonocephalum (Rud., 1808).

Gallo y VOGELSANG, 1951, Bos tauros y Capra hircus (4).

Chabertia ovina (Fabr., 1788).

GALLO y VOGELSANG, 1951, Bos taurus y Capra hircus (4).

Chlamydonema praeputiale (Linstow, 1889).

VOGELSANG y RODRIGUEZ, 1952. Estómago cunaguaro (Felis tigrina) (48).

Choerostrongylus pudendotectus (Wostokow, 1905) Skrjabin 1924.

DIAZ UNGRIA, 1951, en bronquios de Sus scofa (109).

Cooperia sp.

GALLO y VOGELSANG, 1951, Bos taurus y Capra hircus (4).

Cruzia tentaculata (Rud., 1819) Travassos 1917.

CABALLERO y VOGELSANG, 1950, ciego de Didelphis marsupialis (96).

Cylicocercus catinatum (Loos, 1900).

DIAZ UNGRIA y VERGANI, 1951. Equus caballus (100).

Cylicocercus pateratum (Yorke y McFie, 1919).

DIAZ UNGRIA y VERGANI, 1951. Equus caballus (100).

Cylicocyclus insigne (Loos, 1900).

DIAZ UNGRIA y VERGANI, 1951. Equus caballus (110).

Cylicocyclus nassatum (Loos, 1900).

DIAZ UNGRIA y VERGANI, 1951. Equus caballus (100).

Cylicodontophorus bicoronatum (Loos, 1900).

DIAZ UNGRIA y VERGANI, 1951. Equus caballus (100).

Dictyocaulus arnfieldi (Cobb. 1884).

VOGELSANG, 1934, mulo y Equus caballus (71).

Dictyocaulus viviparus Bloch, 1792.

VOGELSANG, 1952, pulmón Bos taurus (103).

Dipetalonema gracilis (Rud., 1809).

CABALLERO y VOGELSANG, 1959, cavidad peritoneal de Cebus sp. (96).

VOGELSANG y RODRIGUEZ, 1952, cavidad Cebus nigrivitatus y Lagothrix lagotricha (48).

Dipetalonema perstans.

DIAZ UNGRIA, 1954, microfilarias en sange de indígenas (108).

Dirofilaria inmitis (Leidy, 1856).

VOGELSANG, E.G., 1934, en Canis familiaris y cunaguaro (Felis pardalis), Zorro (Canis thous thous), Felis catus, Felis onca y Lutra brasiliensis (70).

Enterobius minutus (Schneider 1866) Barreto 1918.

VOGELSANG, 1940, en araguato (Ateles seniculus) (48).

Filaria chitipleuritis.

TEJERA, 1926, intestino blátidos (120).

Gnathostoma spinigerum Owen, 1836.

VOGELSANG, 1939, Felis catus (81), Felis pardalis (81).

VOGELSANG y RODRIGUEZ, 1952, estómago cunaguaro (Felis tigrina) (48).

Gongylonema neoplasticum, (Fiebiger & Ditlevsen, 1914).

TEJERA, 1926, intestino blátidos (120).

E. BRUMPT, 1932, en Rattus norvegicus (80).

Gyalocephalus capitatus (Loos, 1900).
DIAZ UNGRIA y VERGANI, 1951. Equus caballus (110).
Habronema microstoma (Schneider, 1866).
VOGELSANG, 1951, Equus caballus (99).
Habronema muscae (Carter, 1861).
VOGELSANG, 1951. Equus caballus (99).
Keterakis spumosa Sneider, 1866.
VOGELSANG y POTENZA, 1945, intestino de Rattus norvegicus (6).
Kalicephalus subulatus (Molin, 1861).
CABALLERO y VOGELSANG, 1950, intestino delgado de Constrictor constrictor (96).
Mansonella ozzardi.
BRICEÑO ROSSI, 1949, en sangre de indigenas, microfilarias (107).
Metastrongylus apri (Gmelin, 1790).
VOGELSANG, 1939, bronquios de Sus scofa (81).
Neoascaris vitulorum (Goeze, 1786) Travassos, 1927.
VOGELSANG, 1948, en Bos taurus (51).
Oesophagostomum columbianum (Curtice, 1890).
VOGELSANG, 1939, intestino Bos taurus (81).
VOGELSANG y RODRIGUEZ, 1952, intestino nódulos Capra hircus (48).
Oesophagostomum radiatum (Rud., 1803).
VOGELSANG, 1939, colon Sus scofa (81).
Oesopragostomum radiatum (Rud., 1803).
VOGELSANG, 1948, en Bos taurus (51).
Onchocerca bovis (Piettre, 1912).
VOGELSANG, 1940, lig. cerv. Bos taurus (43).
Onchocerca linealis (Stiles, 1892).
VOGELSANG, 1948, en Bos taurus (51).
Onchocerca volvulus (Leuckart, 1893) Railliet y Henry, 1920.
POTENZA, FEBRES CORDERO y ANDUZE, 1948, en el hombre (93).
Ostertagia sp.
GALLO y VOGELSANG, 1951, Bos taurus y Capra hircus (4).
Oxyuris equi (Schrank, 1788).
VOGELSANG, 1951. Equus caballus (99).
Oxyuris gracilis Leyd.
TEJERA, 1926, intestino blátidos (120).
Oxyuris macrura.
TEJERA, 1926, intestino blátidos (120).
Ozolaimus cirratus Linstow, 1906.
LENT y FREITAS, 1948, estómago Iguana tuberculata (119).
Ozolaimus megatyphlon (Rudolphi, 1819).
LENT y FREITAS, 1948, estómago Iguana tuberculata (119).
Physaloptera praeputialis (Linstow, 1889).
VOGELSANG, 1939, Felis catus (81).
Physaloptera retusa Rudolphi, 1819.
CABALLERO y VOGELSANG, 1947, en estómago de Cnemidophorus lemniscatus lemniscatus (44).
Physocephalus sexalatus (Molin, 1860).
VOGELSANG, 1939, Sus scrofa (81).
Protospirura bonnei.
BRUMPT, E., 1931 (76) Rattus norvegicus.
Protospirura muris (Gmelis, 1790).
VOGELSANG y POTENZA, 1945, en estómago Rattus norvegicus (6).
Pseudoaleuris caudatus Lent y Freitas, 1948.
LENT y FREITAS, 1948, intestino grueso de Iguana tuberculata (119).
Pseudoaleuris vogelsangi Lent y Freitas, 1948.

LENT y FREITAS, 1948, estómago de Iguana tuberculata (119).

Setaria equina (Abild, 1856).

VOGELSANG, 1934, Equus caballus, asno, hombre y en serosas y ojo de Bos taurus (70).

Setaria labiato-papillosa (Aless. 1838).

VOGELSANG, 1934, en Bos taurus (70).

Spirocerca lupi (Rud., 1809).

VOGELSANG, 1940, estómago Canis familiaris (63).

Spirocerca sanguinolenta (Rud., 1819).

VOGELSANG, 1948, en Canis familiaris (51).

VOGELSANG y RODRIGUEZ, 1952, zorro (Cerdocyon thous thous) (48).

Spiroptera obtusa.

TEJERA, 1926, intestino blátidos (120).

Stephanurus dentatus Diesing, 1839.

VOGELSANG, 1934, pulmón Sus. scrofa (71).

Otros autores lo han señalado en: hígado y tejido adiposo de Sus Scrofa, 1951 (4).

Tejido adiposo de Bos taurus 1951 (4).

VOGELSANG y RODRIGUEZ, 1952. Adiposo perirrenal váquiro (Tagassu tajacu) (48).

Strongyloides venezuelensis.

ORTIZ, 1948, en Rattus norvegicus (39).

Strongylus edentatus (Loos, 1900).

VOGELSANG, 1951. Equus caballus (99).

Strongylus (Delafondia) vulgaris (Loos, 1900).

DIAZ UNGRIA y VERGANI, 1951, Equus caballus (100).

Strongylus (Strongylus) equinus (Miller, 1780).

DIAZ UNGRIA y VERGANI, 1951. Equus caballus (100).

Syngamus laryngeus (Railliet, 1899).

VOGELSANG, 1934, en Bos taurus (71).

CABALLERO y VOGELSANG, 1950, traquea y bronquios de Panthera onca (96).

Syngamus trachea (Montagu, 1811).

VOGELSANG, 1948, en Gallus gallus (51).

Toxocara canis (Werner, 1872) Stiles 1905.

VOGELSANG 1948, en Canis familiaris (51).

VOGELSANG y RODRIGUEZ, 1952, en intestino zorro (Cerdocyon thous thous) (48).

Trichonema calicatum (Loos, 1900).

DIAZ UNGRIA y VERGANI, 1951. Equus caballus (100).

Trichonema coronatum (Loos, 1900).

VOGELSANG, 1951. Equus caballus (99).

Trichonema laboratum, (Loos, 1900).

VOGELSANG, 1951. Equus caballus (99).

Trichonema longibursatum (Yorke y McFie, 1918).

DIAZ UNGRIA y VERGANI, 1951. Equus caballus (100).

Trichonema poculatum (Loos, 1900).

VOGELSANG, 1951. Equus caballus (99).

Trichonema radiatum (Loos, 1900).

VOGELSANG, 1951. Equus caballus (99).

Trichosomoides crassicauda (Bellingham, 1840).

VOGELSANG y RODRIGUEZ, 1952. Vejiga urinaria rata gris (Mus (E) rattus) (48).

Trichuris oxis (Schrank, 1788).

VOGELSANG y MAYAUDON, 1952, intestino Bos taurus (102).

Trichuris vulpis (Froelich, 1789).

VOGELSANG, 1940, ciego Canis familiaris (63).

Triodontophorus brevicauda, (Boulenger 1916).

DIAZ UNGRIA y VERGANI, 1952. Equus caballus (101).

Triodontophorus minor (Loos, 1900).

DIAZ UNGRIA y VERGANI, 1951. Equus caballus (100).

Triodontophorus serratus (Loos, 1900).

DIAZ UNGRIA y VERGANI, 1951. Equus caballus (100).

Triodontophorus tenuicollis (Boulenger, 1916).

DIAZ UNGRIA y VERGANI, 1951. Equus caballus (100).

PARTE V.

ACANTOCEFALOS

Centrorhynchus tumidulus (Rud., 1819).

VOGELSANG, 1939, garrapatero (Crotophaga ani L.) (81).

Hammanniella microcephala (Rud. 1819).

VOGELSANG, 1939, rabipelado (Didelphis sp.) (81).

Macracanthorhynchus hirudinaceus (Pallas, 1781), Trav., 1916.

VOGELSANG, 1948, en Sus scofa (51).

Oncicola (v. Ihering, 1892).

VOGELSANG, 1939, intestino Felis onca (león americano) (81).

TESIS SOBRE PARASITOLOGIA PRESENTADAS ANTE LA UNIVERSIDAD CENTRAL PARA OPTAR EL TITULO DE DOCTOR EN CIENCIAS MEDICAS, 1945-1955

1945

Orozco, Jiménez, Jesús María: "Parasitosis intestinal en Los Teques".

Pantoja, José Vicente: "Goma sifilítica en el material de autopsia del Hospital Vargas".

Rodríguez, Antonio María: "Estudio comparativo sobre microreacciones (Prueba rural Briceño Rossi, micro-Kahn en lámina, Lieboff y Chediak) en el diagnóstico de sífilis, lepra, buba y TBC".

Rodríguez, Luis Augusto: "Estudio comparativo de la quinina y la quinacrina en la malaria en Venezuela".

Seijas Rivas, Juan Vicente: "Contribución al estudio de la enfermedad de Chagas en el Estado Carabobo (Premiada).

Trujillo, José Manuel: "Flóculo-reacción de Hinton. La comparacíon con la standard de Kahn en más de 600 exámenes de sangre. Su estudio en sífilis, buba, carate, lepra, TBC., cáncer y embarazo. La comparación con la prueba rural Briceño Rossi".

Urdaneta Giacopini, Oswaldo: "Sífilis Pulmonar".

1947

Acevedo Gallegos, Feliciano: "El clorhidrato de emetina en el tratamiento de la schistosomiasis mansoni".

Alliendes M., Juvenal: "Contribución en el estudio de la leishmaniosis tegumentaria".

Acosta Quintero, José León Nelson: "Sífilis y parálisis general".

Cisneros Pérez, Arnaldo: "Contribución al estudio epidemiológico de la schistosomiasis mansoni en Los Teques y sus alrededores".

Cortés Bastidas, Rafael: "Estudio comparativo de los métodos de concentración en diagnósticos coprológicos de la schistosomiasis mansoni".

Dávila, Hugo Trinidad: "Demostración del poder treponemicida de la penicilina en diversas formas de sífilis estudiadas cuidadosamente".

Domínguez C., Henrique: "Leishmania brasilensis Viana 1911. Contribución al estudio de su desarrollo in vitro".

Gathman Hans, J.: "Métodos de concentración de huevos de parásitos en las heces".

Jatens Reyes, José: "Líquido céfalo-raquídeo y sífilis cerebro-espinal antigua".

Ortega de Bustos, María: "Perturbación del líquido céfalo-raquídeo del enfermo de sífilis cardio-vascular".

Pérez R. Miguel Angel: "La escabiosis. Consideraciones generales sobre su tratamiento con benzoato de bencilo".

Zarrameda, Atilio: "Algunas consideraciones sobre la parasitosis intestinal en el Servicio de Gastroenterología del S.S.O."

1948

Carbonell, Luis Manuel: "Investigación de nidos leishmánicos en corazones con miocarditis y xeno-diagnósticos positivos. Descripción de las lesiones anátomopatológicas encontradas".

C. Manuel: "Contribución al estudio de los aspectos cardio-vasculares de la bilharziosis mansoni. Nota previa basada en el estudio de 40 casos (Premiada).

Drayer Brito, Alberto: "Consideraciones sobre la etiología chagásica de algunas miocarditis del Hospital Vargas". (Premiada).

Morales Mora, Luis: "Las Reacciones serológicas cuantitativas en el diagnóstico y pronóstico de la sífilis".

Moreno Orosco, Duilio: "Contribución al estudio de la sífilis adquirida en el medio familiar".

Sánchez Gutiérrez, Alejandro: "Contribución al estudio de la sífilis cardio-vascular en Venezuela".

1949

Benaim Pinto, Carlos: "La insuficiencia hepática, concepto y exploración. Contribución al estudio de la insuficiencia hepática en la bilharziosis mansoni en el hombre" (Premiada).

Moreno Fernández, José: "Tratamiento intensivo de la schistosomiasis mansoni con el emético de sodio".

1950

Rubiño, Josefa María: "Tratamiento de la embarazada sifilítica con penicilina".

1953

Estanga Irigoyen, Ramón: "El parasitismo intestinal en los enfermos del Hospital Vargas".

CAPITULO V.

Para la elaboración de este capítulo nos ha sido de inestimable valor el libro del Dr. Ricardo Archila, "Bibliografía Médica Venezolana", publicada en 1946. Hemos tratado de completar en lo posible lo aparecido en él, agregando lo que hemos podido reunir desde esa fecha hasta el presente. Este trabajo no es completo, lo sabemos, debido a lo difícil que es en nuestro medio realizar una labor de esta naturaleza, la cual, terminada, ha aparecido la segunda edición del libro del Dr. Archila que no hemos podido revisar; los interesados pueden consultarla, con la seguridad que obtendrán magníficas informaciones bibliográficas.

ACOSTA MARTINEZ, Antonio

1942— Algunas observaciones de polineuritis ankilostomiásicas. Rev. San. Mil. I, 3, 222-227 (1).

ACOSTA POLEO, Angel

1930— Anquilostomiasis. Memoria de la I Conferencia Sanitaria Nacional. Págs. 311-313 (2).

1913— El Paludismo en Cristóbal Colón. Memoria de la II Conf. Sanit. Nacional. Págs. 306-311 (3).

1934— La desaparición del paludismo en Cristóbal Colón. Bol. del Minist. de Salub. y de Agric. y Cría. Caracas, II. 12-13, 1012-1015 (4).

ACOSTA SIVA, Manuel

1948— Uncinariosis. Nuevas adquisiciones de Patología y Patogenía. Rev. de la Asoc. Mexicana de Gastro-Enterología, III, N° 13, enero y febrero (5)

1938a— Tratamiento específico de las parasitosis por Giardia intestinal. Gac. Méd. de Car. XLV, 19, 298-300 (6).

ADRIANZA, Luis A.

1935a— La buba en Barlovento. Bol. del Minist. de Salub. y de Agric. y Cría, III, 24, 41-44 (7).

AGUIAR NIETO, R.

1943— Encuesta Sanitaria sobre Porlamar, presentada a la I Conferencia Anual de Médicos Jefes de Unidades Sanitarias. Archivos de la Div. de Unidades Sanitarias M.S.A.S. (8).

1944— La parasitosis infantil en el Estado de Nueva Esparta. Unid. San. Caracas. III, 4-6, 154-161 (9).

ALAMO GUTIERREZ, Enrique

1930— La parasitosis infantil en el Estado de Nueva Esparta. Unid. San. Caracas. III, 4-6, 154-161 (9).

ALAMO GUTIERREZ, Enrique

1939— La infección malárica. Bol. del Minist. de San. y Asist. Social. IV, 4, 191-204 (10).

ALARCON, Carlos Julio y GENATIOS, Tomás

1943— Estudios de 1000 casos de chancros genitales. Valor diagnóstico de la investigación ultramicroscópica. I Jornada de Venereología y Dermatología. Rev. de San. y Asist. Soc. Caracas. VIII, 4 783-796 (11).

ALCALA RANGEL, J.A.

1937— El Paludismo, forma perniciosa. Bol. del Minist. de San. y Asit. Soc. I, 718-720 (12).

ALFONSO BLANCO, Ramón

1928— Bilharziosis en el Estado Zamora, Gac. Méd. de Car. XXXV (13).

1928a— Tratamiento per os de la Bilharziosis. Gac. Méd. de Car. XXXV, 20, 308-309.

1931— Buba. Gac. Méd. de Car. Vol. XXXVIII (15).

ALVARADO, Pedro J.

1928— La Necatoriasis y su tratamiento. Tesis de Doctorado en Ciencias Médicas. Caracas. Edit. Sur-América, 15 p. (16).

POTENZA, L. y ANDUZE, Pablo J.

1942— Kala-azar en el Estado Bolívar. Rev. de la Poli. Car. XI, 67, 312-317 (17).

ANGULO ORTEGA, Rafael

1939— Organización de la campaña antisifilítica en el país. Tesis Doctorado en Ciencias Médicas. Caracas. Tip. Ayacucho, 35 p. (18).

ANZOLA CARRILLO, Antonio

1936— La Sífilis y su influencia en la degeneración de la raza. Diario "El Heraldo". Caracas, N° 4297. Julio 30 (19).

ANZOLA FALCON, Tarsicio

1939— La verdad sobre la fiebre en Lara. Gac. Méd. de Car. XLVI, 2, 26-27 (20).

ARAUJO, Rafael Lorenzo

1927— Un caso de buba. Bol. de los Hosp. Caracas XVII, 13, 499-500 (21).

ARCHILA, Ricardo

1934— Relación sobre la Fiebre Biliosa Hemoglobinúrica en Venezuela. Tesis de Doctorado en Ciencias Médicas. Caracas. Tip. Moderna, 9° p. (22).

1937— La Fiebre Biliosa Hemoglobinúrica en el Estado Bolívar. Bol. Minist. San Asit. Soc. Vol. I, 721-729 (23).

1941— Evaluación del Problema Malárico en las zonas rurales. Acciones originales de la Div. de Malariología; las Comisiones Locales de lucha antimalárica y la distribución organizada de quinina. Diario "El Universal". Car. Mayo, N° 11473 (24).

ARCHILA, Ricardo y NIETO, Miguel

1941— Geografía Médico-Sanitaria del Estado Cojedes con especial referencia al Paludismo Rev. de San y Asist. Soc. VI, 5, 587-785 (25).

ARCHILA, Ricardo

1943-44— La colaboración ciudadana en la lucha antipalúdica. Octubre 6 (26).
La lucha antisifilítica. Condiciones para su éxito. Marzo 18 (27).
Anquilostomiasis: la retrógada. Marzo 27 (28).
Transmisión del Paludismo. El Anófeles Zancudo Vector. Abril 10 (29).
El Enemigo en el Paludismo. Abril 17 (30).
Usted puede evitar el Paludismo. Mayo 10 (31).
La Bancarrota del Paludismo. Mayo 8 (32).
Tratamiento del Paludismo. Mayo 15 (33).
Invasión por Anquilostomos. Mayo 22 (34).
Sífilis y Matrimonio. Junio 5 (35).
Bilharzia. Septiembre 25 (37).
Parásitos solitarios. Octubre 2 (38).

ARMAS ARMAS, Julio C. de

1926— Organización de una lucha antipalúdica. Rev. Ciencias I, 1, 19-30 (39).

1928— La etiología de la fiebre biliosa hemoglobinúrica. Rev. de la Sociedad Médica de Caracas (40).

ARMAS, Julio C. de y CONDE JAHN, Franz

1931— Acerca de un caso de sífilis terciaria uterina. Rev. de Medicina Cirg. Maracay. I, 2 (41).

ARMAS, Julio C. de

1931— A propósito de algunas modalidades nuevas en el tratamiento del paludismo. Rev. de Medic. y Cirug. Maracay I, 3 (42).

1933— Algunas consideraciones sobre etiología y tratamiento de la fiebre biliosa hemoglobinúrica. Rev. de Medic. y Cirug. Maracay, I número extraordinario. Págs. 11-26 (43).

1943— Breve nota sobre algunas modalidades de la amibiasis latente. Rev. de Medic. y Cirug. Maracay II marzo, 11-19 (44).

ARMAS, hijo, Julio C. de

1934— Consideraciones diagnósticas sobre la sífilis osteoarticular hereditaria. Presentación de un caso. Rev. de Medc. y Cirug. Maracay, Julio, 37-47 (45).

ARMAS, hijo, Julio C. de

1934a— Sobre algunos trastornos anafilácticos en las verminosis intestinales. Rev. de Medc. y Cirug. Maracay. Diciembre. Página 117 (46).

1935— El estado actual de la enfermedad de Chagas en Venezuela. Memoria del V Cong. Médico Panamericano (47).

ARMAS, hijo, Julio C. de y VOGELSANG, E.

1941— Notas sobre especies de la flora y de la fauna de nuestros llanos. Rev. Pecuaria, 38-39, 9 11 (48).

AROCHA PINTO, Simón

1927— Un caso de broncoespiroquetos de Castellani y un caso de reumatismo articular agudo. Trabajo presentado al V Congreso Ven. de Medicina. Maracay. Imprenta Oriente 8 p. (49).

ARTEAGA PEREZ, Máximo

1942— Consideraciones sobre la Clínica de la Bilharzosis infantil. Tesis de Doctorado en Ciencias Médicas. Caracas (50).

ARVELO L., ANGULO

1941— Consideraciones sobre el Carate. Tesis de Doctorado en Ciencias Médicas. Caracas (51).

ARREAZA GUZMAN, Alfredo

1935— Contribution experimentale a letude du traitement de la Strongyloidose. París, 78 p. (52).

ARRIA RUIZ, Enrique

1930— Serodiagnóstico de la Anquilostomiasis. Mérida. Tipo de "El Vigilante", 37 p. (53).

1930— La anquilostomiasis en el Estado Mérida. Memoria de la Conferencia Sanitaria Nacional de 1930. Public. del Ministerio de Salub. y de Agric. y Cría. Caracas. Tip. Americana, páginas 225-236 (54).

ASCANIO RODRIGUEZ, J.B.

1930— Estadística de la infestación anquilostomósica en Venezuela de acuerdo a la labor de los técnicos de Laboratorio de la Conf. San. Nac. Memoria de la Conf. San. Nac. de 1930, publicada del Ministerio de Salub. y de Agric. y Cría, 421-497 (55).

1930a— Factores tangibles de la Anquilostomosis y otros parásitos. Rev. de la Conf. Sanit. Nac. I, 3, 72-79 (56).

1931— Estadística malariológica compuesta con los datos de relatores, médicos y técnicos, menos el Distrito Federal. Caracas. Tip. Americana, II vol., ilus. (57).

OTTOLINA C. Y ATENCIO, M.H.

1943— Nuevos caminos para el diagnóstico clínico preciso de la Schistosomiasis mansoni. Rev. de la Poli. Caracas, XII, 73, 348-380 (58).

BAQUERO GONZALEZ, Francisco

1938— Rhodnius prolixus. Tesis de Bachillerato. Caracas. Coop. de Artes Gráficas, 15

p. (59).

BAQUERO GONZALEZ, Ricardo

1939— Un caso de papilomas vulvares y perianales producidos por el Schistosoma mansoni. Rev. de la Clínica Luis Razetti. II, 3, 155-159 y en folleto, Tip. La Nación, 10 p. (60).

VALENCIA PARPARCEN, J. y BAQUERO GONZALEZ, R.

1939— Recto-colitis ulcerosa con amibas en las heces y Schistosoma mansoni en las paredes. Rev. de la Poli. Car. IX, 48, 3, 219 (61).

1939— Apendicitis a Balantidium coli y tricocéfalo. Rev. de la Poli. Car. IX, 48, 3226-3230 (62).

ALEGRIA, Ceferino

1945— Miasis. Consideraciones sobre dos casos. Rev. Soc. Méd. Quirurg. de Zulia, año XIX, N° 4 (63).

ALEGRIA, Ceferino y ARREAZA, Guzmán

1945— Proceso en candente de Brote agudo en Palúdicos crónicos. Rev. Soc. Médic. Quiróg. del Zulia. Año XIX, N° 11 (64).

ACEVEDO GALLEGOS, F.

1949— El clorhidrato de emetina en el tratamiento de la Schistosomiasis mansoni. Rev. Pol. Caracas, vol. XVIII, Nos. 104-105-106, p. 56 (65).

ARENDS, Tulio, RONDON Y GONZALEZ Mijares

1954— Nuevo foco de Oncocercosis humana en Venezuela. Gac. Méd. de Caracas, año LXII, Nos. 11-12 (66).

ANDUZE, Pablo J.

1947— Fauna hematófaga del Distrito Maturín (Estado Monagas). Culícidos. Rev. Méd. Vet. Caracas, p. 121 (67).

ARCHILA, Ricardo

1948— Historia del Paludismo en la antigua provincia de Apure. Rev. S.A.S. vol XIII, Nov. 34, (68).

ARCHILA, Ricardo y NIETO, Caicedo / Miguel

1946— Geografía Médico Sanitaria del Estado Cojedes con especial referencia al Paludismo. Conf. San. Cuaderno amarillo. Número 17 (69).

ARCHILA, D.(S.A.)

El paludismo en la región petrolera de Monagas. Coop. Artes Gráficas, Caracas (70).

ARAUJO, A.M.

1928— La viscosimetría sanguínea en el paludismo crónico y la parasitosis intestinal, págs. 9-25. (Tesis de opción al Doctorado en Ciencias Médicas) (71).

ARTAGAVEYTIA, R. y MONTEMAYOR, Lorenzo

Estudio comparativo de varias cepas de Paracoccidiosis brasiliensis y especies afines (72).

AURRECOECHEA, J.M. y LOVERA, I.

La penicilina en Trat. de las mujeres embarazadas (73).

ADRIANZA, Manuel y RODRIGUEZ, César

1953— "Complicaciones Pleuro-pulmonares de la Amibiasis", Rev. San. y Asis. Social, año 1953, vol XVIII. N° 1-2, pág. 117 (74).

ABREU, A. Carlos, y MEDINA, Rafael

1954— "Campaña contra la Buba en Venezuela". Rev. San. Asist. Soc. Vol. XIX, N° 5 y 6, pág. 345 (75).

ACOSTA MARTINEZ, A. y ANZOLA ESPINOSA, Héctor

1954— "Lucha antivenérea en Venezuela". Rev. San. y Asist. Social. vol. XIX, N° 5 y 6, pág. 309 (76).

BARBARA DE LA TORRE, Armando

1938— Sífilis Nasal. Su referencia en nuestra Consulta Hospitalaria. Tesis de Doctorado en Ciencias Médicas. Caracas. Tip. Americana, 34 p. (78).

BARRETO LIMA, Manuel Salvador

1929— Dermatobia Cyaniventris (Gusano Zancudo). Tesis de Bachillerato en Filosofía. Valencia, Tip. Venezuela, 14 p. (79).

1934— Sobre algunos casos de Paludismo observados. Bol. del Ministerio de Salub. y de Agr. y Cría, I, 8-9, 703-708 (80).

1934a— Las sales de quinina y su acción preventiva para el paludismo. Bol. del Minist. de Salub. y de Agr. y Cría. I, 10-11-817-824 (81).

1935— Un caso de mordedura de serpiente tratado con suero antibotrópico. Bol. del Minist. de Salud. y de Agric. y Cría, II, 22-23, 942-957 (82).

1936— Puntos sobre Paludismo. Bol. del Minist. de San. y Asis. Soc. Págs. 51-57 (83).

1936— 75 días de campaña antipalúdica en Puerto Cabello. Diario "El Heraldo". Caracas, N° 4, 356. Octubre 8 (84).

BARRIOS PADRON, José

1930— La emetina como tratamiento de las supuraciones pulmonares amibianas. Tesis de Doctorado en Ciencias Médicas. Caracas, Tip. Americana, 16 p. (85).

1942— Tratamiento moderno de la sífilis reciente. Crítica y Esquematización. Rev. de la soc. Méd. Quirúrg. del Zuliz, 3-4, 1547 (86).

BASALO, Miguel A.

1934— Las acciones vermífuga de algunos Látex. Rev. de la Soc. Médica Quirúrg. del Zulia. VIII, 11, 416-418 (87).

CAMEJO TROCONIS, Carlos

1940— Un caso de sífilis ingénita complicada con enfermedad de Parrot. Arch. Ven. de Pueric. y Pediat. II, 5, 270-275 (182).

TORREALBA, J.F., CAMEJO TROCONIS, O., e IRAZABAL RON, J.

1937— Primer caso de enfermedad de Chagas tratado en Zaraza por el 7602, Gac. Méd. de Caracas. XLIV, 23, 337-339 (183).

BARROS SAINT, J. Pasteur

1952—Estudio General de la Paracoccidioidosis brasilensis. Su importancie en Odontología. Bol. Lab. Clí. Razetti. Año XIII, N° 37-38 (184).

BALDO, José, IGNACIO, PIFANO, MAYED y GIL Yépez

1946— Investigaciones concernientes a los aspectos pulmonar y cardiovascular de la Schistosomiasis mansoni en un área endémica del país (Conferencia Sanitaria Panamericana. Cuaderno Amarillo. N° 9 (185).

BALDO, José Ignacio

1953— Manifestaciones pulmonares de la bilharziosis. Rev. S.A.S. Vol. XVIII, N° 1-2. Pág. 147 (186).

BRICEÑO ROSSI, A.L.

1950— Trabajo experimental sobre Fasciola hepática, primera comprobación del verdadero huésped intermediario de este parásito en Venezuela. Rev. S.A.S. Vol. XV, N° 6. Pág. 381 (187).

BILBAO LIBANO, Luis

1955— Reacción de Inmovilización del Treponema pallidum (T.P.I.) Nelson Meyer. Edt. Excelsior (188).

BENEROCH, E.I.

1930— Tratamiento del Paludismo. Algunas reflexiones sobre tan grave problema. Of. Cont. San. Nac. Págs. 1-5 (189).

1931— Estudios relativos al Paludismo. IV. Métodos para el estudio del paludismo en Venezuela. S.P.I. p. 7-108 (190)

BERTI, A.L.

1936— Métodos de Ingeniería aplicables al control de la malaria en Venezuela. (Tesis presentada ante la Universidad Central, para optar el título de Doctor en Ciencias Físicas y Matemáticas). (191).

1939— A survey of Anopheline larvae and breeding places at College Station, Texas (A Thesis), p. 1-11 (192).

1942— Control de mosquitos en Venezuela. Atlanta City, N.J. Mosquito exterm. Assoc. pp. 156-158 (193).
1943— Irrigación, Paludismo y Cultivos. Tij. s. mal, 7 (1): 1-10 (194).
1943— Informe sobre el Acueducto de Maracay. 3ª Conferencia Sanitaria Nacional (195).
1945— Acueductos y Cloacas en Relación con la Malaria. Tij. s. mal. 9 (5): 137-142 (196).

BEAUJON, José Dolores
1930— Estudio de la anquilostomiasis en el Puerto de La Vela. Memoria de la Conferencia Sanitaria Nacional. 206-307 (88).
1931— Estudio del paludismo en el Puerto de La Vela, Caracas. Tip. Americana, y en la Memoria de la Conferencia Sanitaria Nacional, 160-161 (89).

BEAUJON, Oscar y RAMIREZ, Fco.
1942— La sífilis en Oftalmología. Ponencia presentada a las Primeras Jornadas de O.R.L., Oftalm. y Neurol. Folleto 3, Imp. La Junta Municipal de Beneficencia, Caracas (90).

BELLARD, E.P. de
1931— Observaciones al trabajo del Dr. Camejo sobre fiebre biliosa hemoglobinúrica. Gac. Méd. de Car. XXXVIII, 8, 109-110 (91).

CHANCIN ITRIAGO, L.G. y BELLO, Carlos J.
1927— Clasificación de las ratas de Caracas. Gac. Méd. de Caracas. XXXIV, 21, 325-327 (92).

BELLO, Carlos J., y SANCHEZ BECERRA, H.
1935— Primeras observaciones de fiebre recurrente en San Cristóbal (reproducción). Bol. del Minist. de Salud y de Agric. y Cría. II, 20, 743-740 (93).
1954a— Sobre Fiebre Recurrente (reproducción). Bol. del Minist. de Salub. y de Agrc. y Cría, II, 20, 731-733 (94).

BELLO, Horacio
1933— Notas de divulgación sobre zancudos trasmisores de paludismo y otras enfermedades. Bol. Minist. Salub. Agric. y Cría. 2, 101-110 (95).

BELLOSOS CHACIN, Rafael
1932b— Sífilis y Embarazo. Rev. de la Soc. Méd. Quirúrg. del Zulia. VI, 10, 121-129 (96).

BENARROCH, E.I.
1926— Distribución geográfica de los zancudos venezolanos del género Anopheles. Caracas, Lit. y Tip. del Comercio. 6 p. (97).

HILL, R.B. y BENARROCH, E.I.
1928— Tratamiento de los portadores de gametocitos por la plasmoquina. Gac. Méd. de Caracas. XXXV, 14, 209-211 (98).

BENARROCH, E.I.
1928— Estudios relativos al paludismo: I. Investigación de los Anófeles malaríferos de Venezuela. II. Persistencia y fluctuaciones de los Gametocitos en la sangre periférica. Tesis de Doctorado en Ciencias Médicas. Caracas. Tip. Americana, 38 p. Reproducida en la Gac. Médica de Caracas. XXXV, p. 369 (99).
1929— La Anquilostomiasis en el Estado Bolívar. Bol. de la Cámara de Comercio. Octubre. Caracas (100).
1929a— El Paludismo en el estado Bolívar. Rev. Cultura Venezolana. XII, 98, 233-238 (101).
1931— Tratamiento del Paludismo. Umfia. Rev. de la Unión Médica Latina. París, 57, 321-329 (102).
1931b— Estudios relativos al Paludismo en Venezuela. El Nuevo Diario. Caracas, N° 6, 591, mayo, 18 (103).

BENARROCH, E.I. y HIERONIMUS, Boos
1930— Proyecto de estudio sobre campaña antipalúdica mediante el uso exclusivo de

medidas directas antiparasitarias. El Nuevo Diario. Caracas, Nº 6, 561. Abril 18 (104).

1931— Tratamiento del Paludismo con plasmoquina. El Nuevo Diario, Nº 6559. Abril 16. Caracas (105).

BENARROCH, E.I.

1931— Studies on Malaria in Venezuela. Amer. Jr. Hyg. XIV, 3, 690-693 (106).

1931a— Métodos para el estudio Paludismo en Venezuela. Caracas. Tip. Americana. 110 p. (1007).

1931b— Acerca de algunos problemas de Anquilostomiasis. "El Universal". Caracas, marzo 14 (108).

1932— Observations sur l'exflagellation des microgametocytos du paludisme humain. Folleto editado por la Industria Tipográfica Romana. Trabajo publicado en la Revista di Malariología. Anno XI, fasc. 5 (1009).

1932d— Bases para una campaña antipalúdica. Caracas. Diario "El Heraldo". Agosto 31 (110).

BERNARROCH, E.I. y HIERONIMUS, Boos

1932— Tratamiento del paludismo con Erion o Atebrina. Comunicación a la Acad. Nac. de Medicina. Julio. Caracas (111).

BENARROCH, E.I.

1933— La Reactivación con Adrenalina (Estudios relativos al Paludismo). Congreso de la Asoc. Méd. Panamericana, Dallas, Tex. U.S.A. Marzo. Pub. en la Revista de la Poli. Caracas 9, 547-552 (112).

1933a— Estudios relativos al Paludismo. Métodos para estudios sobre tratamiento. Congreso de la Asoc. Méd. Panamericana. Dallas, Tex. U.S.A. Marzo. Pub. en la rev. de la Pol. Caracas, 12, 760-764 (113).

1934— Distribución geográfica de los zancudos venezolanos del género Anófeles. Bol. de la Soc. Ven. de Cienc. Nat. 16, 273-274 (114).

1934a— A propos de la reaction de Henry pour le diagnostic du paludisme. Revista di Malariologia. Vol. XIII, Fasc. 6 bis. Página 329 (115).

1934b— Lucha contra la Anquilostomiasis. Rev. Medical. Caracas, 1, 5 (116).

BENARROCH, E.I.

1934c— Observaciones acerca de los zancudos trasmisores. Bol. de la Soc. Ven. de Cienc. Nat. Nº 14, enero 31, Caracas (117).

1934d— Zancudos del Estado Bolívar. Bol. de la Soc. Ven. de Cien. Nat. Caracas, II, 16, 275-276 (118).

1934e— Malarioterapia. Rev. Medical. Caracas, 5, 79181 (119).

1935— Concepto sobre Paludismo. "El Universal". Caracas, Nº 9408. julio 11 (120).

1935— La Campaña contra la Anquilostomiasis. "El Heraldo". Caracas. Nº 4096, Dic. 26 (121).

1936c— El Congreso y el Paludismo. "El Universal". Caracas, Nº 9722 (122).

1936d— Lo Antipalúdico legislable en Venezuela. Diario "Ahora" Número 215 (123).

1936c— La Campaña Antipalúdica. "El Heraldo". Caracas. Enero 7 (124).

1936j— Paludismo. El tratamiento: factor profiláctico. "El Heraldo". Caracas. Febrero 5 (125).

1937— Algunas consideraciones sobre la campaña sanitaria pro letrinas. Rev. S.A.S. de Educ. San. Caracas, I, 6, 4-7 (126).

1941— Métodos para estimar la extensión e intensidad de la anquilostomiasis. Public. del Minist. de San. y Asist. Soc. Talleres Patria. Caracas, 12 p. (este artículo fue publicado en el Bol. de la Ofic. San. Panam. en 1930. I, 7) (127).

BENGOA, José María

1942b— El bocio endémico y la enfermedad de Chagas. Memoria de la Sociedad de Ciencias Naturales La Salle. II, 5, 24-26 (128).

BOCARANDA, Victor M.

1942— Tesis sobre la Malaria en Venezuela, presentada para obtener el grado de Master in Public Health en la Universidad de Michigan, Estados Unidos de Norte-América (129).

BONADIES, Antonio

1944— La quininización y metaquinización obligatoria: bajo del alto porcentaje de fiebre perniciosa en Caripito. Rev. Al Méd. Maturín. I, 1, 19-22 (130).

BORJAS R., Antonio

1940— Treponemas carateum. Rev. del Hosp. Ob. Caracas. I, 6-7, 23-34 (131).

BRICEÑO, Antonio

1933— Tratamiento del paludismo por los nuevos productos sintéticos. Tesis de Doctorado en Ciencias Médicas. Caracas Lit. y Tip. Vargas. 36 p. (32).

BRICEÑO IRAGORRY, Leopoldo

1927— Parasitismo en Hosp. Vargas. Bol. de los Hosp. Caracas. 9, 445-511 (133).

1927b— Un caso de Pie de Madura. Bol. de los Hosp. Caracas, XVII, 10 (134).

1934— Contribución al estudio de los huevos de algunos Reduvideos. Bol. de la Soc. Ven. de Ciencias Naturales. 18, 398-400 y en la Gac. Méd. de Caracas. XLI, 23, 257-358 (136).

1933— Dos casos de miasis. Rev. de la Poli. Caracas. 9, 586 (135).

1934a— Notas sobre Micología. Bol. de .a Soc. Ven. de Cienc. Nat. 19, 407-410 (137).

BRICEÑO IRAGORRY, L. y PLAZA, Gustavo de la

1934— Una nueva especie de flebotomus en Venezuela Rev. Méd. Caracas. 8, 111-113 (138).

BRICEÑO IRAGORRY, L.

1935— Contribución al estudio de la "Piedra" venezolana. Rev. Medical. Caracas. 13 (139).

BRICEÑO IRAGORRY, L.

1935a— Contribución al estudio parasitológico del eczema marginado en Venezuela. Rev. Medical. Caracas. II, 14, 222-223 (14).

1935c— Anquilostomiasis y anemia anquilostomiásica. Rev. Medical. Caracas. II, 15, 243-245 (141).

RUIZ RODRIGUEZ J.M. y BRICEÑO IRAGORRY, L.

1935— Probable caso de Leishmaniosis americana. Rev. de la Poli. Caracas. V, 20, 1335-1338 (14).

BRICEÑO IRAGORRY, L.

1936— La Esporotricosis y el primer caso de Rhinoclaudiosis schenki en Venezuela (en colab. con M. Jiménez Rivero). Rev. Medical. Caracas. 20, 305-312, y en la Gac. Méd. de Caracas. XLIII, 15, 225-236 (143).

1937— Contribución al estudio de la parasitología de la tiña tonsurante en Venezuela. Gac. Méd. de Caracas. XLIV, 8, 115 (144).

1937a— Un nuevo caso de Esporotricosis a Rhinoclaudiosis schenki. Rev. de la Poli. Car. VI, 35, 2346-2349 (145).

1938a— Sobre Cromoblastomicosis. Rev. de la Cli. L.R. I, 2, 108-128 (146).

1939a— Sobre Cromoblastomicosis.Gac. Méd. de Caracas. XLVII, 8, 118-124 y en el N° 9 (147).

1940b— Notas sobre Araecerus fasciculatus de Geer 1775, coleóptero atacante del grano de café. Bol. del Lab. de la Cli. L.R. I, 3, 2-14 (149).

1941— Acerca de dos casos de tiña endotrix. Bol. del Lab. de la Cli. L.R. I, 3, 65-68 (150).

1941a— Notas sobre Simuliidae (Diptera)con citación de una nueva especie para el país y lista de las conocidas en Venezuela. Bol. del Lab. de la Cli. L.R. II, 6, 110-118 (151).

1941c— Breve nota sobre probable foco de schizotripanosomiasis en haciendas vecinas a la laguna de Valencia. Bol. del Lab. de la Cli. L.R. II, 4, 85-86 (152).

1942— Nota sobre Simulium pulverulentum. Nv. sp. para el país. Bol. de la Clí.L.R. II, 7 (153).

1942b— Nota sobre Simulium lutzianus (descripción del adulto) en colab. con G.B. Fairchild. Bol. del Lab. de la Clín. L.R. II, 9, 158-160 (154).

1942c— Notas sobre Simulium clarki Fairchild 1940 (nueva especie para Venezuela). Bol. del Lab. de la Clí. L.R. II, 9, 161 (155).

1943c— Dermato-micosis en Venezuela. Presentado a la Primera Jornada Venezolana de Venereología y Dermatología. Rev. San. Asist. Soc. VIII, 5, 929-935 (156).

1943d— Nota sobre Simúlidos del Valle de Caracas. Bol. del Lab. de Clí. L.R. III, 10, 181-186 (157).

1943e— Nota sobre Simúlidos del Estado Anzoátegui, Citación de una nueva especie para el país. Bol. del Lab. de la Clí. L.R. III, 11 (158).

BRICEÑO IRAGORRY, L., DAO y RODRIGUEZ CABRERA

1943— Asociación Tifo-Malaria. Gac. Méd. de Car. L., 15, 159 (159).

BRICEÑO MAAZ, Tulio

1935a— Estudio del contenido del apéndice. Rev. de la Soc. Méd. Quirúrgica del Zulia. IX, 4, 467-471 (160).

1937— El Paludismo y la Civilización. Rev. de la Soc. Méd. Quirúrg. del Zulia. XI, 9-10, 724-746 (161).

1938— Malaria in its more serious forms. Clí. Arch. Of. Gulf. Hosp. Iv., 4, 4-9 (162).

1943— La enfermedad de Chagas en Venezuela. Rev. S.E.M.X., 95-100, 32-36 (163).

1943b— Histoplasmosis (Citomicosis retículo-endotelial). Rev. de la Poli. Caracas. XIII, 71, 238-243 (164).

BRICEÑO ROSSI, Antonio L.

1926— La espiroquetosis broncopulmonar de Castellani en Ciudad Bolívar. Gac. Méd. de Cd. Bolívar. VIII, 102, 57-62 (165).

1934— El problema del Ofidismo en Venezuela. Bol. Minist. Salub. Agric. y Cría. II, 14, 1079 (166).

1939— Carate or "Mal del Pinto". Reprinted from proceedings of the Sixth Pacific Science Congress. Vol. V, held at Berkeley, Stanford and San Francisco. July 4 to August 12, 1939 (167).

BRICEÑO ROSSI, A.L. e IRIARTE, David R.

1939— Consideraciones sobre el estado actual del Carate y su distribución geográfica en Venezuela. Tip. Americana. Caracas, 39 p., y en la Gac. Méd. de Caracas. XLVI, 5, 68p78 (168).

BRICEÑO ROSSI, Antonio

1941— Algunos datos sobre el Carate en Venezuela, de la Ofic. San. Panam. XX, 3 215-218 (169).

1941a— La frecuencia de la helmintiasis y protozoosis en Caracas como resultado del estudio de 27.746 muestras fecales. Rev. San. Asist. Soc. VI, 4, 523-533 (170).

1941b— Nota preliminar al trabajo del Dr. Pons sobre Kala-Azar. Gac. Méd. de Caracas. XLVIII, 17-18, 328-329 (171).

1942— La coccidiosis en el hombre. Primer caso de Isospora hominis en Venezuela. Rev. de San. y Asist. Soc. VII, 4, 449-458 (172).

1942c.— Nota epidemiológica en disentería amibiana. Rev. San. Asist. Soc. VII, 3, 333-361 (173).

1943— El valor del Verification test en la serología del carate o mal del pinto y buba (pian o yaws). Rev. San. Asist. Soc. VII. 1, 153-165 (174).

1943a.— La serología en el diagnóstico de la sífilis con la reacción "Briceño Rossi". Presentado a la I Journada de Venereología y Dermatología. Rev. San. Asist. Soc. VIII, 4, 587-598 (175).

1943b.— La frecuencia de parásitos en los análisis de materias fecales en la Sección de Coprología del Instituto de Higiene, por grupos de edades. Presentado a las primeras Jornadas Nacionales de Puericultura y Pediatría (176).

BRICEÑO ROSSI, A.L., e IRIARTE, David R.

1943— Breves notas sobre últimas investigaciones verificadas en las zonas pintógenas de

Venezuela en relación al estado actual del conocimiento del carate o mal del pinto. Presentada a la I. jornada Ven. de Venereología y Dermatología. Rev. de San. y Asist. Soc. VIII, 5, 10001-10003 (177).

1944— Recientes adquisiciones técnicas para la interpretación de la inespecificidad serológica de la sífilis. Rev. Ciencias, Caracas, I, 3, 22-24 (178).

BRICEÑO ROSSI, Gualberto

1943— Algo sobre fiebre biliosa hemoglobinúrica. Bol. Minist. Salub. Agric. y Cría. I, 8-9, 735-736 (179).

CALATRAVA, Domingo A.

1937— La trasmisión de la sífilis adquirida. Folleto. La Semana de Venereología. Págs. 59-62 (180).

CAMEJO, Julio

1931— Breves apuntaciones sobre la fiebre biliosa hemoglobinúrica. Gac. Med. de Caracas XXXVIII, 8, 109-110 (181).

1945— Desarrollo de la Ingeniería Antimalárica en Venezuela. Tij. S. mal. 9 (2): 48-51 (197).

BERTI, A.L. & MONTESINOS, M.

1946— Cultivos de arroz en relación con la malaria. El Problema en Venezuela. 3° Conferencia Interamericana de Agricultura. Cuaderno N° 52, pp. 7-33.

BERTI, A.L.

1948— Eliminación de **Anopheles darlingi** por Obras de Ingeniería. Org. Ofic. de la Asoc. Interam. de Ing. San. 2 (2). 103-111 (199).

1949— Control domiciliario de Insectos en Venezuela. Asoc. Interamer. de Ing. San. 2 (4). 327-335 (200).

1950— Observaciones y recomendaciones para una campaña integral de desinfectación en la ciudad de Maracaibo. División de Malariología, pp. 1-12 (202).

1950— Control de insectos y otros vectores de enfermedades del medio rural. División de Malariología, pp. 1-37 (202).

BERTI, A.L. & TAGE, H.H.

1950— Observations on Mosquito and Malaria Control in the Caribbean Area, part 5, Venezuela. Mosquitos News 10 (1): 1-3 (203).

BERTI, A.L., GABALDON, A., COVA GARCIA, P. & GOMEZ, J.

1951— Proyectos de control de moscas de Maracay. Copia hecha a máquina (204).

BERTI, A.L. & JOVE, J.A.

1951— La vivienda en el Medio Rural. III Cong. Méd. Soc. Panameric. Caracas, pp. 107-155 (205).

1951— Saneamiento en el Medio Rural. III Cong. Méd. Soc. Panameric., Caracas, pp. 208-299 (206).

BERTI, A.L.

1952— Almanaque de la lucha Antimalárica en Venezuela. Copia hecha a máquina (207).

BRICEÑO IRAGORRY, L.

1945— Lección inaugural (ct. 1944). Cátedra de Bacteriología y Parasitología. Caracas, Artes Gráficas (208).

1948— Carate o Mal de Pinto. Bol. de Lab. Clí. Razetti. Año VIII, N° 25-26 (209).

1948— Carate o Mal de Pinto (conclusión). Bol. del Lab. Clí. Razetti. Año IX. N° 27-28 (210).

(Trabajos aparecidos en el Boletín del Lab. de la Clí. Razetti del año 46 (211).

BRICEÑO, Iragorry Leopoldo

1946— Nota acerca de culicoides (díptera Cerapogonidae). Descripción de una especie nueva para el país. Boletín del Lab. de la Clínica Luis Razetti. Año VI, N° 19-20 (212).

1947— Nueva especie de foco de Bilharziosis en el Oriente de la República. Boletín del Lab. Clí. Razetti. Año VIII, N° 23-24 (213).

1946— Breve nota acerca de un nuevo simúlido para el país. Boletín del Lab. Clí. Razetti. Año VII. Nº 21-22 (214).

1947— Breve nota acerca de Simúlidos colombianos. Bol. del Lab. de la Clí. Razetti. Año VII. Nº 23-24 (215).

1949— Breve nota sobre Culicoides. Bol. Lab. Clí. Razetti. Año IX Nº 29-30 (216).

BRICEÑO IRAGORRY y COLS

1955— Hemoparásitos y Trichinas de las ratas salvajes en Caracas. Gac. Méd. de Caracas. Año LXII, Nº 34 (217).

BENAIN PINTO, H.

1947— Aspectos cardio-vasculares de la anquilostomiasis, con especial referencia al problema de la miocarditis crónica. (Rev. Pol. Caracas. Vol. XVI. Nº 93, p. 99).

1949— Resultados preliminares de una encuesta de reconocimiento sobre Enfermedad de Chagas y Tripanosomiasis rangeli en un sector del Valle de Caracas (Petare, Edo. Miranda). Rev. Pol. Caracas. Vol. XVIII, Nº 107-108-109, p. 103 (219).

BENAIN PINTO, Carlos

1950— La insuficiencia hepática. Concepto y exploración. Contribución al estudio de la insuficiencia hepático en la Bilharziosis mansoni del hombre. Rev. Pol. Caracas. Vol. 18. Nº 110-111, página (220).

BRUNI CELLI, Blas

1953— Evolución histórica y estado actual del asunto de la toxina anquilostomiástica. Rev. Pol. Caracas, Vol. XXI, Nº 127, p. 237 1 (221).

BALDO, José Ignacio

1953— Paracoccidiosis pulmonar. Rev. S.A.S. Vol. XVIII. Nº 1-2 (22).

BRICEÑO ROSSI, A.L.

1948— Algunas consideraciones sobre la clínica del carate, con estudio de casos de mal de Pinto en la zona de Iguala (México). Gac. Méd. de Caracas. LVI. Nº 13-18 (223).

1952— El problema de la Wuchereriasis en Venezuela. 124 págs. Tip. Vargas (224).

1952— El problema de la Wuchereriasis Bancrofti en Venezuela. Rev. S.A.S. Vol. XVII, Nº 1-2 (225).

1949— Resultados obtenidos con el hetrazan en diferentes modalidades patológicas o clínicas de la Wuchereriasis bancrofti. Arch. Ven. de Pat. y Paras. Med. I. Nº 2 (226).

BRICEÑO ROSSI, A.L. y REDGINAL, Herwit

1949— Treatment of bancroftian filariasis with Hetrazan in Puerto Cabello. Venezuela Southern Med. Jour. Vol. XLII. p. 978 (227).

BRICEÑO, Giménez

1934— Profilaxia del Paludismo. Boletín del Minit. de salub. y de Agri. y Cría. Vol. I, p. 750 (228).

BRICEÑO, Maaz T.

1943— Análisis de 1223 historias clínicas. Edit. Grafolit (229).

1943— La Enfermedad de Chagas en Venezuela. Revista S.E.M. Nº 95-100 (230).

BLAZQUEZ, Vicente, J. & Maier J.

1951— Observaciones sobre el efecto de dosis sub-letales de DDT en el ciclo evolutivo del mosquito. Rev. de San. y Asist. Soc. 15 (6), 1-7 (231).

BRASS-Karl, Polo R. y Montemayor L.

1955— Primer caso. Nota previa. Rev. de la Academia de Medicina Caracas 1955. Enfermedad de Gilchrist en Venezuela. Primer caso. Estudio clínico. Comprobación histológica. Determinación de la primera cepa sudamericana de ''Blastomyces dermatitis'' Rev. San. Asistencia Social (232).

BRICEÑO IRAGORRY y col.

Hemoparásitos y Trichinas de las ratas salvajes en Caracas (233).

BENAIN PINTO, Enrique

1955— Ensayo de la Pentamidina en el tratamiento de la Paracoccidiosis brazilensis. Acta Médica Venezolana. Vol. III. Mayo-junio V3 (234).

BENAIN, Carlos, GOMEZ, Otto, MONTEMAYOR, L., y RIOS, F.

Afecciones pulmonares crónicas con hallazgos del género Geothrichum en los esputos (235).

BORELLI, Dante

Significado de la adenopatía epitroclear en nuestro medio (236).

BRICEÑO ROSSI, A.L.

Primeros casos de filiariasis a Mansonella ozzardi constatados en Venezuela. Revista de Sanidad y Asistencia Social. Vol. XIV. N° 6. Septiembre-diciembre (237).

Trabajos experimentales sobre las reacciones inmunológicas de las treponemosis. Inmunización de los treponemas (238).

BRICEÑO L., y BILBAO LIBANO, Luis

El problema de la Sífilis en Venezuela (239).

BRICEÑO MAAZ, Tulio

1951— Fiebre biliosa hemoglobinúrica. Revista de la Policlínica Caracas. Mayo-junio. N° 118. Vol. XIX (240).

BENARROCH, E.L. y VILLEGAS, J.

1954— "Eficacia comprobada del Hexilresorcinol y de una mezcla de Tetracloretileno y Quenopodio en el Tratamiento de la Helmintiasis intestinal" (241).

BALDO, J.I.

Paracoccidioidomicosis pulmonar. Rev. San. Asit. Soc. Enero de 1953. Vol. XVIII. N° 1-2 (242).

CAMPINS, Humberto

1934— Leucocito-reacción de la Sífilis. Tesis de Doctorado en Ciencias Médicas. Caracas. Lit. y Tip. Casa de Especialidades. 16 p. (243).

CAMPANIS, Humberto, y SILVA ALVAREZ, Alberto

1941— Sífilide pustolosa acneiforme. Rev. de la Soc. Méd. de Lara. I, 1, 16-18 (244).

CAMPO MORENO, R.

1939— Algunos datos epidemiológicos sobre sífilis en Caracas, obtenidos en el Dispensario Venereológico del Suroeste. Bol. Minist. San. Asis. Soc. IV. 2, 30-36 (245).

CARDENAS BECERRA, Héctor

1939— Algunas observaciones sobre Buba y su tratamiento en el Oriente de Venezuela. Tesis de Doctorado en Ciencias Médicas. Caracas. Edit. Bolívar, 21 p. (246).

CARDENAS FARIAS, N.A.

1933— Las diarreas de la primera infancia y la heredosífilis. Rev. de Medic, y Cirug. Diciembre. Págs. 101-106 (217).

CARRILLO, Pedro Emilio

1943— Paludismo larvado. Bol. del Hosp. Nuestra Señora de la Paz Valera. I, 2, 35-38 (248).

CARTENS ECHENIQUE, Rafael

1937— Parasitosis intestinal en San Fernando de Apure. Bol. Minist. San. Asist. Soc. Págs. 1052-1055 (249).

1938— Un caso de paludismo de forma abdominal. Bol. Minist. San. Asist. Soc. Págs. 1154-1156 (250).

1941— Polimorfismo clínico del Paludismo. Rev. de la Poli. Caracas. X 57, 116-120 (251).

CARVALLO. Temístocles

1935c— Anotaciones críticas al estudio "obstrucción intestinal por Ascaris lumbricoides" del Dr. J.R. Hernández d'Empaire. Gac. Méd. de Car. Septiembre 15 (252).

CASTILLO, Carlos E., MAYZ, O. y RODRIGUEZ DELGADO, J.

1943— Parasitosis intestinal en el niño de Maracaibo. IV. Ponencia Oficial. Memorias de las Primeras Jornadas de Pueric. y Pediat. Vol. II, 51-130 (253).

CASTILLO, Demetrio

1942— Datos del pasado. Sobre fiebres palúdicas en las orillas de la Laguna de Valencia. Rev. Tij. Mal. V. 24, 97-89 (254).

CASTILLO PLAZA, Armando

1930— Trabajo sobre la Anquilostomiasis en el Estado Zulia. Memoria de la Conferencia Sanitaria Nacional de 1930. Págs. 354-382 (255).

1931— El Paludismo en el Estado Zulia. Presentado a la Segunda Conferencia Sanitaria Nacional. Memoria de la Conferencia Sanitaria Nacional de 1931. Págs. 363-383 (256).

1939a— Conferencias Sanitarias para maestros, Anquilostomiasis. Rev. S.A.S. de Educ. San. III. 49, 2-7 (257).

CASTILLO REY, Francisco

1940— Estadística de los casos sifilíticos cardiovasculares autopsiados en el Hospital Vargas. Tesis de Doctorado en Ciencias Médicas. Caracas. Emp. El Cojo, 21 p. (258).

CELIS PEREZ, Alfredo

1942b— Un caso de cromoblastomicosis de localización nasal y laríngea. Rev. Poli. Vol. II, 5, 515 y en la Gac. Méd. de Car. L, 1, 8-10 (259).

CELIS SAUNE, Eduardo

1933— Ensayos de Malarioterapia en la Parálisis General. Tesis de Doctorado en Ciencias Médicas. Caracas. Edit. Sur América. 66 p. (260).

Algo sobre profilaxia de las disenterías (conferencia) Bol. Minist. Salub. Agric. y Cría. II. 16, 249-254 (261).

CIFUENTES LABASTIDA, Ricardo

1935d— Divulgaciones Médicas. Enfermedades "inofensivas". El Paludismo. Periódico del Comercio Valerano. Valera-Mayo (262).

CLAVIER G.

1936— Anofelinos de Caracas. Caracas. Mimeografiado (263).

CODECIDO, Luis

1936— Síndrome disentérico febril observado en la ciudad de La Victoria con carácter epidémico. Bol. Ministerial San. Asist. Soc., pp. 204-210 (264).

COLLADO, hijo, Domingo

1936— El reparto gratuito de quinina y antiparasitario necesita una reforma radical. Diario "El Heraldo", Caracas. N° 4.146. Feb. 19 (265).

CONDE JAHN, F., y ARMAS, Julio C. de

1931— Acerca de un caso de sífilis terciaria uterina. Rev. de Medic. y Cirug. Maracay, 1, 2 (266).

CONDE JAHN, Franz

1933— Lesiones sifilíticas en el domino otorrinolaringológico observadas en Maracay. Rev. de Med. y Cirug. Maracay 1, 4 (267).

CONDE JAHN, Y CORRAL, Pedro del

1935— Un caso de faringo-micosis. Rev. de Medic. y Cirug. Mar. II. 2,109-114 (268).

CONDE JAHN, Franz

1937— Cómo se disfraza la sífilis en los oídos y la garganta. Folleto "La Semana de Venéreo". Caracas. Págs. 80-83 (269).

1938— La Sífilis en Otorrinolaringología. Lección Clínica. Rev. S.EM. IV, 37, 17-34 (270).

1938e— La Sífilis en O.R.L. Rev. S.E.M. IV, 37, 17-34 (271).

RIVERO, Fcco. H. y CONDE JAHN, Franz

1942— Las micosis en O.R.L. Memorias de las Primeras Jornadas de O.R.L. Oftalm. y Neurología. Caracas (1944) (272).

CORDOBA, Salvador

1944b— Método diagnóstico de la enfermedad de Chagas. Gac. Méd. de Car. LII, 17, 197-198 (273).

CORRAL, Pedro del

1927— Anotaciones sobre parasitosis intestinal entre nosotros. Memorias del V Congreso Ven. de Medicina. Págs. 111-132, y en la Gac. Méd. de Car. Año 1927. XXXIV, 5, 69-76 (274).

1933— Acerca de un caso de condilomatosis plana heredo-específica; tipo alérgico cutáneo-musculoso. Rev. de Medic. y Cirug. Maracay I, 5, 17-27 (275).

1933a— Actividades de la Clínica de Maracay en la lucha nacional contra el Paludismo. Rev. de Medic. y Cirug. Maracay I. Págs. 27-30. Diciembre (276).

1934— Tópicos Malariológicos. Caracas. Edit. Elite. 78 p. (277).

1934a— Estudios Micológicos. Caracas. Lit. y Tip. Casa de Especialidades. 40 p. (278).

CORRAL, Pedro del

1934b— El biotropismo en la práctica dermosifilopática. Algunos casos observados. Rev. de Medic. y Cirug. Maracay. Julio. Páginas 19-27 (279).

1934c— Dermatomicosis venezolanas observadas en Maracay. Nota preliminar. Rev. de Med. y Cirugía. Maracay. Diciembre. Páginas 35-42 (280).

1934d— Dermatomisosis venezolanas observadas en Maracay. El Trichosporum venezuelensis. Nueva especie de homgo p tógeno. Relación de dos casos de "piedra" provocados por él. Rev. de Med. y Cirug. Maracay. Diciembre. Pág. 43-74 (218).

1934e— Nuestra experiencia sobre Atebrina y otros antipalúdicos conocidos en la malaria. Rev. de Medic. y Cirug. Maracay. II. Págs. 20-42. Marzo (282).

CONDE JAHN, F. y CORRAL, Pedro del

1935— Un caso de faringo-micosis. Rev. de Medic. y Cirug. Maracay II, 2, 109-114 (283).

CORRAL, Pedro del y VOGELSANG, E.G.

1943— Taeniarhynchus saginatus (Goeze 1728), en Venezuela. Rev. de la Pol. Car. XII, 69, 126-128 (284).

CORTE, Agustín La

1935— Anquilostomos libres en el peritoneo. Rev. de la Soc. Med. Quirúrgica del Zulia, IX, 5 (285).

COVA GARCIA, Pablo

1939— Notas sobre los Anofelinos de Venezuela y su identificación. Publ. N° 2 de la Div. de Malar. M.S.A.S. 34 p. (286).

GABALDON, Arnoldo, COVA GARCIA, Pablo y LOPEZ, José Antonio

1940— Anopheles (Nyssorhynchus) rangeli, una nueva especie de la subserie oswaldoi (Diptera, Culicidae) de amplia distribución en Venezuela. Public. de la Div. de Malar. Public. N° 5. Páginas 9-23 (287).

GABALDON, Arnoldo, y COVA GARCIA, Pablo y AREVALO, Ammeris

1940— Observaciones sobre número de huevos, salinidad de criaderos y tiempo de desarrollo de tres especies de la sub-serie oswaldoi. Publi. N° 5 de la Div. de Malar. Págs. 25-32 (288).

GABALDON, Arnoldo, COVA GARCIA, Pablo

1940— Nuevo tipo de clave para la identificación de las larvas de anofelinos venezolanos. Rev. Tij. Mal. III, 10, 76-86 (289).

COVA GARCIA, Pablo

1940— La legislación antimalárica venezolana y proyecto de reglamentación. Publi. N° 6 de la Div. de Malar. 34 p. (290).

GABALDON, Arnoldo, COVA GARCIA, Pablo y LOPEZ, J.A.

1941— Anopheles (Nyssorhynchus) benarrochi, una nueva especie de la sub-serie Triannulatus. Public. N° 7 de la Div. de Malar. Páginas 3-24 (291).

1941— Anopheles (Arthuromya) vargasi, n. sp. y redescripción del sub-género Arthuromya (Galvao 1941). Public. N° 7 de la Div. de Malar. Págs. 25-26 (292).

COVA GARCIA, Pablo y GOMEZ MARCANO, Antonio

1941— Emergencia de Anopheles rangeli de una pupa en estado de sequedad. Publi. N° 7 de la Div. de Malar. Págs. 57-58 (293).

COVA GARCIA, Pablo

1943— Penetración y dispersión en Venezuela de las especies Anopheles (Nyssorhynchus) darlingi y Anopheles (Nyssorhynchus) albimanus. Rev. San. Asist. Soc. VIII, 3, 476-472 (294).

CUENCA, Heberto

1926a— Sobre un caso de actinomicosis pleuro-pulmonar (en colab. con A. d'Empaire). Rev. La Benef. Maracaibo. Julio (295).

CUENCA, Heberto

1927b— Micetoma de granos blancos. Rev. de la Soc. Méd. Quirúrg. del Zulia. I, 5, 56-57 (296).

1927f— Sobre un caso de amibiasis bronquial curado con emetina. Rev. de la Soc. Méd. Quirúrg. del Zulia. I, 2 (297).

1927g— Nota sobre el tratamiento del paludismo por un nuevo específico: la Plasmoquina. Rev. de la Soc. Méd-Quirúrgica del Zulia. I, 3 (298).

1928— Nota sobre la filariosis del Estado Trujillo. Rev. de Soc. Med. Quir. del Zulia.

1929a— Pequeñas notas sobre formas poco frecuentes de la amibiasis. Rev. de la Soc. Médic. Quirúrg. del Zulia. III, 2, 10-11 (300).

1931a— La Atebrina. Nuevo antipalúdico sintético. Relato de las investigaciones realizadas junto con el profesor Mühlens. Gac. Méd. de Car. (301).

1932a— Sobre la importancia de la Atebrina. Rev. de la Socñ. Méd. Quirúrg. del Zulia. VI, 8, 92-95 (302).

1932b— La Atebrina, nuevo antipalúdico sintético. Cac. Méd. de Car. XXXIX (303).

1932c— Profilaxis de las disenterias. Rev. de la Soc. Méd. Quirúrg. del Zulia. Enero. Págs. 22-28 (304).

1935— La forma cardíaca en la enfermedad de Chagas. Gac. Méd. de Car. XLII, 23, 361-365 (305).

1935c— La forma cardíaca de la enfermedad de Chagas con presentación de nuestro primer caso. Arch. Ven. de Cardiol. y Hemat. I, 3, 144-155 (306).

1936— La sífilis hereditaria del corazón y arterias. Diario ''El Heraldo''. Caracas. N° 4.303. Agosto 6 (307).

1936a— Miocarditis subaguada en sifilíticos y bilharzianos sin lesiones anatomopatológicos de sífilis cardíaca. ¿Micorditis bilharziana? Bol. de los Hosp. XXXIV. 3, 111-129 (308).

1937— Sífilis y Aortitis. Folleto ''La Semana del Venéreo''. Caracas. Páginas 128-131 (309).

Plasmoquina. Rev. de la Soc. Méd. Quirúrg. del Zulia.

Un caso de paludismo grave a falciparum curado con Plasmoquina. Rev. de la Soc. Méd. Quirúrg. del Zulia (310).

CURIEL ABENATAR, Darío

1935— Neurosis palúdica. Revista Médica, órgano mensual de la Soc. Méd. del Estado Falcón. N° 6, 7 y 8. Mayo (311).

CURIEL JUVENAL e IRIARTE, David R.

1935— Sobre un caso de cirrosis hipertrófica de origen bilharziano. Rev. de Medic. y Cirug. Caracas. VIII, 91 223-230. (312).

CONVIT J. y LAPENTA P.

1948— Sobre un caso de leihmaniasis tagumentaria de forma diseminada. Rev. Pol. Caracas. Vol 17. N° 100, p. 153 (313).

CARBONELL, L.M.

1949— Investigaciones de nidos leishmánicos en corazones con miocarditis y xenodiagnóstico positivo. Pol. Caracas. Vol. XVII N° 107-108-109 (314).

CARBONELL, Diego

1938— Parasitología en Venezuela y los trabajos del Dr. Núñez Tovar. Caracas. Lit. Tip. Comercio (315).

CORTES, Bastidas J.M.

1949— Absorción de vitamina ''A'' en sujetos parasitados. Rev. Pol. Caracas. Vol.

XVIII. Núms. 107-108-109, p. 129 (316).

COVA GARCIA, Pablo

1946— Nota sobre los anofelinos en Venezuela y su identificación. Com. San. Pan. Cuaderno amarillo N° 1 (317).

1951— Distribución geográfica y datos bionómicos de los anofelinos en Venezuela. M.S.A.S. (318).

CAMPINS y COLS, Humberto

1955— Estudio de una epidemia de Histoplasmosis en el Estado Lara. Gac. Méd. de Caracas. Año LXII. N° 34 (319).

"Examen de exudado rectal mediante el raspado de las mucosas en las enfermedades recto-cólicas". Colmenares Yépez Francisco. Gen. Vol. I. Enero, Febrero y Marzo N° 3 (320).

COVA GARCIA, P.

1938— Penetración y dispersión en Venezuela de las especies Anopheles (Nyssorhynchus) darlingi y Anopheles (Nyssorhynchus) albimanus. Rev. San. Asist. Soc. 8: 467-472 (321).

1948— Distribución geográfica y datos bionómicos de A. albimanus, uno de los principales vectores de la malaria en Venezuela. Arch. Venez. de Patolog. Trop. y Paras. Med. 1 (I): 1-13 (322).

1950— Introducción al estudio de los Insectos. Pub. de la Div. de Malariología. N° 9, pp. 1-141 (323).

1950— Introducción al Estudio de los Insectos. Pub. Div. Malariol. Pub. N° 9: 1-141 (324).

1953— Llave para la Clasificación de los Dípteros más Comunes en Venezuela. II Congreso de Ciencias Naturales y Afines. Pub. N° 9-5-61 (325).

1953— Estudio sobre la Morfología de la Mosca doméstica. Rev. San. y Asist. Soc. 18: 887-919 (326).

1955— Las Moscas, problema de Salud Pública. Conferencia leída en "La Sociedad Médica del Hospital Civil de Maracay". Mimeografiada (327).

CAMPINS H. y SCHARYJ

1953— Cromoblastomicosis. Gaceta Médica de Caracas, marzo a abril, N° 3 y 4 (328)

Corpúsculo calificados en Leishmaniasis tegumentaria americana (329).

El Polimorfismo clínico de las micosis de Lutz (330).

1950— Investigación de la sensibilidad cutánea a la histoplasmina en Venezuela. Arch. Vene. P. Trop. y Parsi. Médica. Enero del 50. Vol. II, N.L. (331).

CONVIT J. y MONTEMAYOR, Lorenzo

Hongos levuriformes (332).

CAMPINS, Humberto

1953— "Coccidioidomicosis pulmonar". Rev. San. Asist. Soc. XVIII, N° 1-2. Pág. 177 (333).

1953— "Histoplasmosis pulmonar". Rev. San. Asist. Soc. XVIII. Números 1-2. 185 (334).

Coccidiomicosis en Venezuela, relación del 2° caso estudiado.

Trab. presentado a la Jornada del Dermatológico. Gac. Méd. Car. 57. 229-238, 1940 (335).

1949— "Coccidiomicosis, un nuevo problema de salud pública en Venezuela". Imprenta del Edo. Lara. Rev. San. Asist. Soc. 15: 18 Enero-abril de 1950 (336).

CAMPINS H., SCHARYJ M., y GLUCK, V.

Coccidioidomicosis (Enfermedad de Posadas), su comprobación en Venezuela". Arch. Pat. Trop. Parasit. Méd. 1 (2) 215-233 (337).

CHACIN, Miguel

1931— Informe que presenta el Médico de Sanidad del Estado Aragua como Relator de la II Conf. Sanit. Nac., cuyo tema en "El Paludismo en Venezuela". Caracas. Tip. Americana y en la Memoria de dicha Conferencia. Págs. 105-109 (338).

CHACIN ITRIAGO, Luis Gregorio

1927— Campaña contra los mosquitos en la ciudad de Caracas. Trabajo presentado a la VIII Conferencia Sanitaria Panamericana reunida en Lima, 1927. Caracas. Tip. Americana, 8 p. (339).

CHACIN ITRIAGO, L.G. y BELLO, Carlos J.

1927— Clasificación de las ratas de Caracas. Gac. Méd. de Car. XXXIV. 21, 325-327, y en folletos. (Trabajo presentado a la VIII Conferencia Sanitaria Panamericana). Caracas. Tip. Americana, 8 p. (340).

CHACIN ITRIAGO, Luis Gregorio

1927— Clasificación de las pulgas que contienen las ratas de Caracas. Gac. Méd. de Car. XXXIV, 21, 327-328 (341).

1927a— Campaña contra el mosquito en 1926. Informe presentado por el Director de Sanidad Nacional al Ejecutivo Federal por órgano del Ministerio de Relaciones Interiores. Caracas. Lit. del Comercio (342).

1927b— Campaña contra el mosquito en 1927. Informe presentado por el Director de Sanidad Nacional al Ejecutivo Federal por órgano del Ministerio de Relaciones Interiores. Caracas. Lit. del Comercio (343).

CHACIN NUÑEZ, Sixto E.

1940— Localizaciones mucosas de la Leishmania tropical (Var. brasilensis) en Venezuela. Tesis de Doctorado en Ciencias Médicas. Caracas, 31 p. (344).

CHACON, Eulogio

1930— La Anquilostomiasis en el Estado Apure. Presentado en calidad de Relator Oficial a la Primera Conferencia Sanitaria Nacional. Memoria de dicha Conferencia. Págs. 41-73 (345).

1931— El Paludismo en el Estado Apure, presentado en calidad de Relator. Memorias de la II Conferencia Sanitaria Nacional. Páginas 49-104 y en follero (346).

1934— Informe sobre la epidemia de paludismo en Margarita. Bol. Ministerial Salb. Agric. y Cría. II, 16, 297-240 (347).

CHACON, Ramón Ignacio

1933a— La fiebre recurrente en el Estado Táchira. Bol. Minist. Salb. Agric. Cría. I, 3, 243-245 (348).

1934— La Buba en el Estado Táchira. Bol. Minist. Salub. Agri. Cría. Págs. 382-384 (349).

CHAUMER, Edmundo

1926— Patología tropical (extracto de un estudio sobre paludismo). Caracas. Tip. Americana 16 p. (350).

CHAVARRIA CH., Manuel

1950— Fasciola hepática. Aparato reproductivo femenino. Rev. de V. de Vet. y Paras. Pág. 69 (351).

DAO L., Luis

1939— Planorbis guadaloupensis (Australorbis glabratus). Tesis de Bachillerato en Filosofía. Caracas. Coop. de Artes Gráficas. 15 páginas (352).

1943— Sobre un caso de hepato-explenomegalia palúdica gigante provocando síndrome de compresión intestinal. Bol. de los Hosp. XLII, 1-2, 26-34 (353).

1943a— Observaciones sobre paludismo congénito. Arch. Ven. de Pueric. y Pediat. V. 17-18, 1002-1005 (354).

1944— La punción esplénica como medio de diagnóstico en un caso de enfermedad de Chagas. Bol. de los Hosp. XLII, 1, 10-17 (355).

1944a— Paludismo pernicioso de la infancia. Arch. Ven. de Pueric. y Pediat. VI, 20-21, 1081-1100 (356).

1944b— Muertes súbitas en la enfermedad de Chagas. Bol. de los Hospitales. Caracas. XVIII, 6, 303 (357).

1944c— Resultados clínicos obtenidos con el Mafarside en el tratamiento del paludismo. Rev. de la Poli. Car. XIII, 78-339-349 (358).

DAO, h., Miguel

1941— Filariasis de Bancrofti en la Ciudad de Puerto Cabello y alrededores. Rev. Sa. Asist. Soc. VI, 3, 336-401 (359).

1941a— Experimentos quimioterapéuticos con guanidinas y amidinas en infecciones tripanosomiásicas. Rev. San. Asist. Soc. VI, 3, 402-424 (360).

BRICEÑO IRRAGORRY, L., DAO y RODRIGUEZ CABRERA

1943— Asociación tifo-malaria. Gac. Méd. de Car. L., 15 159 (361).

PRISCO J. y D'ARAGO FLORES R.

1940— ¿Hepatitis tífica o amibiana? Rev. S.EM. 68-70, 28-33 (262).

D'ASCOLI, Domingo

1940— Contribución al estudio clínico de nuestras parasitosis. Tesis de Doctorado en Ciencias Médicas. Caracas. Emp. El Cojo, 19 p. (363).

DAVILA CELIS, Eloy

1934— El proceso cirrógeno en el paludismo. Contribución a su estudio clínico y patogénico. Tesis de Doctorado en Ciencias Médicas. Caracas. Tip. Casa de Especialidades. 30 p. (364).

DELGADO BLANCO, J. MIR, L. Y TORRES GRATEROL P.

1941— Valor comparativo de las reacciones luéticas en el líquido cefaloraquídeo. Arch. Ven. de O.R.I. Oftalm. Neurol. II 4, 186-190 (365).

DELGADO PALACIOS, Guillermo

Progreso y paludismo. Bol. del Minist. de Fomento. Vol. I, N° 3. Pág. 163 (366).

D;EMPAIRE, Adolfo

1926a— Sobre un caso de actinomicosis pleuropulmonar. Rev. La Benf. Jnio (367).

1928b— Ataque de paludismo que simula una perforación gástrica. Rev. La Benef. Junio. Rev. de la Soc. Méd-Quirúrg. del Zulia, II, 18, 232-234 (368).

1928c— Arteritis cerebral sifilítica. Rev. de la Soc. Méd.-Quirúrgica del Zulia. II, 23, 301-303 (369).

1931— Un caso de fiebre recurrente. Nota clínica. Rev. La Benef. Julio. Rev. de la Soc. Méd.-Quirúrg. del Zulia. V, 3, 29-32 (370).

RIVERO, Luis y DIAZ, Fermín

1928— Sobre esplenomegalia micósica. Rev. de Medic. y Cirug. Caracas. XI, 114, 340-344 (371).

1928a— Esplenectomía por esplenomegalia probablemente de naturaleza micósica. Rev. de Medic. y Cirug. Caracas. XI, 114, 265-273 (372).

DIAZ GUZMAN, J. Alberto

1941— Sífilis pulmonar. Tesis de Doctorado en Ciencias Médicas. Publicada en la Rev. S.E.M. VII, 73-76, 4-54 (373).

DIAZ RUMERO, Isaac

1938a— El paludismo y la serie blanca. Tesis de Doctorado en Ciencias Médicas. Caracas. Tip. Universal. 31 p. (374).

DIAZ SAMANIEGO, Francisco

1936— El método sifilimétrico de Vernes. Tesis de Doctorado en Ciencias Médicas. Caracas. Edit. Athenea (375).

DIEZ DEL CIERVO, Carlos

1933b— El peligro del zancudo y la manera de conjurario. Gac. Médica de Caracas. XL, 22-23 y 24 (376).

1934— Ofidismo en Venezuela. Trabajo presentado a la IX Conferencia Sanit. Panamericana. Buenos Aires. Actas generales de dicha Conferencia. Pág. 516 (377).

DIVISION DE MALARIOLOGIA, M.S.A.S.

1938— Primer informe anual (1937) de la División de Malariología. Publicaciones de la División de Malariología. 1 (378).

1939— Segundo informe anual (1938) de la División de Malariología. Publicaciones de la División N° 4 y en el Bol. Minist. San. Asist. Soc. IV, 4, 3-190 (379).

1939a— La colaboración de los pueblos y caseríos en la lucha antimalárica. Rev. S.A.S.

de Educ. San. II, 52, 6-9 (380).

DIVISION DE VENEREOLOGIA, M.S.A.S.

1941— ¿Qué es la sífilis? Rev. S.A.S. de Educ. San. V, 74, 11-13 (381).

DOMINICI, Santos Aníbal

1943a— De las esquistosomosis hominales y en especial de la bilharziosis americana. Caracas. Escuela Técnica Industrial. Talleres de Artes Gráficas. 219 p. (382).

DOMINGUEZ GALLEGOS, A.

1938— Contribución al estudio clínico del paludismo agudo en Venezuela. Tesis Doctorado en Ciencias Médicas. Caracas. Taller Gráfico. 30 p. (388).

1938a— Algunos datos estadísticos de las aortitis sifilíticas. Rev. S.E.M. IV, 38, 17-21 (384).

DOMINGUEZ GALLEGO, A., y MARRERO, C.

1941— Un caso de Creeping Disease. Rev. de la Poli. Car. X, 60, 347-348 (385).

DOMINGUEZ SISCO, Rafael

1939— Profilaxia y tratamiento de la heredosífilis. Bol. del Minist. San. Asist. Soc. IV, 2, 74-81 (386).

1940— Sífilis reciente y embarazo. Arch. Ven. de Pueric. y Pedia. II, 5, 266-269 (387).

DOMINGUEZ SISCO, R. y MENDOZA ESPIRITU SANTOS

1941— Indice de sífilis prenatal sobre 400 observaciones practicadas en la Maternidad Municipal "Concepción Palacios". Rev. de Obst. y Ginec. I, 4, 183-193 (388).

DOMINGUEZ SISCO, Rafael

1943— Breve comunicación sobre el resultado de la reacción de Kahn con sangre del cordón umbilical de niños cuyas madres han padecido buba. Primera Jornada Venezolana de Venereología y Dermatología. Rev. San. Asist. Soc. VIII, 5, 897-898 (389).

DYAR, H.G. y NUÑEZ TOVAR, M.

1927— Notas sobre nuevos dípteros hematófagos de Venezuela. (Culicidae). Maracay. Oct., 8 p. (390).

1928— Descriptions of new species of Mosquitoes from Venezuela Amer. J. Hyg. 8 N° 1, pp. 89-92 (391).

DOMINICI, Santos A.

1946— Revista de las fiebres con relación a Venezuela. Las fiebres autóctonas: 1° fiebre palúdica. Gac. Méd. Caracas. Año LIV, Números 19-24 (392).

DAO, Luis

1945— La enfermedad de Chagas en el Distrito Aragua (Edo. Anzoátegui). Rev. Pol. Caracas. Vol. XIV, N° 84 (393).

1949— Otros casos de enfermedad de Chagas en el Estado Guárico (Venezuela). Rev. Pol. Caracas. Vol. XVIII. Nums. 104-105-106, p. 17 (394).

1950— Miasis humana en Venezuela. Contribución al estudio de las miasis cutáneas. Dermatobia hominis. Rev. Pol. Caracas. Vol. XVIII, N° 114 (395).

DRAYER, A.

1949— Consideraciones sobre la etiología chagásica de nuestras miocarditis crónicas. Rev. Pol. Caracas. Vol. XVIII. Núms. 107-108-109 (396).

DRAYER, A. y CARBONELL, Luis

1947— Acerca de algunos hallazgos parasitológicos importantes en la región de Baruta. Bol. del Centro Estudiantil. Año I, N° 3 (397).

BORELLI, Dante

1953— Nota técnica sobre el cultivo en lámina de los hongos frágiles. Rev. Pol. Caracas. N° 131 (398).

DIAZ UNGRIA, Carlos y VERGANI, Franco

1951— Contribución al estudio de la Estrongilosis del ciego en equinos de Venezuela. N° 2, 19 Diciembre. Boletín de I, Veteri. (399).

1952— Contribución al conocimiento del género Triodontolus (Nematoda) en los equinos de Venezuela. Boletín del Instituto de Investigaciones Veterinarias. Diciem-

bre. Vol. IV, N° 20 (400).
1954— Nota previa sobre foco filariano entre los indios uniquinas del Delta del Orinoco. Novedades Científicas, 1954, serie zoológica Número 15 (401).

DIEZ, Augusto
1951— Paracoccidiosis esplénica primitiva. Bol. Soc. Ven. de Cirug. IV, 25, 135-142. 1359.

EICHELBAUM, H.R.
1937b— Tropical Mycoses of the foot and hand. A synopsis. Cli. Arch. of Gulf Hosp. Maracaibo. January 15 (402).

ESPIN, José
1941— La sustancia metaplasmática en los nódulos producidos por Schistosoma mansoni. Rev. de la Pol. Car. X, 57, 73-90 (403).
1941a— Mielitis producida por huevos de Schistosoma mansoni. Rev. de la Pol. Car. X, 59, 245-259 (404).
1941b— Hallazgo de corpúsculos semejantes a los de Negri, en un caso de mielitis bilharziana. Rev. de la Pol. Car. X, 60, 327-336 (405).

ESPINOZA, Miguel
1933— Generalidades sobre el Paludismo en el Delta del Orinoco. Bol. Minist. Salub. Agric. Cría, I, 4-6, 367-369 (406).

FERNANDEZ, Alberto
1931— Tripanosomiasis de los bovídeos de Venezuela. Gac. Méd. Pol. Car. I, 1, 31-34 (407).
1931a— Anaplasmosis en el ganado vacuno. Gac. Méd. de Caracas. XXXVII, 3, 34-35 (408).

FERNANDEZ, Alberto J. y VOGELSANG, Enrique G.
1935— Contribución al estudio de la parasitología animal en Venezuela. Rev. de la Pol. Car. 22, 1472-1478 en folleto. Lit. y Tip. del Comercio, 9 p. (409).

FERNANDEZ, Alberto
1935— Notas prácticas sobre tratamiento del paludismo. Rev. de la Pol. Car. 23, 1553-1558 (410).
1956— Puntos de vista de la profilaxia química del paludismo. "El Heraldo". Caracas. N° 4.135. Febrero, 26 (411).
1936a— Proyecto de saneamiento de la región de Ortiz. Diar. "El Heraldo". Caracas. N° 4.181. Marzo 25 (412).
1937a— Tratamiento del Paludismo. Bol. Minist. San. Asit. Soc. I, 19-20. 1207-1222 (413).
1937b— Curso de Malariología: Lecciones orales dictadas por el Doctor A.J. Fernández, Director de la Escuela de Malariología de Caracas, de marzo a junio de 1937. Caracas. 44 p. ilust. (414).
1939— Fiebre biliosa hemoglobinúrica. Lección en la Cátedra de Patología Tropical de la Universidad Central de Venezuela. Gac. Méd. de Car. XLVI, 2, 21-23 y en N° 1. Págs. 10-12 (415).

FERRER VIERA, Miguel
1933— Algo sobre fiebre biliosa hemoglobinúrica. Bol. Minist. Salubridad Agric. Cría. I, 4-6, 396-401 (416).

FERRO, Raúl
1943— Contribución al estudio de la paracoccidioidosis brasilensis en Venezuela. Tesis de Doctorado en Ciencias Médicas. Caracas (417).

FIGARELLA, Jacinto
1933— Un caso de fiebre biliosa hemoglobinúrica tratado con el suero antivenenoso. Bol. Minist. Salub. Agri. Cría. I, 2, 111-114 (418).

FLORES, Manuel Felipe
1930— La anquilostomosis en Cd. Bolívar. Memoria de la Conferencia San. Nac. 1, 7, 195-199 (419).

1930a— Estudio de la anquilostomiasis en Cd. Bolívar. Memoria de la Conferencia Sanitaria Nacional de 1930. Págs. 126-135 (420).

1930b— El paludismo en cirugía. Gac. Méd. de Cd. Bolívar. XVI, 113, 38-43 (421).

FLORES CHACIN, Guillermo

1941— Algunas consideraciones sobre el tratamiento de las anemias (Nécator). Arch. Ven. de Pueric. y Pediat. III, 10, 575-587 (422).

FRANGACHAN, hijo, Carlos

1930— Información del Médico de Sanidad de los Distritos Piar y Roscío del Edo. Bolívar, a la Conferencia San. Nac., sobre las condiciones y grado de infección de la Anquilostomiasis en los mencionados Distritos. Memoria de la Conferencia San. Nac. de 1930. Págs. 136-144 (423).

FRANCO PALACIOS, Miguel

1945— Kala azar infantil en el Estado Carabobo. Rev. Policlínica. Caracas. XVI, 85, pp. 526-531 (424).

FIASSON R., y PIFANO F.

1948— La cariacou (odocoileus gymnotis) porteur de trypanosoma vivax au Venezuela. Bull Soc. de Path. Exot (425).

FUENTEMAYOR, G.F.

1940— Necator Americanus. Tesis Doctoral. Febrero (426).

GABALDON, Arnoldo

1928— Estudios sobre Herpetomonas muscarum. Tesis de Bachillerato. Tip. Americana. Caracas. 17 pp. y en 1929 en la Gac. Méd. de Caracas. XXXVI, p. 10 (427).

1929— Nota sobre el desarrollo "in vitro" del "Chilomastix" mesnili. Gac. Méd. de Caracas. N° extraordinario. Pág. 77 (428).

1930— Nota sobre distribución de protozoos intestinales basada en el examen de 2.000 muestras. Tesis de Doctorado. Tip. Americana. Caracas. 44 p. (429).

1930a— Nota histórica sobre los protozoos señalados en Venezuela de la Gac. Méd. de Caracas. XXXVII, 9, 131-140. Caracas. Tip. Americana, 33 p. (430).

1932— Notas de Viaje. El Curso de Malariología (1931) del Instituto para enfermedades navales y tropicales de Hamburgo y los trabajos antipalúdicos de la estación experimental para la lucha antimalárica de Roma. Exto. de la Gac. Méd. de Caracas, XXXIX, 12 Caracas. Tip. Americana. 40 p. (431).

VOGEL, Hans y GABALDON, Arnoldo

1933— Vestibulosetaria, un nuevo género de filarideos de las ratas. Exto. de la Gac. Méd. de Caracas XL, 3, 39, 43 (432).

GABALDON, Arnoldo

1933— Nota sobre hábitos diurnos, temperaturas de yacimientos larvários y yacimientos larvários artificiales de "anopheles" de Venezuela. Exto. de la Gac. Méd. de Caracas. XL, 5, 72-75 (433).

1933c— Ancylostomiasis y su anemia. Presentación del tratamiento de 15 casos. Exto. de la Gac. Méd. de Caracas. XL, 17, 237-245 (434).

1935— Mollienisia caucana (Steindachner) a larvivorous topminnow from Venezuela. Reprinted from The Journal of Parasitology. August, 1935. Vol. XXI, N° 4 (435).

1935— Balantidium coli: quantitative studies in experimental infections and variations in infectiousness for rats. Reprinted from The Journal of Parasitology. October 1935. Vol. XXI, N° 5. 386-392 (436).

1935b— Balantidium coli, effects of increasisng the viscosity and crytalloid contents of the intestine of an experimental host on the density of infection. Reprinted from The Journal of Parasitology. December, 1935, Vol. 21, N° 6, pages 454-455 (437).

1935c— Experimental lesions caused by trichomonas columbae in the chicken. Reprinted from The Journal of Parasitology. December 1935, Vol. XXI, N° 6. Page 451 (438).

1936a— Carbarsone, its action on the intestinal trichomonads of rats in vivo. Reprinted from The American Journal of Tropical Medicine. Vol. XVI, N° 5. Sep. 1936 (439).

1938— Primer informe anual de la División de Malariología. Public. de la Div. de Malar. M.S.A.S. N° 1, 197 p. (440).

1938a— An Anopheles mattogrossensis from Venezuela with description of the male. Reprinted from The American Journal of Tropical Medicine. Vol. XIX, N° 5. September, 1939. 457-460 (441).

1939— Segundo informe anual (1939) de la División de Malariología Public. de la Div. de Malar. N° 4 M.S.A.S. 184 p. (442).

1939a— Generalidades sobre la Malaria y organización de la lucha antimalárica en Venezuela. Separata del Bol. del Minist. de San. y Asit. Social. IV, 1, 69-76 (443).

1939b— A Method for mounting anopheline eggs. Reprinted from The Journal of Parasitology, June 1939. Vol. 25. N° 3, page 281 (444).

1940— Descripción de Anopheles (Nyssorhynchus) muñeztovari, n. sp. y Consideraciones sobre una sub-división del grupo Nyssorhynchus (Diptera, Culicidae). Public. de la Div. de Malar. N° 5. M.S.A.S., págs. 3-7 (445).

GABALDON, Arnoldo, COVE-GARCIA, Pablo y LOPEZ, José Antonio

1940— Anopheles (Nyssorhynchus) rangeli, una nueva especie de la subserie oswaldoi (Diptera, Culicidae) de amplia distribución en Venezuela. Public. de la Div. de Malar. N° 5. págs. 9-23 (446).

GARBALDON, Arnoldo, COVA-GARCIA, Pablo y AREVALO, Amneris

1940— Observaciones sobre número de huevos, salinidad de criaderos y tiempo de desarollo de tres especies de la subserie oswaldoi, Public, de la Div. de Malar. N° 5. págs. 25-32 (447).

GABALDON, A., LOPEZ, J.A. y OCHOA PALACIOS, Manuel

1940— Variaciones curiosas de cuenta diarias de anofelinos en trampas-establos, Public. de la Div. de Malar. N° 5. págs. 33-39 (471).

GABALDON, A., OCHOA PALACIOS, M. y PEREZ VIVAS, M.A.

1940— Observaciones sobre lecturas de trampas-establos con cebo animal. Public. de la Div. de Malar. N° 5. Págs. 41-56 (472).

GABALDON, A., AGUILERA, Carmen

1940— Variaciones de color de las especies venezolanas de la subserie oswaldoi (Diptera, Culicidae). Public, de la Div. de Malar. N° 5. Páginas 63-82 (473).

GABALDON, Arnoldo y COVA-GARCIA, Pablo

1940— Nuevo tipo de clase para la identificación de las larvas de anofelinos venezolanos. Rev. Tij. Mal. III, 10, 78-86 (474).

GABALDON, Arnoldo, ROZEBOOM, Lloyd E.

1941— A summary of the "Tarsimaculatus" complex of anopheles (Diptera, Culicidae). Reprinted from The American Journal of Hygiene. Vol. XXXIII, N° 33, Sec. C, 88-100, May 1941 (475).

GABLADON, Arnoldo, COVA—GARCIA, Pablo y LOPEZ, José Antonio

1941— Anopheles (Nyssorhynchus) benarrochi, una nueva especie de la subserie Triannulatus. Public. de la Div. de Malar. N° 7. páginas 3-24 (476).

GABALDON, A., COVA-GARCIA, Pablo y LOPEZ, J.A.

1941— Anopheles (Arthuromya) vargasi, n. sp. y redescripción del subgénero. Arthuromyia Galvao, 1941. Publi. de la Div. de Malar. N° 7. págs. 25-26 (477).

GABALDON, A., AGUILERA, Carmen y AREVALO, Amneris

1941— Espinas basales y accesorias anormales en los hipopigios de Anopheles goeldii y Anopheles nuñeztovari. Public. de la Div. de Malar. N° 7. págs. 59-61 (478).

GABALDON, Arnoldo

1941— Métodos a seguir en las labores de entomología requerida en la lucha antimalárica. Rev. Tij. Mal. IV, 1, 2-42 (479).

GABALDON, Fabricio

1931— Estudio sobre tema paludismo en Venezuela por el Médico de Sanidad del Estado Trujillo, Dr. Fabricio Gabaldón. Memoria de la Conferencia Sanitaria Nacional de 1931. Págs. 321-356 (480).
1935— Moscas. Bol. Minist. Salub. Agric. Cría, II, 21, 861-863 (481).
1935a— Anquilostomos, divulgaciones a modo de conferencias a campesinos y analfabetas. Bol. Minist. Salub. Agric. Cría, III, 25, 26, 176-180 (482).

GALLO, Piero
1944— Estudios inmunológicos sobre tripanosoma venezuelensis. Rev. de la Poli. Car. XIII, 79, 407-414 (483).

GARCIA ALVAREZ, Julio
1927— Un caso de miasis del conducto auditivo. Bol. de los Hosp. Caracas. XVII (II Epoca), 9, 440-441 (484).
1934— Sífilis faringea. Rev. de la Poli. Car. 18, 1185, I. 186 (485).
1934c— Sífilis faringea. Rev. de la Poli. Car. 18, 1185-1186 (486).
1939b— El peligro de la sífilis. Rev. S.A. de Educ. San. II, 45, 2-5 (487).

GARCIA, G., MANUEL, A.
1936— Contribución al estudio de las parasitosis intestinales. Tesis Doctoral. Car. Tip. Standard. 20 p. (488).

GARCIA MALDONADO, Leopoldo
1927— Nuevas luces sobre el Paludismo. Rev. de la Soc. Méd.-Quirúrg. del Zulia. 1, 3, 35-39 (489).
1927a— Una nota inglesa sobre biliosa hemoglobinúrica. Rev. de la Soc. Méd.-Quirúrg. del Zulia. 1, 3, 40-41 (490).

GARCIA MALDONADO, Leopoldo
1928— Tratamiento de la balantidiosis. Rev. de la Soc. Méd.-Quirúrg. del Zulia. II, 24, 410-413 (491).
1929a— Paludismo terciario benigno y estovarsol. Rev. de la Soc. Méd.-Quirúrg. del Zulia, III, 12, 109-110 (492).
1931— Sindroma de hemogenia de origen palúdico. Rev. de la Soc. Méd.-Quirúrg. del Zulia. V, 6-7, 65-67 (493).
1932— Notas sobre la actual epidemia palúdica. Rev. de la Soc. Médica-Quirúgica del Zulia, VI, 1, 4-8 (494).
1932a— Reactivación de la sífilis y del paludismo con el Neosalvarsán. Rev. de la Soc. Méd.-Quirúrg. del Zulia. VI, 8, 100-101 (495).
1936— Catecismo venezolano del paludismo. Caracas. Tip. Americana 16 págs. (496).
1942— Sífilis congénita. Arch. Ven. de Pueric. y Pediat. IV, 14, 764-779 (497).
1930— La Anquilostomiasis en el Distrito Pto. Cabello. Memoria de la Conferencia Sanitaria Nacional de 1930. Págs. 151-160 (498).

GARRIDO, Héctor E.
1942— Sobre varios casos de forma atípica de paludismo. Evolución y pronóstico. Folleto. Maracay (499).

GENATIOS, Tomás
1939— Interpretación de la serología en la sífilis y fuera de ella. Revista S.E.M. VI, 47-55, 43-54 (500).
1940b— Reactivación de la serología en la sífilis "Método de Edmond Rajka". Tesis de Doctorado en Ciencias Médicas. Car. Talleres Biogen, 56 páginas (501).

GENATIOS, Tomás y SANCHEZ COVISA, J.
1943— La sífilis ósea (con motivo de una observación interesante). Primera Jornada Venezolana de Venereología y Dermatología. Rev. San. Asist. Soc. VIII, 5, 973-978 (502).

GOMEZ, hijo, Ramón
1931— Arteritis sifilíticas en el Hospital Vargas Tesis de Doctorado en Ciencias Médicas. Caracas. Lit. y Tip. Mercantil, 51 p. (503).
1934— Anotaciones sobre cinco casos de fiebre biliosa hemoglobinúrica. Rev. de la Soc.

Méd.-Quirúrg. del Zulia. VIII, 5, 351-358 (504).

1943— Breves notas sobre la hernia umbilical congénita. Presentación de un caso. Rev. de la Soc. Méd.-Quirúrg. del Zulia. XVII, 8, 2155-2157 (505).

GOMEZ LOPEZ, Luis y LUNA, Guillermo

1938— Primeros casos de quiste hidático del pulmón encontrados en Venezuela. Memoria del 1° Congreso Venezolano de la Tuberculosis. Páginas 573-576 (506).

GOMEZ MARCANO, A.

1942b— Bosquejo de anatomía patológica general de la malaria. Rev. Tij. Mal. V, 5, 100 (507).

1942c— Hematología patológica de la malaria. Rev. Tij. Mal. Caracas. VI, 2, 371 (508).

1942d— Fiebre tifoidea y malaria. Un caso de observación personal. Rev. Tij. Mal. VI, 3, 60 en (colab) (509).

GOMEZ MARCANO, A., y SUAREZ, Miguel

1943— Contribución al estudio de la infección oocística natural del A. darlingi y A. albimanus en Venezuela. Rev. Tij. Mal. VIII, 4, 150 (510).

GOMEZ ALFREDO G.

1941— Acerca del tratamiento de la parasitosis intestinal durante el embarazo, en el Servicio de Higiene Materno-Infantil de San Cristóbal; visitas a través de datos estadísticos. Octubre de 1939 a septiembre de 1941. Arch. Ven. de Pueric. y Pediat. IV, II, 606-610 (511).

GONZALEZ, Eudoro

1949— Sobre Leptospira icterohemorrhagiae. Comentarios al trabajo de la Dra. Pereira Alvarez. Gac. Méd. de Car. XLVI (512).

GONZALEZ, Eudoro

1943— Indice de trabajos de autores venezolanos aparecido en la Gac. Méd. de Car. de Enero 1939 a Marzo 1943 (513).

GONZALEZ, Felipe

1938— Sífilis y embarazo en la Maternidad del Instituto Municipal "Simón Rodríguez" de Caracas. Tesis de Doctorado en Ciencias Médicas. Caracas. Lit. y Tip. Casa de Especialidades. 50 páginas (514).

GONZALEZ, Gaspar

1933— De parasitosis intestinal. Rev. de la Soc. Méd.-Quirúrg. del Zulia. VII, 5, 213-217 (515).

GONZALEZ, Miguel

1936— Paludismo. Modo de hacer profilaxia en el hombre enfermo. Diario "EL Heraldo". Caracas, N° 4350, Octubre 1° (516).

1936a— Profilaxia del paludismo. Lucha contra el zancudo. Diario "El Heraldo". N° 4356. Octubre 8 (517).

1936— Proflaxia médica del paludismo. Diario "El Heraldo". Caracas. N° 4362. Octubre 15 (518).

GONZALEZ, Rafael Emilio

1938— Contribución al estudo clínico de la cirrosis bilharziana. Tesis de Doctorado. Caracas. Tip. Americana, 25 págs. (519).

GONZALEZ RINCONES, Rafael

1930g— Revista sobre Anquilostomosis. Memoria de la Conferencia Sanitaria Nacional de 1930. Págs. 392-399 (520).

1931b— Resumen del método usado en el Instituto de Medicina Tropical de Hamburgo para la diferenciación de las amibas. Rev. Poli. Car. I, a, 100-101 (521).

1931e— Consideraciones acerca del tratamiento de la fiebre hemoglobinúrica. Gac. Méd. de Car. XXXVIII, 9, 126-127 (522).

1939— Esquena evolutivo de la Dermatobia cyaniventris. Bol. de la Academia de Ciencias Físicas Matemáticas y Naturales, IV, 18, 103-107 (523).

1940— Posible diseminación a grandes distancias de los insectos trasmisores de la enfermedad de Chagas por el sistema de los paracaidistas. Gac. Méd. de Car. XLVIII,

10, 113 (524).
1941a— Nociones de parasitología. Apuntes para servir de texto de Curso de Primer Año en la Escuela Nacional de Enfermeras. Imprenta de la Lotería. Caracas. 87 págs. (525).
1942a— Historia abreviada de la Parasitología. Diario "El Universal". Diciembre 24 (526).
1943c— Formas de leishmania del Tripanosoma cruzi y diagnóstico de Kala-Azar. Gac. Méd. de Car. L, I, 2-3 (527).
1943g— Presencia en el Zulia del Anopheles pseudopuntipennis Theobald, 1901. Gac. Méd. de Car. L, 15, 158 (528).
1943i— Encuesta sobre Bilharziosis. La marca del caracol. Gac. Méd. de Caracas. L, 19, 209-210 (529).

GONZALEZ RODRIGUEZ, M.
1936— Los problemas de la profilaxis del paludismo. "El Heraldo". N° 4160. Marzo 4 (530).
1936b— Sugerencias para una campaña antipalúdica. "El Heraldo". N° 4250, Junio 4 (531).

GONZALEZ, V. Carlos Luis
1936— La Microrreacción coloreada de Ide en el diagnóstico de la sífilis. Tesis de Doctorado en Ciencias Médicas. Caracas. Tip. Universal, 62 p. (532).

GRATEROL y MORLES, J.
1930— Estudio sobre la Anquilostomiasis en Venezuela. Memoria de la Conferencia Sanitaria Nacional de 1930. Págs. 385-391 (533).
1931— Algunas apreciaciones sobre génesis del paludismo. Caracas. Tip. Americana (534).

GRANIER, Marcel
1940— Algunas observaciones acerca del estado de las funciones de nutrición en los sujetos parasitados por el Necator americanus. Tesis Doctoral. Caracas (535).

GUERRA, P., RAVAUT, P.
1933— Contribution á l'etude des reactions secondes de la peau. Pityriase versicolor géneralises. Réaction seconde de type lichénoide. Bull. Soc. Franc. Derm. el Syph. 6 juillet (536).

GUERRA, P., LANGERON, M.
1934— Nouvelles méthodes d'etude des champignons lévuriformes. Seme. Reum. Soc. Arg. de Patol. reg. del norte. Santiago del Estero 2 y 3 oct.1936. Buenos Aires, pág. 8105 (537).

GUERRA, Pablo
1935— Role des levures en Dermatologie. Thèse du doctorat. (Premiada en París) (538).

GUERRA, P., FLADIN, H., REBEAU
1936— Levurides desidrosiformes des intranains consécutives a mycose interdigito-plantaire a levures. Intradermo reactions. Bull. Soc. Franc. Derm. et Syph. pág. 462 (539).

GUERRA, P., LANGERON, M.
1938— Remarques sur la Candida stallaoidea (Jones et Martin 1938). Annales de parasitologie humaine et comparée. Tome XVII. N° 3 1er. Mai (540).
1938a— Nouvelles recherches de Zymologie médica. Annales de Parasitologie humaine et comparée. 1er. Janvier, 1938, 1er. Mars. 1938, 1er. sept. 1938, 1er. Nov. (541).
1939— Valeur et nature des variations et dissociations de colonies (542).
1940— Chez les champignons levuriformes. Annales de Parasitologie Humaine et comparée. Tomo XVII, 5 (543).
1939— Orientation de la filamentization des champignons levuriformes (544).
1940a— Cultives sur lames gélosées. Annales de Parasitologie humaine et comparée. Tomo XVII, N° 6 (545).

GUERRA, Pablo

1939— Notas sobre las Epidermicosis de la región caraqueña. Bol. de los Hosp. Caracas. Núms. 7 y 8. Págs. 245-256 (546).

1939a— La "Erosio Interdigitalis" hasta ahora atribuída a la Cándida albicans (Monilia albicans) es en realidad provocada por la asociación de ésta con el parásito del eritrasma. Bol. de los Hospitales. Caracas. Núms. 7 y 9, págs. 257-268 (547).

1940— El granuloma a paraccidioides. Su importancia en patología pulmonar. Primera Jornada Tisiológicas Nacionales. Rev. de San. y Asist. Soc. V, 4, 921-927 (548).

1940a— Un caso de amibiasis cutánea. Rev. de la Poli. Caracas. IX, 54, 3618-3630 (549).

GUERRA, Pablo, SANCHEZ COVISA, P.

1940— La Leishmaniosis tegumentaria en Venezuela. Rev. de la Poli. Car. IX, 54, 3573-3617 (550).

1941— Capilaritis necrosantes de origen sifilítico. Rev. de la Poli. Caracas. X, 59, 227-236 (551).

GUERRA FONSECA, Pedro

1936— Profilaxia antimalárica (552).

1937a— Identificación clínica y bacteri( )gica de la fiebre recurrente en Mérida (553).

1940c— Un caso de Lupoides miliares diseminados (554).

1941— Lecciones de Patología Tropical Venezolana (dactilografiado) (555).

1941a— Un caso de Lambliasis hepato-biliar (556).

GUERRA MENDEZ, Fernando

1935— Un remedio criollo contra la Solitaria. Conferencia en la Soc. de Estudiantes de Medicina. Rev. S.E.M., N° 10 (557).

1941— Obstrucción intestinal por Ascaris. Rev. Poli. Valencia, N° 1 (558).

1942— Absceso hepático amibiano. Folleto, Valencia. 8 págs. y en la Rev. Poli. Val. II, 5 (559).

GUERRA MENDEZ, Rafael

1929— El signo de Paniello en el Paludismo. Gac. Méd. de Caracas. XXXVI (560).

1934— Mosquiticidas. Gac. Méd. de Caracas. XLI (561).

GUEVARA, Francisco A.

1934— Algo sobre tricocefalosis. Bol. de los Hosp. Caracas. XXIII, 24, 110-112 (448).

1943— Anotaciones sobre carate. Rev. del Col. Méd. del Edo. Falcón. I, 1, 20-25 (449).

GUEVARA NUÑEZ, Pedro J.

1927— Un caso de cirrosis hepática ascitógena provocada por la Bilharzia. Rev. Méd. y Quirúrg. Caracas. XI, 102, 25-29 (450).

1934— A propósito de un caso de fiebre biliosa hemoglobinúrica. Bol. de los Hosp. XXIII, 24, 108-110 (451).

GUTFELD, F. J. von, y HENNINGSMEYER, H.

1944— La toma y envío de materiales para exámenes bacteriológicos, serológicos, parasitológicos e histológicos. Rev. S.EM. Caracas, XI, 111-118, 186-194 (452).

GUTIERREZ ALFARO, José J.

1942— Clase de Higiene Práctica (Curso dictado en la Universidad Central de Caracas en el curso 40-41). Cooperativa del Libro. F.E.V. (453).

1944a— Breves consideraciones sobre el cultivo en gasa del Penicilium notatum. Rev. Selecciones Médicas. Caracas. Juli. Págs. 3-5 (454).

1944b— Tricomonas intestinales en pus obtenido por punción toráxica. Rev. Selecciones Médicas. Caracas. Octubre. N° 5 (455).

GONZALEZ RINCONES, Rafael

1941— Nociones de parasitología. Apuntes para servir de texto de Curso de primer año en la Escuela Nacional de Enfermeras. 10-R-G. (456).

1942— Historia abreviada de la Parasitología. Diario "El Universal". Diciembre 24 (457).

1945— A propósito de Bilharzia. Gac. Méd. de Caracas. Año LII. Número 8 (458).

1946— Juicio sobre el trabajo del Dr. David R. Iriarte a la Aca. Nac. de Med. (459).

GABALDON, Arnoldo

1948— De la campaña antimalárica en Venezuela. Rev. S.A.S. Vol. XII. Nº 34 (460).

GAVALLER, Bela de

1950— Toxoplasmosis humana en Venezuela. Presentación de los tres primeros casos congénitos. Arch. Ven. Pat. Trop. Part. Méd. II (1). 265-296 (461).

1951— Algunas consideraciones sobre el primer caso de toxoplasmosis humano comprobado en Venezuela. Bol. de la Mat. Conc. Pal. 2 (3): 43-47 (462).

GARCIA DIAZ, J.

1954— Primer caso publicado en Venezuela. Rev. Soc. Méd. Quirúrg. del Zulia. Año XXVIII. Nº 3 (463).

GABALDON, A.

1933— Presentación de un método para la medición de hepatomegalias. Gac. Méd. de Caracas, 40, 219-220 (464).

1939— De cómo verificar el "Informe sobre condiciones sanitarias de una población". Tij. s. mal. 2: 25-30 (465).

GABALDON A. & BENARROCH, E.I.

1940— Consideraciones sobre el paludismo en Venezuela. Actas IV. Conferencia Panam. Dir. Nac. San. Públ. Nº 192. Of. San. Panam. págs. 181-191 (466).

GABALDON, A.

1945— Adaptability of control measures to regional problems. Neotropical region. Typescriot to Dr. Boyd's book. págs. 1-56 (467).

1945— Métodos estadísticos aplicados en malariología. I. La biometría de la población humana. Tij. s. mal. 9 (2): 26-48 (468).

1945— Métodos estadísticos empleados en malariología. III. La malariologías: Tij. s. mal. 9 (3): 55-86 (469).

1945— Métodos estadísticos empleados en malariología. IV. La selección de muestras. Tij. s. mal. 9 (4): 101-132 (470).

GABALDON, A.

1946— Mortalidad por malaria en Venezuela. I Bases estadísticas y distribución geográficas. Tij. s. mal. 10 (4): 191-237 (562).

GABALDON, A. & GOVA GARCIA

1946— Zoogeografía de los anofelinos en Venezuela: I. Los dos vectores principales. Tij. s. mal. 10 (1): 19-32 (563).

1946— Zoogeografía de los anofelinos en Venezuela: II. Los vectores secundarios y los no vectores. Tij. s. mal. 10 (2): 78-127 (564).

1946— Zoogeografía de los anofelinos en Venezuela: III. Relacciones con el terreno y el clima. Tij. s. mal. 10 (3): 164-179 (565).

GABALDON, A.

1946— Las razones de endemicidad y de epidemicidad: dos nuevas medidas de interés malariométrico. Tij. s. mal. 10 (3):156-160 (566).

1946— Sinopsis aconsejable en la redacción de encuestas malariométricas en Venezuela. Tij. s. mal. 10 (3): 137-148 (567).

1948— The malaria problem in the neotropical region. Proc. 4th. Internat. Congr. Trop. Méd. & Malaria. 1º Ed. págs. 913-931 (568).

1949— Conquistas de la Campaña Antimalárica en Venezuela. Tip. Vargas, Caracas. Págs. 5-30 (569).

1949— Malaria Control in the Neotropi región. Malariology. 2: 1400-1415 (570).

1949— Malaria incedence in the West Indies and South America. "Malariology". 2: 764-787 (571).

1949— The Nation-Wide Campaign against Malaria in Venezuela. Roy Soc. Méd. & Hyg. págs. 113-164 (572).

1952— The effect of DDT on the population of Anopheline vectors in Venezuela. Riv. di Parasitol. 13 (1): 29-41 (573).

1951— Progress of the malaria campaign in Venezuela. Jl. Nat. Mal. Soc. 10: 124-141 (574).

1952— Consideraciones sobre el futuro de la Lucha Antimalárica. Rev. Malariol. e D. Trop., 4: 307-318 (575).

GABALDON, A.

1953— Vector control for Malaria control. (Trabajo presentado en el V. Congreso Internacional de Medicina Tropical y Malaria, Estambul, Turquía). 28 agosto-4 septiembre (576).

1953— Importancia de la mortalidad sin diagnóstico médico en los datos bioestadísticos referentes a la malaria en Venezuela. Bol. Of. San. Panam. 35: 1-10 (577).

GABLADON, A. & BERTI, A.L.

1954— The first large area in the tropical zone to report malaria eradication: North-Central Venezuela. Am. Jl. Trop. Med. & Hyg., 3: 793-807 (578).

GABALDON, A.

1955— Enseñanza para la acción sanitaria en la América Latina derivadas de la lucha antimalárica en Venezuela. Bol. Of. San. Panam: 38: 259-265 (579).

GOMEZ MARCANO, A. & CAPRILES, A.

1944— Esplenomegalia y Parasitemia en la Malaria. Tij. s. mal. 8, (6): 1-10 (580).

GOMEZ MARCANO, A.

1954— Anatomía patológica en la malaria del bazo, hígado y médula ósea. Curso de Malariol. Págs. 1-31 (581).

1945— Anatomía patológica en la malaria, del cerebro, corazón, pulmones, riñón, ganglios linfáticos, páncreas, suprarrenales, estómago, intestino y piel. Curso de Malariol, págs. 1-17 (582).

1946— Malaria y placenta. Curso de Malariol (583).

1948— Infección oocística natural de los anofelinos de Venezuela. Arch. Ven. de Pat. Trop. y Paras. Méd. 1 (1): 1-7 (584).

1950— Quimioterapia general y especial de antimaláricos. Curso de Malariología (585).

1950— Paludrina (Cloroguanida). Farmacología general y aplicación terapéutica en la malaria. Curso de Malariología (586).

1950— Quinina. Farmacología general y aplicación terapéutica en la malaria. Curso de Mal. (587).

1950— Crinacrina: Farmacología general y aplicación terapéutica en la malaria. Curso de Malariología (589).

1950— Cloriquina: Farmacología general y aplicación terapéutica en la malaria. Curso de Malariología (590).

GAVALLER, Bela

Hallazgo anatomopatológico en la sífilis congénita (591).

GALLO, P. y VOGELSANG, E.

1951— La anemia infecciosa de los equinos en Venezuela. Observaciones y estudios experimentales. Vol. II, N° 1 y 4, diciembre. Revista de Medicina Veterinaria y Parasitología (592).

GUERRERO, P.R.A.

1951— Primer caso de Oncocercosis Humana diagnosticado clínicamente en Caracas y proveniente de una probable nueva zona endémica. Gac. Méd. de Caracas. 59-41-53 (1359).

HASE, Albrecht

1931— Resultado de algunas investigaciones parasitológicas en Venezuela. Lit. y Tip. Vargas. Caracas, 19 págs (593).

HEDDERICH ARISMENDI, Henrique

1937— La disentería amibiana, mal endémico en Paraguaná, Estado Falcón. Bol. Minist. San. Asist. Soc. Págs. 1081-1083 (594).

HECHT, Otto

1942— Las pulgas de las ratas en Venezuela. Rev. San. Asit. Soc. VII, 6, 811 (595).

1943a— Las reacciones de la piel contra las picaduras de insectos como fenómeno alérgico. Rev. San. Aist. Sonc. VIII, 4, 545 (597).

1943b— Son todas las reacciones cutáneas contra las picaduras de insectos, chupadores de sangre, manifestaciones alérgicas? Rev. San. Aist. Soc. VIII, 6, 1151 (598).
1943c— Consideraciones entomológicas a la epidemiología de la peste bubónica de los roedores en Venezuela. Rev. San. Asist. Soc. VIII, 6, 1159 (599).
1943d— Algunos consejos técnicos para la cría de pulgas. Rev. San. Asist. Soc. VIII, 6, 1.163 (600).

HERNANDEZ CAMEJO, J.R.
1938a— Hombres y hechos que han contribuído al progreso de la Medicina en Venezuela. Tesis de Doctorado en Ciencias Médicas. Caracas. Coop. de Artes Gráficas. 24 págs. (601).

HERNANDEZ d'EMPAIRE, J.R.
1932— Sindrome hemorrágico en un palúdico. Rev. de la Soc. Méd. Quirúrg. del Zuliz. VI, 1, 34 (602).
1935— Obstrucción intestinal causada por áscaris. Rev. de la Soc. Méd-Quirúrg. del Zuliz. IX, 9, 539-547 y en la Gac. Medic. de Car. XLII (603).

HERNANDEZ, Ramón
1928— El treparsol en la amibiasis crónica. Tesis de Doctorado en Ciencias Médicas. Caracas. Tip. Colón, 43 págs. (604).

HERNANDEZ RODRIGUEZ, Rafael
1935— La Bilharziosis intestinal y sus formas clínicas en San Casimiro. Rev. Méd. II, 7, 385-392 (605).
1937— ¿Espiroquetosis icterohemorrágica? Rev. Mundo Méd. 1, 2, 12-24 (606).
1939— Sindrome Espleno-Hepático. ¿Bilharziano o Palúdico? Rev. Mundo Méd. Ven. II, 5, 14-25 (607).
1939b— Diagnóstico clínico de la Bilharziosis hepato-intestinal. Rev. Car. Méd. VI, 12, 685-708 (608).

HERRERA GUERRERO, Francisco
1930— Informe del Médico de Sanidad de Los Teques sobre Anquilostomiasis. Memoria de la Conferencia Sanitaria Nacional de 1930. Págs. 237-243 (609).

HERRERA PINTO, Adolfo
1937— Trabajos de la Dirección de Malariología. Bol. Minist. San. Asist. Soc. Págs. 982-985 (610).

HILL, R.B.
1928— El paludismo en Venezuela. Gac. Méd. de Car. XXXV, 23, 353-359 (611).

HILL, R.B. y TEJERA, Enrique
1933— Esquistosomiasis en el Rincón de El Valle (Venezuela). Medicina de los Países Cálidos. 6, 450-454 (612).

HILL, R.B. y BENARROCH, E.I.
1940— Anquilostomiasis y Paludismo en Venezuela. Editorial Elite. Caracas. I Vol. 104 págs. (613).

HUNCAL, Fernando
1940— Necesidad del control serológico sistemático en los casos de exámenes ultramicroscópicos negativos o de solo Ducrey positivo. Tesis de Doctorado en Ciencias Médicas. Caracas. Tip. Cosmos. 47 págs. (614).

HERNANDEZ P., Otto
1955— Nuevo foco filarino comprobado en Venezuela entre indios del Territorio Federal Delta Amacuro. Gac. Méd. Caracas. Año LXIII. Núms 1-2 (616).

HOMEZ, Jorge
1954— La dermatitis verminosa serpiginosa (Creeping disease). Rev. Soc. Méd. Quirúrg. Año XXVIII, N° 7 (617).

HOMEZ, Jorge, FERNANDEZ, Carroz y MASO DOMINGUEZ
1954— Diez casos de cromoblastomicosis de los Estados Zulia y Falcón. Rev. Soc. Méd. Quirurg., Zulia. Añp XXVIII. N° 5 (618).

HERNANDEZ GOMEZ, J.G.

Nuevas consideraciones sobre el sindrome febril íctero-hemoglobinúrico. Barcelona (S.P.I.) (619).

HERRERA, J.R.

1943— Nota sobre la inmunidad en la infección palúdica. Pub. Health & Med. 3, 341-346 (620).

1940— Estudios sobre el paludismo en la Rep. de Guatemala. Bol. de la Direc. Gen. de San. Pub., págs. 43-206 (621).

HOMEZ, J.

Contribución al estudio de la dermatitis rampante en Venezuela (622).

HARTZ, P.H.

1954— Auto infección con Strongyloides stercoralis en el niño. Ar. Ven. de P. y P. Méd. Nº 2, Vol. II, 1954 (623).

Complicaciones de la ascaridiosis infantil. Ar. Ven. de P. P. Méd. Nº 2, Vol. II, 1954 (624).

IRAZABAL RON, Jesús, TORREALBA, J.B.

1943— Breve nota sobre triatomideos y schizotrypanum cruzi en el Estado Carabobo. Gac. Méd. de Car. L., 5-59 (625).

IRIARTE, David R.

1927— Algo sobre las flagelosis de las euforbiáceas. Gac. Méd. de Car. XXXIV, 9, 129-130 (626).

IRIARTE, David R.

1927a— Estadística coprológica en el Laboratorio del Hospiral Vargas. Bol. de los Hosp. Caracas (627).

1928— Nota preliminar sobre la otomicosis en Venezuela y sobre un hongo de la Euphorbia hypericifolia. Gac. Méd. de Caracas. XXXV, 17, 258 (628).

1928a— Sobre un caso de Nasomiasis a Chrysomya macellaria Rev. de Medic. y Cirug. Caracas, XI, 116, 307-309 (629).

1928b— Contribución al estudio de la flageliasis de las plantas en Venezuela. Tesis de Doctorado en Ciencias Médicas. Caracas. Taller Gráfico. 21 págs. (630).

1929— Sobre un caso de otomicosis. Rev. de la Soc. Méd. Quirúrg. del Zulia. III, 2, 15-16 (631).

1929a— Pequeña nota sobre la flageliasis de las plantas en el Estado Zulia. Gac. Méd. de Caracas. XXXVI, 19, 271 (632).

1929b— Algunas observaciones sobre enfermedades parasitarias en Maracaibo: paludismo, leishmaniosis, filariosis, mossy foot, otomicosis. Gac. Méd. de Caracas. XXXVI, 19, 271-273 (633).

1930— Un caso de leishmaniosis. Rev. de la Soc. Méd. Quirúrg. del Zulia, IV, 1, 137 (634).

1931— Observaciones sobre el Carate en el Distrito Perija del Estado Zulia. Gac. Méd. de Car. XXXVIII (635).

IRIARTE, David R., BRICEÑO ROSSI, A.L.

1939— Consideraciones sobre el estado actual del carate y su distribución geográfica en Venezuela. Caracas. Tip. Americana. 39 páginas (636).

IRIARTE, David R., BRICEÑO ROSSI, A.L.

1939— Continuación sobre el estudio del Carate en Venezuela (con el hallazgo por primera vez en el país del espiroquete del Carate). Gac. Méd. de Car. XLVI, 5, 74-78 (637).

IRIARTE, David R., y RODRIGUEZ, César

1939— Un caso de granulomatosis paracoccidioica o Blastomicosis brasileña. Rev. de la Clí. L. R. Caracas, II, 4, 209-215 (638).

IRIARTE, David R.

1939— Primer caso de sodoku en Venezuela. Rev. de la Clí. L. R. Caracas, II, 4, 193-202 (639).

1940— Sospecha de focos de bilharziosis en el Oriente de la República. Bol. Lab. Clí. L.

R. I, 15-16 (640).

1940a— El Carate en Venezuela. Bol. Lab. Clí. L. R. Caracas, I, 1, 17-23 (641).

1940b— Datos y clasificación sobre la voraz oruga que azotó el valle de Caracas durante julio y agosto. Bol. Lab. Clí. L. R. I, 2, 39-40 (642).

1940c— Granulomatosis paracoccidioidica o blastomicosis brasileña. Memoria del I Congreso Sudamericano de O.R.L. (643).

1941— Investigaciones parasitológicas y entomológicas sobre la enfermedad de Chagas. Bol. Lab. Clí. L. R. Caracas, I, 3, 45-64 (644).

1941a— Tripanosomiasis caballar. Bol. Lab. L. R. Caracas, II, 5, 91-101 (645).

1941b— Xenodiagnóstico y reacción de Machado Guerreiro en la enfermedad de Chagas. Bol. Lab. Clí. L. R. Caracas, II, 5, 102-107 (646).

1942— La buba o bubas en Venezuela. Rev. de la Facultad de Medicina. Bogotá. Vol. X, N° 12, págs. 767-781 (647).

1942a— Estudios de Patología Tropical. 1. Vol. X, Imprenta de la Lotería. Caracas, 316 págs. (648).

1942c— Estudios sobre epizootia aviaria (espiroquetosis gallinácea) en colab. con A.L. Briceño Rossi. Bol. de la Clí. L. R. Caracas. II, 7, 121-127 (649).

IRIARTE, David R.

1942d— Nota sobre una nueva especie de simulido en el país (Simulium limbatum Knab., 1915-16). Bol. Lab. Clí. L. R. Caracas, II, 2, 134-138 (650).

1942e— Leishmaniosis. Bol. Lab. Clí. L. R. Caracas, II, 8, 141-145 (651).

1943— Aspergilosis auricular por Aspergillus fumigatus Fresenius 1863. Bol. Lab. Clí. L. R. Caracas, III, 10, 173-176 y en arch. Ven. de O.R.L. Oftalm., Neurol., IV, 1, 33-36 (652).

1943a— Faringomicosis a Cándida (monilia) albicans. Bol. Lab. Clí. L. R. Caracas, III, 10, 177-178 (653).

1943b— Infestación experimental por S. cruzi del Triatoma capitata Usinger 1939. Bol. Lab. Clí. L. R. III, 10, 179-180 (654).

IRIARTE, David R., BRICEÑO ROSSI, A.L.

1943— Breves notas sobre últimas investigaciones verificadas en las zonas pintógenas de Venezuela en relación al estado actual del conocimiento del carate o mal del pinto. Primera Jornada Ven. de Venereología y Dermatología. Rev. San. Asit. Soc. VIII, 5, 1001-1014 (655).

IRIARTE, David R.

1944— Consideraciones sobre paracoccidiosis. Arch. Ven. de la Soc. de O.R.L. Oftalm. Neurol. Caracas. V, 3 136-142 (656).

1944b— Sobre una nueva especie de flebotomo en el país (Ph. suis Rozeboom 1940), Bol. Lab. Clí. L. R. Caracas, IV, 15, 268-273 (657(.

ITRIAGO, Pedro Miguel, VEGAS, Martín LLOVERA, Ildemaro y MEDINA, Rafael

1943— La campaña contra la buba en Venezuela. Primera Jornada Ven. de Venereología y Dermatología. Rev. San. Asist. Soc. VIII, 5, 1015-1062 (658).

ITURBE, Juan

1930— Observaciones relativas acerca del diagnóstico biológico de la sífilis. Conferencia en la Sociedad de Biología de Hamburgo con motivo del XXV aniversario del descubrimiento del Spirochaeta pállida, 15-5-30 (659).

1939— Huéspedes invertebrados del Schistosoma mansoni en el Valle de Caracas y algunos otros lugares de Venezuela. Gac. Méd. de Caracas, XLVI, 6, 84-88 y en folleto editado por la Tip. Americana, 14 págs. (660).

1942— I. Nuestros Llanos. Apuntes fisiográficos, biológicos y agropecuarios. II. El Problema de la sífilis en Venezuela. III. Investigaciones experimentales acerca de la rabia paralítica del ganado vacuno en Venezuela y su trasmisión por los murciélagos hematófagos. Caracas. Tip. La Nación. 85 págs. (661).

1943— Comunidad del origen americano de la buba y la sífilis. Discurso de orden. Primera Jornada Venezolana de Venereología y Dermatología. Rev. de San. Asist.

Soc. VIII, 5, 1095-1106 y en folloto Tip. La Nación. Caracas. 18 págs. (662).

1943a— Co-autor del Indice Bibliográfico "400 Trabajos Científicos Venezolanos de Venereología y Dermatología". Caracas. Tip. Americana (663).

IZQUIERDO, Francisco

1928— Luminoso informe del Dr. Llamozas, Médico de Calabozo. Notable encuesta sobre la derrengadera en 1856. Gac. Méd. de Caracas, XXXV, 7, 108-112 (664).

1939— ¿Qué es la fiebre fría en Lara? La Higiene en la Provincia. El Campo es Venezuela y no Caracas. Gac. Méd. de Car. XLVI, 2, 25-26 (665).

1939a— En defensa de la ciencia médica venezolana (sobre la esquistosomiasis). Gac. Méd. de Car. XLVI, 6, 91-91 (66).

IRIARTE, David R.

1946— La familia Simuliidae en Venezuela. Boletín del Lab. de la Clí. Luis Razetti. Año VI, Núms. 19-20 y Año VII, Núms. 21-22 (667).

1946— Contribución al Estudio de la leishmaniosis en Venezuela. Boletín del Lab. de la Clí. Luis Razetti. Año VI, Núms. 19-20 (668).

1946— Las Micosis faríngeas. Bol. del Lab. de la Clí. Luis Razetti. Año VII, Núms. 23-24 (669).

1947— Nuevo simulido para Venezuela. Bol. del Lab. Clínico Razetti. Año VIII, Núms. 23-24 (669).

1948— Pequeñas anotaciones sobre Simulium lutzianus Pinto, 1931. Bol. del Lab. de la Clí. Razetti. Año IX, Núms. 27-28 (671).

1950— Contribución al estudio de las Caratopogoninas hematófacas señaladas en Venezuela. Bol. del Lab. de la Clí. Luis Razetti. Año X, 31-32 (672).

1951— Estadística de Exámenes serológicos practicados en el Laboratorio de la Clí. L. Razetti. Años 1935-49. Bol. de Lab. de la Clí. L. Razetti. Año XI, Núms. 33-34 (673).

1952— Lista de los flebototomos señalados en Venezuela hasta ahora. Bol. del Lab. de la Clí. L. Razetti. Año XII, Núms. 35-36 (674).

1952— Nueva especie de Ceratopogonido para el país Culicoides phlebotomus. Will. Bol. del Lab. de la Clí. L. Razetti. Año XIII, Núms. 37-38 (675).

1956— Un nuevo caso de esporotricosis. Bol. del Lab. de la Clí. L. Razetti. Año XIV, Núms. 39-40 (676).

1954— Apuntes. Bol. del Lab. de la Clí. L. Razetti. Año XVI, Núms. 11-12 (677).

1955— Otomicosis. Bol. del Lab. de la Clí. L. Razetti. Bol. del Lab. A-o XV. Núms. 43-44 (678(.

1948— Estudios Entomológicos y Parasitológicos. Tipografía Americana (obra) (679).

1948— Lecciones de Microbiología y Parasitología. Tip. Americana. (obra) (680).

1954— Bilharziosis-Terapéutica Clínica. Tomo I. Pág. 34 (681). Habana-Cuba.

JAFFE, Rudolf

1936— Comunicación sobre la Bilharziosis (Schistosoma mansoni) sobre todo en lo que respecta a las lesiones hepáticas. Bol. de Los Hospitales. XXXIV, 7, 313.333 (682).

1937c— Comunicaciones sobre las lesiones anatómicas en casos de sífilis en el material de autopsias de un año en Venezuela. Rev. de la Pol. Car. 34, 2269 (683).

1939— Sobre el diagnóstico de la apendicitis y sobre la apendicitis parasitaria. Rev. de la Pol. Car. IX, 46, 3087-3100 (684).

1939a— Lesiones intestinales producidas por la Bilharziosis mansoni encontradas en Venezuela. Rev. de la Pol. Car. IX, 47, 3132-3147 (685).

1939b— Sobre la Bilharziosis en los niños y jóvenes (hasta los veinte años). Rev. de la Pol. Car. IX, 49, 3261-3272 (686).

1939c— Comunicaciones sobre la Bilharziosis pulmonar. Gac. Méd. de Car. XLVII, 19, 390-393 (687).

1940— Sobre la patogenia de las lesiones anátomo-patológicas bilharzianas. Rev. de la Poli. Car. IX, 50, 3321-3345 (688).

1941— Sobre el diagnóstico anatómico de la bilharziosis con comunicación de algunos casos raros. Rev. de la Poli. Car. X, 58, 185-181 (689).

1943b— Las lesiones sifilíticas de la Aorta y su patogenia. Rev. San. Asist. Soc. VIII, 1, 95 (690).

1943e— Observaciones sobre las lesiones pulmonares producidas por el Schistosoma mansoni. Presentado al II Congreso Venezolano de la Tuberculosis (691).

JASO, Roldán L. y SANCHEZ COVISA, José

1943— La sífilis pulmonar y sus analogías y diferencias con la tuberculosis pulmonar. (Primera Jornada Ven. de Venereología y Dermatología). Rev. San. Asist. Soc. VIII, 5, 899 (692).

JELAMBI, Rafael

1928— Parasitismo en la primera edad. Rev. de Medic. y Cirug. Car. XI, 123, 432-442 (693).

JIMENEZ, Juan

1928— Tres casos de Leishmaniosis americana. Rev. de la Soc. Méd. Quirúrg. del Zulia. II, k3, 164-166 (694).

1929— Un caso de bilharziosis. Rev. de la Soc. Méd. Quirúrg. del Zulia. III, 2, 14-15 (695).

JIMENEZ RIVERO, Miguel

1930a— Informe del Médico de Sanidad de La Guaira sobre Anquilostomiasis. Memoria de la Conferencia Sanitaria Nacional de 1930. Págs. 183-194 (696).

1934a— Contribución al estudio de las dermatomicosis en Venezuela. Gac. Méd. de Car. XLI (697).

1934f— Nuevos medicamentos del Paludismo. Rev. Médica Caracas. I, 9, 128-129 (698).

1934h— El origen americano de la sífilis. Rev. Médica. Caracas, I, 5, 70-72 (699).

1935c— Nuevas orientaciones de la Sifiloterapia. La cura de saturación salvarsánica. Gac. Méd. de Car. XLII (700).

JIMENEZ RIVERO, Miguel y FERNANDEZ, Edmundo

1931— Informe que el Médico y el Bacteriólogo de la Oficina Subalterna de Sanidad de La Guaira presentan a la Conferencia Sanitaria Nacional, Caracas, Tip. Americana (701).

JIMENEZ RIVERO, Miguel

1936a— Dermosifilografía venezolana. I Vol. Prólogo del Dr. S. Córdoba. Caracas. Edit. Elite, 183 págs. (702).

JIMENEZ RIVERO, M. y BRICEÑO IRAGORRY L.

1936— La esporotricosis y el primer caso de Rhinoclaudiosis schencki en Venezuela. Rev. Méd. III, 19-20, 305-317 y en la Gac. Méd. de Car. XLIII, 15, 225-236 (703).

JAFFE, Rudolf y FERRO Raúl

1946— El diagnóstico de la bilharzia en el material de autopsia. Rev. de la Poli. Caracas. Vol. XV. N° 88 (764).

JAFFE, R. MAYER M. y PIFANO, Félix

Estudios biológicos y anatomopatológicos con un solo sexo de S. mansoni (705).

LANDAETA PAYARES, Héctor A.

1927a— Disentería balantidiana y Yatren. Rev. de la Soc. Méd. Quirúrg. del Zulia. I, 6, 71-72 (706).

1931— Un caso de sífilis tóraco-pulmonar. Rev. de la Pol. Car. I, 2, 54-57 (707).

1932a— Un caso de hepatitis sifilítica. Rev. de la Pol. Car. 6, 388-389 (708).

1932b— En caso de fiebre biliosa hemoglobinúrica. Rev. de la Pol. Car. 7. 472-475 (709).

1932d— La defensa social contra las enfermedades venéreas. Conferencia. Folleto "Semana Antivenérea". Public. del Minist. de Salub. y de Agric. y Cría (710).

1932e— Los parásitos intestinales en el niño. Folleto "Semana Sanitaria del Niño". Págs. 68-72 (711).

1933— Cuáles son los trasmisores del paludismo. "Folleto Semana Sanitaria contra el Zancudo". Págs. 85-88 (712).

1935— Polineuritis sifilítica. Rev. de la Pol. Car. 20, 1339-1344 (713).
1940a— Sobre un caso de sífilis mediagástrica. Rev. de la Pol. Car. 50, 3347-3353 (714).

LAPEYRE, J.L.

1935b— Un diagnóstico difícil. Perforación intestinal oculta en el curso de una fiebre tifoidea desconocida. Rev. de Medic. y Cirug. Maracay. Abril. Pág. 65 (715).
1936a— Contribución al estudio de la parasitosis intestinal como factor de colitis, apendicitis y oclusión. Rev. de la Pol. Car. Nº 27 (716).

LARES GABALDON, Martín

1934a— La amibiasis crónica en la etiología de las estrecheces rectales. Tesis de Doctorado en Ciencias Médicas. Caracas. Tip. Garrido, 58 págs. (717).

LEON, Alfonso

1943— ¿Debe usarse o no la quinina en la fiebre hemoglobinúrica? Rev. de la Soc. Méd. Quirúrg. del Zulia. XVII, 3-4, 2063-2066 (718).

LEPAGE, Cruz

1934— Gangrena por mordedura de serpiente curada con suero normal de caballo. Rev. de la Pol. Car. 15, 996-1001 (719).

LICCIONI, Horacio

1935— Carlos Chagas, Arch. Ven. de Cardiol. y Hemat. Caracas. I, 2, 92 (720).

LOPEZ, Leopoldo

1943d— Hidatidosis renal. Bol. de los Hosp. XLII, 3, 110-115 (721).

LOPEZ RONDON, Angel

1927— Contribución al estudio de las Bubas en Venezuela. Memorias del V Congreso de Medicina. Vol. I. Págs. 199-238 y en libro. Car. Tip. Americano (722).
1930— Campaña contra la Anquilostomiasis en Venezuela. Memoria de la Conferencia Sanitaria Nacional de 1930. Págs. 251-295 (723).
1931— Informe sobre Paludismo que presenta el Médico de Sanidad del Estado Monagas, Dr. Angel López Rondón a la II Conferencia Naci ›nal. Memoria de la II Conferencia San. Nac. Páginas 202-284 (724).
1933— Trabajo sobre el Paludismo en el Estado Monagas. Caracas. Tip. Americana (725).
1933a— Historia del Paludismo en el Estado Monagas. Rev. "Divulgaciones Científicas". Caracas, I, 8-9, 70-74 (726).

LOPEZ RONDON, Angel

1936— Vulgarizaciones científicas. Faz del Problema del Paludismo en Venezuela. El Hombre Paludígeno como único manantial de contagio. Bol. Minist. San. Asist. Soc. Págs. 643-651 (727).
1939— La fiebre fría. Gac. Méd. de Car. XLVI, 5, 78-80 (728).
1940— Glosas malariológicas. Caracas. Coop. de Artes Gráficas, 137 páginas (729).
1942— Los aspectos de la campaña antipalúdica. Diario "La Esfera". Diciembre 1º (730).
1944— Lucha contra el Mal de Chagas. Diario "La Esfera". Caracas, Julio 12 (731).
1944a— Silabario del Paludismo. Rev. Alma Médica. Maturín. I, 1, 10-18 (732).

LOPEZ VILLORIA, Lisandro

1936— La sífilis de los ojos. Bol. del Minist. de Sanidad y Asist. Soc. Páginas 483-487 (733).
1937— Sífilis del frontal. Observaciones. Gac. Méd. de Car. XLIV, y en el folleto editado por la Tip. Americana, 30 págs. (734).

LOVERA, Ildemaro

1935— La Schizotripanosis en Venezuela y los estudios del Dr. Torrealba. Diario "El Heraldo". Caracas. Agosto 3 (735).
1937— Influencia del anquilostomo sobre la inteligencia. Evolución de la inteligencia en los anquilostomiásicos por diversas pruebas terapéuticas. Trabajo laureado con el Diploma y la Medalla "Luis Razetti, 1937". Caracas, Coop. de Artes Gráficas. 19 p. y en la Rev. S.E.M. IV, 29, 34 Año 1937 (736).

1938— Contribución a los estudios clínicos, serológicos y sanitario de la Buba. Tesis de Doctorado en Ciencias Médicas. Caracas. Impresores Unidos. 55 pág. (737).

1943— Observaciones clínicas de buba. Primera Jornada Venezolana de Venereología y Dermatología. Rev. San. Asist. Soc. VIII, 5, 1073-1092 (738).

1943a— Co-autor del Folleto "400 Trabajos Científicos Venezolanos de Venereología y Dermatología". I Jornada Ven. de Ven. y Dermat. Caracas. Tip. Americana (739).

LOVERA, Ildemaro, VEGAS, Martín, ITRIAGO, Pedro Miguel y MEDINA, Rafael

1943— La campaña contra la buba en Venezuela. Primera Jornada Venezolana de Venereología y Dermatología. Rev. Asist. Soc. VIII, 5, 1015-1062 (740).

LOYNAZ PAEZ, Oscar

1931— Lo que nadie debe ignorar sobre sífilis. Los Nuevos Tratamientos. Prólogo del Dr. Martín Vegas, Folleto de Lit. y Tip. Vargas. Caracas. 48 págs. (741).

1932a— Influencia en los niños del alcoholismo y de la sífilis de los padres. Folleto "Semana Sanitaria del Niño". Public. del Ministerio de Salub. y de Agric. y Cría. Págs. 98-101 (742).

1933— Criaderos de Zancudos y su destrucción. Folleto "Semana Sanitaria contra el Zancudo". Public. del Minist. de Salub. y de Agric. y Cría. Págs. 99-100 (743).

1933a— Crónica Médica. La Sífilis se cura. Rev. Nac. de Medic. Caracas, I, 3, 35-38 (744).

1934— Un tratamiento racional de la Sífilis reciente. Resultados en 102 casos del Dispensario Antivenéreo de la Sanidad Nacional. Caracas. Lit. y Tip. Vargas. 79 págs. (745).

1934b— Uso oportuno y adecuado de los medios de diagnóstico y de control serológico. Bol. Minist. Salub. Agric. y Cría. I, 10-11. 807-816 (746).

1934c— Resultados serológicos del tratamiento contínuo aplicado en el Servicio Antivenéreo en 102 enfermos de sífilis reciente. Bol. Ministerial Salub. Agric. y Cría. I, 12, 13, 983-1006 (747).

1935a— Avariosis. Plan de Lucha Antivenérea. Bol. Minist. Salub. Agric. y Cría II, 24-27-40 (748).

LOZADA, Victor

1927— Anotaciones sobre la radiumterapia de la Leishmaniosis de las mucosas y otras afecciones de la cara. Memoria del V Congreso Ven. de Medic. Vol. II, págs. 197-211 (749).

LUCIANI, Domingo

1944a— Sindrome colo-pericolo-apendicular parasitario. Nota de Introducción. Gac. Méd. de Car. LII, 21, 229-230 (750).

LUCIANI LAIRET, F.

1933— Zancudos que trasmiten enfermedades. Folleto "Semana Sanitaria contra el Zancudo". Public. del Minist. de Salub. y de Agric. y Cría. Págs. 77-84 (751).

LUENGO VALE, J.M.

1936— Paudismo larvado. Bol. del Hosp. Los Andes, I, 1, 19-22 (752).

LUTTERMOSER, W.

1941— Destrucción de caracoles trasnsmisores de Schistosoma mansoni en Venezuela. Rev. San. Asist. Soc. VI, 6, 874-897 (753).

LUTTERMOSER, W. y PIFANO C., Félix

1942— Aspectos epidemiológicos de la Schistomiasis mansoni en San Casimiro (Edo. Aragua). Rev. de San Asist. Soc. VII, 3, 397 (754).

LUTTERMOSER, George W.

1943— Destrucción de caracoles trasnsmisores de Schistosoma mansoni en Venezuela. Rev. San. Asist. Soc. VIII, 1, 3-44 (755).

1946— La campaña anti-bilharziana en Venezuela. Conf. San. Pan. Cuaderno amarillo (756Z(.

LOPEZ RONDON, A.

1933— El paludismo en Venezuela. Tip. Americana. Caracas, págs. 13-131 (757).

LOVERA, Ildemaro

Acción de la Penicilina sobre el Tr. pallidum (758).

LUTTERMOSER G.W.

Estudio sobre el caracol vector del S. mansoni en la ciudad de Maracay y alrededor del estado Aragua, con recomendaciones para lucha contra él (759).

LUTTERMOSER, G.W. y CASTELLANO, J.V.

Observaciones sobre la propaganda y destrucción del caracol Australorbis glabratus vector de la S. mansoni en el Valle D. F. (760).

MACIA ANZOLA, Cristóbal

1942— Sobre la frecuencia de la sífilis congénita de los escolares de Caracas. Tesis de Doctorado en Ciencias Médicas. Caracas. (761).

MACHADO GONZALEZ, Armando

1943— Contribución al estudio del Sodokú en Venezuela. Bol. de los Hosp. Caracas. XLIII, 5-6, 271-290 (762).

MALARET, P.S.

1938— La importancia del examen de la sangre en las regiones maláricas. Bol. Minist. San. Asist. Soc. II, págs. 1895-1902 (763).

MALAVE, Antonio, VIVAS SALAS E. y MEJIA, Abel

1943— Sífilis cardiovascular en Venezuela. Primera Jornada Venezolana de Venereología y Dermatología. Rev. San. Asist. Soc. VII, 4, 711-728 (764).

MANRIQUE TOLEDO, Leopoldo

1938— El parasitismo intestinal en el Valle. Sus causas. Tesis de Doctorado en Ciencias Médicas. Caracas. Emp. El Cojo. 17 páginas (765).

MARCANO CAPDEVIELLA, A.R.

1940— Las especies parásitas del hombre pertenecientes al tipo Nematelmintos. Tip. Mal. Caracas. III, 6, 40-461 (766).

MARMOL LUZARDO, Joaquín

1935— Un interesante caso de absceso hepático amibiano. Rev. de la Soc. Méd. Quirúrg. del Zulia. IX, 5 (767).

MARQUEZ REVERON, Victorino y MARCANO C., Antonio R.

1939— Consideraciones generales sobre clasificación del subreino Protozoos (Lección para el Curso de Capacitación para Inspectores). Rev. Tij. Mal. II, 10, 135 (768).

1939a— Principales especies patógenas y pertenecientes a las clases Rizopodos, Flagelados y Ciliados (Lección para el Curso de Capacitación para Inspectores). Rev. Tij. Mal. II, 10, 140 (769).

MARTINEZ N., Arminio y PONS, Adolfo R.

1941— Primer caso de Kala-azar en Venezuela. Gac. Méd. de Car. XLVIII, Núms. 17 y 18 (5374) (770).

MARTINEZ NIOCHETT A.

1937— Valor y significado del examen de la sangre para la sífilis. Diario "El Heraldo". Octubre 21 (771).

1943— Obstrucción intestinal aguda por ascaris. Presentado a las Primeras Jornadas Nacionales de Puericultura y Pediatría. (772).

MASOS DOMINGUEZ, J.

1944— La prueba rural de Briceño Rossi en el diagnóstico de la sífilis. Memoria de las Primeras Jornadas Venezolanas de Puericultura y Pediatría. Caracas. Vol. III, Págs. 39-64 (773).

MAYER, MARTIN e ORTIZ, Ignacio

1941— Experimentos con Grahamella muris. Rev. San. Asist. Soc. XI, 3, 320-333 (774).

MAYER, Martín y PIFANO C., Félix

1941— Sobre el cultivo de Leishmania tropical en Venezuela e intrarreacciones con Leishmana-antígeno. Rev. San. Asist. Soc. VI, 3, 281-289 (775).

1941a— Reacciones serológicas en Bilharziosis mansoni según el método de Fairley. Rev.

San. Asist. Soc. VI, 3, 290-295 (776).

1941b— Nuevos métodos para el diagnóstico de la enfermedad de Chagas. Rev. San. Asist. Soc. VI, 3, 311-316 (777).

MAYER, Martín

1941— El comportamiento de los gametocitos en la malaria tropical. Rev. San. Asist. Soc. VI, 3, 317-319 (778).

1941a— Algunos puntos de vista para el tratamiento específico del paludismo. Rev. Asist. Soc. VI, 6, 852-862 (771).

1941b— Sobre la etiología de las bartonellosis, especialmente de la fiebre de Oroya. Rev. San. Asist. Soc. VI, 6, 863-873 (780).

MAYER, Martín y PIFANO C., Félix

1942— Estudios biológicos y patológicos en animales infectados con Schistosoma mansoni (infecciones bi y unisexuales). Rev. San. Asist. Soc. VII, 3, 419 (781).

1942a— Sobre el comportamiento de la reacción de Fairley en los estudios clínicos de la Schistosomiasis mansoni. Rev. San. Asist. Soc. VII, 3, 379-396 (782).

MATEO, Alfonso A.

1943— Las formas cerebrales del paludismo. Rev. San. Asist. Soc. VIII, 6, 1167 (783).

MEDINA, Medardo

1931— ¿Qué es la sífilis? Obra de divulgación científica. Caracas. Tip. Universal. 134 págs. (784).

1938— Sífilis y Matrimonio. Rev. S.A.S. de Educ. Sanit. Caracas. II, 24, 7-9 (785).

MEDINA, Rafael, VEGAS, Martín, LOVERA, Ildemaro, ITRIAGO, Pedro Miguel

1943— La campaña contra la buba en Venezuela. Primera Jornada Venezolana de Venereología y Dermatología. Rev. San. Asist. Soc. VIII, 5, 1015-1060 (786).

MEDINA, Rafael

1944— Contribución al estudio de la enfermedad de Chagas en el Estado Yaracuy. Rev. del Col. Médico de Yaracuy.

MEJIAS, Abel

1940— Seroreacción positiva monosintomática. Maracay. Tip. Patria. 10 págs. (788).

1940a— El tratamiento de la sífilis en cinco días. Diario "El Heraldo". 19-10-40 (789).

1941a— Sífilis congénita en Venezuela. Arch. Ven. de Pueric. y Pediat. III, 8, 470-489 y en folleto edit. por los Talleres Biogen, 20 páginas (790).

1941b— El tratamiento moderno de la sífilis reciente. Bol. de Venereología M.S.A.S. Nº 1 Septiembre (719).

1942— ¿Cuántos sifilíticos hay en Venezuela? Rev. de San. Asist. Soc. VII, 5, 745-748 (792).

MEIJAS, Abel, VIVAS SALAS, E, y MALAVE, Antonio

1943— Sífilis cardiovascular en Venezuela. Primera Jornada de Venereología y Dermatología. Rev. San. Asist. Soc. VIII, 4, 711-728 (793).

MEJIAS, Abel, VEGAS, Martín, ITURBE, Juan, SANCHEZ COVISA, José, LOVERA, Ildemaro

1943— Cuatrocientos trabajos Científicos Venezolanos de Venereología y Dermatología. Primera Jornada Venezolana de Venereología y Dermatología. Caracas. Tip. Americana. 68 págs. (794).

MENDEZ, Hernán

1939— Plasmodium ovale. Relación del primer caso observado en Venezuela. Tesis de Doctorado en Ciencias Médicas. Caracas. Editorial Bolívar. 15 págs. y en Public. Div. Malar. Caracas. Nº 3 (5.548) (795).

MENDEZ ESCALANTE, J.A.

1934— Apuntes Entomológicos. Tesis de Bachillerato en Filosofía. Caracas. Tip. Bodoni. 13 págs. (796).

MENDEZ ESCALANTE, J.A. y MILA de la ROCA, F.

1934— Estudios Ofidiología Venezolana. Rev. Caracas. Méd. II, 8, 445 (797).

MENDEZ GIMON, Manuel Vicente

1935— Un caso de Leishmaniosis americana. Rev. de la Pol. Car. 24. 1643-1644 (798).

1936— Algunas experiencias sobre la Schizotrypanosis americana. Estudio experimental y clínico sobre el xeno-diagnóstico. Tesis de Doctorado en Ciencias Médicas. Coop. de Artes Gráficas. 36 páginas (799).

1936a— Pequeñas observaciones, sobre el paludismo y su profilaxia en el Dto. Zaraza. Diario "El Heraldo". Caracas. N° 4309. Agosto 13 (800).

1936b— La úlcera leishmaniósica. Importancia del diagnóstico en esta afección. Diario "EL Heraldo". Caracas. N° 4.309. Agosto 20 (801).

MENDOZA, Delfín

1926— El bismuto en el tratamiento de la Buba. Observaciones. Rev. de Medic. y Cirug. Caracas. IX, 98, 92, 96 y en N° 99, 97, 122 (802).

MENDOZA, Espíritu Santos

1934a— La reacción de Henry. Serodiagnóstico del Paludismo. Tesis de Doctorado en Ciencias Médicas. Caracas. Coop. de Artes Gráficas. 36 págs. (803).

MENDOZA, E.S. y DOMINGUEZ SISCO, R.

1941— Indice de Sífilis Prenatal sobre 400 observaciones practicadas en la Maternidad Municipal "Concepción Palacios". Rev. de Obst. y Ginec. I, 4, 183-193 (804).

MILA DE LA ROCCA, F.

1932— Clasificación de los Ofidios. Tesis de Bachillerato en Filosofia. Caracas. Tip. Americana. 14 págs. (805).

1932a— Introducción al estudio de los ofidios de Venezuela. Bol. de la Soc. Ven. de Cienc. Nat. I, 10, 381-392 (806).

1933a— Clasificación de los ofidios. Gac. Méd. de Car. XL, 10, 134 (807).

1934— Notas sobre seroterapia antiofídica y sobre el desarrollo de la seroterapia antiofídica en el Brasil. Gac. Méd. de Car. XLI, 2, 23, 25 (808).

1934b— Algunas notas sobre el funcionamiento de la Biblioteca del Instituto Vital Brazil. Instucciones para captura y envío de serpientes a dicho Instituto. Gac. Méd. de Car. XLI, 11, 175-176 (809).

1935— Notas sobre Ofidios venenosos. Descripción provisional de la Tigra Mariposa. Rev. Car. Méd. II, 6, 319-333 (810).

1935a— (En colab. con J.A. Méndez Escalante). Estudios de Ofidiología Venezolana. Intoxicación ofídica causada por una Tigra. Rev. Car. Méd. II, 8, 445-453 (811).

1937— Lucha contra los animales ponzoñosos en especial las serpientes. Memoria del Minist. San. y Asist. Soc. Págs. 301-306 (812).

1937a— Informe del viaje hecho al Llano acompañando al Dr. J.A. Vellard. Memoria del Minist. Sanid. y Asist. Social. Págs. 306-308. Fallecimiento del Sr. Vital Brazil, hijo. Notas biográficas. Bol. de la Soc. Ven. de Cienc. Nat. 28, 465-466 (813).

1938— Emponzoñamiento por serpientes venezolanas. Impresos en Mimeógrafo para uso de los alumnos de la Cátedra de Patología Tropical (814).

MINISTERIO DE SANIDAD Y ASISTENCIA SOCIAL

1936— Métodos para estimar la extensión e intensidad de la Anquilostomiasis. Por E.I. Benarroch. Caracas. Tip. Americana, 12 págs. 2° ed, en 1941. Talleres Patria (815).

1937a— Lucha contra la anquilostomiasis; instrucciones para la construcción de escudos de hoyo rurales. Car. Lit. y Tip. del Comercio, 2 h. ilus (817).
Explicaciones referentes a la enfermedad demoninada "anquilostomiasis". Caracas. p. 7 (818).

MINISTERIO DE SALUBRIDAD Y DE AGRICULTURA Y CRIA

1933— Semana sanitaria contra el zancudo. Caracas. Lit. y Tip. Casa de Especialidades. 113 págs. (819).

MONAGAS ORIACH, José Gregorio

1930— Anquilostomiasis en Río Chico. Memoria de la Primera Conferencia Sanitaria Nacional, 1930. Págs. 246-250 (820).

MIR, LEON y MORA, Ramón

1938-39— Conclusión estadística con porcentaje de sífilis hereditaria de 80 escolares. Bol. de los Hosp. Caracas. XXXVIII, 1-3-38-41 (821).

MORENO, Héctor Argenis

1936— Casos de Buba tratados por el Neo-Salvarsán. Tesis de Doctorado en Ciencias Médicas. Caracas. Tip. Millán. 12 págs. (822).

MURILLO, Manuel S.

1939— Valor de la investigación sistemática de la Sífilis en grupos sanos. Rev. Minist. San. Asist. Soc. IV. 2, 82-87 (823).

1941— Un caso de absceso hepático de origen amibiano. Bol. Hosp. Poli. de Los Teques. I, 2, 13-15 (824).

MATHEUS MENDEZ, Noé

1945— Creeping disease. Rev. Gac. Méd. Quirúrg. del Zulia. Año XIX. N° 1 (825).

MEDINA. Mariano

1953— Onicomicosis. Rev. Pol. Caracas. Vol. XXII, 130 (826).

MATEO ALONSO, Alberto

1946— Estudios sobre los cuadros clínicos más graves del paludismo, XII Conferencia San. Pan. Cuadermo Amarillo, N° 33 (827).

MISLE PEÑA, Pedro, PEDRIQUE, Ron y HENRIQUEZ C.

1946— El tercer caso de Kala azar descrito en Venezuela. Gac. Méd. de Caracas. Año LIV. N° 7 a 12 (828).

MONTEMAYOR, Lorenzo

1954— Blastomyces dermatitidis Gilchrist Stolkes 1959 en Venezuela. Gac. Méd. de Caracas. Año LXII. N° 11-12 (829).

MAYER y PIFANO

1946— El diagnóstico de rutina de la Schistosomiasis mansoni. (Experiencias fundamentales en 5.000 intradermos). Conf. San. Panamericana. Cuaderno Amarillo. 18 (830).

MEDINA, Rafael

1954— Reacciones producidas en enfermos de Pınta, Buba o Sífilis por inoculación de Treponemas pertenue, Castellani 1905. Sus posibles aplicaciones de diagnóstico de curación en estas treponematosis. Arc. Ven. Pat. Trop. y pars. Méd. N° 2. Vol. II. (831).

MEDINA, R., BRICEEO, I.L.

— Nota sobre el Cultivo el agente c. (832).

MEDINA, R. y ABREU, Carlos

— Campaña contra la buba en Venezuela (833).

MEDINA, SANCHEZ PEREZ

— Investigación de la Sífilis en las familias bajo control de las Enfermedades polivalentes (834).

MEDINA, R., CONVIT, Jacinto y CONTRERAS, R.

— Formas recientes del Carate. Observaciones clínicas e histopatológicas. A.V. Trop. y, edica. 1950. Vol. II, N° 1 (835).

MORALES MORA, L.A.

— Las reacciones Serológicas cuantitativas en el diagnóstico y pronóstico de la Sífilis (836).

MARCUCCI, Giorgio

1950— Nota sobre la anatomía y la histología Australorbis glabratus. Archivos Venezolanos de Patología Tropical y Parasitología Médica. Vol. II, Enero, N° 1 (837).

1950— Estudio experimental sobre la Miocarditis. A.V. de P. Tropical y Parasilogía Médica. Enero, Vol. II, N° 1 (838).

MIRSA, A.

— El desarrollo del Phebotomus panamensis. Shannon. 1926 y P. gomezi (839).

1931— En condiciones de laboratorio (840).

— Estudios en culicoides (Ceratopoginae) (841).

— Septiembre de 1951 (842).
MIRSA, A., y MIRSA, M.
Primer hallazgo de formas evolutivas de microfilaria en el tórax de culicoides (843).
MIRSA, M.
1949— Sobre hallazgo de Gregarinas (Sporozoas) en el estómago de
1949— Sobre hallazgo de Gregarinas (Sporozoas) en el estómago de y Asistencia Social. Sept.-diciembre. N° 5 y 6 (844).
MOROS, Teófilo
1936— Bilharziosis intestinal en Los Teques. Bol. Minist. San. Asist. Soc. I, 3, 214-221 (845).
MURILLO CHACON, Augusto
1931— Breves apuntaciones acerca del Paludismo en el Estado Táchira. Memoria de la II Conferencia Sanitaria Nacional. Páginas 312-320 (846).
MURZI D'ALTA, Julio
1937-38— Contraste terapéutico en dos casos de anemia por necátor. Bol. de los Hosp. Caracas, XXXVII, 6-8, 324-328 (847).
MACKINNON, J.E., FERRADA-URUZUA, S.V. y MONTEMAYOR, Lorenzo: M a d u r e l l a
Gipsea, n. sp.
A new species fungus producing the black variety of Maduromycosis in South America. Micopathología. Vol. IV. 384-303. 1948 (848).
MACKINNON, J.E., FERRADA-URZUA, L.V. y MONTEMAYOR, Lorenzo
Investigaciones sobre Maduromicosis y sus agentes. Micopathologia. Vol. IV. 356-366. 1948. (849).
MACKINNON, J.E. y MONTEMAYOR, Lorenzo
Observaciones personales sobre la morfología del Paracoddidioides brasiliensis en los tejidos. An. del Instituto de Higiene de Montevideo. 2-(1). 128, 1949. An. Fac. Méd. Montevideo. 34-(1-2-3). 231-300 (850).
MONTEMAYOR, Lorenzo
Estudios de las propiedades biológicas de varias cepas de hongos patógenos causantes de la Cromomicosis y de especies vecinas saprofitas y patógenas. Micopathología. Vol. IV. 379-383 (351).
Propiedades biológicas diferenciales de los agentes de Cromomicosis. An. del Inst. de Hig. Montevideo. 2 (1). 32-35. 1948 (852).
Breve nota del Favus aviarion. Trabajos del Centro de Investigaciones científicas. Caracas. N° 3, 1945. Edt. Grafolit. (853).
Enfermedad de Gilchrist en Venezuela. Gac. Méd. de Caracas. 1955. Primer caso, nota previa (854).
MEYER, Martín y PIFANO, C. Félix
1945— El diagnóstico de la Schistosomiasis por intradermorreacciones con antígeno preparado de vermes adultos de Schistosoma mansoni (Rev. S.A.S. Vol. X, N° 1 pág. 3 (855).
1945— Intradermirreacciones comparativas con extracto de Schistosoma mansoni y Fasciola hepática en el diagnóstico de la bilharziosis. Rev. S.A.S. Vol. X, p. 45 (856).
MEYER, Martín, LUTTERMOSER, George, PIFANO, Félix
1945— Investigaciones diagnósticas sobre la Schistosomiasis mansoni en la ciudad de Maracay y alrededores inmediatos. Rev. S.A.S., Vol. X, p. 165 (857).
MEYER, Martín y PIFANO, Félix
1945— La reacción de desviación del completo según Fairley, en la Schistosomiasis mansoni. Rev. S.A.S., Vol. X, p. 65 (858).
1940-41— Reacciones serológicas en Bilharziosis mansoni, según el Método de Fairley. Rev. S.A.S., Vol. VI, N° 3, p. 290 (859).

MEYER, Martín, PIFANO, Félix y MEDINA, Rafael

1946— Aspectos epidemiológicos de la enfermedad de Chagas en Venezuela. Bases para una compañía de saneamiento a zonas endémicas del medio rural venezolano. XII Conferencia Sanitaria Panamericana, Cuaderno Amarillo, N° 30 (860).

MEYER, Martín y PIFANO, Félix

1951— La cercaria-reacción de Vogel-Minning en la Schistosomiasis mansoni. Rev. S.A.S. Vol. XVI, N° 5 y 6. p. 461 (861).

MEYER, Martín y PIFANO, Félix

1945— La estimación del porcentaje de bilharziosis en una zona endémica por la intro-dermorreacción en niños. Primeras Jornadas Venezolanas de Puericultura y Pediatría. Vol. IV, p. 383 (862).

1941— Nuevos métodos para el diagnóstico de la enfermedad de Chagas. Rev. S.A.S. Vol. VI, p. 311 (863).

1951— Modalidades de la infección producida por el S. mansoni en animales infectados con cercarias provenientes de un solo caracol. R.S. y A.S. diciembre, N° 5 y 6 (864).

MEYER, M., GUERRA y DI PRISCO, J.

Las especialidades de las reacciones con antígeno de S. mansoni y fasciola hepática por el método de Prausnitz-Kustner (865).

MONTEMAYOR, L. de, BRAS, KARL, y POLO, Francisco

1954— "Enfermedad de Gilchrist en Venezuela". Rev. San. Asist. Soc. Vol. XIX. N° 3 y 4. Pág. 217 (866).

MIRSA, María

1954— "Insectos de interés médico en Los Chorros". Edo. Miranda, con referencia especial a los dipteros del género Culicoides Latreille. (Nematocera, Caratopogonidae). Rev. San. Asist. Soc. Vol. XIX. N° 1-2. Pág. 139 (867).

MIRSA, A.

1954— Sobre la biología de algunos Phlebotomos (Díptera Psychodidae) y datos sobre hematófagos colectados en Altagracia de Orituco. Edo. Guárico, Venezuela. Rev. San. Asist. Soc. N° 1-2, 189 (868).

MEDINA, Rafael, MEDINA, Febres, MARIANO, PIFANO, Félix y ROMER, Miguel

1954— "La Leishmaniasis tegumentaria americana". Rev. San. Asist. Soc. N° 5 y 6. Págs. 345 (869).

NEGRETTI DE WINDT, Guillermo

1931a— Sobre algunos moluscos gasterópodos en Venezuela. Tesis de Bachillerato en Filosofía. Caracas. Tip. Mundial. 13 p. (870).

NIETO CAICEDO, M. ARCHILA, Ricardo

1941— Geografía Médico-Sanitaria del Estado Cojedes con especial referencia al Paludismo. Rev. San. Asist. Soc. VI, 5, 587-785 (871).

NIETO CAICEDO M.

1942— Historia clínica de un caso de fiebre biliosa hemoglobinúrica. Tij. Mal. Caracas. VI, 3, 62 (872).

1942a— Epilepsia en la Malaria. Rev. Tij. Mal. Caracas. V, 1, 2 (873).

1943— El índice esplénico: crítica de su signicación en nuestro medio. Rev. Tij. Mal. Caracas. VII, 2, 16 (874).

1943a— La génesis de las epidemias de Malaria. Rev. de la Soc. Méd.-Quirúrg. del Zulia. XVII, 5-6, 2083-2111 (865).

NOGUERA, Antonio

1943a— Un caso de esplenomegalia palúdica seguida de esplenectomía y curación. Arch. Ven. de Pueric. y Pediat. Caracas. V, 15, 839, 842 (876).

NORIEGA TRIGO, Manuel

1943— Tratamiento racional de la fiebre biliosa hemoglobinúrica. Rev. de la Soc. Méd-Quirúrg. del Zulia. XVII, 2, 2035-2043

NUÑEZ PONTE, Filemón

(877).

1930— Estudio de la Anquilostomiasis en el Estado Aragua. Memoria de la Conf. Sanit. Nac. de 1930. Págs. 75-118 (878).

1932— La Anquilostomosis como primordial problema sanitario nacional. Tesis de Doctorado en Ciencias Médicas. Caracas. Tip. Americana. 66 p. (879).

1935— Campaña contra la parasitosis intestinal. Bol. Minist. Salub. Agric. y Cría. III, 25-26, 182-184 (880).

1936— Campaña contra la parasitosis intestinal. Bol. Minist. San. Asist. Soc. I, 1, 30-39 (881).

NUÑEZ TOVAR, M.

1927— Nota dobre insectos hematófagos de Venezuela. Gac. Méd. de Car. XXXIV, 12, 186-187 (882).

1927a— La plasmoquina en el tratamiento del Paludismo. Rev. Cient. de Ven. Caracas. IX, 104, 415 (883).

1928— Contribución para el Estudio de los Dípteros Hematófagos de Venezuela, por los doctores Adolph Lutz y Núñez Tovar. (De la obra "Estudios de Zoología y Parasitología Venezolana". Río de Janeiro, 1928). Reproducida en el libro "La Parasitología en Venezuela, y los trabajos del Dr. Núñez Tovar", por Diego Carbonell, págs. 245-384 (884).

NIETO CAICEDO, M.

1946— Epidemia Regional de Malaria en la Cuenca del Lago de Maracaibo. XII Conferencia Sanitaria Pan. Cuaderno Amerillo. N° 23 (885).

(S.A.) Presente y futuro del paludismo en el Edo. Trujillo. Publ. del Gobierno del Edo. Trujillo, págs. 3-19 (886).

1951— Experiencias venezolanas con las drogas antimaláricas de la serie aminoquinolinas. Rev. de San. Asist. Soc. 16 (3-4) 318-441 (887).

O'DALY, J.A. y DE LA PLAZA, Gustavo

1934— Contribución al estudio de la fiebre biliosa hemoglobinúrica. Gac. Méd. de Car. XLI, 1, 1-7 (889).

O'DALY, J.A. y LANDAETA PAYARES, H.

1934— Sifiloma de la lengua. Rev. Pol. Car. (890).

O'DALY J.A. y JIMENEZ RIVERO, Miguel

1935— El primer caso de Acantosis nigricans en Venezuela. Rev. Medical. Caracas, II, 13, 204-207 (891).

O'DALY, J.A.

1936— Contribución al estudio de la Ascaridosis en el hombre. Bol. de los Hosp. Caracas XXXIV, 7, 334-347 (892).

1937— Las Blastomicosis en Venezuela (Primera Comunicación). Bol. de los Hosp. Caracas XXXVI, 3 127-156 (893).

1938— Un caso de papilomatosis vulvar bilharziana. Rev. de la Poli. Car. 39, 2648-2650 (894).

1938a— Algo sobre Micosis en Venezuela. Micetoma de la mano por Actynomices madurae. Rev. de la Poli. Caracas. N° 41 (895).

1939— La Cromoblastomicosis en Venezuela. Rev. de la Poli. Car. 44 (896).

1941— Estudio anatómico sobre Sífilis cardiovascular en el Hospital Vargas. Trabajo leído en la semana científica destinada a la conmemoración del cincuentenario del Hosp. Vargas (897).

1943a— La Cromoblastomicosis en Venezuela. Primera Jornada Ven. de Venereología y Dermatología. Rev. de San. y Asis. S oc. VIII, 4, 655-680 (898).

ORAA, Espartaco

1943— Encuesta sanitaria sobre la ciudad de Villa de Cura, presentada a la I Conf. Anual de Médicos Jefes de Unidades Sanitarias M.S.A.S. (899).

ORELLANA, Daniel

1934— Contribución al estudio de las Amibiasis latentes. Tesis de Doctorado en Ciencias Médicas. Caracas. Edit. Bolívar, 28 p. (900).

1937— Estudio sobre la Buba en el Distrito Páez del Estado Miranda. Bol. Minist. San. Asist. Soc. Vol. I, págs. 836-854 (901).

1937a— El Problema Social de la Sífilis. Folleto "La Semana del Venéreo". Tip. Americana. Caracas. Págs. 96-104 y en el Bol. Minist. San. Asist. Soc. Págs. 1042-1051, Vol. I (902).

1941— Datos sobre infestación de Triatomideos por Tripanosoma cruzi en la zona de San Juan de los Morros. Rev. San. Asist. Soc. VI, 4, 475-477 (903).

1943— Encuesta Sanitaria sobre la ciudad de Los Teques, presentada a la I Conferencia Anual de Médicos Jefes de Unidades Sanitarias. Arch. de la División de Unidades Sanitarias M.S.A.S. (904).

OROPEZA, Pastor

1935— La necesidad de una gota gruesa en todo caso de pirexia. La fiebre transitoria o criptogenética del recién nacido. Gac. Méd. de Car. XLII (905).

OROPEZA, Pastor y VEGAS, Martín

1939— El tratamiento de la Sífilis en la mujer embarazada y de la heredo-sífilis. Bol. Minist. San. Asist. Soc. IV, 5, 186-191 (906).

ORTIZ, Adelmo

1941— Cuadros febriles bilharzianos. Tesis de doctorado en Ciencias Médicas. Caracas. Tip. Americana. 47 p. y en la Gac. Méd. de Car. Año XLVIII, abril 30 (907).

ORTIZ, C., Ignacio

1942— Insectos hematófagos (Díptera, Heleidae) del Estado Falcón, con citación de una especie nueva (Culicoides variipennis Coq.), para Venezuela. Rev. de la Poli. Car. XI, 66, 258 (908).

OTOLINA, Carlos

1947— El problema clínico de la Schistosomiasis mansoni ante nuevos métodos diagnósticos y sus resultados. (Revista Pol. Car. Vol. 16, N° 93. Pág. 55) (909).

1951— Sobre Schistosomiasis mansoni. Rev. Pol. Caracas. Vol. XIX, N° 121. Pág. 492 (910).

OSECHAS VILLEGAS, Asdrúbal

1930— Contribución al estudio de las parasitosis apendiculares en Venezuela. Tesis de Doctorado en Ciencias Médicas. Caracas. Lit. y Tip. Casa de Espec. (911).

OTOLINA, Carlos

1951— Valor absoluto de la biopsia rectoscópica por transparencia estudiado en 138 rectos humanos enteros preparados con una técnica adecuada. Rev. de la Pol. Caracas. Vol. XIX. N° 117 (912).

OTOLINA, Carlos y ATENCIO, H.

1946— Comentarios al trabajo del Profesor R. Jaffe y del Dr. R. Ferro titulado de la Bilharzia en el material de autopsia. Revista Pol. Caracas. Vol. XV. N° 89 (913).

OTOLINA, Carlos

1946— El diagnóstico de la infección bilharziana con la biopsia rectoscópica por transparencia. Rev. Pol. Caracas. Vol. XV. N° 90 (914).

1947— El problema clínico de la Schistosomiasis mansoni ante nuevo método diagnóstico y sus resultados. Rev. Pol. Caracas. Vol. XVI. N° 93 (915).

ORTIZ, Ignacio

1947— Nota sobre Phlebotomus gomezi Nitzulescu 1921 y Phlebotomus cruciatus. Coq. 1907. Bol. del Lab. Clí. Razetti. Año VII. Núms. 23-24 (916).

ORTIZ, Ignacio, PARDO, Luis E.

1949— Presentación de un caso de Leishmaniosis tegumentaria múltiple con lesiones lepromatoides. Bol. del Lab. Clí. Razetti. Año IX, Núms. 29-30 (917).

ORTIZ, Ignacio

1949— Nota sobre nuevos caratopogonidos hematófagos para Venezuela. Bol. Lab. Clí. Razetti. Año IX. Núms. 29-30 (918).

1951— Estudios en Culicoides. (Díptera-Ceratopogonidae). Año XI. Números 33-34. Boletín del Lab. Clí. Razetti. (919).

ORTIZ, Ignacio y MARIE, Mirsa

1952— Estudios en Culicoides (Diptera-Ceratopogonidae). Año XI. Números 35-36. Boletín del Lab. Clí. Razetti (920).

OROPEZA, R., y RAGA MENDOZA, Miguel

1952— Toxoplasmosis humana en Venezuela. Arch. Ven. Puer. y Ped. XVI (49). 363-368 (921).

OROPEZA, P., VIZCARRONDO, E., GAMEZ, Luis E., ACOSTA M. Antonio y SANCHEZ PEREZ, R.

1950— El problema de la sífilis en Venezuela; pautas para su prevención, diagnóstico y tratamiento. Revista de Sanidad y Asistencia Social. M.S.A. Sep-Octubre 1950. Vol. XV. N° 5. (922).

ORTIZ, Ignacio

1950— Nota de Phlebotomus (Diptera Psychodidae). A.V. de Trop. y P. Medical. Vol. II, N° 1 (923).

Sobre dos nuevos machos del género Phlebotomus de la familia Psychodidae (924).

C. pifanoi, Ortíz, 1951, en Venezuela (925).

Entomología médica. Insectos del género Leptocoptus Diptera Ceratopogonidae. Enero a Abril de 1952. Vol. N° N L y 2 (926).

ORTIZ, Ignacio

1944— Simulium quadrivitatum Loew. Su presencia en Venezuela. Bol. Lab. de la Clí. L.R. IV. 14, 243-246 (927).

OSECHAS VILLEGAS, Aníbal

1930— Contribución al estudio de las parasitosis apendiculares en Venezuela. Tesis de Doctorado en Ciencias Médicas. Caracas. Lit. y Tip. Casa de Especialidades. 44 pç (929).

OTTOLINA, Carlos

1930— Contribución al conocimiento de la parasitosis intestinal en Valencia. Rev. de la Conferencia Sanitaria Nacional. Caracas. I, 8, 227-230 (930).

OTTOLINA, Carlos y ATENCIO M., H.

1943— Nuevos caminos para el diagnóstico clínico preciso de la Schistosomiasis mansoni. Rev. de la Pol. Car. XII, 73, 348-380 (6224) (931).

ORTIZ, Ignacio

1953— Nueva contribución al conocimiento de los caracteres morfológicos externos de las hembras americanas del género. Culicoides. Ltr. (Diptera, Caratopogonidae) con una espermateca. Descripción de dos nuevas especies de Venezuela. Rev. San. Asist. Soc. Vol. XVIII, N° 5 y 6. Pág. 797 (932).

1953— Sobre una nueva especie del género Culicoides (Diptera, Ceratopogonidae) próxima de C. hortícola Lutz 1913. Rev. San. Asist. Soc. Vol. XVIII, N° 5 y 6. Pág. 807 (933).

1954— Sobre dos nuevos Dipteros hematófagos del género Culicoides. Arch. Ven. de P. y P. Med. N° 2, Vol. II (934).

PEÑA, Vicente

1932— Los heredo-sifilíticos. Trabajo de incorporación a la Acad. Nac. de Medicina. Gac. Méd. Car. XXXVII y en folleto. Tip. Americana. 63 p. (935).

1934— Emetino-terapia en la ambiasis de los niños. Gac. Méd. de Car. XLI, 14, 221-223 (936).

1934b— Oportunidad del tratamiento en la sífilis. Gac. Méd. de Car. XL, 18, 273-274 (937).

6315 (OJO).

1938b— Palabras sobre el libro del Dr. D. Carbonell, La Parasitología en Venezuela y los trabajos del Dr. Núñez Tovar. Gac. Méd. de Car. XLV, y en folleto. Car. Tip. Americana. 15 p. (938).

1943— Impaludación relámpago por Plasmodium falciparum. Gac. Méd. de Car. L, 2, 18 (939).

1943a— Las quinas. Gac. Méd. de Car. L, 7, 32-33 (940).

PERDOMO, Raúl

1938— La quinina y sus sales. Tesis de Bachillerato en Filosofía. Caracas. Emp. El Cojo. 18 p. (941).

PERDOMO, Hurtado B.

1937c— Un caso de hepatitis febril de origen bilharziósico. Gac. Méd. de Car. XLIV, 19, 209-291 (942).

PERDOMO, Hurtado B., RUIZ, J.M. y OSUNA, A.

1938— Un caso de cirrosis hipertrófica de origen bilharziano. Gac. Méd. de Car. XLV, 5, 67-71 (943).

PERDOMO, Hurtado B.

1938a— Un caso de hepatitis febril de origen bilharziósico. Gac. Méd. de Car. XLV (944).

1941— Un caso de esplenomegalia insólita de origen bilharziano. Gac. Méd. de Car. XLVIII (945).

PEREIRA ALVAREZ, Virginia

1939— Contribución a la investigación experimental de la Leptospira icterohemorrhagiae en Venezuela. Gac. Méd. de Car. XLVI, 21, 424 (946).

PEREZ CARREÑO, Miguel

1943a— La esplenectomía en la forma hepato-esplénica de la Bilharziosis mansoni. Rev. de la Pol. Car. XII, 69-71-87 (947).

1944— El Síndrome colopericolo-apendicular parasitario. Gac. Méd. de Car. LII, 21, 230-236 (948).

PEREZ CORONEL, R.

1932— Breve disertación sobre el paludismo y su profilaxis en los Llanos. Rev. de la Conf. Sanit. Nac. III, 4, 112-116 (949).

PEREZ GALDOS, I.

1940— Asma bronquial y parasitosis intestinal. Rev. de la Pol. Car. IX, 52, 3493-3500 (950).

PIFANO C., Félix

1934— Las serpientes ponzoñosas del Estado Yaracuy. Tesis de Bachillerato. Imprenta Bolívar. Caracas. 16 p. (951).

1935— Breves notas sobre la terapéutica del emponzoñamiento ofídico. Rev. S.E.M. Caracas. I, 8-9, 13-24 (952).

1935a— Contribución al estudio etio-patológico y clínico del emponzoñamiento bothrópico en Venezuela. Tesis de Doctorado en Ciencias Médicas. Caracas. Coop. de Artes Gráficas. 43 p. (953).

1938— Manera de estudiar un criadero de larvas de Anofelinos. Tij. Mal. Caracas. I, 3, 47-49 (955).

1938a— Enfermedad de Chagas en el Estado Yaracuy. Presentación de caso agudo diagnosticado por el examen directo de la sangre. Rev. de la Pol. Car. 39, 2653-2655 (956).

1938b— Un caso de enfermedad de Chagas en el caserío de Guarativana (Dto. Sucre, Estado Yaracuy), comprobado por el xenodiagnóstico. Estudio de algunos factores epidemiológicos del lugar relacionados con esta dolencia. Rev. Pol. Car. VIII, 43, 2897-2906, en folleto (957).

PIFANO C., Félix

1938c— Anotaciones acerca del Psammolestes arthuri Pinto. 1936 (Hemíptera, Heteróptera, Triatomide), reduvideo hematófago, en un sector de los valles del Yaracuy. Su importancia como probable vector en la naturaleza del Schizotrypanum cruzi Chagas, 1909. Gac. Méd. Car. XLV, 16, 241-251 (958).

1938d— Algunas investigaciones para el estudio de la esquizotripanosis americana o enfermedad de Chagas en los Valles del Yaracuy, resultados del xenodiagnóstico en infecciones experimentales y humanas. Public. de la Asoc. Méd. del Yaracuy,

San Felipe. I, 1, 3-9 (959).

1938e— Corales ponzoñosas de los Valles de Yaracuy. Pesquisas experimentales con la ponzoña del Micrurus lemniscatus (Linneo, 1758). Public. de la Asoc. Méd. del Yaracuy. San Felipe. I, 1, 10-15 (960).

PITANO C., Félix y GOMEZ PERAZA, A.

1938— Infestación natural de Rhodnius prolixus (Stal, 1859) por el Schizotrypanum cruzi en el caserío "Los Yabos", Estado Lara. Presencia del Eutriatoma maculata. (Erichson, 1848; Pinto, 1931) en la región. Public. de la Asoc. Méd. del Yaracuy. San Felipe, I, 1, 15-16 (961).

PIFANO C., Félix

1938— Aspectos clínicos del paludismo pernicioso en los Valles del Yaracuy (962).

1938a— Reduvideos hematófagos de los Valles del Yaracuy. Su infestación en la naturaleza por el Schizotrypanum cruzi. Chagas 1909. Bol. Minist. San. Asist. Soc. I, 3, 1941-1944 (963).

1939— Sobre la colecta de huevos de anofelinos en el campo. Tij. Mal. Caracas. II, 4, 58 (964).

1939a— Breve nota sobre paludismo congenito, presentación de dos casos, Arch. Ven. de Pueric. y Pediat. Caracas, I, 3, 155-157 (965).

1939b— Nota y comentarios sobre un caso agudo de enfermedad de Chagas con edema palpebral unilateral comprobado en el Estado Yaracuy. Arch. Ven. de Pueric. y Pediat. I, 3, 161-167 (966).

1939c— Serpientes venenosas venezolanas. Clínica del emponzoñamiento ofídico (967).

1939d— Breve nota sobre algunos zoo-parásitos observados en el Yaracuy. Bol. Minist. San. Asist. Soc. IV, 4, 186-190 (968).

1939e— Contribución al estudio epidemiológico y clínico de la leishmaniasis cutáneo-mucosa en el Estado Yaracuy. Bol. Minist. San. Asist. Soc. IV, 2, 7-15 (969).

1939f— Sobre un Schizotrypanum de un murciélago del Estado Yaracuy. Venezuela. Rev. de la Pol. Car. 46, 3103-3104 (970).

1939g— Eutriatoma nigromaculata, especie venezolana encontrada infestada por el Schizotrypanum cruzi. Rev. de la Pol. Car. 46, 3115-3118 (971).

1939h— Emponzoñamiento por serpientes venezolanas. Gac. Méd. de Car. XLVI, 12, 184-189 (972).

1939i— Sobre un portador sano de Schizotrypanum cruzi, observado en La Victoria. Gac. Méd. de Car. XLVI, 13-204 (973).

1939j— Nota sobre la infestación experimental y en la naturaleza del Psammolestes arthuri (Pinto, 1926) por el Schizotrypanum cruzi, Chagas 1909. Gac. Méd. de Car. (974).

1939k— Nota sobre Trypanosoma del Myotis nigricans. Wied. murciélago del Estado Yaracuy. Su posible identidad con el Trypanosoma megadermae. Wenyon 1919. Gac. Méd. de Car. (975).

1939l— Nota sobre epidemiología y clínica del paludismo en un sector del Estado Yaracuy. Algunas consideraciones sobre profilaxia antimalárica y tratamiento. Premio A.P. Reverend. Rev. Bol. II, 4, 63-102 (976).

1940— La leismaniosis tegumentaria en el Estado Yaracuy, Venezuela. Rev. de la Poli. Car. XLVIII, 11-12, 292-299 (977).

1941— La epidemiología de la enfermedad de Chagas en el Estado Yaracuy. Rev. San. Asist. Soc. VI, 3, 303-310 (978).

1914a— Investigaciones para el estudio de la fiebre recurrente en Venezuela. Rev. San. Asist. Soc. VI, 6, 787-811 (979).

1940a— La enfermedad de Chagas en Venezuela. Trabajo presentado al VIII Congreso Científico Americano. Rev. de la Ofic. San. Panam. XIX, 10, 984-986 (980).

1940b— Sobre un Trypanosoma del C. prehensilis L. (puerco espín), posible reservorio del Schzotrypanum cruzi en la naturaleza. Gac. Méd. de Car. XLVII, 7, 77-78 (981).

PIFANO C., Félix

1940c— Sobre el desarrollo de la Leishmania trópica brasilensis en flebotomus de Venezuela. Gac. Méd. de Car. XLVII, 10-114-116 (982).

1940d— Sobre un Triatomideo del género Eratyrus comprobado en el Estado Yaracuy, Venezuela. (En colaboración con el Dr. R. Medina). Rev. de Méd. Veterin. y Parasit. II, 1 y 2, 45-47 (983).

1941— La enfermedad de Chagas en Venezuela. Rev. S.E.M. VIII, 71-72-14 (984).

1941b— La enfermedad de Chagas en el Estado Yaracuy. Premio Vargas. Car. Méd. VIII, 19, 1103-1166 y en la Gac. Méd. de Car. XLVIII. Núms. 3 al 7 (985).

1941c— En colab. con H. Lent. Redescripción de Triatoma nigromaculata, su infestación en condiciones naturales por Schizotrypanum cruzi (986).

1941d— En colab. con H. Lent. Redescripción de Panstrongylus rufotuberculatus (987).

1941e— Parasitismo natural de Amblyomma longyrostre Koch 1814 por Schizoytrypanum cruzi, Chagas 1909. Gac. Méd. de Car. XLVIIII, 10, 288-289 (989).

1941f— Nota parasitaria sobre el treponema del carate en Venezuela. Gac. Méd. de Car. XLVIII, 13-14. 313-314 (990).

PIFANO, Félix

1941— La eosinofilia en la Schistosomiasis mansoni. Rev. San. Asist. Social. VI, 3, 296-302 (994).

PIFANO, Félix y LUTTERMOSER, George

1942— Aspectos epidemiológicos de la Schistosomiasis mansoni en San Casimiro (Edo. Aragua). Rev. San. Asist. Soc. VII, 3, 397 (995).

PIFANO, Félix y MAYER, Martín

1941— Nuevos métodos para el diagnóstico de la enfermedad de Chagas. Rev. San. Asist. Soc. VI, 3, 311-316 (991).

1941a— Sobre el cultivo de Leishmania tropica en Venezuela, e intra-reacción con Leishmania-antígeno. Rev. San. Asist. Soc. VI, 3, 281-289 (992).

1941b— Reacciones serológicas en Bilharziosis mansoni según el método de Fairley. Rev. San. Asist. Soc. VI, 3, 390-295 (903).

PIFANO, Félix

1942— En colab. con E. Díaz. Estudios biológicos de un Schizotrypanum de Hemiderma perspicillata (997).

1942— En colab. con E. Díaz. Estudios de un Schizotrypanum de Phyllostoma elongatum del Amazonas (998).

PIFANO, Félix y MAYER, Martín

1942— Estudios biológicos y patológicos en animales infectados con Schistosoma mansoni (infecciones bi y unisexuales). Rev. San. Asist. Soc. VII, 3, 419 (999).

PIFANO, Félix

1943— Phlebotomos transmisores de la leishmaniasis tegumentaria en Venezuela. Rev. de Entomología Venezolana II, 2, 99-102 (1000).

1943a— La schistosomiasis mansoni en un sector del Estado Aragua. Premio J.G. Hernández (1001).

1943b— Trabajos prácticos de la Cátedra: el examen de sangre para la investigación de los parásitos malários. Descripción de la técnica. Coloración según el método de Cliemsa. Public. de la Cátedra de Patología Tropical. Caracas. Tomo I, Fascículo I, páginas 17-21 (1002).

1944— Caracteres diferenciales de los parásitos maláricos del hombre. Public. de la Cátedra de Patología Tropical. Caracas, Tomo I, Fasc. I, págs. 26-32 (1003).

PIÑA DAZA, Mario

1944— Algo más sobre Schistosomiasis Mansoni. Bol. de los Hosp. Caracas. XLIII, 1, 28-46 (1004).

PLANAS TORREALBA, R. y MOLINA G., Jesús

1943— Leishmaniosis en el Estado Yaracuy. Contribución a su estudio. San Felipe. Tip. Moderna, 14 p. (1005).

PLAZA DE LA, Gustavo

1933a— Sifiloma hepático febril (Diagnóstico terapéutico). Bol. de los Hosp. Caracas. XXIII, 21, 14-16 (1006).

PLAZA DE LA, Gustavo y BRICEÑO IRAGORRY, L.

1934— Una nueva especie de flebotomus en Venezuela. Rev. Medical, Caracas, 8, 111-113 (1007).

PLAZA DE LA, Gustavo y O'DALY, J.A.

1934— Contribución al estudio de la fiebre biliosa hemoglobinúrica. Gac. Méd. de Car. XL, 1-7 (1008).

PLAZA IZQUIERDO, L.

1943— La esplenectomía en las enfermedades hepato-esplénicas de la Bilharziosis mansoni. Rev. de la Poli. Car. XII, 72, 280-306 (1009).

POLLAK, Ladislao

1943— Alergia ascaridiana y tuberculosa. Presentado al II Congreso Ven. de Tuberculosis (1010).

PONS, Adolfo R.

1936— La sífilis en el Hospital Vargas. Consideraciones de índole clínica, estadística y profiláctica. Tesis de Doctorado en Ciencias Médicas. Caracas. Coop. de Artes Gráficas. 22 p. (1011).

1936a— Algo más sobre la dolencia de Chagas en Venezuela. Trabajo premiado Concurso Luis Razetti. Año 1936. Gac. Méd. de Car. XLIII y en la Rev. S.E.M. 1936, III, 24-27, 6-8 (1012).

PONS, Adolfo y MARTINEZ NIOCHET, Arminio

1941— Primer caso de Kala-azar en Venezuela. Gac. Méd. de Car. XLVIII, 17-18, 329-331 (1013).

POTENZA, Leandro

1939— Contribución al estudio de la distribución de los huevos de los parásitos intestinales en los diferentes segmentos del tubo digestivo en especial del apéndice. Tesis de Doctorado. Caracas. Lit. y Tip. Casa de Especialidades. 29 p. (1014).

1941a— Estudio comparativo de los pigmentos bilharziano y malárico. Rev. de la Poli. Car. X, 61, 363-373 (1015).

POTENZAL., y ANDUZE, P.J.

1942— Kala-azar en el Estado Bolívar. Rev. de la Poli. CAr. XI, 67, 312-317 (1016).

POTENZA, Leandro

1943— Sífilis en las arterias de calibre mediano. Rev. San. Asist. Soc. VIII, 1103 (1017).

1943a— Sífilis cardiovascular como causa de muerte. Primera Jornada Venezolana de Venereología y Dermatología. Rev. San. Asist. Soc. VIII, 4, 735 (1018).

1943b— Bilharziosis pulmonar. Rev. de la Poli. Car. XII, 69-119-125 (1019).

1944— Cisticercosis cerebral. Rev. de la Poli. Car. XIII, 77-255 (1020).

PRAG, Raúl van

1943a— Breves consideraciones acerca de la anquilostomiasis. Bol. Minist. Salub. Agric. y Cría. I, 8-9. 727-729 (1021).

1936— Notas acerca de un tratamiento de la úlcera fagedénica. Bol. Minist. San. Asist. Soc. I, 2, 116-119 (1022).

PRISCO, J. DI, y D'ARAGO FLORES

1940— ¿Hepatitis tífica o amibiana? Rev. S.E.M. VII, 68-70, 28-33 (1023).

PRISCO, Juan Di

1943— Nota preliminar sobre posibles dermatosis de origen bilharziano y su diagnóstico por la prueba cutánea de la bilharzia. Primeros Jornadas Venezolanas de Venereología y Dermatología. Rev. de San. y Asist. Soc. VIII, 5, 1067-1072 (1024).

POTENZA, Leandro y BARNOLA, José

1950— Leishmaniasis visceral infantil en Venezuela. Arch. Ven. de Puer. y Pediat. XIII: 38, págs. 5-16 (1025).

PIFANO, Félix C.

1947— Primera comprobación del Trypanosoma rangeli en el organismo. Gac. Méd. Car. Año LV. Nos. 10-24. 203 (1026).
1941— La epidemia de la enfermedad de Chagas en el Estado Yaracuy. Rev. S.A.S. Vol. XI, p. 303 (1027).
1947— Aislamiento de Schizotrypanum cruzi en casos crónicos de enfermedad de Chagas. Gac. Méd. Car. Año LV. Nos. 19-24, página 208 (1028).
1953— La resistencia del huésped vertebrado a las re-infecciones por Schistosoma mansoni. Rev. S.A.S. Vol. XVIII, Nos. 5 y 6, página 767 (1029).
1938— Un caso de enfermedad de Chagas en el caserío Guarativana, Distrito Sucre, Estado Yaracuy, comprobado por el xenodiagnóstico (1030).
1940— La enfermedad de Chagas en Venezuela. Trabajo presentado a la IV Conferencia Panamericana F. 27-16 (1031).
1941— La eosinofilia en la Schistosomiasis mansoni. Rev. S.A.S. Vol. VI, pág. 296 (1032).
1938— Reduvidos hematófagos de los Valles del Yaracuy. Bol. S.A.S. pág. 1941. Año 1938 (1033).
1942— Sobre el comportamiento de la reacción de Fairley en los estudios de la Schistosomiasis mansoni. Rev. S.A.S. Vol. VII, página 379 (1034).

PIFANO, Félix y otros

1947— Aislamiento de Schizotrypanum cruzi en casos crónicos de enfermedad de Chagas por cultivo de sangre periférica. Gac. Méd. de Car. (19-24) 208 (1035).
1948— La infección natural del perro por el Trypanosoma rangeli. Gac. Méd. de Car. (7-12): 130-134 (1036).

PIFANO, Félix

1948— La infección uni-sexuada producida por Schistosoma mansoni en condiciones experimentales. Arch. Ven. de Patol. Trop. y Parasit. Mad. I. (1): 63-72 (1037).
1949— Aspectos clínicos del síndrome de Banti bilharziano en Venezuela. Arch. Ven. de Patol. Trop. y Parasit. Med. I (2) 41-72 (1038).
1949— et. al—Estado actual de las investigaciones en Venezuela sobre una nueva trypanosomiasis humana de la región neotrópica producida por el Trypanosoma rangeli. Arch. Ven. de Pat. Trop. Parasit. Med. (1) (2) (1039).

PIFANO, Félix y MAYER, Martín

1949— Conservación por años en la nevera de cerebros con plasmodium falciparum. Arch. Ven. de Pat. Trop. y Parasit. Med. I (2), 327-328 (1040).

PIFANO, Félix y otros

1949— Estudios experimentales con una cepa de Leishmania brasilensis proveniente de un caso de leishmaniasis tegumentaria diseminada de aspecto lepromatoso. Arch. Ven. de Pat. Trip. y Parasit. Med. I (2), 183-291 (1041).

PIFANO, Félix

1949— La leishmaniasis tegumentaria en Venezuela. Arch. Ven. de Pat. Trop. y Parasit. Med. I (2) 170-182 (1044).

PIFANO, Félix, MARCUZZI, Giorgio

1950— Contribución al estudio experimental de las miocarditis parasitarias de la región neotrópica. Arch. Ven. Parasit. Trop. Med. II (1) 175 (1045).

PIFANO, Félix y otros

1950— Investigaciones sobre enfermedad de Chagas y Tripanosomiasis rangeli en el Distrito Roscio, Edo. (1046).

PIFANO, C. Félix

1939— Breve nota sobre algunos zoo-parásitos observados en Yaracuy. Bol. Minist. de San. y Asist. Soc. IV ($) 186-190 (1047).

PIFANO C., Félix y MEYER, Martín

1946— Aspecto epidemiológicos de la Enfermedad de Chagas en Venezuela. Base para una campaña de saneamiento aplicables a zonas endémicas del medio rural venezolano. Conferencia Sanitaria. Cuaderno Amarillo, N° 30 (1048).

PIFANO y MEYER

1951— Modalidades de las infecciones producidas por Schistosoma mansoni en animales de laboratorio infectados con cercarias provenientes de un solo caracol. Rev. S.A.S. Vol. XVI, Nos. 5-6, pág. 445 (1049).

PIFANO, KINNON, MAC, PESSOA y TREJO

1954— Parasitology, 287 pág. (1050).

PIFANO, VOGELSANG, Enrique y ANDUZE, Pablo J.

1947— Nómina de los artrópodos vulnerantes conocidos actualmente en Venezuela. Bol. de Entomología venezolana. Vol. VI, Número extraordinario (1051).

PIFANO, Ortiz Ignacio

1952— Representantes venezolanos del género Phlebotomus rondani 1840 (Diptera-Psychodidae), Rev. S.A.S. Vol. XVII. Nos. 1-2, página 135 (1052).

1952— Cavernícola pilosa Barber, 1937. Hemiptera Heteroptera Triatomidae. Rev. S.A.S. Vol. XVII. Nos. 3-4, pág. 245 (1053).

PIFANO

1951— La cercaría-reacción de Vogel-Minning. Schistosomias mansoni. Rev. S.A.S. N° 5 y 6, pág. 461.
Rev. S.A.S. Vol. XVI, Nos. 5-6, pág. 445 (1054).

1945— Schistosoma mansoni. Rev. S.A.S. Vol. X, pág. 65 (1055).

PRISCO, J. de

1953— Nueva contribución al estudio de la tiña en el medio escolar de Caracas. Vol. XXI, N° 127 (1056).

1948— Las tiñas en el medio escolar de Caracas. Rev. Pol. Caracas. Vol. XVII, Nos. 101-102 (1057).

POTENZA y Alfredo CELIS PEREZ

1947— Rhinosporidiosis nasal humana. Primera observación venezolana. Rev. Pol. Caracas. Vol. XVI. Nos. 95-96 (1058).

POTENZA L., FEBRES CORDERO REYNALDO y ANDUEZA, Pablo

1949— Nuevo foco endémico de oncocercosis humana en el mundo (Venezuela). Bol. Médico. Vol. I, N° 3, pág. 263 (1059).

PUIGBO, J.J.

1949— Estudios comparativos entre los índices hematológicos de Wintrobe y la micrometría directa (curva de Price-Jones) en anemias de sujetos desnutridos y parasitados. Rev. Pol. Caracas. Vol. XVIII. Nos. 107-108-109, pág. 137 (1060).

PEÑA, Vicente

1938— Palabra sobre el libro del Dr. D. Carbonell. La Parasitología en Venezuela y los trabajos del Dr. Núñez Tovar. Gac. Méd. de Car. XLV (1061).

PIFANO y otros

Guárico. Venezuela. Gac. Méd. de Car. (7-12): 85 (1065).

PIFANO, Félix y otros

1950— Estado actual de las investigaciones sobre enfermedad de Chagas en el Valle de Yaracuy, Venezuela. I reunión Panam. sobre enfermedad de Chagas (Julio, 11-16-49. Tucumán, Argentina). Fas. I, 91-95 (1063).

PIFANO, Félix y BENAIN PINTO H.

1950— La miocarditis crónica en Venezuela. Estudio analítico y sintético del problema etio-patogénico de la miocarditis crónica en el medio rural venezolano. Arch. Ven. Pat. Trop. Par. Med. II (1), 223-233 (1065).

PIFANO, Félix y otros

1950— Representantes venezolanos del género Eratryrus (hemiptera, triatomidae) y redescripción del Eratyrus mucronatus Stall. 1859. Arch. Ven. Pat. Med. II (1): 249-244 (1065).

PIFANO, Félix

1954— El diagnóstico parasitológico de la enfermedad de Chagas en la fase crónica. Gac. Med. de Car. (11) 12: 629-637 (1066).

1954— El diagnóstico parasitológico de la enfermedad de Chagas en fase crónica. Estudio comparativo entre la gota gruesa experimentales en animales sensibles. Arch. Ven. Patol. Trop. y Parasit. Med. II (2) 129-156 (1067).

1954— Estado actual del Kala-Azar en Venezuela. Arch. Ven. Pat. Trop. y Parasit. Med. II (2), 213-219 (1068).

1954— Nueva Trypanosomiasis humana de la región neotrópica producida por T. rangeli, con especial referencia a Venezuela. Arch. Ven. de Pat. Trop. y Pars. Med. Vol. II, Nº 2 (1069).

PIFANO, ROMER, Miguel y BR. SANDER, Montilla F.

1950— Serpientes ponzoñosas en Venezuela. Arch. Ven. de Pat. Trop. y Pars. Med. Vol. II, Nº 1 (1070).

PINEDA, A.

1926— Valor diagnóstico del pigmento palúdico en la sangre. Tesis (D.C.M.) Universidad Central de Venezuela. págs. 9-55 (1071).

PRISCO J. Di y MONTEMAYOR, L.

A propósito de un caso de tiña en adulto producida por T. rubrum (1072).

PEÑALVER, Luis M.

1950— Infeccion experimental de moluscos cubanos con S. mansoni A.V.P.T. y Pat. Médica. Enero. Vol. II, Nº 1 (1073).

PARRILLI, Juan Pablo

1951— Corazón pulmonar bilharziano. Primer caso descrito en Venezuela, diciembre 1951 (1074).

PARILLI J.P. y VIVAS SALAS, E.

Ausencia de síntomas en las Aortitis sifilíticas (1075).

PIFANO, Félix

1955— Estado actual del Kala-azar en Venezuela. Revista de San. Asist. Soc. (1076).

PEÑA GARCIA

Presencia A. duodenale Dubini 1843, asociado con necator americanus Stiles 1906, en caso de anquilostomiasis. Maracaibo, Edo. Zulia. Venezuela. Gac. Méd. de Ca- Enero-Febrero 1955. Nº 1, Vol. I y II (1077).

POTENZA, L. y BENAIN PINTO H.

Observaciones en Venezuela de dos casos de Torulopsis cryptococus neoformas del sistema nervioso central 1949. Arch. Ven. de Pat. Trop. y Part. Med. (1078).

POTENZA y FEO M.

Paracoccidiosis infantil en Venezuela, aspecto del parásito a la luz polarizada. Arch. Ven. de Pueric. y Ped. 16-7-22, 1953 (1079).

POLLAK, Ladislao

"Histoplasmosis en Venezuela" (Ensayo Epidemiológico) 3 y 4, 569 (1080).

PIFANO C., Félix, MEDINA FEBRES, Mariano, MEDINA, Rafael y ROMER, Miguel

"La Leishmaniasis tegumentaria americana" (1081/).

QUINTANA, César y SOTO IRIBARREN

1934— Sífilis, Metritis y Aborto. Car. Méd. I, 4, 195 (1082).

QUINTANA LLAMOZAS, Pablo

1931— El paludismo en Puerto Cabello. Caracas. Tip. Americana, 6 h. (1083).

1932— Sífilis ignorada y sífilis sin chancro. Folleto "Semana Antivenérea". Publi. del Minist. de Salub. y de Agric. y Cría. Págs. 81-90 (1084).

1936— Buba. Diario "El Heraldo", Caracas, Nº 4243. Mayo 28 (1085).

QUINTERO LUZARDO, G.

1928— Sobre dos casos de la reavivación de la sífilis por Med.-Quirúrg. del Zul. II, 13, 162-164 (1086).

QUINTERO QUINTERO, J.S.

1929— Parasitosis intestinal en la fiebre tifoidea. Rev. de la Soc. Méd.-Quirúrgica del Zulia. III, pág. 64 (1087).

QUINTINI, José

1929— La defensa contra el Ofidismo. Una serpiente útil. Rev. de la Soc. Méd.-Quirúrg. del Zulia, III, 11, 100-103 (1088).

1935— Apuntes clínicos sobre algunos casos de mordeduras por serpientes ponzoñosas. Rev. Trujillo. I, 1, 12-14 (1089).

1936— El Ofidismo en el Estado Trujillo. Resumen de los éxitos obtenidos con el suero antiofídico. Bol. Minist. San. Asist. Soc. I, 1, 15-21 (1090).

1936a— Contribución al estudio del género Bothrops en el Estado Trujillo. Car. Méd. III, 9, 493 (1091).

1942— Serpientes ponzoñosas o inofensivas. Reglas para diferenciarlas. Rev. Tópicos Shell de Venezuela, Maracaibo, IV. 38, 18-21 (1092).

1942a— Sección Médico-Sanitaria. Tratamiento de los accidentes por mordeduras de serpientes. Rev. Tópicos Shell de Venezuela. Maracaibo. Noviembre (1093).

1943h— La sífilis y otras enfermedades venéreas. Rev. Tópicos Shell de Venezuela. V, 52, 11-12 (1094).

1943i— Las lombrices y otros parásitos intestinales. Rev. Tópicos Shell de Venezuela. Maracaibo. V, 53, 9-11 (1095).

RAMOS SUCRE, Luis

1930— La anquilostomiasis en Cumaná. Mem. de la I Conferencia San. Nac. Caracas. Tip. Americana. Págs. 306-310 (1096).

1931— Paludismo Rev. de Medic. y Cirug. Maracay, I, 3 (1097).

1933— Breves notas sobre amibiasis hepática. Rev. de págs. 59-63. Diciembre (1098).

REYES GONZALEZ, José

1933— Influencia de los climas y de los tratamientos insuficientes en el paludismo. Bol. Minist. Salub. Agric. y Cría. I, 4, 6, 356 (1099).

1934— Lucha contra el paludismo en el Estado Cojedes. Resultados obtenidos en la defensa de la infancia contra el paludismo. Bol. Minist. Salub. Agric. y Cría. II, págs. 355-368 (1100).

1935— Lucha contra el paludismo en el Estado Cojedes. Quininización rural. Bol. Minist. Selub. Agric. y Cría. III, 27, 325-334 (1101).

1936— Campaña antipalúdica en Cojedes. Bol. Minist. San. Asist. Soc. I, 1, 58-62 (1102).

RHODE, Jesús

1932— La sífilis y sus manifestaciones oculares. Folleto "Semana Antivenérea". Public. del Minist. de Salub. y de Agri. y Cría. Caracas. págs. 91-95 (1103).

RISQUEZ, Francisco Antonio

1930b— El pigmento melánico en el paludismo. Gac. Méd. de Car. XXXVII, 10, 149 (1104).

1934— Fiebre biliosa hemoglobinúrica. Gac. Méd. de Car. XLI, 4, 50 (1105).

1934a— Sobre el Paludismo. Gac. Méd. de Car. XLI (1106).

RISQUEZ, Jesús Rafael

1927a— A propósito de Pie de Madura. Bol. de los Hosp. Caracas. XVII (II Epoca), 10, 454-457 (1107).

1927b— Lesiones anátomo-patológicas en un caso de apendicitis parasitaria. Bol. de los Hosp. XVII (II Epoca), 11, 477-481 (1108).

1928— Espiroquetos descritos en Venezuela. Rev. de Medic. y Cirug. Caracas, XI, 1221, 425-427 (1109).

1928a— Estadística acerca de la Bilharziosis. Gac. Méd. de Car. XXXV, 2, 17 (1110).

1929b— Un siglo de Parasitología Nacional, 1828-1928. Gac. Méd. de Car. Núm. especial del 15 de junio. Tomo XXXVI y en folleto Tip. Americana, 43 p. (1111).

1929— Generalidades sobre Micología. Lección para los cursantes de Bacteriología y Parasitología de la Universidad. Gac. Méd. de Car. XXXVI, 1, 1 (1112).

1932— A propósito de Moniliasis. Gac. Méd. de Car. XXXIX, 4, 54 (1113).

1932a— La Sífilis no es una enfermedad vergonzosa. Folleto "Semana Antivenérea". Public. del Minist. de Salub. y de Agric. y Cría. Págs. 54-59 (1114).

1933— Lecciones de Parasitología. Gac. Méd. de Car. XL, Nos. 1, 2, 3, 4, 5, 6 (1115).
1933b— Sobre Tripanosomosis y Rhodnius. Gac. Méd. de Car. XL. (1116).
1933c— Enfermedades trasmitidas por los zancudos. Gac. Méd. de Car. XL, 24 (1117).
1933d— Experimentaciones de la propiedad neurotóxica y hemolítica de los venenos de serpiente de Venezuela. Bol. Minist. Salub. y Cría. I, 4-6, 413 (1118).
1933f— Archivos venezolanos de Medicina Tropical. Publicados bajo la dirección del Dr. Jesús Rafael Rísquez. Vol. 1. Car. Tip. Americana 64 p. (contiene trabajos del Br. Rafael Rangel). (1119).
1933h— Proporción del parasitismo de Caracas. Venezuela. Memoria al IV Congreso de la Asociación Médica Panamericana de Dallas, Texas (1120).
1954— Introducción al trabajo del Dr. Torrealba sobre la Tripanosomosis en Zaraza. Resultados del xenodiagnóstico. Gac. Méd. de Caracas. XLI, 2, 23 (1121).
1934a— Tripanosomosis de los reduvideos de Venezuela. Gac. Méd. de Car. XLI, 7, 97, y en un Bol. Minist. Salub. Agric. y Cría. I, 8, 9, 697, 702 (1122).
1934e— Conferencias de Parasitología. Apuntes tomados en la Cátedra del Prof. Dr. Jesús Rafael Rísquez, por los estudiantes de dicha asignatura en la Universidad Central. Curso 1932-33. Caracas. Tip. Americana (1123).

RISQUEZ, Jesús Rafael

1934g— A manera de Prólogo del "Problema de Ofidismo en Venezuela", trabajo del Dr. A.L. Briceño Rossi. Bol. Minist. Salub. Agric. y Cría. II, 14 (1124).
1934i— La lucha contra el Ofidismo en Venezuela. Diario "La Esfera". Caracas. Marzo (1125).
1935d— Parasitismo por Ascaris lumbricoides. Gac. Méd. de Car XLII, 23-353 (1126).
1938— Sobre Quiste hidático en Venezuela (1127).
1939— Notas para la Historia de la Bilharziosis en Venezuela. Gac. Méd. de Caracas. XLVI, 6, 88-91 (1128).
1939b— La Malaria en Venezuela. Informe al Tercer Congreso Internacional de Medicina Tropical y Paludismo de Amsterdam. Gac. Méd. de Caracas. XLVI (1129).
1939d— Nota sobre el agente causal de la Pinta. Gac. Méd. de Car. XLVI, 5, 16 (1130).

RISQUEZ, J.R. Y VELEZ BOZA, Fermín

1941— Nota preliminar acerca de algunas reacciones alérgicas observadas en caso de bilharziosis mansoni. Bol del Lab. de la Clí. L.R. Caracas. II, 4, 73-75, y en la Gac. Méd. de Caracas. XLVIII, 10, 289-290 (1131).

RISQUEZ, Jesús Rafael

1941— Stiles y Rangel. Gac. Méd. de Car. XLVIII, 15-16, 232-325 (1132).
1941a— Cátedra de Bacteriología y Parasitología. Conferencia 16 y 17. Gac. Méd. de Car. XLVIII (1133).
1941b— Homenaje al Dr. José G. Hernández. Discurso leído con motivo de la conmemoración del L Aniversario de la Fundación de la Cátedra de Histología y Bacteriología y Fisiología Experimental en la Universidad Central de Venezuela. Gac. Méd. de Car. XLVIII, 21, 22, 352, 354 (1134).

RISQUEZ I., Rafael

1934— Quiste Hidatídico en Venezuela. Rev. S.E.M. Caracas. I, 3, 5, 19-23 (1135).

RIVAS LARRALDE, Gustavo

1943— Influencia en la Economía Nacional de los protozoos de la sangre. Tesis de Bachillerato. Caracas. Lit. y Tip. Vargas. 19 p. (1137).

RIVERO SALDIVIA, Hermógenes

1927a— Nota sobre la hematuria bilharziana. Memoria del V Congreso Ven. de Medicina. Vol. I, págs. 109-110, y en la Gac. Méd. de Car. XXXV, 6, 92 (1138).
1931— Observations sur le paludisme au Venezuela C.R. II Cong. Int. Paludisme. Aler. 1930, 1, págs. 289-292 (1139).

RODRIGUEZ, César

1943a— Sifiloma de la amígdala. Sífilis pulmonar. Arch. Ven. de O.R.L. Oftalm., Neurol. Caracas, IV, 2, 65-68 (1140).

RODRIGUEZ, César i IRIARTE, David R.

1939— Un caso de granulomatosis paracoccidioica o Blastomicosis brasilera. Rev. de la Clí. L.R. Caracas, II, 4, 209-215 (1141).

RODRIGUEZ, Miguel

1941— Micosis primitiva endonasal. Rev. de la Soc. Méd. de Lara I, 1, 5 (1142).

RODRIGUEZ BOSCAN, Héctor

1928— Dos casos de fiebre biliosa hemoglobinúrica curados sin quinina. Rev. de la Soc. Méd-Quirúrg. del Zulia. II, 21, 280-282 (1143).

1933— Refutación a los detractores de la quinina. Rev. de la Soc. Méd-Quirúrg. del Zulia. VII, 7, 233-239 (1144).

1934— Anotaciones sobre fiebre biliosa hemoglobinúrica. Rev. de la Soc. Méd-Quirúrg. del Zulia. VIII, 6-7, 363-366 (1145).

1939— La Atebrina en la Leishmaniosis cutánea. Rev. de la Soc. Méd.-Quirúrg. del Zulia. XIII, 3, 873-874 (1146).

1942a— Fiebre biliosa hemoglobinúrica. Rev. de la Soc. Méd.-Quirúrg. del Zulia. XVI, 11 (1147).

RODRIGUEZ CABRERA, J.H., BRICEÑO IRAGORRY L., y DAO M.

1943— Asociación Tifo-Malaria. Gac. Méd. de Car. L. 15, 159 (1148).

RODRIGUEZ NAVARRO, Manuel

1943a— Tratamiento del carate. Presentado a la Primera Jornada Venezolana de Venereología y Dermatología. Caracas. Rev. San. Asist. Soc. VIII, 5, 1093-1094 (1149).

RODRIGUEZ ORTIZ, B.

1934— Campaña contra el anquilostomo realizada por la Oficina de Sanidad Nacional del Estado Lara durante el año 1933. Bol. Minist. Saluᵇ Agric. y Cría, II, págs. 372-374 (1150).

RODRIGUEZ RAMIREZ, Tomás

1939— Datos estadísticos de aortitis sifilítica en el Dispensario Antivenéreo del Noreste. Bol. Minist. San. Asist. Soc. IV, 2, 102-107 (1151).
8.479
8.510

ROMERO LOBO, F.V.

1930a— Contribución al estudio de la anquilostomiasis en Venezuela. Apreciaciones hechas en Calabozo (1151).

ROMERO REVERON, Gustavo

1940— Lesiones cardíacas en la Bilharziosis mansoni. Estudio Experimental. Bol. de los Hosp. Caracas. XXXIX. 3, 73-102 (Tesis de Doctorado en Ciencias Médicas) (1152).

RUIZ G. Miguel

1940— Sífilis secundaria febril. Rev. S.E.M. VI, 60-61. 35-40 (1153).

RUIZ RODRIGUEZ, José María

1932— Consideraciones acerca del tratamiento de la sífilis. Folleto "Semana Antivenérea". Minist. de Salub. y de Agric. y Cría. Caracas. Págs. 109-115 (1153).

RUIZ RODRIGUEZ, J.M. y BRICEÑO IRAGORRI L.

1935— Probable caso de leishmaniosis americana. Rev. de la Poli. Car. 20, 1335-1338 (1154).

RUIZ RODRIGUEZ, J.M., PERDOMO HURTADO, B. y OSUNA, A.

1938— Un caso de cirrosis hipertrófica de origen bilharziano. Gac. Méd. de Car. XLV, 5 (1155).

RUIZ RODRIGUEZ, José María

1938a— Notas de Terapéutica Aplicada. Tratamiento de la amibiasis intestinal (Disentería amibiana). Rev. S.E.M. V, 44-45, 722 (1156).

1939— Notas de Terapéutica Aplicada. Tratamiento de la amibiasis extraintestinal. Rev. S.E.M. V, 46-47. 9-12 (1157).

1939— Notas de Terapéutica Aplicada. Tratamiento de la disentería bilharziana. Rev. S.E.M. VI, 57-59. 7-11 (1158).

1939b— Algo más sobre bilharziosis. Cirrosis y miocarditis bilharzianas. Rev. de la Poli. Car. IX, 44, 2978-2996 (1159).

1943— La Schistosomiasis mansoni en Venezuela. Trabajo de incorporación a la Academia Nacional de Medicina. Rev. San. Asist. Soc. VIII, 2, 169-380 y en folleto (1160).

RISQUEZ IRIBARREN, Rafael y ORTIZ, Ignacio

1947— Consideraciones con motivo del segundo caso de Hymenolepis diminuta en Venezuela. Rev. Pol. Caracas. Vol. XVI. Nos. 95-96 (1161).

RISQUEZ, Jesús Rafael

1933— Lecciones de parasitología. Gac. Méd. de Car. XL (1-6). (1162).

RISQUEZ, Jesús Rafael

1934— Conferencia de Parasitología, apuntes tomados en la Cátedra del Profesor Doctor Jesús Rafael Rísquez, por los estudiantes de dicha asignatura en la Universidad Central. Curso de 1932 a 1933. Caracas. Tip. Americana (1163).

1939— Primera, segunda y tercera conferencia recogidas respectivamente por los alumnos. Drs. Ramón Arrivillaga. R. Cordero Moreno y H. Cedeño Pérez. Gac. Méd. de Caracas. XLVI (1164).

1935— Resumen de os trabajos del laboratorio de bacteriología y parasitología del Ministerio de Salubridad y de Agricultura y Cría durante el año 1934. 9 ah R. (1165).

1941— Cátedra de Bacteriología y Parasitología. Conferencia 16-17. Gac. Méd. de Car. XLVIII (1166).

1940— Cátedra de Bacteriología y Parasitología. Conferencia recogidas por los alumnos. Gac. Méd. de Car. XLVII (1-12) (1167).

1941— Notas estudiantiles. Tip. Americana (1168).

"Hepatitis bilharziana", Dr. M. Ron Pedrique. Gen. Volumen VII. Julio 1952. Junio 1953. N° 1 a 4. Volumen VIII. Enero a Junio 1954. N° 34 (1169).

"Estudio de la biopsia rectal en el diagnóstico de la bilharziosis mansoni", Dr. Miguel Ron Pedrique. Gen. Volumen V. Abril a Junio. 1951. N° 4 (1170).

RISQUEZ, F.A.

1930— El pigmento melánico en el paludismo. Gac. Méd. de Caracas. 37, 149-151 (1171).

RODRIGUEZ, César y ADRIANZA, Manuel

1950— Complicaciones pleuro-pulmonares de la amibiasis A.V.P.T. y P. Méd. N° 1 (1172).

RODRIGUEZ, César, POTENZA MILDRED, DE FEO

1951— Torulopsis neoformans pleural. R.A.M.S., enero a abril de 1951. Vol. XVI. N° 1 y 2 (1173).

ROJAS ANGELINO, Aníbal J.

1940— Tricocéfalos. Tesis Doctoral. Caracas (1174).

RAMIREZ, José

La penicilina en trat. de la queratitis intersticial y la atrofia óptica (1175).

RISQUEZ, Rafael, VIVAS SALAS, E. SANCHEZ PEREZ, R.

El tratamiento de la Sífilis cardio-vascular con Penicilina (1176).

SALAS, César Armando

1638— Contribución al estudio de la Schistosomiasis en Venezuela. Emp. El. Cojo. Tesis de Doctorado en Ciencias Médicas. Caracas. 22 p. (1177).

SALAS, Luis M.

1628— Apuntes para el estudio de la Terapéutica de la Neuro-Sífilis. Tesis de Doctorado en Ciencias Médicas. Caracas. Tip. Americana. 65 p. (1178).

SALMERON OLIVARES, José Manuel

1936a— Algo acerca del zancudo y sus peligros (Divulgación). Bol. Minist. San. Asist.

Soc. I, 2, 120-116 (1179).

SALMON, Carlos E.

1930a— Apreciaciones clínicas sobre Anquilostomosis. Rev. de la Conferencia San. Nac. I, 9, 276-288 (1180).

1931c— Sobre algunos Ofidios y Reptiles de la Guayana Venezolana. Gac. Méd. de Cd. Bol. (1181).

1936— Secuelas de blenorragia y sífilis en los padres observados en algunos de los niños que concurren a la Clínica de Niños Pobres. (Conferencia). Gac. Méd. de Cd. Bol. XXI, 128, 10-13 (1182).

1940a— Apreciaciones clínicas sobre el paludismo. Gac. Méd. de Cd. Bol. XXV. 140, 273-285 (1183).

SANCHEZ BECERRA, Héctor y BELLO Carlos José J.

1935— Primeros observaciones de fiebre recurrente en San Cristóbal (reproducción). Bol. Minist. Salb. Agric. y Cría. II, 20, 734-740 (8.937) (1184).

SANCHEZ COVISA, José y GUERRA, Pablo

1940a— Las Leishmaniosis tugumentarias en Venezuela. Rev. de la Poli. Car. IX, 54, 3573-3617 (1185).

SANCHEZ COVISA, José

1940— Acantosis nigricans y linfosarcoma difuso del vientre. Rev. de la Poli. Car. IX, 52, 3473-3484 (1186).

SANCHEZ COVISA, José y GUERRA Pablo

1941— Capilaritis necrosantes de origen sifilítico. Rev. de la Poli. Car. X, 59, 227-236 (1187).

SANCHEZ COVISA, José

1942— Diagnóstico de la sífilis. Bol. de Venereología. Caracas. N°. 2 (1188).

1942a— Diagnóstico de los chancros genitales. Rev. San. Asist. Soc. VII, 5, 749 (1189).

1943— Un caso notable de sífilis de los huesos craneales. Rev. San. Asist. Soc. VIII, 5, 973-978 (en Colab. con Tomás Genatios). (1190).

SANCHEZ PEREZ, Rafael

1935— Las Reacciones de Wasserman y Kahn en la sangre del cordón umbical. Tesis de Doctorado en Ciencias Médicas. Caracas. Coop. Artes Gráficas. 38 pág. (1191).

1942— Algunos aspectos de la lucha antisifilítica en el Dispensario de San Juan, durante el trienio 1938 a 1940. Rev. Minist. San. Asist. Soc. VII, 5, 761-770 (1192).

1943— El Mafarside en los Dispensarios Antivenéreos de Caracas. Primera Jornada Venezolana de Venereología y Dermatología. Rev. San. Asist. Soc. VIII, 5, 979-988 (1193).

SCANNONE, Francisco

1939— Sobre un caso de superinfección sifilítica. Rev. de la Clí. L.R. Caracas, II, 3, 147-154 (1194).

SCOTT, J. Allen

1938— La Esquistosomiasis o Bilharziosis. Bol. Minist. San. Asis. Soc. Págs. 1057-1519 (1195).

1939— La Helmintiasis en Venezuela. Bol. Minist. San. Asist. Soc. IV, 1, 85-87 (1196).

1941— Horizontes helmintológicos. Rev. San. Asist. Soc. VI, 509-522 (1197).

1941a— Los caracoles venezolanos del género Australorbis. Rev. San. Asist. Soc. VI, 2, 237-349 (1198).

1941b— La Esquistosomiasis en los Valles irrigados de las montañas de Venezuela. Rev. San. Asist. Soc. VI, 2, 250-279 (1199).

1942— La epidemiología de la Schistosomosis en Venezuela. Rev. San. Asist. Soc. VII, 6, 771-809 (1200).

SILVA, Antonio Ramón

1930— Anotaciones clínicas de algunos casos de nefritis parasitarias. Tesis de Doctorado. Caracas. Edif. Sur-América. 28 p. (1201).

1934— Dos casos de flebitis sifilíticas. Car. Méd. I, 17-24 (1202).

SILVA ALVAREZ, Alberto

1939a— La Anquilostomiasis. Charla radiofundida. Rev. S.A.S. de Educ. San. II, 43, 10-13 (1203).

1939o— La campaña antianquilostomiásica. Rev. S.A.S. de Educ. San. II, 44-12, 15 (1204)

SILVA BRAVO, José M.

1943— El aneurisma sifilítico de la aorta. Estudio estadístico y comunicaciones sobre dos aneurismas perforados en la arteria pulmonar. Tesis de Doctorado. Bol. de los Hosp. Caracas, XLII, 4, 156-166 (1205).

SMITH, Antonio

1931— Informe sobre el Paludismo en el Estado Falcón. Memoria de la II Conferencia San. Nac. Caracas. Tip. Americana. Páginas 148-159 (1206).

1932— Instrucciones para los que tengan Sífilis. Instrucciones para los que padecen Blenorragia. En el folleto "Divulgaciones Sanitarias. Semana Antivenérea". Publicado por la Oficina Subalterna de Sanidad de Coro. Edo. Falcón. Págs. 27-35 (1207).

SOCIEDAD VENEZOLANA DE SIFILOGRAFIA Y LEPROLOGIA

1939— Pautas para el tratamiento standard de la sífilis reciente de menos de cuatro años. Bol. Minist. San. Asist. Soc. IV, 2, 61-63 (1208).

SORIANO R., Humberto

1944— Un caso de leishmaniasis. Rev. de la Poli. Valencia. III, 12-14-22.

1944a— Sobre un caso de leishmaniasis americana. Rev. Policlínica. Valencia, IV, 13 (1209).

SOTO, Víctor R.

1932— Tratamiento insuficiente de la sífilis. En el folleto "Divulgaciones Sanitarias. Semana Antivenérea", publicado por a Oficina Subalterna de Sanidad de Coro. Estado Falcón. Páginas 5-8 (1210).

SOTO Iribarren, R. y QUINTANA, César

1934— Sífilis, metritis y aborto. Car. Méd. I, 4, 195 (1211).

SANCHEZ BEAUJON, R.A. y SHARY, M.

1953— Rhinosporidiosis. Rev. Pol. Caracas. Vol. XXI. N° 124 (1212).

SCORZA, José Vicente y Cols

1955— Exploraciones de la acción de la Actinomicina C sobre Schizotrypanum cruzi y otros. Méd. de Caracas. Año LXII. N° 34 (1213).

SANCHEZ, R.

Prevalencia de la Sífilis en Venezuela (1214).

SCORZA, José Vicente

1954— Contribución al estudio de los escorpiones venezolanos. Clave para identificaciones de peces y consideraciones generales sobre los escorpiones domiciliarios. Arch. Ven. de Pat. y P. Med. N° 2, Vol. II (1215).

SCORZA, José Vicente

1953— "Contribución al estudio de los Peripatus caribes (Epiperipatus) de Venezuela con adición de una nueva especie. Rev. San. Asist. Soc. Vol. XVIII, N° 5 y 6. Pág. 7.3 (1216).

SUAREZ, Octavio y COVA GARCIA, P.

1953— "Estudio sobre la morfología de la mosca doméstica". Rev. San. Asist. Soc. Vol. XVIII, N° 5 y 6. Pág. 887 (1217).

TALAMO, Salvador

1935— Tres casos de leishmaniosis de las mucosas. Rev. Truxillo, Trujillo, I, 1, 10-11 (1218).

TEJERA, Enrique

1932a— El Paludismo en el Distrito Federal y distribución de los anofeles en esta región. Memoria de la II Conf. San. Nac. Caracas. Tip. Americana. Págs. 383-416 (1219).

1936— Exposición ante la Cámara del Senado sobre la Ley de Defensa contra el Paludismo. Diario "El Universal". Caracas. Nº 9742 (1220).

TOLEDO ROJAS, M.

1932— Algunas consideraciones sobre la sífilis. Folleto "Semana Antivenérea". Págs. 24-30 (1221).

TORREALBA, José Francisco

1932— Breves notas para el estudio de algunas parasitosis intestinales en Zaraza y otras poblaciones de Guárico y Anzoátegui. Gac. Méd. de Car. XXXIX, 23, 355-358 (1222).
Divulgaciones sobre Profilaxia de la Anquilostomiasis. El Unare. Divulgaciones sobre Ascaridiosis y Disenterías. "El Sembrador" (1224).
Nota sobre el Mal de Chagas en Zaraza. "El Sembrador" (1225).

1933b— Tripanosomosis y Rhodnius. Gac. Méd. de Car. XL, 13-178 (1226).

1934— Algo más sobre tripanosomosis, xenodiagnóstico. Gac. Méd. de Car. XLI, 3, 33 (1227).

1934a— El primer caso de tripanosomosis americana diagnosticado en el Estado Guárico por el examen directo de la sangre. Gac. Méd. de Car. XLI, 18, 275 (1228).

1935— La Maladie de Chagas. Trypanosomose americaine ou Schizotripanose au Venezuela. Decouverte et Recherches (1932-34), dans la región de Zaraza, Estado Guárico. Caracas. Lit. y Tip. Vargas. 46 p. (1229).

1935a— Pequeñas notas sobre relaciones biológicas experimentales entre algunos reduvidos y el Tripanosoma venezuelense de la derrengadera de los equideos de Venezuela. Gac. Méd. de Car. XLII, 9, 140-141 (1230).

1935c— Sobre la enfermedad de Chagas en Zaraza. Gac. Méd. de Car. XLII, 23 (1231).

1935d— La Enfermedad de Chagas. Una segunda serie de xenodiagnóstico. El primer caso de forma cardíaca pura descrito en Venezuela. Gac. Méd. de Car. XLII, 24 (1232).

1936a— En colab. con Díaz Emmanuel. Infección del T. maculata, por el Schizotrypanum cruzi. Gac. Méd. de Car. XLIII, 24-377 (1233).

1937— Más investigaciones para el estudio de la enfermedad de Chagas en el Distrito Zaraza. Caracas. Coop. de Artes Gráficas, 45 p. (1234).

1937a— Breves investigaciones sobre la enfermedad de Chagas (varios). Gac. Méd. de Car. XLIV, 14 (1235).

1937b— Algo acerca de hemoglobinuria en Zaraza. Gac. Méd. de Car. XLIV, 20, 311 (1236).

TORREALBA, J.F. CAMEJO TROCONIS, R. e IRAZABAL, Ron

1937— El primer caso de enfermedad de Chagas tratado en Zaraza por 7602. Gac. Méd. de Car. XLIV, 22, 337-339 (1237).

TORREALBA, J.F.

1937e— Reservorios. Gac. Méd. de Car. XLIV, Nos. 20-21 (1238).

1937f— El primer caso de enfermedad de Chagas diagnosticado en Zaraza por despistaje debido al edema ocular, conjuntivitis esquizotripanósica o "signo de Romaña". Gac. Méd. de Car. XLIV, 21, 321 (1239).

TORREALBA, J.R. y EMMANUEL DIAZ

1938— Infeccao natural do Eutriatoma maculata pelo Schizotrypanum cruzi, no Brasil e na Venezuela. Memorias do Instituto Oswaldo Cruz. Tomo 33. Fac. 2. Río de Janeiro (1240).

TORREALBA J.F. y GONZALEZ RODRIGUEZ M.

1939— Pequeños apuntes epidemiológicos sobre la enfermedad de Chagas en el Estado Guárico. Gac. Méd. de Car. XLVII, 24, 456-458 y en folleto (1241).

TORREALBA, J.F.

1939a— La enfermedad de Chagas. Gac. Méd. de Car. XLVII, Nos. 20 al 24 (1242).

1939c— Otros pequeños apuntes acerca de la Peste de Chagas. Casos agudos mortales. Referencias biográficas. Gac. Méd. de Car. XLVI (1243).

1939b— Otros pequeños apuntes acerca de la Peste de Chagas. Trabajo de la Medicatura de Sanidad de Zaraza. Gac. Méd. de Caracas. XLVI, Nos 3 y 4 (1244).

TORREALBA, J.F.

1940— Resumen de la labor xenodiagnóstica para enfermedad de Chagas realizada en Zaraza hasta 1939. 66 pruebas con 22 positivos. Rev. de Medicina Veterinaria y Parasitología. Caracas. Números 1 y 2 (1245).

1941— Notas clínicas y epidemiológicas acerca de la enfermedad de Chagas. Gac. Méd. de Car. XLVIII, Nos. 6 y 7 (1246).

1942— Investigaciones sobre enfermedad de Chagas en Zaraza. Rev. de la Poli. Valencia. 1, 4, 161-178 (1247).

1942a— Investigaciones sobre enfermedad de Chagas en el Estado Guárico, Venezuela. Resultados de xenodiagnósticos en San Juan de los Morros. Otras notas. Gac. Méd. de Car. (1248).

1942b— Resumen de la práctica del xenodiagnóstico para enfermedad de Chagas en Zaraza (Guárico), Venezuela. Sesenta y seis pruebas con veintidós positivas. Gac. Méd. de Car. (1249).

TORREALBA, IRAZABAL RON y GALINDEZ TORRES, Félix

1943— Breves notas sobre Triatomideos y Schizotripanum cruzi en el Estado Carabobo. Gac. Méd. de Car. L, 5, 59 (1250).

TORREALBA, J.F.

1943d— Investigaciones sobre enfermedad de Chagas en Zaraza (Estado Guárico, Venezuela). Otras notas científicas. Recopilación. Fascículo 1°. Caracas. Lit. del Comercio, 167 págs. (1251).

1943e— Resumen de la labor xenodiagnóstica para enfermedad de Chagas, en animales, realizada en Zaraza hasta diciembre de 1941. Gac. Méd. de Car. L, 21, 225 (1252).

1944— Breves notas sobre xenodiagnóstico para enfermedad de Chagas y muy especialmente sobre su aplicación en el país. S.E.M. XI, 107-108, 20-23 (1253).

1944a— Enfermedad de Chagas. Rev. S.E.M. XI, 109-110, 127-137 (1254).

TORREALBA, J.F., SANTAELLA, Victorino, URDANETA, Enrique y ROJAS MARROQUIN, Fernando

1944— Pequeñas notas sobre investigaciones de patología regional venezolana. Rev. S.E.M. XI, 107-108, 7-19 (1255).

TORREALBA, J.F.

1944a— Informaciones sobre enfermedad de Chagas en el Estado Guárico. Gac. Méd. de Car. LI, 4, 31-36 (1256).

1944b— Nota preliminar sobre Penicilina y Schizotrypanum cruzi. Gac. Méd. de Car. LII, 16, 188-189 (1257).

TROMPIZ, Gabriel

1932— La Sífilis y su contagio. Educación sexual. En el folleto "Divulgaciones Sanitarias. Semana Antivenérea", publicado por la Oficina Subalterna de Sanidad de Coro. Edo. Falcón. Páginas 9-13 (1258).

1943— Conducta del médico ante ciertos problemas sifilográficos. Primera Jornada Venezolana de Venereología y Dermatología. Rev. San. Asist. Soc. VIII, 4, 599 (1259).

TORREALBA, J.F.

1944— Enfermedad de Chagas. Conferencia leída en el Anfiteatro del Hospital Vargas. "El Nacional". 19 de febrero de 1944 (1260).

1944— Nota preliminar sobre Penicilina y Schizotrypanum cruzi. Gaceta Médica de Caracas, 1944 (1261).

1944— Xenodiagnóstico de miocardíticos rurales. Una segunda nota sobre Penicilina y S. Cruzi. Gaceta Médica de Caracas (1262).

1944— Investigaciones sobre Enfermedad de Chagas, en Zaraza. Estado Guárico, Venezuela. Otras notas científicas. Caracas. Tip. del Comercio.

(Recopilación-Fascículo 1) (1263).
1944— Breves consideraciones sobre la choza venezolana y la enfermadad de Chagas. Prensa capitalina (1264).

TORREALBA, J.F. y PIERETTI, Rafael Vicente

1946— Otros casos de Chagas comprobados en San Juan de los Morros. Gac. Méd. de Caracas (1265).

1946— Investigaciones sobre la Enfermedad de Chagas en Zaraza, Estado Guárico, Venezuela. Recopilación. Fascículo 2° Car. Tip. Garrido (1266).

1947— J.F. Torrealba. Cartilla Antichagásica. Imprenta Nacional. Caracas, 20.000 ejemplares (1267).

TORREALBA, J.F., PIERETTI, Rafael Vicente Bra. RAMOS, Italia (laboratorista).

1947— Investigaciones sobre Enfermedad de Chagas en el Estado Guárico. Otros 39 casos comprobados. Estudios de la Escuela Rural de Cantagallo. Estudio de la familia Cerdeño. Un caso agudo. Gaceta Médica de Caracas (1268).

1947— Palabras en la Unidad Sanitaria de San Juan de los Morros en el día de la Salud. Inéditas. Fascículo IV. 1953. Muchos trabajos de divulgaciones científicas sobre Ascaris, disenterías, tuberculosis, vivienda rural, peligro venéreo, etc. Prensa de Zaraza. "El Unare", "Tierra", "El Sembrador" (1269).

1949— Una pequeña nota sobre el primer caso de Tripanosomosis rangeli o Tripanosomosis de Tejera, descrito en el país. Gac. Méd. de Caracas (1270).

1949— Otra pequeña nota sobre las Tripanosomosis en San Juan de los Morros. Gaceta Médica de Caracas (1271).

1949— Sobre Tripanosomosis en el Distrito Roscio, en el Estado Guárico, Venezuela, Pífano, Römer, Gaceta Médica de Car. Fasc. III, 1951 (1272).

1949— Informe solicitado por el Ministerio de Sanidad, Dr. Antonio Martín Araujo. San Juan de los Morros, 16 de septiembre de 1949. Fasc. IV, 1952 (1273).

TORREALBA, J.F. y VARADI, F.

1949— Otro caso agudo de Chagas. Caso 121 de las comprobaciones en el "Laboratorio del Dr. Torrealba". Fasc. III, 1951, Revista de Medicina Veterinaria y Parasitología. Nos. 1 al 4, diciembre 1949. Caracas (1274).

TORREALBA, J.F., Bra, RAMOS Italia, Br. RICCARDI, Blas

1949— Dos casos más agudos de Tripanosomosis de Tejera. Tripanosomosis rangeli o Tripanosomosis de la región caribeana. Revista de Medicina Veterinaria y Parasitología. Nos. 1 al 4. Diciembre de 1949. Caracas, Fasc. III, 1951 (1275).

1951— Investigaciones sobre Enfermedad de Chagas en Zaraza. Estado Guárico. Venezuela. Otras notas científicas. Recopilación. Fascículo III. Tip. Garrido (1276).

1951— Más investigaciones sobre Enfermedad de Chagas en el Estado Guárico. Gaceta Médica de Caracas. Set. oct. Nov. Dic. 1951 (1277).

1952— Prólogo del Folleto "Enfermedad de Chagas en el Estado Cojedes", de J.R. López Gómez y Hermana San Tarsicio de San José (1278).

TORREALBA, J.F. Bra. RAMOS Italia y Br. RICARDI, Blas

1952— Otra nota de Enfermedad de Chagas en el Estado Guárico. Nuevos casos comprobados. (Comprobaciones desde el 144 hasta el 163, de las investigaciones en Guárico) (1279).

TORREALBA, J.F.

1953— La Enfermedad de Chagas. Divulgación CIentífica. Rev. Agustín Codazzi, Maracay (1280).

TORREALBA, J. y CLAVO, C.E.

1953— Sobre un caso de absceso tropical del hígado. Gaceta Médica de Caracas (1281).

TORREALBA, J.F. y DIAZ VASQUEZ, Angel

1953— Traducción del portugués de la obra del sabio Dr. Francisco S. Laranja. Evolución de los Conocimientos sobre la Cardiopatía de la Enfermedad de Chagas. Revisión crítica de la literatura. Impresnta Nacional. Editado por el Presidente Perez Jiménez y Ministro Vallenilla Lanz (1282).

TORREALBA, J.F., Prof., SCORZA, Vicente, ZERPA, Mariano Bres., RAMOS, Italia, RICCARDI, Blas y JORDAN, Luis Segundo

1953— Nota preliminar sobre la acción malaquicida del fruto del parapara (Sapindusa onaria L.) Gaceta Médica de Caracas (1283).

1953— Los mismos. La Iloticina y la Enfermedad de Chagas. Otros experimentos con el mismo antibiótico. Gaceta Médica de Caracas (1284).

TORREALBA, J.F.

1953— Investigaciones sobre Enfermedad de Chagas en Zaraza, Estado Guárico, Venezuela. Recop. Fasc. IV. Tip. Garrido (1285).

TORREALBA, J.F., RICARDI B. RAMOS, Italia

1953— Otras notas sobre Enfermedad de Chagas en el Estado Guárico. Casos del 144 al 163. Repetido en el N° 75 (1286).

1953— Los mismos: Distribución geográfica de las especies de tritomideos en el Estado Guárico, por municipios y caseríos. Gaceta Médica de Caracas (1287).

TORREALBA, J.F., RAMOS, Italia

(92)— Casuística Clínica. Mansonella ozzardi, Tricocefalosis Rectal. Pénfigo, Balantidiosis. Gaceta Méd. de Car. 1954 (1288).

TORREALBA, J.F., RICCARDI, Italia Ramos, A. DIAZ VAZQUEZ, TORREALBA, P.A., J.W. TORREALBA

1954— Nota preliminar sobre un tripanosoma del grupo lewisi comprobado en roedor Dasyprocta rubrata de Venezuela. Enero Febrero 1954. N° 1 y 2 (1289).

1939b— Con relación al problema hepato-esplénico de la Schistosomiasis mansoni. Rev. Poli. Car. IX, 48, 2187-3218 (1301).

TORREALBA, J.F. y COLS

1954— Breve nota sobre un nuevo Tripanosoma infectante para Triatomidos comprobado en un mono. Cebus nigrivittattus. Gac. Méd. Caracas. Año LXII. Nos 3-4 (1290).

TORREALBA, J.F. y GONZALEZ RODRIGUEZ

1955— Pequeñas consideraciones sobre la enfermedad de Chagas. Gac. Méd. Caracas. Año LXII. Nos. 3-4 (1291).

TORREALBA, J.R., BRICEÑO L. PIERETTI Vte., RAMOS, Julia

1949— Investigaciones sobre enfermedad de Chagas en el Estado Guárico, Gaceta Médica de Caracas. Enero-Marzo, N° 6 (1292).

TORREALBA, J.F. Y GONZALEZ RODRIGUEZ, Miguel

Breve nota sobre un nuevo Tripanosoma infectante para Triatominos comprobado en un mono en Venezuela. Pág. 1. Gac. Méd. de Caracas (1293).

URRUTIA, Ivaiza

1954— Ascaridiosis de las vías biliares. G.E.N. Julio-Septiembre. N° 1-2 Vol. IX (1294).

VALDIVIESO O., Agustín

1928— La úlcera fagedénica de los países tropicales. Consideraciones clínicas y terapéuticas. Tesis de Doctorado en Ciencias Médicas. Caracas. Tip. Universal. 25 p. (1295).

VALDIVIESO, Martín E.

1939— Ileo por Ascaris. Bol. de los Hosp. Caracas. XXXVIII, 5, 205-109 (1296).

VALDIVIESO, Humberto

1942— Contribución al estudio de la Prueba rural Briceño Rossi. Tesis de Doctorado en Ciencias Médicas. Caracas (1297).

VALENCIA PARPARCEN, Josel

1938a— Contribución a la Clínica de la Bilharziosis. Rev. de la Poli. Car. VIII, 42, 8841-8894 (1298).

1939— Consideraciones a propósito de la sintomatología gastro-intestinal causada por el Ascaris lumbricoides y el Tricocefalus hominis principalmente en adultos. Bol. de los Hosp. Caracas. XXXVIII, 5, 186-203 (1299).

1939a— Observaciones sobre la forma intestinal de la Schistosomiasis mansoni. Rev. de la Poli. Car. IX, 45, 3039-3054 (1300).

1939c— Con relación al problema hepato-esplénico de la Schistosomiasis mansoni. II parte. Rev. de la Poli. Car. IX, 49, 3287-3312 (1302).

VALENCIA PARPARCEN, J. y BAQUERO GONZALEZ, R.

1939— Recto-Colitis ulcerosa con amibas en las heces y Schistosoma mansoni en las paredes. Rev. de la Poli. IX, 48, 3219-3225 (1303).

VALENCIA PARPARCEN, Joel

1940— La estadística en la clínica de la Schistosomiasis mansoni digestiva. Rev. de la Poli. IX, 52, 3447-3466 (1304).

1942a— Tratamiento médico de la Schistosomiasis mansoni en los adultos. Rev. de la Poli. Car. XI, 67, 293-307 (1305).

VALENCIA PARPARCEN, Joel y BAQUERO GONZALEZ, R.

1939— Encuesta sanitaria de la ciudad de Maturín presentada a la Primera Conferencia Anual de Médicos Jefes de Unidades Sanitarias. Archivos de la División de Unidades Sanitarias M.S.A.S. (1307).

VALLADARES GONZALEZ, Rogelio

1940— Anotaciones sobre los protozoarios. Tesis de Bachillerato. Caracas. Edit. Venezuela. 12 p. (1380).

1943a— Encuesta Sanitaria de la ciudad de El Tocuyo presentada a la Primera Conferencia Anual de Médicos Jefes de Unidades Sanitarias. Archivos de la División de Unidades Sanitarias M.S.A.S. (1309).

VASQUEZ, Nicomedes

1930— La Anquilostomosis en Carúpano, Memoria de la I Cong. San. Nac. Págs. 314-322 (1310).

1931— Paludismo en el Estado Sucre. Caracas. Tip. Americana, 6 h. num. y en la Memoria de la II Conf. Nac. Págs. 301-305 (1311).

VEGAS, Martín

1935— Primer caso de esporotricosis en Venezuela. Rev. de la Poli. Car. 21, 1377 y en folleto. Caracas. Lit. y Tip. del Comercio. 15 págs. (9674) (1312).

1936a— Necesidad urgente que tiene Venezuela de intensificar su campaña contra la sífilis. Diario "El Heraldo". N° 1115. Enero 15 (1313).

1938— Sífilis reciente y sífilis antigua. Bol. Cient. Caracas. I, 3, 6-9 (1314).

VEGAS, M. y GUERRA, P.

1938— Una observación de Creeping Disease. Rev. de la Poli. Car. VIII, 41, 2793-2795 (1315).

VEGAS, Martín

1938b— Información acerca del valor y significación del examen de la sangre de la Sífilis. Rev. S.A.S. de Educ. San. II, 26, 33-37 (1316).

VEGAS, Martín

1939— Las bases del actual tratamiento de la sífilis reciente. Bol. Minist. San. Asist. Soc. IV, 2, 53-60 (1317).

1939a— Peligros y Prevención de la Sífilis. Del Ciclo de "Conferencias Sanitarias para Maestros". Rev. S.A.S. de Educ. San. III, 48, 2-5 (1318).

1939b— Comentarios acerca de las esporotricosis en Venezuela, con motivo de una nueva observación. Bol. de los Hosp. Caracas. XXXVIII, págs. 237-244 (1319).

VEGAS, Martín, LOVERA, Ildemaro, ITRIAGO, Pedro Miguel y MEDINA, Rafael

1943— La campaña contra la buba en Venezuela. Primera Jornada Venezolana de Venereología y Dermatología. Rev. San. Asist. Soc. VIII, 5, 1015-1062 (1320).

VELEZ BOZA, Fermín

1942— Contribución al estudio de las reacciones cutáneas alérgicas en la Schistosomiasis mansoni. Tesis de Doctorado en Ciencias Médicas. Caracas. Coop. de Artes Gráficas. 64 p. y en la Rev. Far. y Méd. Caracas (1321).

1943— El Dypilidium caninum en Venezuela. Gac. Méd. de Car. L. (1322).

VERA, Rafael

1943— Sífilis congénita. Presentado a las Primeras Jornadas Nacionales de Puericultura y Pediatría. Caracas. Vol. III, págs. 143-146 (1323).

VETANCOURT RAVARD, Rafael

1928a— La Reacción de Kahn, Tesis de Doctorado en Ciencias Médicas. Empresa Guttemberg, 27 p. y en la Gac. Méd. de Car. XXXV, 15 (1324).

VIANA CASTILLO, Bruno

1931— Informe que presenta el médico de sanidad del Estado Guárico a la Conferencia Sanitaria Nacional de 1931 (Paludismo) Caracas. Tip. Americana. 4 h. y en la Memoria de dicha Conferencia (1325).

1936— Lucha efectiva contra el Paludismo, Anquilostomiasis, Tuberculosis, Enfermedades venéreas y otras. Bol. Minist. San. Asist. Soc. I, págs. 222-224 (1326).

1939— Gusano de zancudo. Un caso de localización rara en el hombre. Rev. Poli. Car. 47, 3183-3185 (1327).

VISO PITTALUGA, Raf. A.

1938— Subfamilia de los anofelinos. Tesis de Bachillerato. Lit. y Tip. Vargas. 16 págs. (328).

1938a— Contribución al estudio biológico del Paludismo. Tesis de Doctorado en Ciencias Médicas. Caracas. Lit. y Tip. Vargas. 20 páginas (9911) (1329).

VIVAS, SALAS, E. MEJIAS, Abel y MALAVE, Antonio

1943— Sífilis cardiovascular en Venezuela. Primera Jornada Venezolana de Venereología y Dermatología. Rev. San. Asist. Soc. VIII, 4, 711 (1330).

VIZCARRONDO, Ernesto, CUENCA, Heberto, H.A. y O'DALY, J.A.

1934— Un caso de endo-aortitis maligna que simula la endocarditis de tipo Osler. Bol. de los Hosp. Caracas. XXXIII, 34-35, 390 (1331).

VIZCARRONDO, Ernesto

1936— Sobre un caso de Bilharziosis mansoni que simula clínicamente una leucemia aguda. Bol. de os Hosp. Caracas. XXXIV, 3, 123-129 (1332).

VIZCARRONDO, R. Oswaldo

1934— Notas sobre la Biología de los Moluscos del Género Planorbis. Tesis de Bachillerato en Filosofía. Caracas (1333).

1934a— Contribucíon al estudio de la Bilharziosis en Venezuela (Observaciones clínicas). Tesis de Doctorado en Ciencias Médicas. Caracas. Edit. Bolívar, 38 págs. (1334).

1935b— Un caso de Mielosis crónica post-palúdica. Rev. de Méd. y Cirug. Maracay, II, 2, 131-136 (1335).

1935c— Dos nuevas especies de Rhodnius para Venezuela. Rev. de Méd. y Cirug. Maracay. Págs. 155-156 (1336).

1935d— Temas de Patología Tropical (La Bilharziosis). Car. Méd. II, 8455-9941 (1337).

VOGELSANG, E.G. y CAMPO, Rafael Martín del

1947— Parasitología de los Nahoas. Rev. Méd. Vet. Parasit. IV (1-4), 47-52 (1338).

VALLE ALI, del

1947— Papel del Ascaris en las conplicaciones quirúrgicas. Rev. Poli. Caracas. Vol. XVI, N° 94 (1339).

VELUTINI, Luis A.

1949— Sobre un caso de leishmaniasis americana tratada con éxito por estreptomicina. Rev. Poli. Caracas. Vol. XVIII, Nos. 104-105-106, pág. 56 (1340).

"El Priodax como tenifugo", por J. Valencia Parpacen. GEN. Vol. I. Enero, Febrero y Marzo, N° 3, 1947 (1341).

"El diagnóstico de la Bilharziosis mansoni. La biopsia rectal en la búsqueda de los huevos de schistosomas", por Joel Valencia Parparcen. Gen. Volumen I. Abril, Mayo y Junio. N° 4, 1947 (1342).

"Pólipos rectales bilharzianos", por Joel Valencia Parparcen. Echandía y E. Bruni Celli. Vol. N° 36 (1334).

"La ascaridiosis intestinal y la enteritis ascaridiana, imágenes radiológicas del ascaris adulto y la enteritis". Doctores Joel Valencia y F. Lechín. Gen. Volumen

V. Abril a Junio de 1951. N° 4 (1344).
"Las várices del esófago en la bilharziosis hepato-esplénica", por el Dr. Joel Valencia Parparcen y C. Mizrahi H. Gen. Vol. V. Enero a Marzo, 1951, N° 3 (1345).

VIVAS BERTHIER, E.
1941— Gusano de monte de zancudo o de mosquito Dermatobia hominis Linn (1781). Revista Médica Veterinaria y Parasitología. Vol. II, N° 1 y 44 Diciembre (1346).

VIVAS SALAS E., y DAO, Miguel
Ausencia de Complicaciones en el Trat. de la Sífilis cardiovascular con Penicilina (1347).

VEGAS ALVARADO, A.
1941— Observaciones sobre Tripanosomiasis bovina. Varios casos de una forma nerviosa presentada en el Estado Zulia. R. de M. Vet. Diciembre (1348).

VILLALOBOS, Tulio
Variaciones serológicas en enfermos sifilíticos tratados con el esquema de Eagle (1349).

VILLEGAS, J. y BENARROCH, E.I.
Eficacia comparada del Hexilresorcinol y de una mezcla de Tetracloretileno y Quenopodio en el tratamiento de la Helmintiasis intestinal" (1350).

VELUTINI, L.A.
1953— Primer caso de tiña por M. ardouini en Venezuela. Acta Médica Venezolana (1351).
1951— Actinomicosis primitiva del abdomen. Memoria II Jornada Venezolana de Ven. y Le. (1352).
1955— Histoplasmosis de la boca. Gac. Méd. de Caracas (1353).

VANES OLAVARRIETA, M.
1938— Apuntes sobre Sanidad Regional en el Distrito Infante. Estado Guárico. Tip. Guariqueña. Valle de la Pascua, 11 p. (1354).

YERENA, Jesús Antonio
1944— Tricomoniasis vaginal. Tesis de Doctorado en Ciencias Médicas. Rev. Ciencias, I, 1, 25-31 y en los Nos. 2, 3 y 4 (1355).

ZAPATA GONZALEZ, Luis
1944b— El problema del diagnóstico clínico-serológico de la sífilis congénita. Micro-reacción de Chediak. Memoria de las Primeras Jornadas Nacionales de Puericultura y Pediatría. Vol. III, páginas 17-38 (1356).

ZERPA MORALES, R.
1940— Ensayo sobre el valor de la microreacción de Chediak en el diagnóstico de confirmación de la sífilis congénita. Tesis de Doctorado en Ciencias Médicas. Caracas. Talleres Patria, 51 p. (1351).
"Blastomicosis del ciego", por el Dr. J.R. Zerpa Morales, Gen. Vol. V. Julio a Diciembre 1950. N° 1 y 2 (1358).

SUPLEMENTO PRIMERO
BIBLIOGRAFIA DE PROTOZOOS

45. FERNANDEZ, A.J., 1931.—"Anaplasmosis en el ganado vacuno de Venezuela". Gaceta Médica de Caracas.

3. VOGELSANG y OTROS, 1948.—"Babesia argentina. Localización cerebral en el bovino". Rev. Grancolombiana de Zootecnia, Higiene y Medicina Veterinaria. Caracas. Vol. 00, pp. 269.

2. GALLO y VOGELSANG, 1940.—"La anaplasmosis en Venezuela". Rev. Méd. Vet. y Paras. II, 3-4; 3-22.

4. GALLO, P., y VOGELSANG., E.G., 1951.—"Nosografía veterinaria venezolana". Rev. Med. Vet. y Paras." Caracas, X, 1-4; 3-47.

5. VOGELSANG, E.G. y ESPIN, C., 1949.—"Bartonella canis Kikuth, 1928, en caninos de Venezuela". Rev. Med. Vet. y Paras. Caracas, VIII, 1-4; 135-137.

6. VOGELSANG, E.G. y POTENZA, 1945.—"Endoparásitos de las ratas salvajes de Caracas". Publicaciones Biogen, Caracas, III, 21-30.

1. GABALDON, ARNOLDO, 1930.—"Nota histórica sobre los protozoos señalados en Venezuela". Gaceta Médica de Caracas, XXXVII, 132-140.

8. VOGELSANG, E.G., 1937.—"Contribución al estudio de la parasitología animal en Venezuela, VI. Infección por Costia necatrix Henneguy (Flagellata) en el Plecostomus". Rev. Pol. de Caracas. 1937, N° 35, pp. 2352.

9. NOVISZKY.—"La coccidiosis de los cerdos en Venezuela". III Conferencia Interamericana de Agricultura, cuaderno N° 12, 1945.

48. VOGELSANG, E.G. y RODRIGUEZ, C.C., 1952—"Ecto y endoparásitos de animales en cautiverio del Jardin Zoológico de Maracay". Rev. Méd. Vet. y Paras., XI, 3-4; 311-316.

10. ORTIZ, C., IGNACIO, 1940.— "Epherytrozoon coccoides en ratas grises (Mus norvegicus) en Venezuela". Rev. Med. Vet. y Paras. Caracas, II; pp. 77.

11. VOGELSANG, E.G., y GALLO, PIERO, 1941.—"Globidium besnoitti Marotel, 1912) y habronemosis cutánca en bovinos de Venezuela". Rev. Med. Vet. y Paras. Caracas, III pp. 153.

38. MARTIN MAYER e IGNACIO ORTIZ, 1941.—"Experimentos con Grahamella muris". Rev. San. y Asistencia Social, Caracas, VI, 3; 320.

17. MIRSA, M., 1950.—"Sobre el hallazgo de gregarinas (Sporozoa) en el estómago de las pulgas Ctenocephalides felis Bouche (Aphaniptera)". Rev. San. Asist. Soc. XV, 5-6; 745.

18. JOSE V. SCORZA y CECILIA DAGERT.—"Notas sobre una nueva Herpetomonas parásita de un Phoridae (Diptera) de Venezuela". Acta Científica Venezolana, V, 127-31; 1954.

37. A.L. BRICEÑO ROSSI, 1945.—"La coccidiosis en el hombre. Primer caso de Isospora hominis en Venezuela". Rev. de San. y Asist. Social, VII, 4; 449-455.

31. PONS, A.R. y MARTINEZ, N., 1941—"Primer caso de kala-azar en Venezuela". Academia de Medicina de Caracas.

35. GOLDMAN, CARLOS y ESPIN, JOSE, 1951.—Leptospirosis canícola. Primer caso comprobado en Venezuela. "Acta Científica Venezolana". Caracas, II, 1; 23.

16. VOGELSANG, E.G., 1938.—"Contribución al estudio de la parasitología animal en Venezuela. VIII. Sarcocystis iturbeí. n. sp., del bovino (Bos. taurus L.)". Bol. Soc. Venez. Cienc. Nat. IV. 32; 279.

24. DIAZ, ENMANUEL, y PIFANO, FELIX, 1940.—"Parasitismo natural de morcego "Carolilia persenpillata" por un Schizotrypanum Venezuela". "Médico, LIV, 42; 5-6.

22. BRICEÑO ROSSI, A.L., e IRIARTE, DAVID, R., 1942.—"Estudios sobre una epizootia aviaria (espiroquetosis)". "Bol. del Laboratorio de la Clínica Luis Razetti", II, 7; 121-128.

14. RIVAS LARRALDE, 1939.—"Un caso de durina en Venezuela". Rev. Med. Vet. y Paras. I, 2-3-4; 119-123.
29. PIFANO, C., FELIX, y BUSTAMANTE, F.E., 1939.—"Nota sobre un Trypanosoma de Miotis nigricans (Wied) murciélago del Estado Yaracuy. Venezuela. Su posible identidad con Trypanosoma megalodermal Wenyon 1939". Gaceta Médica de Caracas, XLVII, 435.
300. TORREALBA, I.F., RICARDI, B., RAMOS, I., DIAZ VASQUEZ, A., TORREALBA, P.A.—Breve nota sobre un nuevo Tripanosoma infectante para Triatominos comprobado en un mono en Venezuela: El Cebús nigrivitatus. Gaceta Médica, Caracas. Año LXII, Nos. 1-2, 1955.
978. PIFANO, FELIX.—Sobre un Schizotrypanum de un murciélago del Estado Yaracuy. Venezuela. Rev. Poli. Car., 46, 3101-3104, 1039.
983. PIFANO, FELIX.—Nota sobre un Trypanosoma del Myotis nigricans Wied Murciélago del Estado Yaracuy. Su posible identidad con el Trypanosoma megaderma Wenyon, 1919. Gaceta Médica de Caracas, 1939.
989. PIFANO, FELIX.—Sobre un Trypanosoma del C. prehensilis L. (puerco espín), posible reservorio de S. cruzi en la naturaleza. Gac. Med. de Caracas, XLVII, 7, 77-78.
1004. PIFANO, FELIX y E. DIAZ.—Estudio biológico de un Schizotrypanum del Hemiderma perspicillata, 1942.
1005. PIFANO, FELIX y E. DIAZ.—Estudio de un Schizotrypanum de Phyllostoma elongatum del Amazonas, 1942.
1032. TORREALBA, J.F., B. RICCARDI, I. RAMOS, A. DIAZ, V. SCORZA y TORREALBA.—Nota preliminar sobre un tripanosoma del grupo lewisi comprobado en un roedor Dasyprocta rubrata de Venezuela. Gac. Med. de Caracas. Enero-Febrero de 1954.

SUPLEMENTO SEGUNDO
BIBLIOGRAFIA DE TREMATODES

52. LUTZ, ADOLPHO, 1928.—"Estudios de Zoología y Parasitología Venezolana". R'o de Janeiro, + 133 págs.
42. CORDERO, E.H. y VOGELSANG, E.F., 1940—"Nuevos trematodos, II". Rev. Med. Vet. y Paras., II, 1-2; 3-14.
40. CABALLERO, C., EDUARDO, y VOGELSANG, E.G., 1949.—"Fauna helmintológica venezolana, II. Algunos trematodos de aves y mamíferos". Rev. de Med. Vet. y Paras. Caracas, VIII; 43-65.
48. VOGELSANG, E.G. y RODRIGUEZ, C.C., 1952.—"Ecto y endoparásitos de animales en cautiverio del Jardín Zoológico de Maracay". Rev. Med. Vet. y Paras., XI, 3-4; 311-316.
43. VOGELSANG, E.G., 1940.—Contribución al estudio de la parasitología animal en Venezuela (XIII)". Rev. Med. Vet. y Paras. II, 3-4; 37-40.
49. CABALLERO, E., VOGELSANG, E.G. y ZERECERO, M.C., 1953.—"Fauna helmintológica venezolana, IV. Algunos trematodes de batracios y mamíferos". Rev. Med. Vet. y Paras., XII; 195-209.
39. ORTIZ, IGNACIO, 1949.—"Contribución al estudio de la parasitología de las ratas de la ciudad de Caracas". Apuntes Científicos, Cabimas, I, 2; 9.
44. CABALLERO, C., EDUARDO, y VOLGELSANG, E.G., 1947.—"Fauna helmintológica venezolana". Rev. Med. Vet. y Paras., VI; 53-62.
54. VOGELSANG, E.G., 1935.—"Contribución al estudio de la parasitología animal venezolana". Rev. de Med. y Cirugía. Maracay, 67-88.
41. CORDERO, E.H. y VOGELSANG, E.G., 1939.—"Nuevos trematodos". Rev. Med. Vet. y Paras., I, 2-3-4; 95-101.
53. TRAVASSOS & DARRIBA, O. CRUZ, XXIII: 237-253.

SUPLEMENTO TERCERO
BIBLIOGRAFIA DE CESTODES

4. GALLO, P. y VOGELSANG, E.G., 1951.—"Nosografía venezolana". Rev. Med. Vet. y Paras. Caracas. X, 1-4; 3-47.

118. VOGELSANG, E.G., 1935.—"Contribución al estudio de la parasitología animal en Venezuela."IV. Rev. Med. y Cirugía, Maracay; 285.

116. FERNANDEZ, A.J. y VOGELSANG, E.G., 1935.—"Contribución al estudio de la parasitología animal en Venezuela. III. Formas larvales de cestodes". Rev. Policlínica, Caracas 22; 1472.

51. VOGELSANG, E.G., 1948.—"Ecto y endoparásitos de animales domésticos y salvajes de la Guayana venezolana". Rev. Med. Vet. y Paras. Caracas, VIII; 144-151.

48. VOGELSANG, E.G. y RODRIGUEZ, C.C., 1952.—"Ecto y endoparásitos de animales en cautiverio del Jardín Zoológico de Maracay". Rev. Med. Vet. y Paras., XI, 3-4; 311-316.

61. HORACE W. STUNKARD, 1953.—"Raillietina demerariensis (Cestoda) from Proechimys cayennensis of Venezuela". J. of Parasitol., XXIX, 3; 272-279.

56. IGNACIO ORTIZ, 1945.—"Comunicación preliminar sobre una posible nueva parasitosis intestinal en Venezuela". Bol. Lab. Clín. Luis Razetti, Caracas, VI, 16; 287-291.

67. VOGELSANG y GALLO, 1949.—"Contribución al estudio de la parasitología animal en Venezuela. XVII. Dos nuevos Sparganum". Rev. Med. Vet. y Paras., VIII, 1-4; 79-83.

6. VOGELSANG, E.G., y POTENZA, L., 1945.—"Endoparásitos de las ratas salvajes de Caracas". Publicaciones Biogen. Caracas; III; 21-30.

207. DIAZ UNGRIA, C., 1955.—"Un nuevo cestode (Citottaenia pectinata) (Goeze), del conejo (Sylvilagus floridanus margaritae) de la isla Margarita, "Mem. S.C.N. La Salle".

SUPLEMENTO CUARTO
BIBLIOGRAFIA DE NEMATODES

97. VOGELSANG, E.G., 1950.—"Contribución al estudio de la parasitología animal en Venezuela". Rev. Med. Vet. y Paras., IX, 1-4; 121-122.

48. VOGELSANG, E.G. y RODRIGUEZ, C.C., 1952.—"Ecto y endoparásitos de animales en cautiverio del Jardín Zoológico de Maracay". Rev. Med. Vet. y Paras., XI, 3-4; 311-316.

81. VOGELSANG, E.G., 1939.—"Contribución al estudio de la Parasitología animal en Venezuela". X. Notas parasitológicas". Rev. Med. Vet. y Paras. I, 1; 51-54.

102. VOGELSANG, E.G., y H. MAYAUDON T., 1952.—"Nematodes parasitos intestinales de bovinos de Venezuela". Rev. de Med. Vet. y Paras., XI, 3-4; 279-301.

4. GALLO, P., y VOGELSANG, E.G., 1951.—"Nosografía veterinaria venezolana". Rev. Med. Vet. y Paras., Caracas, X, 1-4; 3-47.

100. DIAZ UNGRIA, C., 1951.—"Estrongilosis broncopulmonar del cerdo de Venezuela". Mem. Soc. Cienc. Nat. La Salle, XI, 29; 183-194.

96. CABALLERO y VOGELSANG, 1950.—"Fauna helmintológica venezolana". Rev. Med. Vet. y Paras., IX, 1-4; 55-69.

100. DIAZ UNGRIA, C., y FRANCO VERGANI, 1951—"Contribución al estudio de la estrongilosis del ciego en los equidos de Venezuela". Bol. Inst. Vet. 1951, IV, 19; 617-643.

71. VOGELSANG, E.G., 1934.—"Nematodes del tracto respiratorio de los animales domésticos en Venezuela". Rev. Med. y Cirugía. Maracay, II, marzo 1934; 91-94.

103. VOGELSANG, E.G., 1952.—"Estrongilosis pulmonar de los bovinos en Venezuela

(Dictyocaulosis)''. Rev. Med. Vet. y Paras., XI, 3-4; 205-210.

108. DIAZ UNGRIA, C.—''Nota previa sobre un foco filariano entre los indios uiniquinas del Delta del Orinoco''. Novedades Científicas, 1954, serie zoológica N° 15.

70. VOGELSANG, E.G., 1934.—''Contribución al estudio de la parasitología animal en Venezuela''. Rev. Med. y Cirugía, Maracay, dice 1934; 137-138.

120. TEJERA, E., 1926.—''Les blattes envisagées comme agents de disemination des germes pathogenes''. Comp. Rend. Sociedad. Biol., LXXXVIII; 1382-1384.

80. BRUMPT, E., 1932.—''Nemathelminthes parasites des rats sauvage (Epimys norvegicus) de Caracas, II. Gongylonema neoplasticum''. Ann. Paras. Hum. et. Comp., X, 5; 414-24.

99. VOGELSANG, E.G., 1951.—''Nematodes parásitos de los equinos de Venezuela''. Rev. Med. Vet. y Paras., X, 1-4; 119-124.

6. VOGELSANG, E.G., y POTENZA, 1945.—''Endoparásitos de las ratas salvajes de Caracas''. Publicaciones Biogen, Caracas, III; 21-30.

107. BRICEÑO ROSSI, A.L., 1949.—''Primeros casos de filiariasis M. ozzardi constatados en Venezuela''. Rev. San. y Asist. Social, XIV, 5-6; 671.

51. VOGELSANG, E.G., 1948.—''Ecto y endoparásitos de animales domésticos y salvajes de la Guayana venezolana''. Rev. Med. Vet. y Paras. Caracas, VII; 144-151.

43. VOGELSANG, E.G., 1940.—''Contribución al estudio de la parasitología animal en Venezuela (XIII)''. Rev. Med. Vet. y Paras. II, 3-4; 37-40.

93. POTENZA, FEBRES CORDERO, y ANDUZE, 1949.—''Oncocercosis humana en Venezuela''. Gaceta Médica de Caracas, 46; 219.

119. LENT, H. e J.F.T. de PREITAS, 1948.—''Uma colecao de Nematódeos, parásitos salvajes de la Guayana venezolana''. Rev. Med. Vet. y Paras., Caracas, VIII; de vertebrados, do Museu de Historia Natural de Montevideo''. Mem. Inst. O. Cruz, XLVI, 1; 1-71.

44. CABALLERO y C., EDUARDO, y VOGELSANG, E.G.—''Fauna helmintológica venezolana''. Rev. Med. Vet. y Paras., 1147, VI; 53-62.

76. BRUMPT, E., 1931.—''Nemathelmintes parasites des rats sauvages (Epimys norvegicus) de Caracas, I. Protospirura bonnel''. Ann. Parasit, IX, 4; 344-358.

63. VOGELSANG, E.G., 1940.—''Ecto y endoparásitos de los caninos (Canis fam.) de Caracas. Rev. Med. Vet. y Paras., II, 3-4; 65-69.

39. ORTIZ, IGNACIO, 1948.—''Contribución al estudio de la parasitología de las ratas de la ciudad de Caracas''. Apuntes Científicos. Cabimas, I, 2; 9.

101. DIAZ UNGRIA, C., y FRANCO VERGANI, 1952.—''Contribución al conocimiento del género Triodóntophorus (Nematoda) en los equinos de Venezuela''. Bol. Inst. Ins. Vet., IV, 20; 673-710.

SUPLEMENTO QUINTO
BIBLIOGRAFIA DE ACANTOCEFALOS

81. VOGELSANG, E.G., 1939.—''Contribución al estudio de la Parasitología animal en Venezuela''. X. ''Notas parasitológicas''. Rev. Med. Vet. y Paras., I, 1; 51-54.

51. VOGELSANG, E.G., 1948.—''Ecto y endoparásitos de animales domésticos y 144-151.

INDEX

CHAPTERS

BOOKS OF THE SAME AUTHOR

Trabajos Científicos - Editorial Elite - Caracas - 1938.

Oídos, nariz y garganta - Editorial Ercilla - Chile - 1941.

Estudios de Medicina Tropical - Imprenta de la Lotería - Caracas - 1942.

Lecciones de Microbiología y Parasitología - Tipografía Americana - Caracas - 1948.

Estudios Entomológicos y Parasitológicos - Tipografía Americana - Caracas - 1948.

Historia de la Aviación Civil en Venezuela - Primera Edición - Gráfica Americana - Caracas - 1967.

Historia de la Aviación Civil en Venezuela - Segunda Edición - Imprenta Nacional - Caracas - 1971.

Trayectoria de una Vida - Madrid - 1981.